W9-AXR-071

Transcultural Concepts in Nursing Care

Margaret M. Andrews, PhD, RN, CTN, FAAN
Director and Professor of Nursing
School of Health Professions and Studies
University of Michigan—Flint

Flint, Michigan

Joyceen S. Boyle, PhD, RN, MPH, FAAN
Adjunct Professor of Nursing
College of Nursing
University of Arizona
Tucson, Arizona

Adjunct Professor of Nursing
School of Nursing
Medical College of Georgia
Augusta, Georgia

SIXTH EDITION

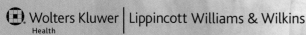
Wolters Kluwer | Lippincott Williams & Wilkins
Health
Philadelphia · Baltimore · New York · London
Buenos Aires · Hong Kong · Sydney · Tokyo

Acquisitions Editor: Hilarie Surrena
Product Manager: Eric Van Osten
Editorial Assistant: Jacalyn Clay
Design Coordinator: Joan Wendt

Illustration Coordinator: Brett MacNaughton
Manufacturing Coordinator: Karin Duffield
Prepress Vendor: Thomson Digital

6th edition

Copyright © 2012 Wolters Kluwer Health | Lippincott Williams & Wilkins.
Copyright © 2008, 2003, 1999 Lippincott Williams & Wilkins
All rights reserved. This book is protected by copyright. No part of this book may be reproduced or transmitted in any form or by any means, including as photocopies or scanned-in or other electronic copies, or utilized by any information storage and retrieval system without written permission from the copyright owner, except for brief quotations embodied in critical articles and reviews. Materials appearing in this book prepared by individuals as part of their official duties as U.S. government employees are not covered by the above-mentioned copyright. To request permission, please contact Lippincott Williams & Wilkins at Two Commerce Square, 2001 Market Street, Philadelphia, PA 19103, via email at permissions@lww.com, or via our website at lww.com (products and services).

9 8 7 6 5 4 3 2 1

Printed in China

Library of Congress Cataloging-in-Publication Data

Transcultural concepts in nursing care / editors, Margaret M. Andrews, Joyceen S. Boyle. — 6th ed.
    p. ; cm.
  Rev. ed. of: Transcultural concepts in nursing care / Margaret M. Andrews,
Joyceen S. Boyle. 5th ed. c2008.
    Includes bibliographical references and index.
    ISBN 978-1-60831-075-3 (pbk. : alk. paper)
1. Transcultural nursing.   I. Andrews, Margaret M.   II. Boyle, Joyceen S.   III. Andrews, Margaret
M. Transcultural concepts in nursing care.
[DNLM: 1. Transcultural Nursing. WY 107]
RT86.54.A53 2012
362.17'3—dc23

                                                                    2011015477

Care has been taken to confirm the accuracy of the information presented and to describe generally accepted practices. However, the authors, editors, and publisher are not responsible for errors or omissions or for any consequences from application of the information in this book and make no warranty, expressed or implied, with respect to the currency, completeness, or accuracy of the contents of the publication. Application of this information in a particular situation remains the professional responsibility of the practitioner; the clinical treatments described and recommended may not be considered absolute and universal recommendations.

The authors, editors, and publisher have exerted every effort to ensure that drug selection and dosage set forth in this text are in accordance with the current recommendations and practice at the time of publication. However, in view of ongoing research, changes in government regulations, and the constant flow of information relating to drug therapy and drug reactions, the reader is urged to check the package insert for each drug for any change in indications and dosage and for added warnings and precautions. This is particularly important when the recommended agent is a new or infrequently employed drug.

Some drugs and medical devices presented in this publication have Food and Drug Administration (FDA) clearance for limited use in restricted research settings. It is the responsibility of the health care provider to ascertain the FDA status of each drug or device planned for use in his or her clinical practice.

LWW.com

CONTRIBUTORS

Martha B. Baird, PhD, RN, ARNP, CTN
Clinical Assistant Professor
Kansas University Medical Center
The University of Kansas
Kansas City, Kansas

Joanne T. Ehrmin, PhD, RN, CNS
Professor
Department of Health Promotion
College of Nursing
University of Toledo
Toledo, Ohio

Patricia A. Hanson, PhD, RN, APRN, GNP
Professor
College of Nursing and Health
Madonna University
Livonia, Michigan

Paula Herberg, PhD, RN
Professor and Acting Associate Vice President,
    International Programs
California State University, Fullerton
Fullerton, California

Jana Lauderdale, PhD, RN
Assistant Dean for Cultural Diversity
School of Nursing
Vanderbilt University
Nashville, Tennessee

Patti Ludwig-Beymer, PhD, RN, CTN,
    NEA-BC, FAAN
Chief Nursing Officer
Edwards Hospital and Health Services
Naperville, Illinois

Margaret A. McKenna, PhD, MPH, MN
Clinical Associate Professor
Department of Health Services
University of Washington
Seattle, Washington

Dula F. Pacquiao, EdD, RN, CTN
Associate Professor
Director
Stanley Bergen Center for Multicultural
    Education, Research, and Practice
University of Medicine and
    Dentistry of New Jersey
School of Nursing
Newark, New Jersey

Barbara C. Woodring, EdD, CPN, RN
Professor and Director
Byrdine F. Lewis School of Nursing
College of Health and Human Services
Georgia State University
Atlanta, Georgia

Shirlee Cohen, MS, MPH, NP/NPP, CCRN
Lecturer
Lehman College of the University of New York
Bronx, New York

Emerson E. Ea, DNP, APRN, BC, CEN
Clinical Assistant Professor of Nursing
New York University College of Nursing
New York, New York

Susan Gaskins, DSN, ACRN
Professor
Capstone College of Nursing
University of Alabama
Tuscaloosa, Alabama

Barbara King, RN
Clinical Instructor
University of Texas Health Science Center
San Antonio, Texas

Susan Price Lofton, RN, PhD,
  PHCNS/BC
Professor of Nursing
University of Mississippi
Jackson, Mississippi

Jenny Radsma, PhD, RN
Professor
University of Maine at Fort Kent
Fort Kent, Maine

Ardith L. Sudduth, PhD, MSN,
  FNP-BC, RN
Associate Professor
College of Nursing and Allied Health
  Professions
University of Louisiana at Lafayette
Lafayette, Louisiana

Dianne C. Swantz, RN, BN, MSA
Nurse Consultant
Internationally Educated Nurses Assessment
  Centre
Mount Royal University
Calgary, Alberta, Canada

Quincy J. Tharps, RN, PHD, LPC
Psychiatric Consultant and Therapists
Milwaukee, Wisconsin

Marshelle Thobaben, RN, MS,
  PMHNP, FNP
Professor and Chair, Department of Nursing
Humboldt State University
Arcata, California

Cynthia A. Watson, RN, MSN
Nursing Instructor
Delaware Technical and Community College,
  Stanton Campus
Stanton, Delaware

FOREWORD

The 21st century is a time when nurses and other health care professionals are eager to learn about different cultures of the world and to provide effective, safe, and culturally competent health care. In the last three decades, transcultural nursing has been soundly established, with theories and guidelines to provide culturally competent health care to immigrants, refugees, and people of many different cultural backgrounds. Transcultural nursing is acknowledged by many nurse leaders and others as the first recognized discipline in nursing with the research findings to support and direct transcultural nursing practice. This has been a major breakthrough in nursing and in the health care disciplines.

This sixth edition of *Transcultural Concepts in Nursing Care* by Professors Andrews and Boyle is a significant and major contribution to transcultural nursing to advance and affirm the discipline of transcultural nursing. The authors have updated the content to help nurses function in different clinical contexts using theory-based research findings and principles in order to practice transcultural nursing. Most importantly, new trends and standards of transcultural nursing have been included in the book to guide nurses and other professionals to practice effectively and appropriately with diverse cultures. These additions and incorporations are most encouraging. In this textbook, the chapter authors demonstrate their leadership in teaching, writing, and practice. They are also well-known leaders who are advancing transcultural nursing in today's multicultural world through their scholarship. Moreover, they are transmitting these insights to future teachers and students of nursing. Most assuredly, the authors in this text have based the content of their

chapters on culturally based practices and on transcultural concepts, principles, and research in many areas of nursing. Providing culturally based care that accommodates and respects different cultures' care values are major and important new contributions to health care.

Most importantly, this edition reflects the authors' scholarly ability to draw upon past historical developments in transcultural nursing and to draw upon important concepts, principles, and new research findings to promote and sustain culturally competent care. This book reveals the cumulative growth and use of transcultural nursing knowledge by the authors. It is most encouraging to witness the use of accumulative transcultural nursing knowledge and to see this knowledge transmitted intergenerationally as former students transmit transcultural nursing knowledge to the latest generation of professional nurses. Scholarship, wisdom, and creative thinking are reflected throughout this book in commendable ways. These are truly hallmarks of genuine transcultural nursing scholars as they build upon and advance transcultural nursing knowledge in significant ways over time and worldwide. Among the highly valuable and special features of this book is that the authors have incorporated comparative culture care practices in community and clinical settings using ethical values and research findings based on contextual data.

New standards of transcultural nursing practice are also introduced and discussed by the authors. A unique feature of this book is that different cultural contexts are emphasized to increase nurses' knowledge of the importance of context. Undoubtedly, the readers will find this sixth edition enormously helpful as they teach and mentor undergraduate students in transcultural nursing courses and clinical settings. This book is also an important foundation to guide students who pursue graduate study because it provides both sound and broad foundations for transcultural nursing. This book will complement other texts and evidence-based articles as researchers pursue further theoretical, clinical, and research studies in transcultural nursing. Professors Andrews and Boyle are to be highly commended for their creative and diligent efforts to update and expand transcultural nursing knowledge, research, and clinical practices with this most recent edition. This publication is indeed a major and important contribution to advance transcultural nursing and to guide students in providing culturally competent, safe, and meaningful care to people of diverse cultures. These are hallmarks of scholarship in this valuable, timely, and updated publication.

Madeleine M. Leininger, PhD, LHD, DS, RN, CTN, FAAN, FRCN
Founder and Leader of Transcultural Nursing and Human Care Theory and Research
Professor Emeritus of Nursing, Wayne State University, Detroit, Michigan
Clinical Professor of Nursing, University of Nebraska, Omaha, Nebraska
Transcultural Global Nursing Consultant and Lecturer, residing in Omaha, Nebraska

In the mid 1950s, nurse-anthropologist Dr. Madeleine M. Leininger envisioned transcultural nursing as a formal area of study and practice for nurses. Her first book, *Nursing and Anthropology*, was published in 1970 urging nurses to draw upon the concepts and principles of anthropology in their nursing practice. Since that time, there has been national attention and keen interest by health professionals in culturally competent health and nursing care. The influence of transcultural nursing has spread to many countries in the world. In addition, transcultural nursing has influenced other health disciplines, including medicine, pharmacy social work, and other fields as well. Culturally competent care is now an expected standard of care for individuals, families, groups, and communities, and many state and national accrediting bodies include criteria related to the cultural needs of patients.

Our major contribution to transcultural nursing in all six editions of *Transcultural Concepts in Nursing Care* has been a synthesis of transcultural theories, models, and research studies compiled into a comprehensive text. Our primary goal has been to advance the use of transcultural knowledge in nursing practice and to develop cultural competence in the care of individuals and groups. We have deliberately emphasized incorporating cultural knowledge in nursing practice and urged nurses and others reading this text to consider the cultural context when providing care. We believe that over the years, we have made a significant contribution to the theories, concepts, and practice of transcultural nursing.

Initially published in 1989, *Transcultural Concepts in Nursing Care* began as a collegial effort among faculty and doctoral students at the University of Utah College of Nursing to help us expand and clarify our view of transcultural nursing. Many of the chapter authors were teaching undergraduate students and we were looking for articles and textbooks to help us in both the classroom and clinical practice settings. We had strong clinical backgrounds and an interest in solving clinical problems, so we wanted a textbook that would apply transcultural nursing concepts to clinical practice. In particular, we wanted a textbook that undergraduate students would find interesting, challenging, and, above all, helpful in providing culturally competent nursing care to patients/clients of diverse cultural backgrounds. We also had (and still retain) a strong commitment to theory development in nursing. In this sixth edition, we have many of the same contributors, but are always pleased to welcome other transcultural nursing experts who join us. As we have completed each edition of this text, we are impressed at the significant progress that has been made by our colleagues in terms of research and publications as well as refinement of concepts and theories that we are able to use in our writing.

Many contributors teach in baccalaureate, masters, and/or doctoral programs in nursing. Over the years, we have explored ways to creatively and effectively teach our students how to apply transcultural concepts to practice, with the goal of developing their knowledge and skills in providing culturally competent and culturally congruent nursing care. The Commission on Collegiate Nursing Education, the National League for Nursing, most state boards of nursing, and other accrediting and certification bodies require or strongly encourage the inclusion of cultural aspects of care in nursing curricula. This, of course, underscores the importance of the purpose, goal, and objectives for *Transcultural Concepts in Nursing Care, Sixth Edition*.

Purpose: To contribute to the development of theoretically based transcultural nursing knowledge and the advancement of transcultural nursing practice.

Goal: To increase the delivery of culturally competent care to individuals, families, groups, communities, and institutions.

Objectives:

1. To apply a transcultural nursing framework to guide nursing practice in diverse health care settings across the life span.
2. To analyze major concerns and issues encountered by nurses in providing transcultural nursing care to individuals, families, groups, communities, and institutions.
3. To expand the theoretical bases for using concepts from the natural and behavioral sciences and from the humanities to provide culturally competent nursing care.

We believe that cultural assessment skills, combined with the nurses' critical thinking abilities, will provide the necessary knowledge on which to base transcultural nursing care. Using this approach, nurses have the ability to provide culturally competent and contextually meaningful care for clients—individuals, groups, families, communities, and institutions.

Given that nurses are likely to encounter people from literally hundreds of different cultures, we believe this approach is more effective than simply memorizing the esoteric beliefs and practices of a litany of different groups. Thus, we believe that nurses must acquire the knowledge and skills needed to assess and care for clients from any and all cultural groups that they might encounter in their professional careers.

We would like to acknowledge that extensive progress has been made in nursing education, practice, and research in terms of cultural awareness, sensitivity, and competence during the last two decades. Although much remains to be done, we are pleased that many clinicians, educators, researchers, administrators, and consultants have integrated transcultural nursing concepts into their respective areas of expertise with increasing success. In addition, the authors of nursing and health care textbooks and other publications often integrate transcultural nursing into their work or invite expert transcultural nurses to do so. While we are pleased with this trend, we also recognize that there remains a need for a comprehensive text that provides nurses with the theoretical foundations for transcultural nursing, develops competence in cultural assessment, and systematically applies transcultural concepts across the life span. We are also committed to the notion that contemporary health care issues, problems, and challenges warrant critical analysis and dialogue, thus making a text such as *Transcultural Concepts in Nursing Care, Sixth Edition*, a useful and necessary adjunct to general and specialty nursing textbooks.

The editors and chapter authors share a commitment to:

- Foster the development and maintenance of a disciplinary knowledge base and expertise in culturally competent care.
- Synthesize existing theoretical and research knowledge regarding nursing care of different ethnic/minority/marginalized and other disenfranchised populations.
- Identify and describe evidence-based practice and best practices in the care of diverse individuals, families, groups, communities, and institutions.
- Create an interdisciplinary and interprofessional knowledge base that reflects heterogeneous health care practices within various cultural groups.
- Identify, describe, and examine methods, theories, and frameworks appropriate for developing knowledge that will improve health and nursing care to minority, underserved, underrepresented, disenfranchised, and marginalized populations.

Recognizing Individual Differences and Acculturation

When consulting transcultural nursing issues, nurses and other health care professionals are, with increasing frequency, referring to the federally defined population categories (i.e., White, Black, Hispanic, Asian/Pacific Islander, and American Indian/Alaska Native). The creation of these defined population categories by the United States government has had a tremendous impact on our conceptualization of the various groups that constitute our society. The unique characteristics and individual differences of the five cultural groups have often been ignored, along with the impact acculturation has had on these groups. The outcomes are reminiscent of the melting pot metaphor; only now we have five pots instead of just one. While the most recent census enabled citizens to self-identify with more than one group, the data remain far from perfect in describing the multicultural, multiethnic, and multiracial composition of contemporary society in the United States. Canada, Australia, the United Kingdom, western Europe, and other nations continue to struggle with the challenges of diversity in their societies, as well.

We believe that it is tremendously important to recognize the myriad of health-related beliefs and practices that exist within the population categories. For example, the differences are rarely recognized among people who identify themselves as Hispanic/Latino: this group includes people from along the U.S.–Mexico border, Puerto Rico, Mexico, Spain, Guatemala, or "little Havana" in Miami, as well as other Central and South American countries, who may share some similarities (speaking Spanish, for example) but who may also have distinct cultural differences.

We would like to comment briefly on the terms *minority* and *ethnic minorities*. These terms are perceived by some to be offensive because they connote inferiority and marginalization. Although we have used these terms occasionally, we prefer to make reference to a specific subculture or culture whenever possible. We refer to categorizations according to race, ethnicity, religion, or a combination, such as ethnoreligion (e.g., Amish), but we make every effort to avoid using any label in a pejorative manner. We do believe, however, that the concepts or terms *minority* or *ethnicity* are limiting, not only for those to whom the label maybe applies, but also for nursing theory and practice. We believe that concept of *culture* is richer and has more theoretical usefulness. In addition, we all have cultural attributes while not all are from a minority group or claim a particular ethnicity.

Critical Thinking Linked to Delivering Culturally Competent Care

We believe that cultural assessment skills, combined with the nurse's critical thinking ability, will provide the necessary knowledge on which to base transcultural nursing care. Using this approach, we are convinced that nurses will be able to provide culturally competent and contextually meaningful care for clients from a wide variety of cultural backgrounds, rather than simply memorizing the esoteric health beliefs and practices of any specific cultural group. We believe that nurses must acquire the skills needed to assess clients from virtually any and all groups that they encounter throughout their professional life.

New to the Sixth Edition

All content in this edition has been reviewed and updated to capture the nature of the changing health care delivery system, new research studies, and theoretical advances and to explain how nurses and other health care providers can use culturally competent skills to improve the care of clients, families, groups, and communities. In writing this sixth edition, we have been impressed with the developments in the field of transcultural nursing. The Transcultural

Nursing Society and the American Academy of Nursing (AAN) have moved ahead with developing Standards of Practice for Culturally Competent Care that nurses around the world will use as guides in clinical practice, research, education, and administration. In addition, a special task force from the Transcultural Nursing Society has developed a Core Curriculum for Transcultural Nursing that can be used as a basis for certification in transcultural nursing and by faculty and students in educational programs. The recognition of the Standards of Practice and Core Curriculum for transcultural nursing will enhance the development of cultural competence in nursing, thus improving the care of clients.

New Chapter

We welcome a new colleague, Joanne Ehrmin, PhD, RN, CNS, who is currently Professor, Department of Health Promotion at the College of Nursing, University of Toledo. Dr. Ehrmin has a strong background in Psychiatric/Mental Health Nursing and many readers will be familiar with her work with African American women undergoing treatment for chemical dependencies. Dr. Ehrmin obtained her PhD from Wayne State University under the tutelage of Dr. Madeleine Leininger. We were delighted when she agreed to write a new chapter "Transcultural Perspectives in Mental Health Nursing."

In addition, Barbara Woodring, EdD, CPN, RN, currently Professor and Director of the Byrdine F. Lewis School of Nursing has collaborated with Margaret Andrews to update and revise Chapter 6, "Transcultural Perspectives in the Nursing Care of Children." Dr. Woodring has a strong clinical background in pediatric nursing and many years of experience in working with diverse cultural groups.

Martha B. Baird, PhD, ARNP, CTN, who is currently a faculty member at the School of Nursing, University of Kansas Medical Center, collaborated with Joyceen Boyle to update and add to Chapter 11, "Culture, Family, and Community." Dr. Baird completed her dissertation research with Sudanese refugee women and their children; her study focused on health and wellness of refugee women experiencing cultural transitions and we have incorporated aspects of her research findings in Chapter 11.

We have maintained the same conceptual framework for the text; focusing on the life span first and then on specialty areas within transcultural nursing. We have updated all chapters, reorganized and revised to make the content current and more readable and succinct. We are excited about the new research and theoretical work that transcultural nurses are publishing. This makes the field very exciting.

Chapter Pedagogy

Learning Activities

All of the chapters include review questions as well as learning activities to promote critical thinking. In addition, each chapter includes chapter objectives and key terms to help readers understand the purpose and intent of the content. Many chapters include up-to-date case studies that present cultural knowledge as well as content on cultural competencies.

Evidence-Based Practice

Current research studies related to the content of the chapter are presented as Evidence-Based Practice Boxes. We have included a section in each box describing appropriate clinical applications derived from the research.

Case Studies Based on Actual Clinical or Research Experiences

Case Studies based on the authors' actual clinical experiences and research findings are presented to make conceptual linkages and to illustrate how concepts are applied in health care settings. Case studies are oriented to assist the reader to begin to develop cultural competence with selected cultures.

Text Organization

Part One: Historical and Theoretical Foundations of Transcultural Nursing

This first section focuses on the historical and theoretical aspects of transcultural nursing.

The development of transcultural nursing frameworks that include concepts from the natural and behavioral sciences are described as they apply to nursing practice. Because nursing perspectives are used to organize the content in *Transcultural Concepts in Nursing Care*, the reader will not find a chapter purporting to describe the nursing care of a specific cultural group. Instead, the nursing needs of culturally diverse groups are used to illustrate cultural concepts used in nursing practice. Chapter 1 provides an overview of the historical and theoretical foundations of transcultural nursing, and Chapter 2 introduces key concepts associated with cultural competence. In Chapter 3, we discuss the domains of cultural knowledge that are important in cultural assessment and describe how this cultural information can be incorporated into all aspects of care. Chapter 4 provides a summary of the major cultural belief systems embraced by people of the world with special emphasis on their health-related and culturally based values, attitudes, beliefs, and practices.

Part Two: Transcultural Nursing: Across the Life Span

Chapters 5 through 8 use a developmental framework to discuss transcultural concepts across the life span. The care of childbearing women and their families, children, adolescents, middle-aged adults, and the elderly is examined, and information about cultural groups is used to illustrate common transcultural nursing issues, trends, and concerns.

Part Three: Nursing in Multicultural Health Care Settings

In the third section of the text, we explore the components of cultural competence in mental health and in family and community health care settings. We also examine cultural competence in health care organizations and cultural diversity in the health care workforce, two very critical and current topics of concern. The clinical application of concepts throughout this section uses situations commonly encountered by nurses and describes how transcultural nursing principles can be applied in diverse settings. The chapters in this section are intended to illustrate the application of transcultural nursing knowledge to nursing practice.

Part Four: Contemporary Challenges in Transcultural Nursing

In the fourth section of the text, Chapters 13 to 15, we examine selected contemporary issues and challenges that face nursing and health care. In Chapter 13, we review major religious traditions of the United States and the interrelationships among religion, culture, and nursing. Recognizing the numerous moral and ethical challenges in contemporary health care as well as within the transcultural nursing, Chapter 14 discusses cultural competence in ethical and moral dilemmas from a transcultural perspective. Chapter 15 provides a global perspective of what is occurring in the international areas to promote human and health. This chapter is slightly different from the rest of the chapters as it highlights the field of international nursing and the ways in which nurses from the United States can contribute to the global efforts to improve the health status of people across the world.

Margaret M. Andrews, PhD, RN, FAAN, CTN
Joyceen S. Boyle, PhD, RN, MPH, FAAN

ACKNOWLEDGMENTS

We are pleased to acknowledge the assistance and support of our families, friends, and colleagues in once again making this book possible. We also appreciate the help of the many nursing faculty members, practitioners, and students who have offered helpful comments and suggestions. We have found it very gratifying to be able to call upon many of our colleagues for help and advice in this new edition. Particular appreciation is extended to Joanne Ehrmin, Barbara Woodring, and Martha Baird who contributed new ideas and much work on this sixth edition. We would like to especially thank our colleague Patti Ludwig-Beymer who provided some "heavy lifting"—helping us out when we needed it. Larry Purnell readily shared information and advice. Once again we are indebted to Teresa and Neil Cooper who provided another memorable photograph for us.

We would like to acknowledge Hilarie Surrena, Senior Acquisitions Editor, Wolters Klower Health. Hilarie worked with us during the preparation for the fifth edition and we were pleased to be able to work with her again on this sixth edition. Eric Van Osten, Product Manager, stepped in during the second half of the project; he has supported and encouraged us through the process of "getting things together" as well as helped with editorial advice along the way. Karen Ettinger, Project Manager at O'Donnell and Associates, helped put the final touches on this book. We thank her for her expertise, guidance, and patience. It has been our pleasure to work with such pleasant and supportive professionals.

We gratefully acknowledge the support of our friends, too numerous to list by name, who often wrote encouraging emails or phoned to express their interest and encouragement. We thank all of our colleagues who have purchased our book in the past and the many who have expressed interest in the sixth edition. We are always appreciative of their support.

Last of all, we would once again like to thank each other for what has been a lifetime of friendship that has withstood the test of time and now six editions of this book! We can't say that it has become any easier with time. We started this course in 1983 with sharpened pencils and yellow legal pads with our first edition and now we have progressed to emails, electronic documents, computers, and fax machines. Through it all, we have found our professional endeavors in transcultural nursing and the friends that we have made along the way to be both satisfying and rewarding.

CONTENTS

PART ONE
Historical and Theoretical Foundations of Transcultural Nursing   1

CHAPTER 1
Theoretical Foundations of Transcultural Nursing   3
Margaret M. Andrews and Joyceen S. Boyle

CHAPTER 2
Culturally Competent Nursing Care   17
Margaret M. Andrews

CHAPTER 3
Cultural Competence in the Health History and Physical Examination   38
Margaret M. Andrews

CHAPTER 4
The Influence of Cultural and Health Belief Systems on Health Care Practices   73
Margaret M. Andrews

PART TWO
Transcultural Nursing: Across the Lifespan   89

CHAPTER 5
Transcultural Perspectives in Childbearing   91
Jana Lauderdale

CHAPTER 6
Transcultural Perspectives in the Nursing Care of Children   123
Barbara C. Woodring and Margaret M. Andrews

CHAPTER 7
Transcultural Perspectives in the Nursing Care of Adults   157
Joyceen S. Boyle

CHAPTER 8
Transcultural Perspectives in the Nursing Care of Older Adults   182
Margaret A. McKenna

PART THREE
Nursing in Multicultural Health Care Settings 209

CHAPTER 9
Creating Culturally Competent Organizations 211
Patti Ludwig-Beymer

CHAPTER 10
Transcultural Perspectives in Mental Health Nursing 243
Joanne T. Ehrmin

CHAPTER 11
Culture, Family, and Community 277
Joyceen S. Boyle and Martha B. Baird

CHAPTER 12
Cultural Diversity in the Health Care Workforce 316
Margaret M. Andrews and Patti Lugwig-Beymer

PART FOUR
Contemporary Challenges in Transcultural Nursing 349

CHAPTER 13
Religion, Culture, and Nursing 351
Patricia A. Hanson and Margaret M. Andrews

CHAPTER 14
Cultural Competence in Ethical Decision Making 403
Dula F. Pacquiao

CHAPTER 15
Perspectives on International Nursing 421
Paula Herberg

APPENDIX A
**Andrews/Boyle Transcultural Nursing Assessment Guide for
   Individuals and Families   451**
Joyceen S. Boyle and Margaret M. Andrews

APPENDIX B
**Andrews/Boyle Transcultural Nursing Assessment Guide for
   Groups and Communities   456**
Joyceen S. Boyle and Margaret M. Andrews

APPENDIX C
**Andrews/Boyle Transcultural Nursing Assessment Guide for
   Health Care Organizations and Facilities   459**
Joyceen S. Boyle, Margaret M. Andrews, and Patti Ludwig-Beymer

APPENDIX D
Components of a Cultural Assessment: Traditional Native American Healing   462
Joyceen S. Boyle

INDEX   465

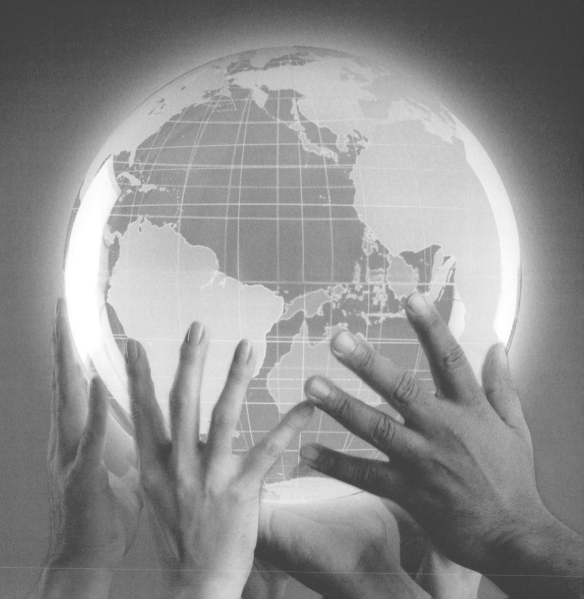

PART ONE

Historical and Theoretical Foundations of Transcultural Nursing

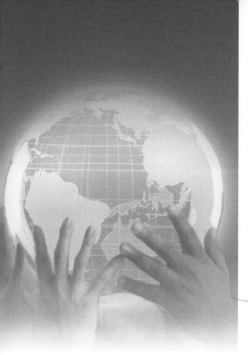

Theoretical Foundations of Transcultural Nursing

Margaret M. Andrews and
Joyceen S. Boyle

KEY TERMS

Andrews/Boyle Transcultural
    Nursing Assessment Guide
Anthropology
Campinha-Bacote Model of Cultural
    Competence in the Delivery of
    Healthcare Services
Cultural competence
Cultural congruence
Culturally congruent care
Culture-specific nursing care
Culture-universal nursing care
Diversity
Ethnocentric
Giger and Davidhizar Transcultural
    Assessment Model
Leininger's Sunrise Model
Leininger's Theory of Culture Care
    Diversity and Universality
Panethnic minority groups
Purnell Model for Cultural
    Competence
Transcultural nursing
Transcultural nursing certification
Transcultural nursing standards

LEARNING OBJECTIVES

1. Examine the historical origins of transcultural nursing with special emphasis on its roots in anthropology.
2. Critically analyze the need for transcultural nursing in contemporary society.
3. Critically analyze prevailing nursing paradigms and nursing theories from a transcultural nursing perspective.
4. Identify resources available in transcultural nursing and health care.

During the last six decades, the founder of transcultural nursing, Dr. Madeleine M. Leininger, and thousands of other nurses from around the world have worked diligently to establish **transcultural nursing** as a formal area of academic study and practice. Since its initial conception in the 1950s to its formal creation as a specialty and new discipline within the profession in the 1960s and 1970s, a substantial and important body of transcultural theoretical, research-, and evidence-based knowledge has been generated by nurse scholars on every continent.

The term *transcultural nursing* is sometimes used interchangeably with *cross-cultural, intercultural,* or *multicultural nursing.* In analyzing the Latin derivations of the prefixes associated with these terms, you will notice that *trans* means *across, inter* means *between*, and *multi* means *many*. Given these derivations, it is understandable that various words have been used with similar connotative meaning (Andrews, 1992, 1995). In the 1970s, after Leininger established transcultural nursing, other nurse authors who were writing about ethnicity and/or culture used the term *ethnic nursing care* (Orque, Bloch, & Monrroy, 1983) or referred to *caring for people of color* (Branch & Paxton, 1976).

Approximately 50 years ago, nurse-anthropologists debated the conceptual differences between transcultural and cross-cultural nursing, and debate has continued (Lipson, 1999). We have chosen to use transcultural nursing in this book in recognition of the historical and theoretical contributions of Dr. Madeleine M. Leininger, a nurse-anthropologist who, in the mid-1950s, envisioned transcultural nursing as a formal area of study and practice for nurses and coined the term *transcultural nursing* (Andrews & Boyle, 1997; Leininger, 1995, 1999; Leininger & McFarland, 2002, 2006). In her classic work, *Nursing and Anthropology: Two Worlds to Blend*, Dr. Leininger notes that the fields of anthropology and nursing must be interdigitated so that each field will profit from the contribution of the other. ". . . It is apparent that if these two fields were sharing their special knowledge and experiences, both would undoubtedly see new pathways in thinking and research" (Leininger, 1970).

As the name implies, transcultural nursing transverses cultural boundaries, usually those between the nurse or health care provider and patient. Transcultural nursing is the blending of anthropology and nursing in both theory and practice (Dougherty & Tripp-Reimer, 1985; Lipson & Bauwens, 1988; McKenna, 1984; Osborne, 1969). **Anthropology** refers to the study of humans and humankind, including their origins, behavior, social relationships, physical and mental characteristics, customs, and development through time and in all places in the world. Recognizing that nursing is an art and a science, transcultural nursing enables us to view our profession from a cultural perspective.

Transcultural nursing is not just for immigrants, people of color, or members of the federally defined **panethnic minority groups**, that is, Blacks, Hispanics, Asians/Pacific Islanders, and American Indians/Alaska Natives. Everyone has a cultural heritage, including nurses, patients, and other members of the health care team; the latter groups might be referred to as being members of occupational or professional cultures (Andrews & Boyle, 1997, 2002). There are also many other examples of *nonethnic cultures*, such as the culture of poverty or affluence, culture of the deaf or hearing impaired and the blind or visually impaired, and the gay, lesbian, and transgender cultures.

Transcultural nursing is a specialty within nursing focused on the comparative study and analysis of different cultures and subcultures. These groups are examined with respect to their caring behavior, nursing care, and health–illness values, beliefs, and patterns of behavior. The goal of transcultural nursing is to develop a scientific and humanistic body of knowledge in order to provide **culture-specific** and **culture-universal nursing care** practices to individuals, families, groups, and communities from diverse backgrounds. *Culture-specific* refers to particular values, beliefs, and patterns of behavior that tend to be special or unique to a group and that do not tend to be shared with members of other cultures. *Culture-universal* refers to the commonly shared values, norms of behavior, and life patterns that are similarly held among cultures about human behavior and lifestyles (Leininger, 1978, 1991, 1995; Leininger & McFarland, 2002).

Transcultural nursing requires sophisticated assessment and analytic skills and the ability to plan, design, implement, and evaluate nursing care for individuals, families, groups, and communities representing various cultures. In addition, nurses with transcultural expertise must also be able to apply that knowledge to the culture of organizations, institutions, and agencies, especially those concerned with health and nursing.

The Importance of Transcultural Nursing

Leininger (1995) cites eight factors that influenced her to establish transcultural nursing:

1. There was a marked increase in the migration of people within and between countries worldwide. Transcultural nursing is needed because of the growing diversity that characterizes our national and global populations. In its broadest sense, **diversity** refers to differences in race, ethnicity, national origin, religion, age, gender, sexual orientation, ability or disability, social and economic status or class, education, and related attributes of groups of people in society.
2. There has been a rise in multicultural identities, with people expecting their cultural beliefs, values, and lifeways to be understood and respected by nurses and other health care providers.
3. The increased use of health care technology sometimes conflicts with cultural values of clients, such as Amish prohibitions against using certain apnea monitors, intravenous equipment, and other such health care technologic devices in the home.
4. Worldwide, there are cultural conflicts, clashes, and violence that have an impact on health care as more cultures interact with one another.
5. There was an increase in the number of people traveling and working in many different parts of the world.
6. There was an increase in legal suits resulting from cultural conflict, negligence, ignorance, and imposition of health care practices.
7. There has been a rise in feminism and gender issues, with new demands on health care systems to meet the needs of women and children.
8. There has been an increased demand for community and culturally based health care services in diverse environmental contexts.

Let's examine a few clinical examples of ways in which transcultural nursing can be used in the care of people with diverse backgrounds. Transcultural nursing enables nurses to communicate more effectively with clients from diverse cultural and linguistic backgrounds and to assist those with mental health problems. Transcultural nursing enables nurses to more accurately assess the cultural expression of pain and to provide culturally appropriate interventions to prevent or alleviate discomfort. Last, incidents have been reported in which parents have been arrested for child abuse because culturally based child-rearing practices were poorly understood. Transcultural nursing is a vehicle for assessing the parent–child relationship and for encouraging forms of parental discipline that promote the health and well-being of children and prevent physical or emotional harm (Andrews, 1992, 1995; Flaskerud, 2000; Leininger, 1997; Leininger & McFarland, 2002, 2006; Mahoney & Engebretson, 2000).

Throughout this book, we shall examine various ways in which transcultural nursing facilitates nurses' knowledge and skill in caring for people from diverse backgrounds. Although much of the emphasis will be on diversity, we shall also explore the universal attributes that we have in common with other members of the human race, such as the need for food, sleep, shelter, safety, and human interaction. Let us now examine some key developments in transcultural nursing from a historical perspective.

History of Transcultural Nursing

In the 1950s, Dr. Madeleine M. Leininger noted cultural differences between patients and nurses while working with emotionally disturbed children. This clinical experience led her in 1954 to study cultural differences in the perceptions of care, and in 1965 she earned a doctorate in cultural anthropology from the University of Washington (Leininger, 1995; Leininger & McFarland, 2002, 2006; Reynolds & Leininger, 1993). Leininger recognized that one of anthropology's most important contributions to nursing was the realization that health and illness states are strongly influenced by culture. Table 1-1 gives a summary of Dr. Leininger's contributions to the development of transcultural nursing.

To help develop, test, and organize the emerging body of knowledge in transcultural nursing, it is necessary to have a specific conceptual framework from which various theoretical statements can emerge. **Leininger's Sunrise Model** (Figure 1-1) is based on the concept of cultural care and shows three major nursing modalities that guide nursing judgments and activities to provide **culturally congruent care**—that is, care that is beneficial and meaningful to the people being served (Leininger, 1991, 1995; Leininger & McFarland, 2002).

Leininger's Theory of Culture Care Diversity and Universality focuses on describing, explaining, and predicting nursing similarities and differences focused primarily on human care and caring in human cultures. Leininger uses worldview, social structure, language, ethnohistory, environmental context, and the generic (folk) and professional systems to provide a comprehensive and holistic view of influences in culture care. Culturally based care factors are recognized as major influences on human expressions and experiences related to health, illness, and well-being or on facing disabilities or death. The three modes of nursing decisions and actions—culture care preservation and/or maintenance, culture care accommodation and/or negotiation, and culture care repatterning and/or restructuring—are presented to demonstrate ways to provide culturally congruent nursing care (Leininger, 1991, 1995; Leininger & McFarland, 2002). Among the strengths of Leininger's theory is its flexibility for use with individuals, families, groups, communities, and institutions in diverse health systems. Leininger's Sunrise Model depicts components of the Theory of Cultural Care Diversity and Universality, and it provides a visual schematic representation of the key components of the theory and the interrelationships among its parts. As the world of nursing and health care has become increasingly multicultural, the theory's relevance has increased as well. For further information about Dr. Leininger and her Theory of

Culture Care Diversity and Universality, visit either Dr. Leininger's Web site (http://www.madeleine-leininger.com) or the Transcultural Nursing Society's Web site (http://www.tcns.org).

Other Models to Provide Nursing Care to Culturally Diverse Clients

While this text has chosen to focus on the work of Leininger and the Theory of Cultural Care Diversity and Universality, there are other models that assist nurses to provide culturally competent care. The **Giger and Davidhizar Transcultural Assessment Model** was developed in 1988 to help nursing students provide care to patients who were culturally diverse. The model includes six cultural phenomena that are used as a framework for patient assessment and to provide culturally competent care to clients. The six cultural phenomena are communication, time, space, social organization, environmental control, and biological variations. This model is especially helpful for nursing students and other nurses or health care professionals who are developing an interest in providing care that is appropriate for patients from diverse cultures (Giger & Davidhizar, 1991, 2002).

The **Purnell Model for Cultural Competence** is an organizing framework of 12 domains as well as the primary and secondary characteristics of culture, which determine the beliefs, values, and practices of an individual's cultural heritage. The model can be used by multidisciplinary members of the health care team in a variety of primary, secondary, and tertiary settings. Purnell (2002, 2005) emphasizes that culture is an extremely demanding and complex concept, requiring providers to look at themselves, their patients, their communities, their colleagues, and their employment settings from multiple perspectives. He suggests that culture is learned first in the family, then in the school, and later in the community and social organizations such as churches, workplaces, and other group associations (Purnell & Paulanka, 2008).

TABLE 1-1

Contributions of Madeleine Leininger to the Development of Transcultural Nursing

DATE	ACHIEVEMENT AND CONTRIBUTION
1954	Dr. Madeleine Leininger noticed and studied the cultural differences in the perception of care
1965	Leininger earned a doctorate in cultural anthropology (University of Washington)
1965–1969	Leininger offered first courses and telelectures offered in transcultural nursing (University of Colorado School of Nursing)
	Established first PhD nurse–scientist program combining anthropology and nursing (University of Colorado School of Nursing)
1973	First academic department in transcultural nursing established (University of Washington School of Nursing)
1974	Transcultural Nursing Society established as the official organization of transcultural nursing
1975	First national transcultural nursing conference, *Care of Infants and Children*, held at Snowbird, Utah; thereafter annual conferences held at various locations in the United States, Canada, the Netherlands, Finland, Australia, Spain, and United Kingdom
1978	First advanced degree programs (master's and doctoral) established (University of Utah School of Nursing) Dr. Leininger published *Transcultural Nursing: Concepts Theories, Research and Practices* (1st ed.)
1988	Transcultural Nursing Society initiated certification examinations: Certified Transcultural Nurse (CTN)
1989	*Journal of Transcultural Nursing* (JTN) first published as official publication of the Transcultural Nursing Society with Dr. Madeleine Leininger as founding editor. Goal of the *JTN*: to disseminate transcultural ideas, theories, research findings, and/or practice experiences
1991	Dr. Leininger published *Culture Care Diversity and Universality: A Theory of Nursing*, in which she outlined her theory (Culture Care Diversity and Universality and the Sunrise Model) and its research applications
1995	Dr. Leininger published *Transcultural Nursing: Concepts Theories, Research and Practices* (2nd ed.)
2000	As part of a longstanding history of collaboration with Madonna University (Livonia, Michigan), Dr. Leininger negotiated to build the Transcultural Nursing Society's World Headquarters as part of a new wing of the building that houses the College of Nursing and Health
2002	Dr. Leininger (with co-author Dr. Marilyn McFarland) published *Transcultural Nursing: Concepts, Theories, Research, and Practices* (3rd ed.)
2004	Installation of the Founder and Presidential Photos in the Global Transcultural Nursing Headquarters and induction as a charter member of the Transcultural Nursing Scholars (TNS)
2006	Dr. Leininger (with co-author Dr. Marilyn McFarland) published *Culture Care Diversity and Universality: A Worldwide Theory for Nursing*
2006	Dr. Leininger released a series of three DVDs: *The Life Career of Leininger*, *The Theory of Culture Care*, and *Conversation with a Legend*
2007 to present	A member of the Transcultural Nursing Society's Board of Directors and Professor Emerita at Wayne State University and the University of Nebraska, Dr. Leininger continues to be active as a transcultural nurse consultant, scholar, researcher, speaker, and leader in the field of transcultural nursing

Table based, in part, on Transcultural Nursing Society. (2007). Transcultural Nursing Society: Historical moments. *Transcultural Nursing Society Newsletter*, *16*(1), 9.

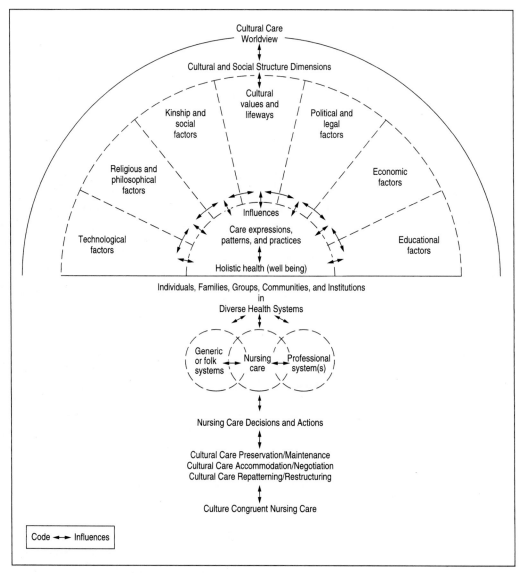

FIGURE 1-1   Leininger's Sunrise enabler to depict the Theory of Cultural Care Diversity and Universality. (Reprinted by permission from Leininger, M. M., & McFarland, M. R. [2006]. *Culture care diversity and universality: A worldwide theory for nursing* [2nd ed., p. 25]. Sudbury, MA: Jones & Bartlett, Publishers.)

The **Andrews/Boyle Transcultural Nursing Assessment Guide** (Appendix A) provides a comprehensive and practical overview of key assessment areas and the foundation for culturally competent care.

Campinha-Bacote (2002, 2007) developed a practice model for nurses and other health care providers to use to develop cultural competence. The **Campinha-Bacote Model of Cultural Competence in the Delivery of Healthcare Services**

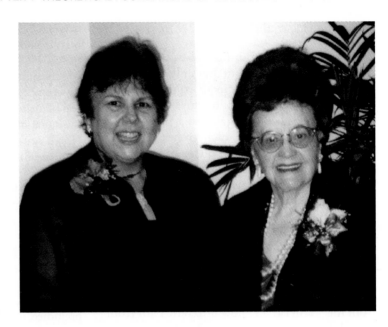

FIGURE 1-2 Author Dr. Margaret Andrews (*left*) and Transcultural Nursing Foundress, Dr. Madeleine Leininger (*right*), at a meeting of The American Academy of Nursing.

has five encompassing concepts that depict the process for developing cultural competence. The concepts are cultural awareness, cultural knowledge, cultural skill, cultural encounter, and cultural desire. Campinha-Bacote (2009) emphasizes that a cultural assessment should be conducted on every client as each client has values, beliefs, and practices that must be taken into consideration when delivering health and nursing care. A graphic display and additional information about the Campinha-Bacote Model can be found at Dr. Campinha-Bacote's Web site (http://www. transculturalcare.net/).

In addition, other nurse researchers have focused on generating their own descriptive theories that focus on nursing phenomena or specific cultural groups. Lipson and other researchers' extensive work with Afghan refugees (1991, 1992, 1993, 1994, 1995, 1997) has provided nurses and other health care professionals with the theoretical foundation and cultural knowledge to provide care to Afghan refugees living in the United States. Boyle, Ferrell, Hodnicki, and Muller (1996) and Boyle, Hodnicki, and Ferrell (1999) focused on African American caregiving while Shambley-Ebron and Boyle (2006a, 2006b)

examined caregiving and mothering in African American mothers with HIV/AIDS. Baird's (2009) study of Dinka Sudannese refugee women helps us understand the transition experiences of Dinka women who have immigrated to the United States and how these experiences influence health and well-being. There are countless other examples in the current nursing literature of research studies that focus on cultural phenomena and nursing care; the major goal is to help nurses and other health care professionals provide culturally competent care.

Critical Analysis of Transcultural Nursing

Transcultural nursing has been criticized for its definitional, theoretical, and practical limitations. You are encouraged to think critically as you examine some of the major criticisms of transcultural nursing. Recognizing that all nursing theories have limitations, you are urged to critically reflect on ways in which the limitations can be addressed or overcome.

Major Criticisms

Let us begin by examining the criticism that transcultural nursing contains ambiguous terminology and lacks clarity in describing key concepts (Habayeb, 1995; Mulholland, 1995). For example, nurses have struggled to achieve clarity in concepts such as cultural awareness, cultural sensitivity, **cultural competence**, and **cultural congruence**. Color, religion, and geographic location are most often used to narrowly define culture and highlight cultural diversity, which is often portrayed as a minority/majority issue. Discrepancies in definition arise when one fails to recognize that every person has a cultural heritage. Talabere (1996) suggests that cultural diversity is itself an **ethnocentric** term because it focuses on "how different the other person is from me" rather than "how different I am from the other." In using the term *cultural diversity*, the White panethnic group is frequently viewed as the norm against which the differences in everyone else (ethnocentrically referred to as non-Whites) are measured or compared.

Another criticism of transcultural nursing models is their failure to recognize the relationship between knowledge and power and their inattention to the complexities associated with prejudice, discrimination, and racism (cf. Gustafson, 1999; Price & Cortis, 2000). Although Leininger and other transcultural nurses address the need to consider the political, economic, and social dimensions in their theoretical formulations, transcultural nursing has been criticized for doing too little to encourage nurses to be actively involved in setting political, economic, and social policy agendas.

Culley (1996) criticizes transcultural nursing for failing to recognize the power relations that exist between groups. When clients from traditionally underrepresented groups fail to behave as a nurse expects, the behavior is sometimes referred to as *noncompliant*, a term with a negative connotation that is sometimes used synonymously with *different, deviant, abnormal,* or *pathologic*. Problems are thought to be generated by customs or traditions

deemed by the nurse to be "inappropriate," a judgment that may be the result of personal bias, lack of knowledge concerning the cultural context in which these customs are practiced, the nurse's inexperience, or other factors. As a result, complex sociocultural phenomena are often reduced to overgeneralized stereotypes. For example, some North American nurses are critical of the role of women in traditional African and Middle Eastern cultures. In concentrating on culturally determined gender issues, you might ignore or minimize the significance of power, gender inequality, and racism as embedded in structures or institutions (Gustafson, 1999; Price & Cortis, 2000), factors that fundamentally affect the health of cultural groups and their members' access to quality health care. The same criticism might be applied to nursing's failure to address other forms of bias, prejudice, discrimination, and social injustice.

Juntunen (2007) has criticized Leininger for generalizing her research by creating lists of the culture care values, meanings, and action modes of each of the cultures that she and others have studied. These generalizations foster stereotyping and fail to consider the variations within cultures that influence the ways in which people express their cultural orientation. Lastly, every belief and practice has both cultural and individual or familial determinants.

Finally, transcultural nursing has been criticized for embracing models based on the assumption that understanding one's own culture and the culture of others creates tolerance and respect for people from diverse backgrounds. It has become apparent that the mere awareness of one's own culture and that of others is insufficient for the alleviation and potential eradication of prejudice, bigotry, racial, ethnic, or cultural conflicts, discrimination, or ethnic violence. Rather, nursing students, nurses, and other health care providers must have positive experiences with members of other cultures and learn to genuinely value the contributions all cultures make to our multicultural society. Nevertheless, becoming aware of one's own culture and that of others is a starting pointing for developing the sensitivity, skills, and knowledge necessary to provide cultur-ally competent health and nursing care.

Response to Criticisms

In the remainder of this book, we, the authors, will attempt to address these criticisms of transcultural nursing through our approach to topics. It should be noted, however, that many of the issues raised by critics have deeply rooted historical, socioeco-nomic, religious, cultural, and political origins. Because the nursing profession is a microcosm of society, it mirrors the biases and prejudices found in the larger social order. It is unrealistic to expect that transcultural nursing can reverse all the in-equalities cited by the critics. It is realistic, however, to expect more definitional, conceptual, and theo-retical clarity. It also is realistic to expect nurses to become increasingly active in setting political, economic, and social policy agendas at the local, state/provincial, national, and international levels.

For example, you can empower yourself and your profession by running for elected offices; supporting candidates with health-related agen-das congruent with your own; voting for candi-dates from diverse cultural backgrounds; using print, broadcast, and Web-based media to influ-ence public opinion; and joining professional or-ganizations or unions that employ professional lobbyists to represent them. You have the power to confront prejudice and discrimination by re-fusing to tolerate ethnic jokes and other expres-sions of prejudice in health care or educational settings. You can use peer pressure to change cul-turally insensitive or offensive behavior by oth-ers. You can also work with others to ensure that medical and surgical procedures, health-related appointments, and schedules are congruent with the religious and cultural calendars of clients, staff, and students.

Nurse educators can examine admission and re-cruitment policies, curricula, pedagogy, academic calendars, and teaching strategies from a transcul-tural nursing perspective. Nurse researchers need to ensure that diversity is represented in the popu-lation studied, that appropriate translation and interpretation have been used for non–English-speaking informants or subjects, and that research instruments are appropriate for use with diverse populations. Finally, nurses in key administrative positions can critically assess the organizational climate and culture for its encouragement of di-versity, examine the organization's administrative hierarchy for the presence of diversity in leadership positions, evaluate its commitment to culturally sensitive and appropriate personnel policies, and foster an openness to different perspectives on leadership and management. The examples cited are intended to be illustrative, not exhaustive.

A variety of organizations, professional publi-cations, and electronic resources support the de-velopment of transcultural nursing and health. With the proliferation of electronic resources available to search for subjects related to trans-cultural nursing and health, it is important for you to keep abreast of computer-based tools that enable you to obtain the information you need on a wide variety of transcultural subjects. Andrews, Burr, and Janetos (2004) provide sug-gestions for narrowing and focusing your search using important research databases such as Med-line, Cumulative Index to Nursing and Allied Health Literature (CINAHL), Educational Re-sources Information Center (ERIC), and Psycho-logical Abstracts (PsycINFO). Selected Web sites for U.S. government agencies, organizations, and commercial groups that concern transcul-tural nursing and health care are also described in brief annotations. Table 1-2 provides some basic information on selected resources.

Standards for Transcultural Nursing

Under the leadership of the Minnesota Chap-ter of the Transcultural Nursing Society, stan-dards for transcultural nursing have been developed based on Leininger's Theory of Cul-ture Care Diversity and Universality (Leininger, 1991, 1995, 1998; Leininger & McFarland,

TABLE 1-2
Selected Resources for Transcultural Nursing

PROFESSIONAL RESOURCES	DESCRIPTION	REMARKS
Professional Organizations	Council on Nursing and Anthropology Association (CONAA) (1968)	Organization for nurse–anthropologists, transcultural nurses, and anthropologists Purpose: promotes interdisciplinary research exchange
	Transcultural Nursing Society (TNS) (1974)	Organization of transcultural nurses Purpose: to promote transcultural nursing knowledge and competencies globally through education, research, consultation, and clinical services
	Council on Cultural Diversity of the American Nurses' Association (ANA, 1978)	ANA council of transcultural nurses Purpose: to focus on diversity issues in clinical practice
	International Association of Human Caring (1987)	Organization of qualitative researchers, some of whom are nurses Purpose: to explore the cultural similarities and differences in expressions of human care
	Committee on Cultural Diversity	Committee established by the American Academy of Nursing Purpose: to develop guidelines for culturally competent nursing
Refereed Printed Materials on Transcultural Nursing and Health	*Journal of Transcultural Nursing*	Only publication focused on transcultural nursing theory, research methods, consultation, teaching, and clinical community practices
	Journal of Multicultural Nursing and Health (JMCNH)	Interdisciplinary; addresses multiculturalism in nursing education and/or health
	Journal of Cultural Diversity	Focuses on cultural diversity theory and principles from a variety of perspectives
	Association of Black Nursing Faculty (ABNF) *Journal*	Documents the distinct nature and health care needs of the Black patient
	International Nursing Review *International Journal of Nursing Studies*	Both published by the International Council of Nurses
Nonrefereed Print Materials	*Minority Nurse Newsletter*	Examines minority issues affecting patient care and nursing education
	Closing the Gap (newsletter)	Published by the Federal Office of Minority Health; focuses on federal interventions aimed at improving the health of panethnic groups
	IHS Primary Care Provider (newsletter)	Published by the Federal Indian Health Service; free to nursing and medical students and health care providers

PROFESSIONAL RESOURCES	DESCRIPTION	REMARKS
Electronic Resources	http://www.ojccnh.org	Official Web site for the *Online Journal of Cultural Competence in Nursing and Healthcare*
	http://www.tcns.org	Official Web site for the Transcultural Nursing Society, provides information about membership in the organization, conferences, regional workshops, transcultural nursing certification, and the *Journal of Transcultural Nursing*; useful links to other Web sites of relevance to transcultural nursing

2002) and Campinha-Bacote's Model of Cultural Competence (Campinha-Bacote, 2002). The Standards for Transcultural Nursing were developed to foster excellence in transcultural nursing practice, provide criteria for the evaluation of transcultural nursing, create a tool for teaching and learning, increase the public's confidence in the nursing profession, and advance the field of transcultural nursing. The general membership of the Transcultural Nursing Society subsequently reviewed and approved the standards, which, effective fall 2008, will form the foundation for the Transcultural Nursing Certification Exam. Each of the eight **transcultural nursing standards** is accompanied by rationale, process criteria, and outcome criteria. The eight standards are (1) Theoretical Foundations of Transcultural Nursing, (2) Cultural Information Gathering, (3) Caring and Healing Systems, (4) Cultural Health Patterns and Caring Practices, (5) Health Care Planning, (6) Evaluation, (7) Research, and (8) Professional Development. These eight standards were developed to assist nurses in providing culturally competent and culturally congruent care, a topic that will be discussed in more depth in Chapter 2. Standards provide clarity in direction for nursing practice, reflect values and priorities in professional practice, define accountability to the public, and provide a clear framework for evaluation of transcultural nursing practice (Leuning, Swiggum, Wieger, &

McCullough-Zander, 2002; Transcultural Nursing Certification Committee, 2007).

Certification in Transcultural Nursing

Transcultural nursing certification represents a professionally recognized credentialing process. Certification sets apart those professional graduate nurses who have achieved a level of understanding of diverse cultures and had clinical experiences to provide knowledgeable and competent care to clients of diverse cultural backgrounds. In addition, the transcultural nurse identifies the necessary concepts and has the skills to assess and implement care that is congruent with the values, beliefs, and life ways of the clients being served. Professional certification in transcultural nursing is paramount to the advancement of the discipline (Marilyn R. McFarland, personal communication, April, 4, 2010).

Initial credentialing of transcultural nurses took place at the annual meeting of the Transcultural Nursing Society in Edmonton, Alberta, Canada in 1988. In the early days of certification, applicants had to make application, including documented qualifications, though a portfolio of credentials attesting academic and experiential understanding of transcultural nursing theory, principle, concepts, and research. An oral examination was also administered. The ensuing years have brought changes in the certification application and process. Applicants today still have to compile a portfolio of qualifying documentation to authenticate their educational and experiential background, but have the flexibility of taking an examination online at multiple dates throughout the year. The oral examination is no longer required. Successful applicants earn the CTN-A (Certified Transcultural Nurse-Advanced) credential. Plans are also underway to initiate a basic certification process in 2011 for associate degree and baccalaureate degree nurses. Basic certification is recognition by the Transcultural Nursing Certification Commission that cultural competence should be practiced by all nurses.

SUMMARY

In this introductory chapter, we have examined the historical origins of transcultural nursing as a blending of two fields: anthropology and nursing. Founded by nurse–anthropologist Dr. Madeleine M. Leininger, transcultural nursing has provided a theoretical foundation to guide nurses in the provision of culturally congruent and competent care for individual clients and patients of all ages, families, groups, and communities. Transcultural nursing also enables nurses to examine the cultural dimensions of health and nursing organizations, institutions, and agencies. Leininger's Theory of Culture Care Diversity and Universality and her Sunrise Model were introduced. Others models for developing Cultural Competence were presented. Selected resources in transcultural nursing and health care were identified. Standards for Transcultural Nursing and Certification in Transcultural Nursing were briefly discussed.

REVIEW QUESTIONS

1. Conceived in the early 1950s by nurse–anthropologist Dr. Madeleine M. Leininger, the term *transcultural nursing* was coined in 1970 with her seminal work *Nursing and Anthropology: Two Worlds to Blend*. Define transcultural nursing in your own words.
2. Summarize the historical development of transcultural nursing since its founding by Dr. Madeleine Leininger.
3. Review the limitations of transcultural nursing cited by critics. What can be done to address the criticisms?
4. Identify electronic and print resources in transcultural nursing and health.

CRITICAL THINKING ACTIVITIES

1. Visit the Transcultural Nursing Society's official Web site (http://www.tcns.org).

   a. Briefly summarize the information you found at the Web site.
   b. Critically evaluate the strengths and limitations of this information source and the data available.
   c. What clinical relevance does the electronic information on transcultural nursing have for you as a nurse?
   d. Visit links to other related Web sites on transcultural nursing.

2. Using CINAHL, enter the words *transcultural nursing* and search for references cited during the past year. How many references are identified? What are the subcategories under which you can narrow your search? If you want information about a specific cultural, ethnic, or minority group, what keywords will help you to narrow the search? Consult a reference librarian for assistance if you need help.

REFERENCES

Andrews, M. M. (1992). Cultural perspectives on nursing in the 21st century. *Journal of Professional Nursing, 8*(1), 1–9.

Andrews, M. M. (1995). Transcultural nursing: Transforming the curriculum. *Journal of Transcultural Nursing, 6*(2), 4–9.

Andrews, M. M., & Boyle, J. S. (1997). Competence in transcultural nursing care. *American Journal of Nursing, 97*(8), 16AAA–16DDD.

Andrews, M. M., & Boyle, J. S. (2002). Transcultural concepts in nursing care. *Journal of Transcultural Nursing, 13*(3), 178–180.

Andrews, M. M., Burr, J., & Janetos, D. H. (2004). Searching electronically for information on transcultural nursing and health subjects. *Journal of Transcultural Nursing, 15*(3), 242–247.

Baird, M. B. (2009). *Resettlement transition experiences among Sudanese refugee women.* Doctoral Dissertation, University of Arizona, Tucson, Arizona.

Boyle, J. S., Ferrell, J., Hodnicki, D., & Muller, R. (1996). Going home: African American caregiving for adult children with human immunodeficiency virus disease. *Holistic Nursing Practice, 11,* 27–35.

Boyle, J. S., Hodnicki, D. R., & Ferrell, J. A. (1999). Patterns of resistance: African American mothers and adult children with HIV disease. *Scholarly Inquiry for Nursing Practice, 13,* 111–133.

Branch, M. F., & Paxton, P. P. (Eds.). (1976). *Providing safe nursing care for ethnic people of color.* New York: Appleton-Century-Crofts.

Campinha-Bacote, J. (2002). The process of cultural competence in the delivery of healthcare services: A model of care. *Journal of Transcultural Nursing, 13*(3), 181–184.

Campinha-Bacote, J. (2007). *The process of cultural competence in the delivery of health care services: The journey continues* (5th ed.). Cincinnati, OH: Transcultural C.A.R.E. Associates.

Campinha-Bacote, J. (2009). A culturally competent model of care for African Americans. *Urologic Nursing, 29*(1), 49–54.

Culley, L. (1996). A critique of multiculturalism in health care: The challenge for nursing education. *Journal of Advanced Nursing, 23,* 564–570.

Dougherty, M. C., & Tripp-Reimer, T. (1985). The interface of nursing and anthropology. *Annual Review of Anthropology, 14,* 219–241.

Flaskerud, J. H. (2000). Ethnicity, culture and neuropsychiatry. *Issues in Mental Health Nursing, 21*(5), 5–29.

Giger, J. N., & Davidhizar, R. E. (1991). *Transcultural nursing: Assessment and intervention.* St. Louis: C. V. Mosby.

Giger, J. N., & Davidhizar, R. E. (2002). The Giger and Davidhizar transcultural assessment model. *Journal of Transcultural Nursing, 13*(3), 185–188.

Gustafson, D. L. (1999). Toward inclusionary practices in the education of nurses: A critique of transcultural nursing theory. *The Alberta Journal of Educational Research, 45*(4), 468–470.

Habayeb, G. L. (1995). Cultural diversity: A nursing concept not yet reliably defined. *Nursing Outlook, 43*(5), 224–227.

Juntunen, A. (2007). *Professional and lay care in the Tanzanian village of Ilembula* (Doctoral dissertation, University of

Oulu). Retrieved March 18, 2007, from http://herkules. oulu.fi/isbn9514264312/isbn9514264312.pdf.

Leininger, M. M. (1970). *Nursing and anthropology: Two worlds to blend.* New York: John Wiley & Sons.

Leininger, M. M. (1978). *Transcultural nursing: Concepts, theories and practices.* New York: John Wiley & Sons.

Leininger, M. M. (1991). *Culture care diversity and universality: A theory of nursing.* New York: National League for Nursing.

Leininger, M. M. (1995). *Transcultural nursing: Concepts, theories, research and practices.* New York: McGraw-Hill.

Leininger, M. M. (1997). Future directions in transcultural nursing in the 21st century. *International Nursing Review, 44*(1), 19–23.

Leininger, M. M. (1998). Twenty five years of knowledge and practice development transcultural nursing society annual research conferences. *Journal of Transcultural Nursing, 9*(2), 72–74.

Leininger, M. M. (1999). What is transcultural nursing and culturally competent care? *Journal of Transcultural Nursing, 10*(1), 9.

Leininger, M. M., & McFarland, M. R. (2002). *Transcultural nursing: Concepts, theories and practices.* New York: McGraw-Hill.

Leininger, M. M., & McFarland, M. R. (2006). *Culture care diversity and universality: A worldwide theory for nursing* (2nd ed.). Sudbury, MA: Jones & Bartlett, Publishers.

Leuning, C. J., Swiggum, P. D., Wieger, H. M. B., & McCullough-Zander, K. (2002). Proposed standards for transcultural nursing. *Journal of Transcultural Nursing, 13*(1), 40–46.

Lipson, J. (1991). Afghan refugee health: Some findings and suggestions. *Qualitative Health Research, 1,* 349–369.

Lipson, J. (1993). Afghan refuges in California: Mental health issues. *Issues in Mental Health Nursing, 14,* 411–423.

Lipson, J. G. (1999). Cross-cultural nursing: The cultural perspective. *Journal of Transcultural Nursing, 10*(1), 7.

Lipson, J., & Bauwens, E. (1988). Uses of anthropology in nursing. *Practicing Anthropology, 10,* 4–5.

Lipson, J., & Miller, S. (1994). Changing roles of Afghan refugee women in the U.S. *Health Care for Women International, 15,* 171–180.

Lipson, J., & Omidian, P. (1992). Afghan refugees: Health issues in the United States. *Western Journal of Medicine, 157,* 271–275.

Lipson, J., & Omidian, P. (1997). Afghan refugee issues in the U.S. social environment. *Western Journal of Nursing Research, 19*(1), 100–116.

Lipson, J., Omidian, P., & Paul, S. (1995). Afghan health education project: A community survey. *Public Health Nursing, 12,* 143–150.

Mahoney, J. S., & Engebretson, J. (2000). The interface of anthropology and nursing guiding culturally competent care in psychiatric nursing. *Archives of Psychiatric Nursing, 14*(4), 183–190.

McKenna, M. (1984). Anthropology and nursing: The interaction between two fields of inquiry. *Western Journal of Nursing Research, 6*(4), 423–431.

Mulholland, J. (1995). Nursing humanism and transcultural theory: The "bracketing out" of reality. *Journal of Advanced Nursing, 22,* 442–449.

Orque, M. S., Bloch, B., & Monrroy, L. S. (1983). *Ethnic nursing care.* St. Louis: C.V. Mosby.

Osborne, O. (1969). Anthropology and nursing: Some common traditions and interests. *Nursing Research, 18*(3), 251–255.

Price, K. M., & Cortis, J. D. (2000). The way forward for transcultural nursing. *Nurse Education Today, 20*(3), 233–243.

Purnell, L. (2002). The Purnell model for cultural competence. *Journal of Transcultural Nursing, 13,* 193–196.

Purnell, L. (2005). The Purnell model for cultural competence. *Journal of Multicultural Nursing & Health, 11*(2), 7–15.

Purnell, L., & Paulanka, B. J. (Eds.). (2008). Transcultural health care: A culturally competent approach. Philadelphia: F. A. Davis.

Reynolds, C. L., & Leininger, M. M. (1993). *Madeleine Leininger: Cultural care diversity and universality theory.* Newbury Park, NJ: Sage.

Shambley-Ebron, D., & Boyle, J. S. (2006a). Self-care and the cultural meaning of mothering in African American women with HIV/AIDS. *Western Journal of Nursing Research, 28,* 42–60.

Shambley-Ebron, D. & Boyle, J. S. (2006b). In our grandmothers' footsteps: Perceptions of Being Strong in African *American women with HIV/AIDS.* Advances in Nursing Science, 29(3), 195–206.

Talabere, L. R. (1996). Meeting the challenge of culture care in nursing: Diversity, sensitivity, and congruence. *Journal of Cultural Diversity, 3*(2), 53–61.

Transcultural Nursing Certification Committee. (2007, March 23–25). *Transcultural Nursing Certification revision.* Conducted at Transcultural Nursing Certification Committee Meeting, Fenton, Michigan.

Transcultural Nursing Society. (2007). Transcultural Nursing Society: Historical moments. *Transcultural Nursing Society Newsletter, 16*(1), 9.

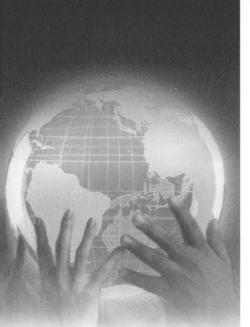

Culturally Competent Nursing Care

Margaret M. Andrews

KEY TERMS

Collateral relationships
Cross-cultural communication
Cultural code
Cultural competence
Culturally and linguistically
    appropriate services (CLAS)
Culturally congruent care
Cultural self-assessment
Distance
Environmental context
Eye contact
Individual cultural competence
Linguistic competence
Nonverbal communication
Proxemics
Sick role behavior
Silence
Space
Touch

LEARNING OBJECTIVES

1. Analyze the complex integration of knowledge, attitudes, and skills needed for cultural competence.
2. Explore cross-cultural communication as the foundation for the provision of culturally competent nursing care.
3. Identify strategies for promoting effective cross-cultural communication in multicultural health care settings.

Cultural competence has been a subject of considerable interest during the past two decades. Health care professionals, educators, social workers, and others are all concerned that their services be acceptable and appropriate for those they serve. Cultural competence can be divided into two major categories: (1) *organizational cultural competence* and (2) *individual cultural competence*, which refers to nurses, physicians, social workers, or others in health care, education, or social services professionals.

According to the National Center for Cultural Competence (Georgetown University Center for Child and Human Development, n.d.), cultural competence requires that *organizations* have the following characteristics:

• A defined set of values and principles and demonstration of behaviors, attitudes, policies, and structures that enable them to work effectively cross-culturally.

- The capacity to (1) value diversity, (2) conduct self-assessment, (3) manage the dynamics of difference, (4) acquire and institutionalize cultural knowledge, and (5) adapt to diversity and the cultural contexts of the communities they serve.
- Incorporation of the previously mentioned items in all aspects of policy making, administration, practice, and service delivery, and systematic involvement of consumers, key stakeholders, and communities.

Individual cultural competence refers to a complex integration of knowledge, attitudes, beliefs, skills, and encounters with those from cultures different from one's own that enhances cross-cultural communication and appropriate and effective interactions with others (American Academy of Nursing, 1992, 1993; Campinha-Bacote, 2000, 2002, 2003; Geron, 2002). Cultural competence has been defined as a process, as opposed to an end point, in which the nurse continuously strives to work effectively within the cultural context of an individual, family, or community from a diverse cultural background (Andrews & Boyle, 1997; Campinha-Bacote, 2000, 2002, 2003; Campinha-Bacote & Munoz, 2001; Wells, 2000; Smith, 1998). Campinha-Bacote (2003) defines cultural competence as "the ongoing process in which the health care professional continuously strives to seek the ability and availability to work effectively within the cultural context of the client (individual, family, community). This process involves the integration of cultural desire, cultural awareness, cultural knowledge, cultural skill and cultural encounters" (Campinha-Bacote, 2003, p. 14).

Cultural competence is one of the main ingredients in closing the health disparities gap as health care services that are respectful and responsive to the health care beliefs, practices, cultural, and linguistic needs of diverse patients can help bring about positive health outcomes. It is becoming increasingly clear that the health care provider who views the world through his or her own limited set of values can compromise access for patients from other cultures. Health care organizations that do not respect the values of the communities they serve also compromise the services they provide.

In addition to cultural competence, some experts have noted the considerable impact that **linguistic competence** by health care providers has on clients' access and response to health care services. Cultural and linguistic competence refers to the ability of health care providers and health care organizations to understand and effectively respond to the cultural and linguistic needs brought by clients to the health care encounter. Summarized in Box 2-1 are the 14 recommended standards for **culturally and linguistically appropriate health care services (CLAS)** proposed by the U.S. Department of Health and Human Services, Office of Minority Health (2007). These 14 standards include a definition of culturally competent care, as well as standards concerning language access, required organizational support, implementation guidelines, the relationship between the standards and existing laws, diverse and culturally competent staff, data collection, and information dissemination.

Instead of using the term *cultural competence*, Leininger (1991, 1995, 1999) and Leininger and McFarland (2002, 2005) prefer **culturally congruent care**, which they define as the provision of care that is meaningful and fits with cultural beliefs and lifeways. Leininger's early definition of culturally congruent care is holistic and focuses on the complex interrelationship of lifeways, religion, kinship, politics, law, education, technology, language, **environmental context**, and worldview—all factors that contribute to culturally congruent care.

Because you may encounter clients from literally hundreds of cultures in your professional career and clients of mixed cultural heritage, it is virtually impossible to know about the culturally based, health-related beliefs and practices of them all. It is, however, possible to master the knowledge and skills associated with cultural assessment and learn about some of the cultural dimensions of care for clients representing the groups most frequently encountered. In-depth knowledge of several cultures is often a reasonable goal if you live in a large urban center characterized by a high degree of diversity. You can also learn about other cultures by reading

> ### BOX 2-1
>
> ## Office of Minority Health Standards for Culturally and Linguistically Appropriate Services (CLAS) by Health Care Organizations
>
> - Health care organizations should ensure that patients/consumers receive from all staff members effective, understandable, and respectful care that is provided in a manner compatible with their cultural health beliefs and practices and preferred language.
> - Health care organizations should implement strategies to recruit, retain, and promote at all levels of the organization a diverse staff and leadership that are representative of the demographic characteristics of the service area.
> - Health care organizations should ensure that staff at all levels and across all disciplines receive ongoing education and training in culturally and linguistically appropriate service delivery.
> - Health care organizations must offer and provide language assistance services, including bilingual staff and interpreter services, at no cost to each patient/consumer with limited English proficiency at all points of contact, in a timely manner during all hours of operation.
> - Health care organizations must provide to patients/consumers in their preferred language both verbal offers and written notices informing them of their right to receive language assistance services.
> - Health care organizations must assure the competence of language assistance provided to limited English proficient patients/consumers by interpreters and bilingual staff. Family and friends should not be used to provide interpretation services (except on request by the patient/consumer).
> - Health care organizations must make available easily understood patient-related materials and post signage in the languages of the commonly encountered groups and/or groups represented in the service area.
> - Health care organizations should develop, implement, and promote a written strategic plans that outlines clear goals, policies, operational
>
> plans, and management accountability/oversight mechanisms to provide culturally and linguistically appropriate services.
> - Health care organizations should conduct initial and ongoing organizational self-assessments of CLAS-related activities and are encouraged to integrate cultural and linguistic competence-related measures into their internal audits, performance improvement programs, patient satisfaction assessments, and outcomes-based evaluations.
> - Health care organizations should ensure that data on the individual patient's/consumer's race, ethnicity, and spoken and written language are collected in health records, integrated into the organization's management information systems, and periodically updated.
> - Health care organizations should maintain a current demographic, cultural, and epidemiological profile of the community as well as a needs assessment to accurately plan for and implement services that respond to the cultural and linguistic characteristics of the service area.
> - Health care organizations should develop participatory, collaborative partnerships with communities and utilize a variety of formal and informal mechanisms to facilitate community and patient/consumer involvement in designing and implementing CLAS-related activities.
> - Health care organizations should ensure that conflict and grievance resolution processes are culturally and linguistically sensitive and capable of identifying, preventing, and resolving cross-cultural conflicts or complaints by patients/consumers.
> - Health care organizations are encouraged to regularly make available to the public information about their progress and successful innovations in implementing the CLAS standards and to provide public notice in their communities about the availability of this information.

Source: Office of Minority Health (April, 2007). National standards on culturally linguistically appropriate services (CLAS). *Federal Register* 65(247), 80865–80879. Department of Health and Human Services, U.S. Public Health Service. Washington, D.C. Retrieved February 2, 2010 from *http://www.omhre.gov/clas/ds.htm.*

books and professional journals that discuss other cultures and culturally competent care, participating in cultural celebrations, ceremonies, and related activities, eating food from diverse cultures, attending museums, theatre, and various cultural or ethnic events. Schools, television, churches, and political and social organizations all offer opportunities for multicultural exposure.

Cultural Self-Assessment

Before you can provide culturally competent care for people from diverse backgrounds, it's important to engage in a **cultural self-assessment**. When interacting with clients from various cultural backgrounds, you must be aware of your own cultural values, attitudes, beliefs, and practices. To gain insight into the way you relate to various groups of people in society, describe your level of response to the groups identified in Box 2-2.

Through self-assessment, it is possible to gain insights into the health-related values, attitudes, beliefs, and practices that have been transmitted to you by your own family and your own life experiences. These insights also enable you to overcome ethnocentric tendencies and cultural stereotypes, which are vehicles for perpetuating

---

BOX 2-2

How Do You Relate to Various Groups of People in the Society?

Described below are different levels of response you might have toward a person.

Levels of Response

1. Greet: I feel I can greet this person warmly and welcome him or her sincerely.

2. *Accept*: I feel I can honestly *accept* this person as he or she is and be comfortable enough to listen to his or her problems.

3. *Help*: I feel I would genuinely try to *help* this person with his or her problems as they might relate to or arise from the label-stereotype given to him or her.

4. *Background*: I feel I have the *background* of knowledge and/or experience to be able to help this person.

5. *Advocate*: I feel I could honestly be an *advocate* for this person.

The following is a list of individuals. Read down the list and place a checkmark next to anyone you would *not* "greet" or would hesitate to "greet." Then move to response level 2, "accept," and follow the same procedure. Try to respond honestly, not as you think might be socially or professionally desirable. Your answers are only for your personal use in clarifying your initial reactions to different people.

Level of Response

Individual	1 Greet	2 Accept	3 Help	4 Background	5 Advocate
1. Haitian	☐	☐	☐	☐	☐
2. Child abuser	☐	☐	☐	☐	☐
3. Jew	☐	☐	☐	☐	☐
4. Person with hemophilia	☐	☐	☐	☐	☐
5. Neo-Nazi	☐	☐	☐	☐	☐
6. Mexican American	☐	☐	☐	☐	☐
7. IV drug user	☐	☐	☐	☐	☐
8. Catholic	☐	☐	☐	☐	☐

BOX 2-2 (continued)

9. Senile, elderly person	☐	☐	☐	☐	☐
10. Teamster Union member	☐	☐	☐	☐	☐
11. Native American	☐	☐	☐	☐	☐
12. Prostitute	☐	☐	☐	☐	☐
13. Jehovah's witness	☐	☐	☐	☐	☐
14. Cerebral palsied person	☐	☐	☐	☐	☐
15. ERA proponent	☐	☐	☐	☐	☐
16. Vietnamese American	☐	☐	☐	☐	☐
17. Gay/lesbian	☐	☐	☐	☐	☐
18. Atheist	☐	☐	☐	☐	☐
19. Person with AIDS	☐	☐	☐	☐	☐

How Do You Relate to Various Groups of People in the Society?

Level of Response

Individual	1 Greet	2 Accept	3 Help	4 Background	5 Advocate
20. Communist	☐	☐	☐	☐	☐
21. Black American	☐	☐	☐	☐	☐
22. Unmarried expectant teenager	☐	☐	☐	☐	☐
23. Protestant	☐	☐	☐	☐	☐
24. Amputee	☐	☐	☐	☐	☐
25. Ku Klux Klansman	☐	☐	☐	☐	☐
26. White Anglo-Saxon	☐	☐	☐	☐	☐
27. Alcoholic	☐	☐	☐	☐	☐
28. Amish person	☐	☐	☐	☐	☐
29. Person with cancer	☐	☐	☐	☐	☐
30. Nuclear armament proponent	☐	☐	☐	☐	☐

Scoring Guide: The previous activity may help you anticipate difficulty in working with some clients at various levels. The 30 types of individuals can be grouped into five categories: ethnic/racial, social issues/problems, religious, physically/mentally handicapped, and political. Transfer your checkmarks to the following form. If you have a concentration of checks within a specific category of individuals or at specific levels, this may indicate a conflict that could hinder you from rendering effective professional help.

(box continues on page 22)

BOX 2-2

How Do You Relate to Various Groups of People in the Society? (continued)

Level of Response

Individual	1 Greet	2 Accept	3 Help	4 Background	5 Advocate
Ethnic/racial					
1. Haitian American	☐	☐	☐	☐	☐
6. Mexican American	☐	☐	☐	☐	☐
11. Native American	☐	☐	☐	☐	☐
16. Vietnamese American	☐	☐	☐	☐	☐
21. Black American	☐	☐	☐	☐	☐
26. White Anglo-Saxon	☐	☐	☐	☐	☐
Social issues/problems					
2. Child abuser	☐	☐	☐	☐	☐
7. IV drug user	☐	☐	☐	☐	☐
12. Prostitute	☐	☐	☐	☐	☐
17. Gay/lesbian	☐	☐	☐	☐	☐
22. Unmarried expectant teenager	☐	☐	☐	☐	☐
27. Alcoholic	☐	☐	☐	☐	☐
Religious					
3. Jew	☐	☐	☐	☐	☐
8. Catholic	☐	☐	☐	☐	☐
13. Jehovah's Witness	☐	☐	☐	☐	☐
18. Atheist	☐	☐	☐	☐	☐
23. Protestant	☐	☐	☐	☐	☐
28. Amish person	☐	☐	☐	☐	☐

How Do You Relate to Various Groups of People in the Society?

Level of Response

Individual	1 Greet	2 Accept	3 Help	4 Background	5 Advocate
Physically/mentally handicapped					
4. Person with hemophilia	☐	☐	☐	☐	☐
9. Senile elderly person	☐	☐	☐	☐	☐
14. Cerebral palsied person	☐	☐	☐	☐	☐

BOX 2-2 *(continued)*

19. Person with AIDS	☐	☐	☐	☐	☐
24. Amputee	☐	☐	☐	☐	☐
29. Person with cancer	☐	☐	☐	☐	☐
Political					
5. Neo-Nazi	☐	☐	☐	☐	☐
10. Teamster Union member	☐	☐	☐	☐	☐
15. ERA proponent	☐	☐	☐	☐	☐
20. Communist	☐	☐	☐	☐	☐
25. Ku Klux Klansman	☐	☐	☐	☐	☐
30. Nuclear armament proponent	☐	☐	☐	☐	☐

Reproduced with permission of the Association for the Care of Children's Health, 7910 Woodmont Avenue, Suite 300, Bethesda, MD 20814, from E. Randall-David (1989). *Strategies for Working with Culturally Diverse Communities and Clients*, pp. 7–9.

prejudice and discrimination against members of certain groups.

After you have engaged in a cultural self-assessment, it is possible to conduct a cultural assessment of others.

Cultural Assessment

The author believes that cultural assessment is the foundation for culturally competent and culturally congruent nursing care. Appendix A contains the Andrews/Boyle Transcultural Nursing Assessment Guide for Individuals and Families, an instrument that is intended to help you to ask key questions during your assessment interview. Please refer to Chapter 3, Cultural Competence in the Health History and Physical Examination, for a complete discussion of cultural assessment. Attaining competence in conducting a cultural assessment is a developmental process that occurs along a continuum. As you work and learn about people from another cultural group, you gain the skills and knowledge necessary for cultural competence.

Skills Needed for Cultural Competence

The term *cultural competence* implies that you have developed certain psychomotor or behavioral skills. Box 2-3 contains selected examples of these skills, and others will be presented throughout the text. It should be noted that mastery of some skills, such as the assessment of cyanosis in people with darkly pigmented skin, might be critical for a patient's survival. Other skills may be helpful in promoting hygiene or comfort, but they do not have such dire consequences. Because communication is a skill foundational to all nursing interactions, the remainder of this chapter will focus on this important topic.

Cross-Cultural Communication

Communication is an organized, patterned system of behavior that regulates and makes possible all nurse–client interactions. It is the exchange of messages and the creation of meaning. Because

BOX 2-3
Selected Examples of Psychomotor Skills Useful in Transcultural Nursing

Assessment

- Techniques for assessing biocultural variations in health and illness,for example, assessing cyanosis, jaundice, anemia, and related clinical manifestations of disease in darkly pigmented clients; differentiating between mongolian spots and ecchymoses (bruises)
- Measurement of head circumference and fontanelles in infants using techniques not in violation of taboos for selected cultural groups
- Growth and development monitoring for children of Asian heritage, using culturally appropriate growth grids
- Cultural modification of the Denver II and other developmental tests used for children
- Conducting culturally appropriate obstetric and gynecologic examinations of women from various cultural backgrounds

Communication

- Speaking and writing the language(s) used by clients
- Using alternative methods of communicating with non–English-speaking clients and families when no interpreter is available (e.g., pantomime)

Hygiene

- Skin care for clients of various racial/ethnic backgrounds
- Hair care for clients of various ethnic/racial backgrounds, for example, care of African American clients' hair

Activities of Daily Living

- Assisting Chinese American clients to regain use of chopsticks as part of rehabilitation regimen after a stroke
- Assisting paralyzed Amish client with dressing when buttons and pins are used
- Assisting West African client who uses "chewing stick" with oral hygiene

Religion

- Emergency baptism and anointing of the sick for Catholics
- Care before and after ritual circumcision by *mohel* (performed 8 days after the birth of a male Jewish infant)

---

communication and culture are acquired simultaneously, they are integrally linked. In effective communication there is mutual understanding of the meaning attached to the messages. Barriers to communication include differences in language, worldview, and values. It is estimated that up to 90% of all difficulties in nurse–client interactions have resulted from miscommunication.

To begin the discussion on **cross-cultural communication**, it is necessary to examine the ways in which people from various cultural backgrounds communicate with one another. In addition to oral and written communication, messages are conveyed nonverbally through gestures, body movements, posture, tone of voice, and facial expressions (Figure 2-1).

Frequently overlooked is the context in which communication occurs. The environmental context imparts its own message and is influenced by the

setting, the purposes of the communication, and the perceptions of the nurse and client concerning time, space, distance, touch, modesty, and other factors. For example, let us imagine you know that a Mexican American patient is extremely anxious about having a mammogram. After the procedure, you intend to send an empathetic, caring message by remarking, "It's all over, Señora Garcia." Señora Garcia bursts into tears because she believes she has been diagnosed with terminal breast cancer. Needless to say, even communication between individuals having the same cultural background may be fraught with pitfalls. When you communicate with others from cultural backgrounds different from your own and with those for whom English is a second language, the probability of miscommunication increases significantly. In promoting effective cross-cultural communication, you should avoid technical jargon, slang, colloquial expressions,

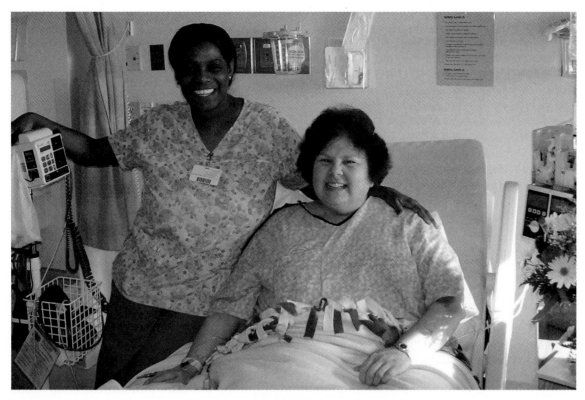

FIGURE 2-1 Effective cross-cultural communication is vital to the establishment of a strong nurse–patient relationship. It is important to understand both verbal and nonverbal cues when communicating with people from various cultural backgrounds (© Copyright M. Andrews).

abbreviations, and excessive use of medical terminology. This requires a very conscious effort on the part of the nurse.

There are numerous factors that are important to consider in cross-cultural communication. Certainly respect for the other cultural group, appreciation and comfort with cultural differences; enjoyment of learning through the cultural exchanges and ability to observe behavior without judging are all important ways to enhance cross-cultural communication. The ability to speak slowly and distinctly and without the use of slang are all very important, as anyone who has tried to learn and understand a foreign language has experienced. Success in cross-cultural communication includes the ability to communicate sincere interest in others, patience, and the ability to intervene

or start over when misunderstandings occur. Important factors to consider for cross-cultural communication include communication with family members and significant others; space, distance, and intimacy; nonverbal communication; language; and sick role behaviors (Figure 2-2).

Communication with Family Members and Significant Others

Knowledge of a client's family and kinship structure helps you to ascertain the values, decision-making patterns, and overall communication within the household. It is necessary to identify the significant others whom clients perceive to be important in their care and who may be responsible for decision making that affects their

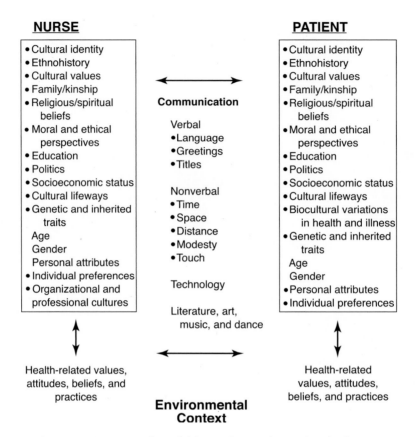

FIGURE 2-2   Conceptual model for understanding cultural influences on nurse–patient interactions.

health care. For example, for many clients, familism—which emphasizes interdependence over independence, affiliation over confrontation, and cooperation over competition—may dictate that important decisions affecting the client be made by the family, not the individual alone. When you work with clients from cultural groups that value cohesion, interdependence, and collectivism, you may perceive the family as being overly involved and usurping the autonomy of the client. At the same time, clients are likely to perceive the involvement with family as a source of mutual support, security, comfort, and fulfillment.

The family is the basic social unit in which children are raised and where they learn culturally based values, beliefs, and practices about health and illnesses. The essence of family consists of living together as a unit. Relationships that may seem obvious sometimes warrant further exploration when the nurse interacts with clients from culturally diverse backgrounds. For example, most European Americans define siblings as two persons with either the same mother, the same father, the same mother and father, or the same adoptive parents. In some Asian cultures, a sibling relationship is defined as any infants breast-fed by the same woman. In other cultures, certain kinship patterns, such as maternal first cousins, are defined as sibling relationships. In some African cultures, anyone from the same village may be called brother or sister.

Members of some ethnoreligious groups (e.g., Roman Catholics of Italian, Polish, Spanish, or Mexican descent) recognize relationships such as godmother or godfather, in which an individual who is not the biologic parent promises to assist with the moral or spiritual development of an infant and agrees to care for the child in the event of parental death. The godparent makes these promises during the religious ceremony of baptism and often the relationship is strong and supportive throughout the life of the godparents and/ or child. In communicating with the parent or parent surrogate of infants and children, it is important to identify the primary provider of care and the key decision maker who acts on behalf of the child. In some instances, this person may not be the biologic parent. Among some Hispanic groups, for example, female members of the nuclear or extended family such as sisters and aunts are primary providers of care for infants and children. In some African American families, the grandmother may be the decision maker and primary caretaker of children. To provide culturally congruent care, you must be certain that you are effectively communicating with the appropriate decision maker(s).

When making health-related decisions, some members of culturally diverse backgrounds in which lineal relationships predominate may seek assistance from other members of the family. It is sometimes culturally expected that a relative (e.g., parent, grandparent, eldest son, or eldest brother) will make decisions about important health-related matters. For example, in many Asian cultures, it is the obligation and duty of the eldest son and his spouse to assume primary responsibility for his aging parents and to make health care decisions for them. If **collateral relationships** are valued, decisions about the client may be interrelated with the impact of illness on the entire family or group. For example, among the Amish, the entire community is affected by the illness of a member because the community pays for health care from a common fund, members join together to meet the needs of both the sick person and his or her family throughout the illness, and the roles of dozens of people in the community are likely to be affected by the illness of a single member. The individual values orientation concerning relationships is predominant among the dominant cultural majority in North America. Although members of the nuclear family may participate to varying degrees, decision making about health and illness is often an individual matter. Sometimes decisions are made after consultation with family members, but the individual is the primary decision maker.

Cultural Perspectives on Intimacy

Interactions between you and your client are influenced by the degree of intimacy desired, which may range from very formal interactions to close personal relationships. For example, some clients of Asian origin expect you and other health care providers to be authoritarian, directive, and detached. In seeking health care, some clients of Chinese descent may expect you to know intuitively what is wrong with them, and you may actually lose some credibility by asking a fairly standard interview question such as, "What brings you here?" The Asian American patient may be thinking, "Don't you know why I'm here? You're supposed to be the one with all the answers." The reserved interpersonal behavioral characteristics of many Asian Americans may leave you with the impression that the client agrees with or understands your explanation. Nodding or smiling by Asians may simply reflect their cultural value for interpersonal harmony, not agreement with what you have said. The emphasis on social harmony among Asian American clients may prevent their full expression of concerns or feelings.

In Thai culture, a high value is placed on *kreeng-caj*, or awareness and anticipation of the feelings of others by kindness and the avoidance of interpersonal conflict. By obtaining validation of assumptions, you may distinguish between genuine concurrent and socially compliant client responses aimed at maintaining harmony. This may be accomplished by inviting the client to respond frankly to suggestions or by giving the client "permission" to disagree.

By contrast, Appalachian clients often have close family interaction patterns that lead them to expect close personal relationships with health care providers. The Appalachian client may evaluate your effectiveness on the basis of interpersonal skills rather than professional competencies. Some Appalachian clients may be uncomfortable with the impersonal orientation of most health care institutions.

Among some Hispanic groups, such as Mexican Americans and Cuban Americans, *simpatia* and *personalismo* should be considered. *Simpatia* refers to the need for smooth or harmonious interpersonal relationships, characterized by courtesy, respect, and the absence of critical or confrontational behavior. The concept of *personalismo* emphasizes intimate personal relationships. Persons of Latin American or Mediterranean origins often expect a high degree of intimacy and may attempt to involve you in their family system by expecting you to participate in personal activities and social functions. These individuals may come to expect personal favors that extend beyond the scope of what you believe to be professional practice, and they may feel it is their privilege to contact you at home during any time of the day or night for care or advice. If your cultural value system emphasizes a high level of personal privacy, you may choose to give clients the agency's phone number and address rather than disclose information about your personal residence.

Because initial impressions are so important in all human relationships, cross-cultural considerations concerning introductions warrant a few brief remarks. To ensure that a mutually respectful relationship is established, you should introduce yourself and indicate to the client how you prefer to be called: by first name, last name, and/or title. You should elicit the same information from the client because this enables you to address the person in a manner that is culturally appropriate.

Nonverbal Communication

Because **nonverbal communication** patterns vary widely across cultures, nurses must be alert for cues that convey cultural differences in the use of silence, eye contact, touch, space, distance, and facial expressions. Cultural influences on appropriate communication between individuals of different genders also need to be considered.

Silence

Wide cultural variations exist in the interpretation of **silence**. Some individuals find silence extremely uncomfortable and make every effort to fill conversational lags with words. By contrast, many Native Americans consider silence essential to understanding and respecting the other person. A pause following your question signifies that what has been asked is important enough to be given thoughtful consideration. In traditional Chinese and Japanese cultures, silence may mean that the speaker wishes the listener to consider the content of what has been said before continuing. Other cultural meanings of silence may be found. English persons and Arabs may use silence out of respect for another's privacy, whereas French, Spanish, and Russian persons may interpret it as a sign of agreement. Asian cultures often use silence to demonstrate respect for elders. Among some African Americans, silence is used in response to a question perceived as inappropriate. Because many Americans may find silences uncomfortable, it is important that we as health professionals understand our own cultural values and learn to respond in culturally appropriate ways with our clients.

Eye Contact

The use of **eye contact** is among the most culturally variable nonverbal behaviors that clients will use to communicate with you. Although most nurses have been taught to maintain eye contact when speaking with clients, individuals from culturally diverse backgrounds may attribute other culturally based meanings to this behavior. Asian, Native North American, Indochinese, Arab, and Appalachian clients may consider direct eye contact impolite or aggressive, and they may avert their own eyes when talking with you. Native Americans often stare at the floor during conversations—a culturally appropriate behavior indicating that the listener is paying close attention to the speaker. Some African Americans use oculistics (eye rolling) in response to what is perceived to be an inappropriate question. Among Hispanic clients, respect dictates appropriate deferential behavior in the form of downcast eyes toward others on the basis of age, sex, social position, economic status, and position of authority. Elders expect respect from younger individuals, adults from children, men from women, teachers from students, and employers from employees. In the nurse–client relationship with Hispanic clients, eye contact may be expected of you but will not necessarily be reciprocated by the client.

In some cultures, including Arab, Latino, and African American groups, modesty for both women and men is interrelated with eye contact. Muslim-Arab women achieve modesty, in part, by avoiding eye contact with males (except for one's husband) and keeping the eyes downcast when encountering members of the opposite sex in public situations. In many cultures, the only woman who smiles and establishes eye contact with men in public is a prostitute. Hasidic Jewish males also have culturally based norms concerning eye contact with females; you may observe a Hasidic Jewish man avoiding direct eye contact and turning his head in the opposite direction when walking past or speaking to a woman. The preceding examples are intended to be illustrative, not exhaustive.

Touch

You are urged to give careful consideration to issues concerning **touch**. While we recognize the often-reported benefits in establishing rapport with clients through touch, including the promotion of healing through therapeutic touch, physical contact with clients conveys various meanings cross-culturally. In many Arab and Hispanic cultures, male health care providers may be prohibited from touching or examining part or all of the female body. Adolescent girls may prefer female health care providers or may refuse to be examined by a male. You should be aware that the client's significant others also may exert pressure by enforcing these culturally meaningful norms in the health care setting. If in doubt about these cultural norms, it is always appropriate to inquire about preferences from the client or family members.

In some cultures, there are strict norms related to touching children. Many Asians believe that

touching the head is a sign of disrespect because it is thought to be the source of a person's strength. You need to be aware that patting a child on the head or examining the fontanelles of a Southeast Asian infant should be avoided or done only with parental permission. Whenever possible, you should explore alternative ways to express affection or to obtain information necessary for the assessment of the client's condition. For example, you might ask the mother to hold the child on her lap while you observe for other manifestations of increased intracranial pressure or signs of premature fontanelle closure. You might also try placing your hand over the mother's while asking for a description of what she feels. In all instances, it is important that you describe the purpose of your actions to the parents before touching an infant or a child.

Space and Distance

The concepts of **space** and **distance** are significant in cross-cultural communication. The perception of appropriate distance zones varies widely among cultural groups. Although there are individual variations in spatial requirements, people of the same culture tend to act in similar ways. For example, if you are of European North American heritage, you may find yourself backing away from clients of Hispanic, East Indian, or Middle Eastern origins who frequently seem to invade your personal space. Such behavior by these clients is probably an attempt to bring you closer into the space that is comfortable to them. Although you may be uncomfortable with close physical proximity to these clients, they are perplexed by your distancing behavior and may perceive you as aloof and unfriendly.

Because individuals are usually not consciously aware of their personal space requirements, they frequently have difficulty understanding a different cultural pattern. For example, sitting in close proximity to another person may be perceived by one client as an expression of warmth and friendliness but by another as a threatening invasion of personal space. According to Watson (1980), Americans, Canadians, and British require the most personal space, whereas Latin Americans, Japanese, and Arabs need the least.

In the early 1960s, Edward T. Hall pioneered the study of **proxemics**, which focuses on how people in various cultures relate to their physical space. Although there are intercultural variations, the intimate distance in interpersonal interactions ranges from 0 to 18 inches. At this distance, people experience visual detail and each other's odor, heat, and touch. Personal distance varies from 1.5 to 4 feet, the usual space within which communication between friends and acquaintances occurs. Nurses frequently interact with clients in the intimate or personal distance zones. Social distance refers to 4 to 12 feet, whereas anything greater than 12 is considered public distance (Hall, 1963).

Sex and Gender

Nonverbal behaviors are culturally significant, and failure to adhere to the **cultural code** (set of rules or norms of behavior used by a cultural group to guide behavior and to interpret situations) is viewed as a serious transgression. Violating norms related to appropriate male–female relationships among various cultures might jeopardize your therapeutic relationship with clients and their families. Among Arab Americans, you may find that adult males avoid being alone with members of the opposite sex (except for their wives) and are generally accompanied by one or more male companions when interacting with females. The presence of the companion(s) conveys that the purpose of the interaction is honorable and that no sexual impropriety will occur. Some women of Middle Eastern origin do not shake hands with men, nor do men and women touch each other outside the marital relationship. Given that clients who have recently immigrated are in various stages of assimilation, traditional customs such as these may or may not be practiced. If in doubt, you should ask the client or observe the client's behaviors, preferably at the time of admission.

A brief comment about same-sex relationships is warranted. In some cultures, it is considered an acceptable expression of friendship

and affection to openly and publicly hold hands with or embrace members of the same sex without any sexual connotation being associated with the behavior. For example, you may note that although a Nigerian American woman may not demonstrate overt affection for her husband or other male family members, she will hold hands with female relatives and friends while walking or talking with them. You may find that clients display similar behaviors toward you, and you should feel free to discuss cultural differences and similarities openly with the client. The discussion should include how each person feels about the cultural practice and exploration of mutually acceptable—and unacceptable—avenues for communicating.

Language

In the United States, nearly 47 million people, age 5 years or older, speak a language other than English at home (U.S. Census Bureau, 2000). Summarized in Table 2-1 are the numbers of Americans who speak other languages and who report that they have difficulty speaking English well.

According to the U.S. Census Bureau (U.S. Department of Commerce [DOC], U.S. Census Bureau, 2003), nearly 1 in 5 people, or 47 million U.S. residents age 5 and older, speak a language other than English at home. Fifty-five percent of the people who spoke a language other than English at home reported they spoke English "very well."

Other than English, Spanish is the major language spoken in the United States, and it is spoken by 31 million U.S. citizens age 5 and older; 11 million of those individuals indicated that they speak *only* Spanish. The Western states are home to more than one-third (37%) of all those who spoke a language other than English at home, the highest proportion of any region. California led the states (39%), followed by New Mexico (37%) and Texas (31%). After English (215.4 million speakers) and Spanish (31 million), Chinese (2 million) was the language most commonly spoken at home, eclipsing French, German, and Italian during the decade of the 90s (U.S. DOC, U.S. Census Bureau, 2003).

TABLE 2-1
Summary of Languages Spoken at Home

LANGUAGE SPOKEN AT HOME	ESTIMATE
Population 5 years old and older	268,110,961
English only	216,176,111
Language other than English	51,934,850
Speak English less than "very well"	23,142,029
Spanish or Spanish Creole	32,184,293
Speak English less than "very well"	15,396,674
Other Indo-European languages	9,929,004
Speak English less than "very well"	3,302,077
Asian and Pacific Islander languages	7,769,500
Speak English less than "very well"	3,828,819
Other languages	2,052,053
Speak English less than "very well"	614,459

Adapted from: U.S. Census Bureau (2005). *2005 American Community Survey*. Retrieved from http://www.factfinder. census.gov.

Use of Interpreters

One of the greatest challenges in cross-cultural communication occurs when you and your client speak different languages. After assessing the language skills of non–English-speaking clients, you may find yourself in one of two situations: either struggling to communicate effectively through an interpreter or communicating effectively when there is no interpreter (see Box 2-4).

Non–English-Speaking Patients and Interpreters

Interviewing the non–English-speaking person requires a bilingual interpreter for full communication. Even a person from another culture or country who has a basic command of English (someone for whom English is a second language) may need an interpreter when faced with the anxiety-provoking situation of entering a hospital, encountering a strange symptom, or discussing a sensitive topic such as birth control or gynecologic or urologic concerns. Ideally, a trained medical interpreter should be used. This person knows interpreting techniques, has a health care background,

and understands patients' rights. The trained interpreter is also knowledgeable about cultural beliefs and health practices. This person can help you to bridge the cultural gap and can give advice concerning the cultural appropriateness of your recommendations.

Although you will be in charge of the focus and flow of the interview, the interpreter should be viewed as an important member of the health care team. It can be tempting to ask a relative, a friend, or even another client to interpret because this person is readily available and likely is anxious to help. However, this violates confidentiality for the client, who may not want personal information shared. Furthermore, the friend or relative, though fluent in ordinary language usage, is likely to be unfamiliar with medical terminology, hospital or clinic procedures, and health care ethics.

Whenever possible, work with a bilingual member of the health care team. In ideal circumstances, you should ask the interpreter to meet the client beforehand to establish rapport and to obtain basic descriptive information about the client such as age, occupation, educational level, and attitude toward health care. This eases the interpreter into the relationship and allows the client to talk about aspects of his or her life that are relatively nonthreatening.

When using an interpreter, you should expect that the interaction with the client will require more time than is needed in the care of English-speaking clients. It will be necessary to organize nursing care so that the most important interactions or procedures are accomplished first before any of the parties (including yourself) becomes fatigued.

Both you and the client should speak only a sentence or two and then allow the interpreter time to translate. You should use simple language, not medical jargon that the interpreter must simplify before it can be translated. Summary translation—allowing a person to speak in his or her native language and then having an interpreter summarize what was said—goes faster and is useful for teaching relatively simple health techniques with which the interpreter is already

BOX 2-4

Overcoming Language Barriers

Use of an Interpreter

- Before locating an interpreter, be sure that the language the client speaks at home is known, considering it may be different from the language spoken publicly (e.g., French is sometimes spoken by well-educated and upper-class members of certain Asian or Middle Eastern cultures).
- Avoid interpreters from a rival tribe, state, region, or nation (e.g., a Palestinian who knows Hebrew may not be the best interpreter for a Jewish client).
- Be aware of gender differences between interpreter and client. In general, same gender is preferred.
- Be aware of age differences between interpreter and client. In general, an older, more mature interpreter is preferred to a younger, less experienced one.
- Be aware of socioeconomic differences between interpreter and client.
- Ask the interpreter to translate as closely to verbatim as possible.
- Expect an interpreter who is not a relative to seek compensation for services rendered.

Recommendations for Institutions

- Maintain a computerized list of interpreters who may be contacted as needed.
- Network with area hospitals, colleges, universities, and other organizations that may serve as resources.
- Utilize the translation services provided by telephone companies (e.g., American Telephone and Telegraph Company).

What to Do When There Is No Interpreter

- Be polite and formal.
- Greet the person using the last or complete name. Gesture to yourself and say your name. Offer a handshake or nod. Smile.
- Proceed in an unhurried manner. Pay attention to any effort by the patient or family to communicate.

- Speak in a low, moderate voice. Avoid talking loudly. Remember that there is a tendency to raise the volume and pitch of your voice when the listener appears not to understand. The listener may perceive that the nurse is shouting and/or angry.
- Use any words known in the patient's language. This indicates that the nurse is aware of and respects the client's culture.
- Use simple words, such as *pain* instead of *discomfort*. Avoid medical jargon, idioms, and slang. Avoid using contractions. Use nouns repeatedly instead of pronouns. Example: Do *not* say, "He has been taking his medicine, hasn't he?" Do say, "Does Juan take medicine?"
- Pantomime words and simple actions while verbalizing them.
- Give instructions in the proper sequence. Example: Do *not* say, "Before you rinse the bottle, sterilize it." Do say, "First, wash the bottle. Second, rinse the bottle."
- Discuss one topic at a time. Avoid using conjunctions. Example: Do *not* say, "Are you cold and in pain?" Do say, "Are you cold [while pantomiming]?" Are you in pain?"
- Validate whether the client understands by having him or her repeat instructions, demonstrate the procedure, or act out the meaning.
- Write out several short sentences in English, and determine the person's ability to read them.
- Try a third language. Many Southeast Asians speak French. Europeans often know three or four languages. Try Latin words or phrases, if the nurse is familiar with that language.
- Ask who among the client's family and friends could serve as an interpreter.
- Obtain phrase books from a library or bookstore, make or purchase flash cards, contact hospitals for a list of interpreters, and use both formal and informal networking to locate a suitable interpreter.

Adapted from M. Andrews (2004). Transcultural considerations in health assessment. In C. Jarvis, *Physical Examination and Health Assessment* (p. 69). Philadelphia: W.B. Saunders. Reprinted by permission.

familiar. Be alert for nonverbal cues as the client talks; he or she can give valuable data. A skilled interpreter also will note nonverbal messages and pass them on to you (Nailon, 2004, 2006). Evidence-Based Practice 2-1 examines a series of articles about the use of translators/interpreters in studies with the Dinka tribe of Southern Sudan, Samoans in Hawaii, and the culturally Deaf. These articles discuss the "lessons learned" while working with translators and interpreters. An important "lesson" throughout these articles is that cultural values, norms, and traditions influence communication between the patient, the nurse, and the translator/interpreter.

The Joint Commission on Accreditation of Healthcare Organizations and the American Hospital Association both require that accommodations be made for patients who lack proficiency in English, and some states have passed laws requiring health care organizations to provide interpreters for their non–English-speaking patients. Box 2-5 provides a summary of suggestions for the selection and use of an interpreter and for overcoming language barriers when an interpreter is unavailable. It is important that a certified interpreter be used in health care situations as they are trained and certified in medical terminology. Although the use of an interpreter is ideal, you will need a strategy for promoting effective communication when none is present.

Sick Role Behaviors

If you find yourself feeling uncomfortable because a client is asking too many questions, assuming a defensive posture, or otherwise showing discomfort, it might be appropriate to pause for a moment to examine the source of the conflict from a transcultural perspective. During illness, culturally acceptable **sick role behavior** may range from aggressive, demanding behavior to silent passivity. Researchers have found that complaining, demanding behavior during illness is often rewarded with attention among Jewish and Italian

EVIDENCE-BASED PRACTICE 2-1

Working with Translators and Interpreters: Lessons Learned

This series of articles describes culturally competent approaches for working with translators or interpreters who participate in transcultural studies. However, the lessons learned have wide applicability for health care professionals in clinical situations. The introductory article by Jones and Boyle provides background for the three exemplars of lessons learned in working with translators. The examples provided in the three exemplars offer fascinating glimpses into the cultures of the Dinka (Baird), Samoan (Siaki), and culturally Deaf (Sheppard).

Baird describes working with translators and interpreters from the Dinka tribe of southern Sudan during an ethnographic study with refugee Dinka women who were resettled with their children to the United States. Navigating the cultural differences between the researcher and translator and interpreters provided a deeper understanding about the culture of the Dinka. The lessons learned included the importance of cultural congruence between the interpreters and participants; the education, training, and experience of the interpreters; and the difficulties encountered in preparing interpreters according to university IRB requirements. Cultural differences such as time perception and communication and literacy styles were negotiated throughout the study. The most valuable lesson learned from this experience was the importance of the relationship between the researcher and translator and

(Evidence-Based Practice continues on page 34)

EVIDENCE-BASED PRACTICE 2-1

Working with Translators and Interpreters: Lessons Learned (*continued*)

interpreters, as well as between the interpreters and participants to achieve credibility and trustworthiness of the study results. This would also be applicable to a clinical situation wherein the relationship between the health care provider and the translator/interpreter would facilitate culturally competent care.

Siaki conducted her research with Samoans who were at risk for heart disease and live in Oahu, Hawaii. Perceptions of risk are those beliefs or value judgments about personal vulnerability to specific health threats and their consequences. Therefore it is important to understand perceptions of risk from the cultural standpoint of those most affected. Samoan sociocultural customs, beliefs, values, and practices are referred to by Samoans as *fa'a Samoa*, or the Samoan way. Spirituality, respect, balance, and harmony are major aspects of *fa'a Samoa*. Siaki found that showing respect for *fa'a Samoa* enhanced her interactions with the Samoan community and helped her establish rapport and build trust. Allowing for family and/or group participation, rather than focusing on individuals, was a culturally important way to show respect for Samoan traditions and practices.

Sheppard was interested in how Deaf adults described depressive symptoms. Health care providers commonly discuss depressive symptoms with clients, enabling early interventions, however such discussions rarely occur between providers and Deaf clients. Most culturally Deaf adults have experienced early-onset hearing loss; they self-identify as part of a unique culture, and communicate in the visual language of American Sign Language (ASL). Communication barriers are common and depression screening instruments may be unreliable when used with culturally Deaf clients. Sheppard believed that using trained interpreters was vital to the success of her research; she was surprised to learn that there was no central ASL registry within the state where her

study was conducted. She eventually located two interpreters who acted as gatekeepers to the local Deaf community but Sheppard had to gain their trust and respect before her study could proceed. Fortunately, Sheppard was able to carry on simple conversations in ASL and this ability greatly enhanced her relationship with the interpreters and her study participants.

The four articles in this translation series reinforce that working with interpreters often adds expense, time, and challenges to research or practice situations. However, the benefits are worth the effort. Interpreters can serve as helpful bridges between the researchers or health care providers and the cultural community. Interpreters can be valuable members of the health care team, contributing understanding and meaning to health care encounters.

Clinical Application: To ensure cultural competence in the nurse–patient relationship when an interpreter is needed.

1. Plan for adequate time for the translation process. Using an interpreter can be time consuming and the encounter with the patient and family members cannot be hurried or abbreviated.
2. Learn about the preferred qualifications of translators, including cultural background and linguistic skills, professional credentials, and even usual pay before working with or employing translators. Learn about the role of translators in the targeted community; what their relationship is with others in their community.
3. Arrange meetings with potential translators to discuss the health care goals. Discuss the usual translation procedures, the role of the translator as a colleague and collaborator, time commitment, and timeline. Lay translators may be required to complete human subjects training for research purposes or if employed by health

EVIDENCE-BASED PRACTICE 2-1 (*continued*)

care organizations, they may be required to complete HIPAA training.

4. Plan adequate time for mutual learning between the nurse and the translator in preparation for beginning the translation process. The translator can help health care professionals understand cultural values, social structures including family and community

organization. Their skills and expertise are absolutely essential in providing culturally competent care to patients.

5. Last, but certainly not least, learn a few words ("hello," "how are you?") from the patient, family members, or translators. Your interest and willingness to learn will be appreciated by all involved.

Reference: Baird, M. B. (2011). Lessons learned from translators and interpreters from the Dinka tribe of Southern Sudan. *Journal of Transcultural Nursing, 22*(2), 116-121.

Jones, E. G. & Boyle, J. S. (2011). Working with translators and interpreters in research: Lessons learned. *Journal of Transcultural Nursing, , 22*(2), 109-115.

Sheppard, K. (2011). Using American Sign Language interpreters to facilitate research among deaf adults: Lessons learned. *Journal of Transcultural Nursing, 22*(2), 129-134.

Siaki, L. (2011). Translating a questionnaire for use with Samoan adults: Lessons learned. *Journal of Transcultural Nursing, 22*(2), 122-128.

groups. Because Asian and Native North American patients are likely to be quiet and compliant during illness, they may not receive the attention they need. Children are socialized into culturally acceptable sick role behaviors at an early age.

Clients of Asian heritage may provide you with the answers that they think are expected. This behavior is consistent with the dominant cultural value for harmonious relationships with others. Thus, you should attempt

---

BOX 2-5

National Council for Interpreters in Health Care

The National Council on Interpreting in Health Care (2002) has developed the first set of national standards for medical interpreting professionals in the United States. The 32 national standards provide guidelines on the following nine issues:

- Accuracy: To enable other parties to know precisely what each speaker has said.
- Confidentiality: To honor the private and personal nature of the health care interaction and maintain trust among all parties.
- Impartiality: To eliminate the effect of interpreter bias or preference.

- Respect: To acknowledge the inherent dignity of all parties in the interpreted encounter.
- Cultural Awareness: To facilitate communication across cultural differences.
- Role Boundaries: To clarify the scope and limits of the interpreting role to avoid conflicts of interest.
- Professionalism: To uphold the public's trust in the interpreting profession.
- Professional Development: To attain the highest possible level of competence and service.
- Advocacy: To prevent harm to parties whom the interpreter serves.

Source: National Council on Interpreting in Health Care. (2002). Models for the provision of health care interpreter training. http://www.ncihc.org

to phrase questions or statements in a neutral manner that avoids foreshadowing an expected response.

SUMMARY

In this chapter, we have explored culturally competent and culturally congruent nursing care as well as the importance of linguistic competence. We have discussed cultural self-assessment and encouraged you to gain insights into your own attitudes and beliefs about different ethnic, religious, and social groups.

Most of the chapter has focused on the complex, multifaceted topic of cross-cultural communication, including aspects of verbal and nonverbal communication that enable nurses to provide culturally competent and culturally congruent nursing care.

REVIEW QUESTIONS

1. Summarize the key standards for culturally and linguistically competent health care (CLAS) recommended by the Office of Minority Health, U.S. Department of Health and Human Services. Why are these standards helpful?
2. Critically examine the strategies for promoting effective cross-cultural communication between nurses and clients. Identify actions that you can take to overcome communication barriers when caring for non–English-speaking clients.
3. Propose strategies for using translators/interpreters successfully in health care encounters. Identify problems that might arise in a cross-cultural communication.
4. What are the major languages spoken in households in the United States and Canada?

CRITICAL THINKING ACTIVITIES

1. After critically analyzing the definitions of cultural competence presented in the chapter, craft a definition of the term in your own words.

2. To provide culturally competent nursing care, you should engage in a cultural self-assessment. Answer the questions in Box 2-2, How Do You Relate to Various Groups of People in the Society? and score your answers using the guide provided. What did you learn about yourself? How would you learn more about the background of those groups mentioned, including information about their health-related beliefs and practices? What resources might you use in your search for information?

3. At the request of the Bureau of Primary Health Care, Health Resources and Services Administration, in the U.S. Department of Health and Human Services, staff at the National Center for Cultural Competence (NCCC) developed the *Cultural Competence Health Practitioner*

Assessment which is available online. Visit the Web site at http://www11.Georgetown.edu/research/gucchd/nccc/ features/CCHPA.html and complete this assessment.

4. After identifying someone for whom English is a second language, ask the person what he or she believes (a) promotes effective communication and (b) sets up barriers to effective communication. What has the person found to be most challenging in communicating health-related needs to physicians, nurses, and other health care providers?

5. Interview a nurse with experience in caring for clients whose primary language is not English. What challenges does the nurse report in communicating with these clients? What strategies does the nurse use to promote effective cross-cultural communication? How effective does the nurse believe these strategies have been in the care of these clients?

REFERENCES

American Academy of Nursing. (1992). AAN expert panel report: Culturally competent health care. *Nursing Outlook, 40*, 277-283.

American Academy of Nursing. (1993). *Promoting cultural competence in and through nursing education.* New York: Subpanel on Cultural Competence in Nursing Education, American Academy of Nursing.

Andrews, M. M., & Boyle, J. S. (1997). Competence in transcultural nursing care. *American Journal of Nursing, 98*(8), 16AAA-16DDD.

Baird, M. B. (2011). Lessons learned from translators and interpreters from the Dinka tribe of Southern Sudan. *Journal of Transcultural Nursing , 22*(2), 116-121.

Campinha-Bacote, J. (2000). A model of practice to address cultural competent health care in the home. *Home Care Provider, 5*(6), 213-219.

Campinha-Bacote, J. (2002). The process of cultural competence in the delivery of healthcare services: A model. *Journal of Transcultural Nursing, 13*, 181-184.

Campinha-Bacote, J. (2003). *The process of cultural competence in the delivery of healthcare services* (4th ed.). Cincinnati, OH: Transcultural C.A.R.E. Associates.

Campinha-Bacote, J., & Munoz, C. (2001). A guiding framework for delivering culturally competent services in case management. *The Case Manager, 12*(2), 48-52.

Georgetown University Center for Child and Human Development, National Center for Cultural Competence (NCCC). (n.d.). *Foundations of cultural and linguistic competence.* Retrieved February 3, 2010, from http://www.gucchd.georgetown.edu/nccc.

Geron, S. M. (2002). Cultural competency: How is it measured? Does it make a difference? *Generations, 26*(3), 39-45.

Hall, E. (1963). Proxemics: The study of man's spatial relationships. In I. Gladstone (Ed.). *Man's image in medicine and anthropology* (pp. 109-120). New York: International University Press.

Jones, E. G. & Boyle, J. S. (2011). Working with translators and interpreters in research: Lessons learned. *Journal of Transcultural Nursing , 22*(2), 109-115.

Leininger, M. M. (1991). *Culture care diversity and universality: A theory of nursing.* New York: National League for Nursing Press.

Leininger, M. M. (1995). *Transcultural nursing: Concepts, theories, research and practices.* New York: McGraw-Hill.

Leininger, M. M. (1999). What is transcultural nursing and culturally competent care? *Journal of Transcultural Nursing, 10*(1), 9.

Leininger, M. M., & McFarland, M. R. (2002). *Transcultural nursing: Concepts, theories, research and practices.* New York: McGraw-Hill.

Leininger, M. M., & McFarland, M. R. (2005). *Culture care diversity & Universality: A worldwide nursing theory.* Sudbury, MA: Jones & Bartlett.

Nailon, R. E. (2004). Expertise in the care of Latinos: An interpretive study of culturally congruent nursing practices in the emergency department. *Dissertation Abstracts International, 65,* 12B (UMI No. 3158546).

Nailon, R. E. (2006). Nurses' concerns and practices with using interpreters in the care of Latino patients in the emergency department. *Journal of Transcultural Nursing, 17*(2), 119-128.

National Council on Interpreting in Health Care. (2002). *Models for the provision of health care interpreter training.* Retrieved February 3, 2010, from http://www.ncihc.org.

Siaki, L. (2011). Translating a questionnaire for use with Samoan adults: Lessons learned. *Journal of Transcultural Nursing , 22*(2), 122-128.

Sheppard, K. (2011). Using American Sign Language interpreters to facilitate research among deaf adults: Lessons learned. *Journal of Transcultural Nursing , 22*(2), 129-134.

Smith, L. S. (1998). Concept analysis: Cultural competence. *Journal of Cultural Diversity, 5*(1), 4-10.

U.S. Census Bureau. (2000). *2000 census of population and housing.* Washington, DC: U.S. Government Printing Office. http://www.census.gov. Retrieved February 2, 2010.

U.S. Department of Commerce, U.S. Census Bureau. (2003, October 8). Nearly 1-in-5 speak a foreign language at home. Press release retrieved on August 19, 2006, from http://www.census.gov/Press-Release/www/releases.language3.pdf.

U.S. Department of Health and Human Services, Office of Minority Health. (April, 2007). National standards on culturally and linguistically appropriate services (CLAS), *Federal Register, 65*(247), 80865-80879. Retrieved from http://www.omhrc. gov/clas/ds.htm.

Watson, O. M. (1980). *Proxemic behavior: A cross-cultural study.* The Hague, Netherlands: Mouton Press.

Wells, M. I. (2000). Beyond cultural competence: A model for individual and institutional cultural development. *Journal of Community Health Nursing, 17*(4), 189-199.

Cultural Competence in the **Health History** and **Physical Examination**

Margaret M. Andrews

KEY TERMS

Biocultural variations
Clinical decision making
Cultural assessment
Cultural care accommodation or
    negotiation
Cultural care repatterning or
    restructuring
Cultural preservation or
    maintenance
Culture-bound syndromes
Cyanosis
Ecchymotic lesions
Erythema
Ethnohistory
Evaluation
Jaundice
Leukoedema
Mongolian spots
Nursing actions
Oral hyperpigmentation
Pallor
Petechiae
Plant-derived medications
TCN Assessment Guide for Groups
    and Communities
TCN Assessment Guide for
    Individuals and Families

LEARNING OBJECTIVES

1. Explore the process and content needed for the comprehensive cultural assessment of individuals, families, and groups from diverse cultures.
2. Identify biocultural variations in health and illness for individuals, families, and groups from diverse cultures.
3. Discuss biocultural variations in common laboratory tests.
4. Critically review transcultural perspectives in the health history and physical examination.
5. Examine cultural factors that influence clinical decision making, nursing actions, and evaluation.

Cultural assessment, or *culturologic nursing assessment*, refers, first of all, to a systematic, comprehensive examination of individuals, families, groups, and communities regarding their health-related cultural beliefs, values, and practices, and, second, to a plan and interventions that are culturally congruent and culturally relevant. The goal of cultural assessment is to determine the explicit nursing and health care needs of people and to intervene in ways that are culturally congruent and meaningful (cf. Leininger, 1995; Leininger & McFarland, 2002). Because they deal with cultural values, belief systems, and lifeways, cultural assessments tend to be broad and comprehensive, although it is possible to focus on smaller segments. Cultural assessment consists of both *process* and *content*. *Process* refers to your approach to the client, consideration of verbal and nonverbal communication, and the sequence and order in which data are gathered. The *content* of the cultural assessment consists of the actual data categories in which information about clients is gathered.

This chapter will be divided into two major sections: (1) transcultural perspectives on the health history and (2) transcultural perspectives on the physical examination. Ideally, the cultural assessment should be integrated into the overall assessment of the client, family, group, and/or community. It is usually impractical to expect that nurses will have the time to conduct a separate cultural assessment, so questions aimed at gathering cultural data should be integrated into the overall assessment.

In Appendix A, you will find the Andrews and Boyle **Transcultural Nursing Assessment Guide for Individuals and Families**. The major categories in this guide include cultural affiliations, values orientation, communication, health-related beliefs and practices, nutrition, socioeconomic considerations, organizations providing cultural support, education, religion, cultural aspects of disease incidence, biocultural variations, and developmental considerations across the life span. Appendix B contains the Andrews and Boyle **Transcultural Nursing Assessment Guide for Groups and Communities**. The major categories in this guide include family and kinship systems, social life and networks, political or government systems, language and traditions, worldview, values, norms, religious beliefs and practices, health beliefs and practices, and health care systems.

Transcultural Perspectives on the Health History

The purpose of the health history is to gather *subjective data*—a term that refers to things that people say or relate about themselves. The health history provides a comprehensive overview of a client's past and present health, and it examines the manner in which the person interacts with the environment. The health history enables the nurse to assess health strengths, including cultural beliefs and practices that might influence the nurse's ability to provide culturally competent nursing care. The history is combined with the *objective data* from the physical examination and the laboratory results to form a diagnosis about the health status of a person. Both kinds of data, subjective and objective, are important and necessary for a complete health history.

For the well client, the history is used to assess lifestyle, which includes activity, exercise, diet, and related personal choices that enable you as the nurse to identify potential risk factors for disease. For the ill client, the health history includes a chronologic record of the health problem(s). For both well and ill clients, the health history is a screening tool for abnormal symptoms, health problems, and concerns. The health history also provides you with valuable information about the coping strategies, health-related behaviors and responses used previously by clients and family members.

In many health care settings, the client is expected to fill out a printed history form or checklist. From a transcultural perspective, this approach has both positive and negative aspects. On the positive side, this approach provides the client with ample time to recall details such as relevant family history and the dates of health-related events such as surgical procedures and illnesses. It is expedient for nurses because it takes less time to review a form or a checklist than to elicit the information in a face-to-face or telephone interview.

However, this approach has limitations. First, the form is likely to be in English. Those whose primary language is not English might find the form difficult or impossible to complete accurately. Although some health care facilities provide forms translated into Spanish, French, or other languages known to be spoken by relatively large numbers of people who use the facility, it is costly to translate forms into multiple languages.

In some instances, the literal translation of medical terms is not possible. In other instances, the symptom or disease is not recognized in the culture with which the client identifies. For example, in asking about symptoms of depression, there might be many cultural factors that influence the client's interpretation of the question. In Chinese languages, there is no literal translation for the word *depression*. In Chinese culture it is more acceptable to somaticize emotional pain with expressions of physical discomfort such as chest pain or "heaviness of the heart." In rural Guatemala, Mayan Indians might refer to *"dolar de corazon"* or pain in the heart. If health care providers fail to understand the cultural meaning of the symptom "heaviness of the heart," or "pain in the heart," unnecessary, invasive, and costly tests might be performed to rule out cardiovascular disease. In some instances, clients might be unable to read or write in any language; thus, an assessment of the client's literacy level should precede the use of printed history forms or checklists.

Although there is wide variation in health history formats, most contain the following categories: *biographic data, reason for seeking care, present health or history of present illness, past history, family and social history,* and *review of systems.* This chapter will not cover a comprehensive overview of all data categories in a health history; it will present only those relative to the provision of culturally congruent and culturally competent nursing care.

Biographic Data and Source of History

In addition to the standard descriptive information about clients (name, address, phone, age, gender, and so forth), it is necessary to record who has furnished the data. Whereas this is usually the client, the source might be a relative or friend. Note whether an interpreter is used and indicate his or her relationship to the client. Be sure to document the *specific language* spoken by the client, for example, Mandarin Chinese (compared with Cantonese Chinese or other dialects).

Although the biographic information might seem straightforward, several cultural variations in recording age are important to note. In some Asian cultures, an infant is considered to be 1 year old at birth. Among some South Vietnamese immigrants who migrated to the United States during the Vietnam War, there might be inaccuracies in the reported age. These inaccuracies occurred in response to U.S. immigration laws in the 1960s and 1970s, which attempted to limit the numbers of Southeast Asians entering the United States. For many reasons, age may not be reported correctly. Some clients may not wish to report their correct age, others may not know (by our standards) their exact age.

One of the first areas that you should assess is the client's cultural affiliation. With what cultural group(s) does the client report affiliation? Where was the client born? What is the **ethnohistory** of the client? Knowledge of the client's ethnohistory is important in determining his or her risk factors for genetic and acquired diseases and in understanding the client's cultural heritage. How many years have the client and his or her family lived in this country? If the client is a recent immigrant, ask him or her to describe what the migration experience was like and what his or her life has been like in this country.

Reason for Seeking Care

The *reason for seeking care* refers to a brief statement describing in clients' own words why they are visiting a health care provider. In the past, this statement has been called the *chief complaint,* a term that is now avoided because it focuses on illness rather than wellness and tends to label the person as a complainer. All symptoms are believed to have cultural meanings, and the nurse should realize that they are usually more than manifestations of a biologic reality.

Symptoms are defined as phenomena experienced by individuals that signify a departure from normal function, sensation, or appearance and that might include physical aberrations.

By comparison, *signs* are objective abnormalities that the examiner can detect on physical examination or through laboratory testing. As individuals experience symptoms, they interpret them and react in ways that are congruent with their cultural norms. Symptoms cannot be attributed to another person; rather, individuals experience symptoms from their knowledge of bodily function and sociocultural interactions. Symptoms are perceived, recognized, labeled, reacted to, ritualized, and articulated in ways that make sense within the cultural worldview of the person experiencing them (Good & Good, 1980; Wenger, 1993).

Symptoms are defined according to the client's perception of the meaning attributed to the event. This perception must be considered in relation to other sociocultural factors and biologic knowledge. People develop culturally based explanatory models to explain how their illnesses work and what their symptoms mean. The search for cultural meaning in understanding symptoms involves a translation process that includes both the nurse's worldview and the client's. You need to assess the symptoms within the client's sociocultural and ethnohistorical context. It is important to use the same terms for symptoms that clients use. For example, if the client refers to "swelling" of the leg, refrain from medicalizing that to "edema." Knowledge of the cultural expression of symptoms will influence the decisions you make and will facilitate your ability to provide culturally congruent or culturally competent nursing care (Wenger, 1993).

Present and Past Illnesses

Table 3-1 provides an alphabetic listing of selected diseases and their increased or decreased prevalence among members of certain cultural groups. Accurate assessment and evaluation of the present and past illnesses requires knowledge of the biocultural aspects of acute and chronic diseases.

Culture-Bound Syndromes

Although all illnesses might be culturally defined, the term **culture-bound syndromes** refers to disorders restricted to a particular culture or group of cultures because of certain psychosocial characteristics of those cultures. Culture-bound syndromes are often referred to as folk illnesses or folk diseases in which alterations of behavior and experience are prominent features. More than 200 culture-bound syndromes have been identified. For example, anorexia nervosa is believed to be a Western culture-bound syndrome because the condition is largely confined to Western cultures or to non-Western cultures undergoing the process of westernization, such as Japan. Culture-bound syndromes are thought to be illnesses created by personal, social, and cultural reactions to malfunctioning biologic or psychologic processes and can be understood only within defined contexts of meaning and social relationships (Kleinman, 1980). When you encounter clients with culture-bound syndromes, it is important to find out what they and other concerned individuals believe is happening. What prior efforts for help or cure have been tried? What were the results? It is impossible to produce a definitive list of all culture-bound syndromes, but Table 3-2 summarizes selected examples that are found in specific cultural groups. For a more comprehensive list of culture-bound syndromes and descriptions of them, see the well-known classic book, Simons, R. & Hughes, C. (1986) *Introduction to Culture-Bound Syndromes* or go to http://www.psychiatrictimes.com/display/article/10168/54246?verify=0. Chapter 10 (Transcultural Perspectives in Mental Health Nursing) also includes an extensive list and description of culture-bound syndromes.

Current Medications

In the health history you should note the name, dose, route of administration, schedule, frequency, purpose, and length of time of each medicine that has been taken. It is also important to note all prescription and over-the-counter medications, including herbs that clients might purchase or grow in home gardens. Because of cultural differences in people's perception of what substances are considered medicines, it is important to ask about specific items by name. For example, you should inquire about vitamins, birth control pills,

TABLE 3-1
Biocultural Aspects of Disease

DISEASE	REMARKS
Alcoholism	American Indians have double the rate of Whites; lower tolerance to alcohol among Chinese and Japanese Americans
Anemia	High incidence among Vietnamese because of the presence of infestations among immigrants and low iron diets; low hemoglobin and malnutrition found among 18.2% of Native Americans, 32.7% of Blacks, 14.6% of Hispanics, and 10.4% of White children under 5 years of age
Arthritis	*Increased incidence among Native Americans*
	Blackfoot 1.4%
	Pima 1.8%
	Chippewa 6.8%
Asthma	Six times greater for Native American infants < year; same as the general population for Native Americans aged 1–44 years
Bronchitis	Six times greater for Native American infants < year; same as the general population for Native Americans aged 1–44 years. Main cause of death for Aboriginal Canadian infants in the postnatal period
Cancer	Nasopharyngeal: high among Chinese Americans and Native Americans
	Breast: Black women 1 1/2 times more likely than White
	Colorectal: Blacks 40% higher than Whites
	Esophageal: No. 2 cause of death for Black men aged 35–54 years
	Incidence:
	White men 3.5/100,000
	Black men 13.3/100,000
	Liver: Highest among all ethnic groups are Filipino Hawaiians Latinos have twice the rate of Whites
	Stomach: Black men twice as likely as White men; low among Filipinos
	Cervical: 120% higher in Black women than in White women
	Mexican American and Puerto Rican women 2 to 3 times higher than Whites
	Uterine: 53% lower in Black women than White women
	Prostate: Black men have highest incidence of all groups
	Most prevalent cancer among Native Americans: biliary, nasopharyngeal, testicular, cervical, renal, and thyroid (females) cancer
	Lung cancer among Navajo uranium miners 85 times higher than among White miners
	Most prevalent cancer among Japanese Americans: esophageal, stomach, liver, and biliary cancer
	Among Chinese Americans, there is a higher incidence of nasopharyngeal and liver cancer than among the general population

DISEASE	REMARKS
Cholecystitis	*Incidence:*
	Whites 0.3%
	Puerto Ricans 2.1%
	Native Americans 2.2%
	Chinese 2.6%
Colitis	High incidence among Japanese Americans
Diabetes mellitus	Three times as prevalent among Filipino Americans as Whites; higher among Hispanics than Blacks or Whites
	Death rate is 3–4 times as high among Native Americans aged 25–34 years, especially those in the West such as Utes, and Tohono O'odham (Pimas and Papagos)
	Complications
	Amputations: Twice as high among Native Americans vs. general U.S. population
	Renal failure: 20 times as high as general U.S. population, with tribal variation,for example, Utes have 43 times higher incidence
G-6-PD deficiency	Present among 30% of Black males
Influenza	Increased death rate among Native Americans aged 45+
Ischemic heart disease	Responsible for 32% of heart-related causes of death among Native Americans; Blacks have higher mortality rates than all other groups
Lactose intolerance	Present among 66% of Hispanic women; increased incidence among Blacks and Chinese
Myocardial infarction	Leading cause of heart disease in Native Americans, accounting for 43% of death resulting from heart disease; low incidence among Japanese Americans
Otitis media	7.9% incidence among school-aged Navajo children versus 0.5% in Whites
	Up to 1/3 of Eskimo children <2 years have chronic otitis media
	Increased incidence among bottle-fed Native Americans and Eskimo infants
Pneumonia	Increased death rate among Native North Americans aged 45+
Psoriasis	Affects 2%–5% of Whites but <% of Blacks; high among Japanese Americans
Renal disease	Lower incidence among Japanese Americans
Sickle cell anemia	Increased incidence among Blacks
Trachoma	Increased incidence among Native Americans and Eskimo children (3 to 8 times greater than general population)

(table continues on page 44)

TABLE 3-1
Biocultural Aspects of Disease (*continued*)

DISEASE	REMARKS	
Tuberculosis	Highest among Asian Americans & Pacific Islanders;	
	Increased incidence among Native Americans	
	Apache	2.0%
	Sioux	3.2%
	Navajo	4.6%
	Aboriginals living on Canadian reserves are 10 times more likely to have TB than non-Aboriginal Canadians	
	Non-Whites 5.2 times more than Whites	
Ulcers	Decreased incidence among Japanese Americans	

Table based on data accessed on February 10, 2010, at American Cancer Society (http://www.cancer.org); American Diabetes Association (http://www.diabetes.org); American Heart Association (http://www. americanheart.org); Office of Minority Health (http://www.omhrc.gov/omh/whatsnew/2pgwhatsnew/special128a.htm); National Center for Health Statistics (http://www.cdc.gov/nchs); National Center on Minority Health & Health Disparities, National Institutes of Health (ncmhd.nihgov); Spotlight on Minority Health (http://www.cdc.gov/omh/populations/populations.htm).

aspirin, antacids, herbs, teas, inhalants, poultices, vaginal and rectal suppositories, ointments, and any other items taken by the client for therapeutic purposes.

Plant-Derived Drugs
In particular, it is important to be aware of the widespread use of **plant-derived medications** among various cultures (Table 3-3). Since prehistoric times, people have attempted to identify plants, marine organisms, arthropods, animals, and minerals with healing properties. According the World Health Organization, 80% of people residing in less developed countries use traditional medicine, including medicinal plants, for their major primary health care needs. Although the exact number of plants being used medicinally worldwide is unknown, approximately 5% of the 250,000 known species of plants have ever been studied for bioactive compounds that might have healing effects. (It is estimated that approximately 75% of the plant-derived drugs currently used in the United States and Canada were

discovered as a result of chemical studies designed to isolate the active ingredients responsible for the use of the plants in traditional medicine. These drugs are derived from approximately 90 of the 250,000 known species of plants on this planet.) The global market for plant-derived drugs is worth an estimated $18 billion and is projected to grow to $26 billion by 2011. Currently, respiratory problems such as asthma represent the largest medical application of plant-derived drugs, accounting for 24% of total sales of plant-derived medicines. In the future, cancer treatment is expected to become the largest application of plant-derived drugs, capturing 24% of the market by 2011 (BCC Research, 2009; Ma et al., 2005) (Figure 3-1).

Many of the active ingredients in plant-derived drugs or herbs are unknown and remain largely unregulated by government agencies, except for customs officials who make efforts to control the flow of illegal drugs. Fresh or dried herbs are usually brewed into a tea, with the dosage adjusted according to the chronicity or acuteness of the illness, age, and size of the patient.

TABLE 3-2
Selected Culture–Bound Syndromes

GROUP	DISORDER	REMARKS
Blacks, Haitians	Blackout	Collapse, dizziness, inability to move
	Low blood	Not enough blood or weakness of the blood that is often treated with diet
	High blood	Blood that is too rich in certain things because of the ingestion of too much red meat or rich foods
	Thin blood	Occurs in women, children, and old people; renders the individual more susceptible to illness in general
	Diseases of hex, witchcraft, or conjuring	Sense of being doomed by spell; gastrointestinal symptoms, for example, vomiting; hallucinations; part of voodoo beliefs
Chinese/ Southeast Asians	*Koro*	Intense anxiety that penis is retracting into body
Greeks	Hysteria	Bizarre complaints and behavior because the uterus leaves the pelvis for another part of the body
Hispanics	*Empacho*	Food forms into a ball and clings to the stomach or intestines, causing pain and cramping
	Fatigue	Asthma-like symptoms
	Mal ojo, "evil eye"	Fitful sleep, crying, diarrhea in children caused by a stranger's attention; sudden onset
	Pasmo	Paralysis-like symptoms of face or limbs; prevented or relieved by massage
	Susto	Anxiety, trembling, phobias from sudden fright
Japanese	*Wagamama*	Apathetic childish behavior with emotional outbursts
Korean	*Hwa-byung*	Multiple somatic and psychologic symptoms; "pushing up" sensation of chest; palpitations, flushing, headache, "epigastric mass," dysphoria, anxiety, irritability, and difficulty concentrating; mostly afflicts married women
Native Americans	Ghost	Terror, hallucinations, sense of danger
North India Indians	Ghost	Death from fever and illness in children; convulsions, delirious speech (or incessant crying in infants); choking, difficulty breathing; based on Hindu religious beliefs and curing practices
Whites	Anorexia nervosa	Excessive preoccupation with thinness; self-imposed starvation
	Bulimia	Gross overeating and then vomiting or fasting

Traditional Chinese medicine usually is used only as long as symptoms persist. Some patients extend the same logic to Western biomedicine. For example, they might stop taking an antibiotic as soon as the symptoms subside instead of completing the course of treatment for the prescribed length of time. Be sure to consider the potential interaction of herbs with Western biomedicines. The root of the shrub *ginseng*, for example, is widely used for the treatment of arthritis, back and leg pains, and sores.

TABLE 3-3
Herbal Remedies

Aloe Vera

Source	Leaf of *Aloe barbadensis* Mill. (family Liliaceae)
Action	Topical analgesic, anti-inflammatory, antibacterial, and antifungal agent
Traditional uses	Applied topically for treatment of inflammation, minor burns, sunburn, cuts, bruises, and abrasions
	Orally, aloe juice was used for gastrointestinal upset, arthritis, diabetes mellitus, and gastric ulcers
Current uses	Promotes wound healing in soft tissue injuries
	Prevents wound pain by inhibiting the action of the pain-producing agent bradykinin
	May prevent progression of skin damage from electrical burns and frostbite
	Prevention of wound infection because of its antibacterial and antifungal properties
	Used in a wide variety of ointments, creams, lotions, and shampoos
Dosage	Apply topically as needed
Warnings	Rarely, skin rash follows topical application
	May cause burning if applied after removal of acne scars
	To avoid deterioration of active ingredients, use the fresh gel and avoid diluted extracts
	When taken internally as aloe latex, it causes intestinal cramping and may lead to ulcers and bowel irritation

Dong-Quai (Chinese Angelica)

Angelica sinensis

Source	Dried root of a member of the parsley family
Action	Smooth muscle relaxant; antispasmodic
Traditional uses	A highly regarded herb in Chinese medicine, dong-quai means "proper order"; used to suppress menstruation, cleanse the blood, and promote harmony in the body
	In the West, used to regulate menstrual periods, symptoms of menopause, and premenstrual syndrome (PMS)
Current uses	Relaxes uterine muscle and improves circulation to the uterus. Improves circulation and lowers blood pressure; reduces inflammation, pains, and spasm; increases number of red blood cells and platelets.
	Protects liver from toxins
Dosage	5–12 g (1–3 teaspoons) daily
Warnings	Contraindicated for pregnant and breast-feeding women and persons with abdominal distention or diarrhea
	Large doses may cause contact dermatitis and photodermatitis

Echinacea

Echinacea angustifolia, E. pallida, E. pururea

Source	Member of the daisy family; also known as purple coneflower
Action	Reduces cold symptoms
Traditional uses	Used by Native Americans in poultices, mouthwashes, and teas for colds, cancer, and other disorders
	Some herbalists consider it a blood purifier and an aid to fighting infections
Current uses	Enhances the immune system by stimulating the production of white blood cells needed to fight infection or cancer
Dosage	Follow directions on label; needed at onset of symptoms; usually taken for no longer than 2 weeks
Warnings	Contraindicated for pregnant or breast-feeding women, children, and those who are allergic to ragweed. Not recommended for people with severely compromised immune systems such as those with HIV/AIDS, tuberculosis, or multiple sclerosis
	Look for reputable suppliers, because a high percentage of the root currently marketed is adulterated with less expensive inactive substitutes

Evening Primrose Oil

Oenothera biennis

Source	Seeds of the wildflower evening primrose
Action	Antihypertensive, immunostimulant, weight reduction
Traditional uses	Used by Native Americans for food; in eastern North America, used to treat obesity and hemorrhoids; new settlers to North America used the plant for gastrointestinal upsets and sore throats
Current uses	Used as a dietary supplement for essential fatty acids; believed to help asthma, migraine headaches, inflammations, PMS, diabetes mellitus, and arthritis; also believed to lower blood pressure and lower cholesterol, slow the progression of multiple sclerosis, promote weight loss without dieting, alleviate hangovers, and moisturize dry eyes, brittle hair, and fingernails
Dosage	Follow directions on label; will take at least 1 month to experience benefits
Warnings	Side effects include occasional reports of headache, nausea, and abdominal discomfort; not recommended for children
	Some capsules may be altered with other types of oil such as soy or safflower

(table continues on page 48)

TABLE 3-3
Herbal Remedies (*continued*)

Ginger

Current uses	Effective in reducing morning sickness and postoperative nausea for some people; used in China to treat first- and second-degree burns
Dosage	Boil 1 oz dried ginger root in 1 cup water for 15 to 20 minutes
	Follow label directions on ginger supplements
Warning	Large doses may cause central nervous system depression and cardiac arrhythmias
	Side effects include heartburn
	Contraindicated in the presence of gallbladder disease

Ginkgo

Ginkgo biloba

Source	Extract from leaves of the ginkgo tree, a living fossil, believed to be more than 200 million years old
Action	Antioxidant; improves blood circulation
Traditional uses	Used in China since the 15th century for cough, asthma, diarrhea, skin lesions, and removal of freckles
Current uses	Promotes vasodilation and improves circulation of blood; may be an effective free radical scavenger or antioxidant; improves short-term memory, attention span, and mood in early stages of Alzheimer's disease by improving oxygen metabolism in the brain
Dosage	Range: 120–160 mg TID
	May take 6–8 weeks before results are evident
Warnings	Large doses may cause irritability, restlessness, diarrhea, nausea, and vomiting
	Some people (who are also sensitive to poison ivy) are unable to tolerate even low doses
	Contraindicated for women who are pregnant or breast-feeding
	Contraindicated for persons with clotting disorders
	Not recommended for children

Ginseng (American And Asian)

Panax quinquefolius (American)

Panax ginseng (Asian)

Source	Dried root of several species of the genus *Panax* of the family Aralaceae

Action	Tonic
Traditional uses	Treatment of anemia, atherosclerosis, edema, ulcers, hypertension, influenza, colds, inflammation, and disorders of the immune system (American)
	In traditional China, used for treatment of shock, diaphoresis, dyspnea, fever, thirst, irritability, diarrhea, vomiting, abdominal distention, anorexia, and impotence; considered a "heat-raising" tonic for the blood and circulatory system (Asian)
Current uses	Used to enhance sexual experience and treat impotence, though there is no current research to support this claim (American)
	In Germany may be labeled as a tonic to treat fatigue, reduced work capacity. In some parts of Asia, used for lack of concentration and for convalescence (Asian)
	Improved sense of well-being (Asian)
Dosage	American: Follow directions on label
	Asian: 100 mg BID
Warnings	American: May cause headaches, insomnia, anxiety, breast tenderness, rashes, asthma attacks, hypertension, cardiac arrhythmias, and postmenopausal uterine hemorrhage
	Should be used with caution for the following conditions: pregnancy, insomnia, hay fever, fibrocystic breasts, asthma, emphysema, hypertension, clotting disorders, and diabetes mellitus
	Asian: Same as American
Gotu Kola	
Centella asiatica	
Source	Dried and powdered leaves of a member of the parsley family
Action	Improves memory
Traditional uses	In ancient India, considered a rejuvenating herb that increases intelligence, longevity, and memory while slowing the aging process
	In China, used as a tea for colds and for lung and urinary tract infections, and topically for snakebite, wounds, and shingles
	Recommended for treatment of mental disorders, hypertension, abscesses, rheumatism, fever, ulcers, skin lesions, and jaundice
Current uses	Acceleration of wound healing, diuretic, treatment of phlebitis
Dosage	Follow directions on label; lower dose needed for children and older adults
Warnings	Sides effects include headaches and skin rash

(table continues on page 50)

TABLE 3-3
Herbal Remedies (*continued*)

	Contraindicated for pregnant or breast-feeding women and children younger than 2 years
	Contraindicated when using tranquilizers or sedatives

Saint John's Wort

Hypericum perforatum

Source	Tea made from the leaves and flowering tops of the perennial *Hypericum perforatum*, which is particularly abundant on June 24th, the feast of St. John the Baptist
Action	Antidepressant
Traditional uses	Used in 1st-century Greece for wound healing and menstrual disorders, and as a diuretic
	In 19th-century North America, used for its astringent, wound healing, diuretic, and mild sedative effects
Current uses	Treatment of mild to moderate depression; effects are linked to various substances that act as monoamine oxidase (MAO) inhibitors
Dosage	300 mg daily
Warnings	Fair-skinned people may experience urticaria or vesicular skin lesions upon exposure to sunlight
	Reduces effectiveness of some anticancer agents
	Clinical manifestations of depression should be considered seriously
	Encourage client to see a mental health care provider

Valerian

Valeriana officinalis

Source	Dried rhizome and roots of the tall perennial *Valeriana officinalis*
Action	Mild tranquilizer and sedative
Traditional uses	Used by the ancient Greeks for the treatment of epilepsy and menstrual disorders, and as a diuretic
	Used by 17th- and 18th-century Europeans as an antispasmodic and sedative
	Listed as an official remedy in the *United States Pharmacopoeia* from 1820 to 1936
Current uses	Used as a mild tranquilizer and sedative; relieves muscle spasms
	Especially effective for insomniac persons and older adults

Dosage	300–400 mg daily; take 1 hour before bedtime as a sleeping aid
Warnings	Reported side effects include headache, gastrointestinal upset, and excitability
	Signs of overdose include severe headache, restlessness, nausea, morning grogginess, or blurred vision
	Must not be taken in combination with other tranquilizers or sedatives
	Client should be cautioned against operating a motor vehicle after ingesting

Table based on data accessed on February 10, 2010, at The Alternative Medicine Home Page (http://www.pitt.edu/˷cbw/herb. html); MedlinePlus Herbal Medicine (http://www.nlm.nih.gov/medlineplus/herbalmedicine.html); National Center for Complementary and Alternative Medicine (http://www.nccam.gov); Sloan-Kettering: About Herbs, Botanicals and Other Products (http://www.mskcc.org/mskcc/html/11570.cfm).

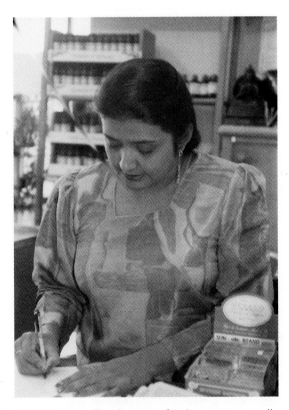

FIGURE 3-1 Shopkeeper of Indian ancestry sells herbal remedies used in Ayurvedic healing in a neighborhood store that attracts recent immigrants from India. People from diverse backgrounds who embrace Ayurvedic medicine also patronize the store, which sells prepackaged herbal remedies and dried herbs used to brew teas.

Because ginseng is known to potentiate the action of some antihypertensive drugs, you must ask the patient whether he or she is experiencing side effects or toxicity, and monitor blood pressure frequently. It might be necessary to withhold doses of the prescribed antihypertensive medicine if the blood pressure is low or to ask the client to discontinue or reduce the strength of the ginseng. When assessing the patient's use of traditional Chinese medicine, you should be aware that some Chinese Americans who use herbs topically do not consider them to be drugs. For further information about herbs, the nurse should ask the patient and family, consult a herbalist, search for reputable sources on the Internet; or check reference books on herbal remedies.

Dosage Modifications

As indicated in Table 3-4, there is growing evidence-based data indicating that modifications in dosages of some drugs should be made for members of selected racial and ethnic groups. It might be difficult to develop ethnic-specific norms for drug dosages because of intermarriage, individual differences (e.g., weight and body fat index), and related factors. It is possible, however, to alert nurses to the variations that occur in side effects, adverse reactions, and toxicity so that clients from diverse cultural backgrounds can be monitored for possible untoward clinical manifestations.

TABLE 3-4
Cultural Differences in Response to Drugs

DRUG CATEGORY	REMARKS
Arab Americans	
Antiarrhythmics	Some may need lower dosage
Antihypertensives	Some may need lower dosage
Neuroleptics	Some may need lower dosage
Opioids	Some may require higher dosage because of diminished ability to metabolize codeine to morphine
Psychotropics	Some may need lower dosage
Asian/Pacific Islanders	Be aware that drugs are part of the yin/yang belief system embraced by some Asian Americans and that herbal remedies may be used in addition to prescription drugs.
	Be sure to consider lower body weight and mass when calculating doses
Narcotic analgesics	Chinese may be less sensitive to the respiratory depressant and hypotensive effects of morphine but more likely to experience nausea; Chinese have a significantly higher clearance of morphine
Antihypertensives	Respond best to calcium antagonists
Neuroleptics	Require lower dose
Psychotropics	Require lower dose, sometimes as little as half the normal dose for tricyclic antidepressants (TCAs) and lithium
Fat-soluble drugs	On average, Asian Americans have a lower percentage of body fat, so dosage adjustments must be made for fat-soluble vitamins and other drugs, for example, vitamin K used to reverse the anticoagulant effect of Coumadin (warfarin); consider dietary intake of vitamins when calculating doses
Blacks	
Analgesics	Despite decreased sensitivity to pain-relieving therapeutic action of drugs, there are increased gastrointestinal side effects, especially with acetaminophen
Antihypertensives	Respond best to treatment with a single drug (vs. combined antihypertensive therapy)
	Research suggests favorable response to diuretics, calcium antagonists, and alpha-blockers
	Less responsive to beta-blockers (e.g., propranolol) and angiotensin-converting enzyme (ACE) inhibitors (e.g., enalapril, imidapril)
	Increased side effects such as mood response (e.g., depression) to thiazides (e.g., hydrochlorothiazide), which may explain reluctance to take drug as prescribed
	There is little justification to use racial profiling to avoid drug classes. Current research is focusing on differences in the causes of hypertension in Blacks to explain differences in drug responses
Mydriatics	Less dilation occurs with dark-colored eyes

DRUG CATEGORY	REMARKS
Psychotropics	Increased extrapyramidal side effects with TCAs such as haloperidol
Steroids	When methylprednisolone is used for immunosuppression in renal transplant patients, there is increased toxicity such as steroid-associated diabetes; although Blacks are four times as likely to develop end-stage renal disease as Whites, they have the poorest long-term graft survival of any ethnic group
Tranquilizers	15%–20% are poor metabolizers of Valium (diazepam)
Hispanics	
Psychotropics	May require lower dosage and experience higher incidence of side effects with TCAs
Greeks, Italians, And Others Of Mediterranean Descent With G-6-Pd Deficiency	
Oxidating drugs	The following drugs may precipitate a hemolytic crisis: primaquine, quinidine, thiazolsulfone, furazolidone, haloperidol, nitrofural, naphthalene, toluidine blue, phenylhydrazine, chloramphenicol, aspirin
Jewish North Americans (Ashkenazi)	
Psychotropics	Agranulocytosis develops in 20% when clozapine is used to treat schizophrenia; thus, the granulocyte count should be checked before the drug is administered
Native North Americans	
Muscle relaxants	Native Alaskans may experience prolonged muscle paralysis and an inability to breathe without mechanical ventilation for several hours postoperatively when succinylcholine has been administered in surgery

Table based partially on data from

Bloche, M. G. (2006). Race, money, and medicines. *The Journal of Law, Medicine, and Ethics, 34*(3), 555–558.

Davies, S. (2006). Pharmacogenetics, pharmacogenomics and personalized medicine: Are we there yet? *Hematology,* 2006, 111–117.

Harty, L., Johnson, K., & Power, A. (2006). Race and ethnicity in the era of emerging pharmacogenomics. *Journal of Clinical Pharmacology, 46,* 405–407.

Lin, K., Anderson, D., & Poland, R. (1995). Ethnicity and psychopharmacology: Bridging the gap. *Psychiatric Clinics of North America, 18*(3), 635–647.

Ma, J. K., Chikwamba, R., Sparrow, P., Fischer, R., Mahoney, R., & Twyman, R. M. (2005). Plant-derived pharmaceuticals—the road forward. *Trends in Plant Science, 10*(12), 580–585.

Mathis, A. S., & Knipp, G. T. (2002). Do sex and ethnicity influence drug pharmacokinetics in solid organ transplantation? *Graft, 5*(50), 294–302.

Overfield, T. (1995). *Biologic variation in health and illness.* New York: CRC Press.

Schultz, J. (2003). FDA guidelines on race and ethnicity: Obstacle or remedy? *Journal of the National Cancer Institute, 95*(6), 425–426.

Zhou, H. H., Sheller, J. R., Nu, H., Wood, M., & Wood, A. J. J. (1993). Ethnic differences in response to morphine. *Clinical Pharmacology and Therapeutics, 54*(3), 507–513.

Medication Administration

If the medication prescribed, its route of administration, or the substances given with it conflict with clients' adherence to the yin/yang, hot/cold, or other belief system, it is unlikely that they will follow your advice concerning the medication. The nurse should be aware that some clients of Latino, Middle Eastern, and Asian heritage believe that it is important to take medicine with certain beverages or foods to provide the necessary balance for health. If clients give cues that they are uncomfortable with the beverage or food being used in the health care setting, discuss alternatives. For example, in most health care facilities, medications are given with cold water, but they could be given with hot water, tea, coffee, or a similar beverage if the client believes that such a beverage would promote healing. Some Mexican Americans believe that grapefruit juice has healing properties, so you might contact the dietary department to ensure that this juice is available when medications are administered. If the cultural healing beliefs and practices of the client are incorporated into medication administration, there is a higher probability that the client will believe in the healing properties of the drugs and will continue to take them as prescribed after discharge.

Family and Social History

In addition to diagramming a family tree to identify familial relationships and the presence of disease conditions among those related to the client, you should assess the broader socioeconomic factors influencing the client. The health history should include in-depth data pertaining to the client's family and/or close social friends, including identification of *key decision makers*. Although personal financial information is often a sensitive topic, it is important to determine the overall economic factors that influence a client. For example, regardless of race or ethnicity, people from lower socioeconomic categories have poorer health and shorter lives. Unfortunately, there is a disproportionately high level of poverty among Blacks, Latinos/Latinas, First Nation People of Canada, and American Indians/Alaska Natives. Economic factors have been identified as causes of less favorable outcomes among clients with cancer. Research suggests that this is caused by a lack of health insurance and/or diminished access to health care services, both of which contribute to a situation in which less affluent clients receive diagnosis and treatment later in the course of the disease. See Appendix A for suggested interview topics aimed at eliciting information about family and social history.

Review of Systems

The purposes of the review of systems are to evaluate the past and present health state of each body system, to provide an opportunity for the client to report symptoms not previously stated, and to evaluate health-promotion practices. Knowledge of current research on diseases prevalent in specific ethnic and racial groups might be useful in asking appropriate questions in the review of systems. For example, if the nurse is gathering review of systems information from a middle-aged African American man, it is useful to know that there is a statistically higher incidence of hypertension, sickle cell anemia, and type 2 diabetes in this group than in counterparts from other racial and ethnic groups. This will assist in customizing the review of systems questions and ensuring that symptoms of disease specific to the client's ethnic or racial heritage are included.

Transcultural Perspectives on the Physical Examination

The purpose of this discussion is to identify selected **biocultural variations** that nurses sometimes encounter when conducting the physical examination of clients from different cultural backgrounds. Accurate assessment and evaluation of clients require knowledge of normal biocultural variations among healthy members of selected populations. You must also possess assessment skills that will enable you to recognize variations that occur in illness. The following remarks are intended to be helpful and illustrative, not exhaustive. As more research on biocultural variations is conducted, undoubtedly there will be additions and perhaps some modifications. The author would like to note that the data in the following section is evidence-based and reflects the findings of classic studies that have been conducted over a period of years. The work of Dr. Theresa Overfield, a renowned nurse–anthropologist who published extensively on biological variations in health and illness, has been cited frequently in the discussion of biocultural variations that follows.

Biocultural Variations in Measurements

Height

Summarized in Table 3-5 are average heights for men and women from selected cultural groups that have been studied. In all groups, height increases up to 1.5 inches as socioeconomic status improves. First-generation immigrants might be up to 1.5 inches taller than their counterparts in the country of origin because of (1) better nutrition and (2) decreased interference with growth by infectious diseases. During the past decade, the overall height of men from the United States increased by 0.7 inches, whereas women from the United States grew an average of 0.5 inches taller (Overfield, 1995).

Body Proportions

Biocultural variations are found in the body proportions of individuals, largely because of differences in bone length. In examining sitting/standing height ratios, you will notice that Blacks of both genders have longer legs and shorter trunks than Whites. Because proportionately most of the weight is in the trunk, White men appear more obese than their Black counterparts. The reverse is true of women. Clients of Asian heritage are markedly shorter, weigh less, and have smaller body frames than their White counterparts and/or the overall population (Overfield, 1995).

Weight

Biocultural differences exist in the amount of body fat and the distribution of fat throughout the body. As a general rule, people from the lower socioeconomic class are more obese than those from the middle class, who are more obese than members of the upper class. On average, Black men weigh less than their White counterparts throughout adulthood (166.1 pounds vs. 170.6 pounds). The opposite is true of women. Black women are consistently heavier than White women of every age (149.6 pounds vs. 137 pounds). Between the ages of 35 and 64 years, Black women weigh on average 20 pounds more than White women. Mexican Americans weigh more in relation to height than non-Hispanic Whites because of differences in truncal fat patterns. Most differences in the amount of body fat are related to socioeconomic factors, which in turn influence nutrition and exposure to communicable diseases. Around the world, people in cold climates tend to have more body fat, whereas those residing in warmer areas have less. Blacks have smaller skinfold thicknesses on their trunks and arms than do their White counterparts. Bottle-fed infants are heavier on average than those who are breast-fed, although their lengths are similar (Overfield, 1995).

Biocultural Variations in Vital Signs

Although the average pulse rate is comparable across cultures, there are racial and gender differences in *blood pressure*. Black men have lower systolic blood pressures than their White counterparts from ages 18 to 34, but between the ages of 35 and 64 it reverses: Blacks have an average systolic blood pressure 5 mmHg higher. After age 65 there is no difference between the two races. Black women have a higher average systolic blood pressure than their White counterparts at every age. After age 45, the average blood pressure of Black women might be as much as 16 mmHg higher than that of White women in the same age group (Overfield, 1995).

Biocultural Variations in General Appearance

In assessing general appearance, you should survey the person's entire body. You will want to note the general health state and any obvious physical characteristics and readily apparent biologic features unique to the individual. In assessing the client's general appearance, you should consider four areas: physical appearance,

TABLE 3-5
Biocultural Variations in Height for Selected Groups

HEIGHT (IN INCHES) FOR ALL GROUPS				
All groups of men (n)	White American	African American	Mexican America	Asian
69.1	69.1	69.2	67.2	65.7
All groups of women				
63.7	63.8	63.8	61.8	60.3

Table developed using data from Overfield, T. (1995). *Biologic variation in health and illness.* New York: CRC Press.

body structure, mobility, and behavior. *Physical appearance* includes age, gender, level of consciousness, facial features, and skin color (evenness of color tone, pigmentation, intactness, and presence of lesions or other abnormalities). *Body structure* includes stature, nutrition, symmetry, posture, position, and overall body build or contour. *Mobility* includes gait and range of motion. *Behavior* includes such variables as facial expression, mood and affect, fluency of speech, ability to communicate ideas, appropriateness of word choice, grooming, and attire or dress.

In assessing a client's hygiene, it is useful to ask about typical bathing habits and customary use of various hygiene-related products. People in most cultures in the United States and Canada make a great effort to disguise their natural body odors by bathing frequently, using douches, or applying antiperspirants, colognes, and/or perfumes with scents that are deemed to be desirable. Ironically, some colognes and perfumes such as those with musk oil are marketed in the United States and Canada because of their more "natural" odor, which is alleged to give the wearer more sex appeal. Recent immigrants from some arid nations where water is scarce might bathe less frequently than those from countries where water is more abundant.

Bicultural Variations in Skin

An accurate and comprehensive examination of the skin of clients from culturally diverse backgrounds requires that you possess knowledge of biocultural variations and skill in recognizing color changes, some of which might be subtle. Awareness of normal biocultural differences and the ability to recognize the unique clinical manifestations of disease are developed over time as you gain experience with clients having various skin colors.

The assessment of a client's skin is subjective and is highly dependent on your observational skill, ability to recognize subtle color changes, and repeated exposure to individuals having various gradations of skin color. *Melanin* is responsible for the various colors and tones of skin observed in different people. Melanin protects the skin against harmful ultraviolet rays—a genetic advantage accounting for the lower incidence of skin cancer among darkly pigmented Black and Native American clients.

Normal skin color ranges widely. Some health care practitioners have made attempts to describe the variations by labeling their observations with some of the following adjectives: *copper, olive, tan,* and various shades of *brown (light, medium, and dark).* In observing pallor in clients, the term *ashen* is sometimes used. Of most clinical significance, particularly for clients whose health condition might be linked to changes in skin color, is your ability to establish a reliable description of a baseline color and subsequently to recognize when variations occur in the same individual.

Mongolian Spots

Mongolian spots are irregular areas of deep blue pigmentation usually located in the sacral and gluteal areas but sometimes occurring on the abdomen, thighs, shoulders, or arms. During embryonic development, the melanocytes originate near the embryonic nervous system in the neural crest. They then migrate into the fetal epidermis. Mongolian spots consist of embryonic pigment that has been left behind in the epidermal layer during fetal development. The result looks like a bluish discoloration of the skin.

Mongolian spots are a normal variation in children of African, Asian, or Latin descent. By adulthood, these spots become lighter but usually remain visible. Mongolian spots are present in 90% of Blacks, 80% of Asians and Native Americans, and 9% of Whites (Overfield, 1995). If you are unfamiliar with Mongolian spots, it is important to exercise caution so as to not confuse them with bruises. Recognition of this normal variation is particularly important when you are dealing with children who might be erroneously identified as victims of child abuse, causing much anguish to the parents or guardians.

Vitiligo

Vitiligo, a condition in which the melanocytes become nonfunctional in some areas of the skin, is characterized by unpigmented skin patches. Vitiligo affects an estimated 2 to 4 million Americans, primarily dark-skinned individuals. Clients with vitiligo also have a statistically higher-than-normal risk for pernicious anemia, diabetes mellitus, and hyperthyroidism. These factors are believed to reflect an underlying genetic abnormality. There are numerous online sites with information about vitiligo including Vitiligo Support International (http://www.vitilgosupport.org) and the National Vitiligo Foundation (http://www.nvfi.org).

Hyperpigmentation

Other areas of the skin affected by hormones and, in some cases, differing for people from certain ethnic backgrounds are the sexual skin areas, such as the nipples, areola, scrotum, and labia majora. In general, these areas are darker than other parts of the skin in both adults and children, especially among African American and Asian clients. When assessing these skin surfaces on dark-skinned clients, you must observe carefully for erythema, rashes, and other abnormalities because the darker color might mask their presence.

Cyanosis

Cyanosis is the most difficult clinical sign to observe in darkly pigmented persons. Because peripheral vasoconstriction can prevent cyanosis, you need to be attentive to environmental conditions such as air conditioning, mist tents, and other factors that might lower the room temperature and thus cause vasoconstriction. For the client to manifest clinical evidence of cyanosis, the blood must contain 5 g of reduced hemoglobin in 1.5 g of methemoglobin per 100 ml of blood (Overfield, 1995).

Given that most conditions causing cyanosis also cause decreased oxygenation of the brain, other clinical symptoms, such as changes in the level of consciousness, will be evident. Cyanosis usually is accompanied by increased respiratory rate, use of accessory muscles of respiration, nasal flaring, and other manifestations of respiratory distress. You must exercise caution when assessing persons of Mediterranean descent for cyanosis because their circumoral region is normally dark blue.

Jaundice

In both light- and dark-skinned clients, **jaundice** is best observed in the sclera. When examining culturally diverse individuals, exercise caution to avoid confusing other forms of pigmentation with jaundice. Many darkly pigmented people, for example, African Americans, Filipinos, and others, have heavy deposits of subconjunctival fat that contains high levels of carotene in sufficient quantities to mimic jaundice. The fatty deposits become denser as the distance from the cornea increases. The portion of the sclera that is revealed naturally by the palpebral fissure is the best place to accurately assess color. If the palate does not have heavy melanin pigmentation, jaundice can be detected there in the early stages (i.e., when the serum bilirubin level is 2 to 4 mg/100 ml). The absence of a yellowish tint of the palate when the sclerae are yellow indicates carotene pigmentation of the sclerae rather than jaundice. Light- or clay-colored stools and dark golden urine often accompany jaundice in both light- and dark-skinned clients. If you are to distinguish between carotenemia and jaundice, it will be necessary to inspect the posterior portion of the hard palate using bright daylight or good artificial lighting (Overfield, 1995).

Pallor

When assessing for **pallor** in darkly pigmented clients, you might experience difficulty because the underlying red tones are absent. This is significant because these red tones are responsible for giving brown or black skin its luster. The brown-skinned individual will manifest pallor with a more yellowish brown color, and the black-skinned person will appear ashen or gray. Generalized pallor can be observed in the mucous membranes, lips, and nail beds. The palpebrae, conjunctivae, and nail beds are preferred sites for assessing the pallor of anemia. When inspecting the conjunctiva, you should lower the lid sufficiently so you can see the conjunctiva near the inner and outer canthi. The coloration is often lighter near the inner canthus.

In addition to changes seen on skin assessment, the pallor of impending shock is accompanied by other clinical manifestations, such as increasing pulse rate, oliguria, apprehension, and restlessness. Anemia, particularly chronic iron deficiency anemia, might be manifested by the characteristic "spoon" nails, which have a concave shape. A lemon-yellow tint of the face and slightly yellow sclerae accompany pernicious anemia, which is also manifested by neurologic deficits and a red, painful tongue. Also, fatigue, exertional dyspnea, rapid pulse, dizziness, and impaired mental function accompany the most severe anemia (Overfield, 1995).

Erythema

You might find that it is difficult to assess **erythema** (redness) in darkly pigmented clients. Erythema is frequently associated with localized inflammation and is characterized by increased skin temperature. The degree of redness is determined by the quantity of blood in the subpapillary plexus, whereas the warmth of the skin is related to the rate of blood flow through the blood vessels. In the assessment of inflammation in dark-skinned clients, it is often necessary to palpate the skin for increased warmth, tautness, or tightly pulled surfaces that might indicate edema, and hardening of deep tissues or blood vessels. You will find that the dorsal surfaces of your fingers will be the most sensitive to temperature sensations. The erythema associated with rashes is not always accompanied by noticeable increases in skin temperature. Macular, papular, and vesicular skin lesions are identified by a combination of palpation and inspection. In addition, it is important that you listen to the client's description of symptoms. For example, persons with macular rashes usually will complain of itching, and evidence of scratching will be apparent. When the skin is only moderately pigmented, a macular rash might become recognizable if the skin were gently stretched. Stretching the skin decreases the normal red tone, thus providing more contrast and making the macules appear brighter. In some skin disorders with a generalized rash, you will observe that the rash is most readily visible on the hard and soft palates (Overfield, 1995).

The increased redness that accompanies carbon monoxide poisoning and the blood disorders collectively known as *polycythemia* can be observed on the lips of dark-skinned clients. Because lipstick masks the actual color of the lips, you should ask the client to remove it prior to inspection.

Petechiae

In dark-skinned clients, **petechiae** are best visualized in the areas of lighter melanization, such as the abdomen, buttocks, and volar surface of the forearm. When the skin is black or very dark brown, petechiae cannot be seen in the skin. Most of the diseases that cause bleeding and the formation of microscopic emboli, such as thrombocytopenia, subacute bacterial endocarditis, and other septicemias, are characterized by petechiae in the mucous membranes and skin. Petechiae are most easily seen in the mouth, particularly the buccal mucosa, and in the conjunctiva of the eye (Overfield, 1995).

Ecchymoses

In assessing **ecchymotic lesions** caused by systemic disorders, you will find them in the same locations as petechiae, although their larger size makes them more apparent on dark-skinned individuals. When you are differentiating petechiae and ecchymoses from erythema in the mucous membrane, pressure on the tissue will momentarily blanch erythema but not petechiae or ecchymoses.

Normal Age-Related Skin Changes

Although aging is accompanied by the growing presence of wrinkles in all cultures, Blacks, Asian Americans, American Indians, and Eskimos wrinkle later in life than their Anglo American counterparts. Light skin shows the effects of sun damage more than dark skin, regardless of race or ethnicity. The area of the skin that is exposed to the sun shows the effects of aging more than protected skin, such as those parts covered by clothing. Regardless of climate, dry skin is inevitable in individuals older than 70 years of age. In part, dry skin is caused by transepidermal water loss, which decreases in older adults. African Americans have a significantly higher transepidermal water loss than Whites, which correlates with the water content of the stratum corneum layer of the skin. Because the number of moles increases with age, they are thought to be the result of long-term exposure to the sun. People with lighter skin have more moles than those with darkly pigmented skin. Whites have more moles than Asian Americans or African Americans (Overfield, 1995).

Nurses and other health care providers often overestimate or underestimate age when dealing with clients whose cultural heritage is different from their own. Whites tend to underestimate the age of Africans, Asians, and American Indians, whereas African Americans, Asians, and American Indians tend to overestimate the age of White clients (Overfield, 1995).

Biocultural Variations in Body Secretions

The *apocrine* and *eccrine sweat glands* are important for fluid balance and for thermoregulation. Approximately 2 to 3 million glands open onto the skin surface through pores and are responsible for the presence of sweat. When they are contaminated by normal skin flora, odor results. Most Asians and Native Americans have a mild to absent body odor, whereas Whites and African Americans tend to have strong body odor.

Eskimos have made an environmental adaptation whereby they sweat less than Whites on their trunks and extremities but more on their faces. This adaptation allows for temperature regulation without causing perspiration and dampness of their clothes, which would decrease their ability to insulate against severe weather and would pose a serious threat to their survival.

The amount of chloride excreted by sweat glands varies widely, and African Americans have lower salt concentrations in their sweat than do Whites. A study of Ashkenazi Jews (of European descent) and Sephardic Jews (of North African and Middle Eastern descent) revealed that those of European origin had a lower percentage of sweat chlorides (Levin, 1966). This variation might be significant in the care of clients with renal or cardiac conditions or of children with cystic fibrosis (Overfield, 1995).

Biocultural Variation in the Head, Eyes, Ears, and Mouth

Hair

Perhaps one of the most obvious and widely variable cultural differences occurs with assessment of the hair. African Americans' hair varies widely in texture. It is very fragile and ranges from long and straight to short, spiraled, thick, and kinky. The hair and scalp have a natural tendency to be dry and require daily combing, gentle brushing, and the application of oil. By comparison, clients of Asian backgrounds generally have straight, silky hair.

Obtaining a baseline hair assessment is significant in the diagnosis and treatment of certain disease states. For example, hair texture is known to become dry, brittle, and lusterless with inadequate nutrition. The hair of Black children with severe malnutrition, as in the case of marasmus, frequently changes not only in texture but also in color. The child's hair often becomes straighter and turns a reddish copper color. Certain endocrine disorders are also known to affect the texture of hair.

Although gray hair correlates with age for both men and women, there are cultural differences in the rate of hair graying. Whites gray significantly faster than any other group. The hair of 66% of fair-haired individuals, but only 37% of dark-haired persons, is fully white by age 60 (Overfield, 1995). Among Asian Americans, graying might be delayed significantly, with some in their eighth or ninth decade of life showing little or no graying.

Eyes

Biocultural differences in both the structure and the color of the eyes are readily apparent among clients from various cultural backgrounds. Racial differences are evident in the palpebral fissures. Persons of Asian background are often identified by their characteristic epicanthal eye folds, whereas the presence of narrowed palpebral fissures in non-Asian individuals might be diagnostic of a serious congenital anomaly known as Down syndrome or trisomy 21.

There is culturally based variability in the color of the iris and in retinal pigmentation: Darker irises are correlated with darker retinas. Clients with light retinas generally have better night vision but can experience pain in an environment that is too light. The majority of African Americans and Asians have brown eyes, whereas many individuals of Scandinavian or northern European descent have blue eyes (Overfield, 1995).

It is clinically relevant that differences in visual acuity occur among people from different cultures. Blacks have poorer corrected visual acuity than Whites. The visual acuity of Hispanic Americans is between that of Blacks and Whites. American Indians are comparable to Whites in visual acuity, whereas Japanese and Chinese Americans have the poorest corrected visual acuity because of a high incidence of myopia (Overfield, 1995).

Ears

It does not take long to notice that ears come in a variety of sizes and shapes. Earlobes can be freestanding or attached to the face. Ceruminous glands are located in the external ear canal and are functional at birth. Cerumen is genetically determined and comes in two major types: (1) dry cerumen, which is gray and flaky and frequently forms a thin mass in the ear canal, and (2) wet cerumen, which is dark brown and moist. Asians and Native Americans (including Eskimos) have an 84% frequency of dry cerumen, whereas African Americans have a 99% frequency and Whites have a 97% frequency of wet cerumen (Overfield, 1995). The clinical significance of this occurs when you are examining or irrigating the ears. You should be aware that the presence and composition of cerumen are not related to poor hygiene, and caution should be exercised to avoid mistaking flaky, dry cerumen for the dry lesions of eczema.

Hearing gradually declines with age, especially in the high frequencies. After age 40, men have poorer hearing than women. Blacks have better hearing at high and low frequencies, whereas Whites have better hearing at middle frequencies. Blacks are less susceptible to noise-induced hearing loss (Overfield, 1995).

Mouth

Oral hyperpigmentation also shows variation by race. Usually absent at birth, hyperpigmentation increases with age. By age 50, 10% of Whites and 50% to 90% of African Americans will show oral hyperpigmentation, a condition believed to be caused by a lifetime of accumulation of postinflammatory oral changes (Overfield, 1995).

Cleft uvula, a condition in which the uvula is split either completely or partially, occurs in 18% of some Native American groups and 10% of Asians. The occurrence in Whites and Blacks is rare. *Cleft lip* and *cleft palate* are most common in

Asians and Native Americans and least common in African Americans (Overfield, 1995).

Leukoedema, a grayish white benign lesion occurring on the buccal mucosa, is present in 68% to 90% of Blacks but only 43% of Whites. Care should be taken to avoid mistaking leukoedema for oral thrush or related infections that require treatment with medication (Overfield, 1995).

Teeth

Because teeth are often used as indicators of developmental, hygienic, and nutritional adequacy, you should be aware of biocultural differences. Although it is rare for a White baby to be born with teeth (1 in 3,000), the incidence rises to 1 in 11 among Tlingit Indian infants and to 1 or 2 in 100 among Canadian Aboriginal infants. Although congenital teeth are usually not problematic, extraction is necessary for some breast-fed infants (Overfield, 1995).

The size of teeth varies widely, with the teeth of Whites being the smallest, followed by Blacks and then Asians and Native Americans. The largest teeth are found among Native Alaskans and Australian Aborigines. Larger teeth cause some groups to have prognathic (protruding) jaws, a condition that is seen more frequently in African and Asian Americans. The condition is normal and does not reflect a serious orthodontic problem.

Agenesis (absence of teeth) varies by race, with missing third molars occurring in 18% to 35% of Asians, 9% to 25% of Whites, and 1% to 11% of Blacks. Throughout life, Whites have more tooth decay than Blacks, which might be related to a combination of socioeconomic factors and biocultural variation. Complete tooth loss occurs more often in Whites than in African Americans despite the higher incidence of periodontal disease in Blacks (Overfield, 1995). Overfield (1995) noted that approximately one third of Whites 45 years or older have lost all their teeth, compared with 25% of Blacks in the same age group. There is reason to believe that as dental care is more advanced and accessible, both Whites and Blacks will retain more of their original teeth over their life spans.

The differences in tooth decay between African Americans and Whites can be explained by the fact that African Americans have harder and denser tooth enamel, which makes their teeth less susceptible to the organisms that cause caries. The increase in periodontal disease among African Americans is believed to be caused by poor oral hygiene. When obvious signs of periodontal disease are present, such as bleeding and edematous gums, a dental referral should be initiated (Overfield, 1995).

Biocultural Variations in the Mammary Venous Plexus

Regardless of gender, the superficial veins of the chest form a network over the entire chest that flows in either a transverse or a longitudinal pattern. In the transverse pattern, the veins radiate laterally and toward the axillae. In the longitudinal pattern, the veins radiate downward and laterally like a fan. These two patterns occur with different frequencies in the two populations that have been studied. The recessive longitudinal pattern occurs in 6% to 10% of White women and in 30% of Navajos. The only known alteration of either pattern is produced by breast tumor. Although this variation has no clinical significance, it is mentioned so that if nurses note its presence during physical assessment, they will recognize it as a nonsignificant finding (Overfield, 1995).

Biocultural Variation in the Musculoskeletal System

Many normal biocultural variations are found in clients' musculoskeletal systems. The long bones of Blacks are significantly longer, narrower, and denser than those of Whites. Bone density measured by race and gender shows that Black males have the densest bones, thus accounting for the relatively low incidence of osteoporosis in this population. Bone density in Chinese, Japanese, and Native Alaskans is below that of Whites (Overfield, 1995).

TABLE 3-6
Biocultural Variations in the Musculoskeletal System

DRUG CATEGORY	REMARKS
BONE	
Frontal	Thicker in Black males than in White males
Parietal occiput	Thicker in White males than in Black males
Palate	Tori (protuberances) along the suture line of the hard palate
	Problematic for denture wearers
	Incidence:
	Blacks 20%
	Whites 24%
	Asians Up to 50%
	Native Americans Up to 50%
Mandible	Tori (protuberances) on the lingual surface of the mandible near the canine and premolar teeth
	Problematic for denture wearers
	Most common in Asians and Native Americans; exceeds 50% in some Eskimo groups
Humerus	Torsion or rotation of proximal end with muscle pull
	Whites > Blacks
	Torsion in Blacks is symmetric; torsion in Whites tends to be greater on right side than left side
Radius	Length at the wrist variable
Ulna	Ulna or radius may be longer
	Equal length
	Swedes 61%
	Chinese 16%
	Ulna longer than radius
	Swedes 16%
	Chinese 48%
	Radius longer than ulna
	Swedes 23%
	Chinese 10%
Vertebrae	Twenty-four vertebrae are found in 85% to 93% of all people; racial and sex differences reveal 23 or 25 vertebrae in select groups
	Vertebrae Population
	23 11% of Black females
	25 12% of Native Alaskan and Native American
	Related to lower back pain and lordosis

DRUG CATEGORY	REMARKS	
Pelvis	Hip width is 1.6 cm (0.6 in) smaller in Black women than in White women; Asian women have significantly smaller pelvises	
Femur	Convex anterior	Native American
	Straight	Black
	Intermediate	White
Second tarsal	Second toe longer than the great toe	
	Incidence:	
	Whites	8–34%
	Blacks	8–12%
	Vietnamese	31%
	Melanesians	21–57%
	Clinical significance for joggers and athletes	
Height	White males are 1.27 cm (0.5 in.) taller than Black males and 7.6 cm (2.9 in.) taller than Asian males	
	White females = Black females	
	Asian females are 4.14 cm (1.6 in.) shorter than White or Black females	
Composition of long bones	Longer, narrower, and denser in Blacks than in Whites; bone density in Whites > Chinese, Japanese, and Native Alaskan	
	Osteoporosis lowest in Black males; highest in White females	
Muscle		
Peroneus tertius	Responsible for dorsiflexion of foot	
	Muscle absent:	
	Asians, Native Americans, and Whites	3%–10%
	Blacks	10%–15%
	Berbers (Sahara desert)	24%
	No clinical significance because the tibialis anterior also dorsiflexes the foot	
Palmaris longus	Responsible for wrist flexion	
	Muscle absent:	
	Whites	12%–20%
	Native Americans	2%–12%
	Blacks	5%
	Asians	3%
	No clinical significance because three other muscles are also responsible for flexion	

Based on data reported by T. Overfield. (1995). *Biologic variation in health and illness: Race, age, and sex differences.* New York: CRC Press.

TABLE 3-7
Distribution of Selected Genetic Traits and Disorders by Population or Ethnic Group

ETHNIC OR POPULATION GROUP	GENETIC OR MULTIFACTORIAL DISORDER PRESENT IN RELATIVELY HIGH FREQUENCY
Aland Islanders	Ocular albinism (Forsius–Eriksson type)
Amish	Limb girdle muscular dystrophy (IN—Adams, Allen counties)
	Ellis–van Creveld syndrome (PA—Lancaster county)
	Pyruvate kinase deficiency (OH—Mifflin county)
	Hemophilia B (PA—Holmes county)
Armenians	Familial Mediterranean fever
	Familial paroxysmal polyserositis
Blacks (African)	Sickle cell disease
	Hemoglobin C disease
	Hereditary persistence of hemoglobin F
	G-6-PD deficiency, African type
	Lactase deficiency, adult
	β-thalassemia
Burmese	Hemoglobin E disease
Chinese	α-thalassemia
	G-6-PD deficiency, Chinese type
	Lactase deficiency, adult
Costa Ricans	Malignant osteopetrosis
Druze	Alkaptonuria
English	Cystic fibrosis
	Hereditary amyloidosis, type III
Eskimos	Congenital adrenal hyperplasia
	Pseudocholinesterase deficiency
	Methemoglobinemia
French Canadians (Quebec)	Tyrosinemia
	Morquio syndrome
Finns	Congenital nephrosis
	Generalized amyloidosis syndrome, V
	Polycystic liver disease
	Retinoschisis

ETHNIC OR POPULATION GROUP	GENETIC OR MULTIFACTORIAL DISORDER PRESENT IN RELATIVELY HIGH FREQUENCY
	Aspartylglycolsaminuria
	Diastrophic dwarfism
Gypsies (Czech)	Congenital glaucoma
Hopi Indians	Tyrosinase-positive albinism
Icelanders	Phenylketonuria
Irish	Phenylketonuria
	Neural tube defects
Japanese	Acatalasemia
	Cleft lip/palate
	Oguchi disease
Jews	
Ashkenazi	Tay-Sachs disease (infantile)
	Niemann–Pick disease (infantile)
	Gaucher disease (adult type)
	Familial dysautonomia (Riley–Day syndrome)
	Bloom syndrome
	Torsion dystonia
Sephardi	Factor XI (PTA) deficiency
	Familial Mediterranean fever
	Ataxia–telangiectasia (Morocco)
	Cystinuria (Libya)
	Glycogen storage disease III (Morocco)
Orientals	Dubin–Johnson syndrome (Iran)
	Ichthyosis vulgaris (Iraq, India)
	Werdnig–Hoffman disease (Karaite Jews)
	G-6-PD deficiency, Mediterranean type
	Phenylketonuria (Yemen)

(table continues on page 66)

TABLE 3-7
Distribution of Selected Genetic Traits and Disorders by Population or Ethnic Group (*continued*)

ETHNIC OR POPULATION GROUP	GENETIC OR MULTIFACTORIAL DISORDER PRESENT IN RELATIVELY HIGH FREQUENCY
	Metachromatic leukodystrophy (Habbanite Jews, Saudi Arabia)
Lapps	Congenital dislocation of hip
Lebanese	Dyggve–Melchoir–Clausen syndrome
Mediterranean people (Italians, Greeks)	G-6-PD deficiency, Mediterranean type β-thalassemia
	Familial Mediterranean fever
Navajo Indians	Ear anomalies
	Joseph disease
Polynesians	Clubfoot
Poles	Phenylketonuria
Portuguese	Joseph disease
Nova Scotia Acadians	Niemann–Pick disease, type D
Scandinavians (Norwegians, Swedes, Danes)	Cholestasis-lymphedema syndrome (Norwegians)
	Sjögren–Larsson syndrome (Swedes)
	Krabbe disease
Scots	Phenylketonuria
	Phenylketonuria
	Cystic fibrosis
	Hereditary amyloidosis, type III
Thoi	Lactase deficiency, adult
	Hemoglobin E disease
Zuni Indians	Tyrosinase-positive albinism

From Cohen, F. L. (1984). *Clinical Genetics in Nursing Practice* (pp. 23–24). Philadelphia: J.B. Lippincott. Reprinted by permission.

Curvature of the body's long bones varies widely among culturally diverse groups. Native Americans and First Nation People of Canada have anteriorly convex femurs, whereas Blacks have markedly straight femurs, and Whites have intermediate femurs. This characteristic is related to both genetics and body weight. The femurs of thin Blacks and Whites have less curvature than average, whereas those of obese Blacks and Whites display increased curvatures. It is possible that the heavier density of the bones of Blacks helps to protect them from increased curvature caused by obesity (Overfield, 1995). Table 3-6 summarizes biocultural variations occurring in the musculoskeletal system that have been identified through observation and study of people from various cultures and subcultures.

Biocultural Variations in Illness

Researchers have abundant evidence that there is a relationship between ethnicity and the incidence of certain diseases across the life span, from infancy to old age. Table 3-7 provides an alphabetical listing of selected diseases and their increased or decreased prevalence among members of certain cultural groups. A knowledge of normal biocultural variations and those occurring during illness helps nurses to conduct more accurate, comprehensive, and thorough physical examinations of clients from diverse cultures.

Laboratory Tests

You should be aware that biocultural variations occur with some laboratory test results, such as measurement of *hemoglobin, hematocrit, cholesterol, serum transferrin,* and *blood glucose.* You also will want to consider cultural differences in the results of tests conducted during pregnancy. The *multiple-marker screening* test and two tests of *amniotic fluid constituents* are used to screen pregnant women for potential fetal problems.

TABLE 3-8
Biocultural Variations and Clinical Significance for Selected Laboratory Tests

TEST	REMARKS	
Hemoglobin/hematocrit	1 g lower for Blacks than other groups; Blacks < counterparts in other groups	
Serum transferrin	Biocultural variation in children aged 1–3 1/2 years	
	Mean for Blacks 22 mg/100 ml > Whites	
	Note: May be due to lowered hemoglobin and hematocrit levels found in Blacks	
	Clinical significance: Transferrin levels increase in the presence of anemia, thus influencing the diagnosis, treatment, and nursing care of children with anemia	
Serum cholesterol	Biocultural variation across the life span	
	Birth	Blacks = Whites
	Childhood	Blacks 5 mg/100 ml > Whites
	Tohono O'odham (Pima) Indians 20–30 mg/100 ml > Whites	
	Adulthood	Blacks < Whites
	Tohono O'odham (Pima) Indians 50–60 ml/100 ml < Whites	

(table continues on page 68)

TABLE 3-8
Biocultural Variations and Clinical Significance for Selected Laboratory Tests (*continued*)

TEST	REMARKS
	Clinical significance: Prevention, treatment, and nursing care of clients with cardiovascular disease
High-density lipoproteins (HDLs)	Biocultural variation in adults Blacks > Whites Asians ≥ Whites, Mexican Americans < Whites
Ratio of HDL to total cholesterol	Blacks < Whites
Low-density lipoproteins (LDLs)	Biocultural variation in adults
	Blacks < Whites
	Clinical significance: Prevention, treatment, and nursing care of clients with cardiovascular disease
Blood glucose	Biocultural variation in adults
	North American Indians, Hispanics, Japanese > Whites
	Blacks = Whites (for equivalent socioeconomic groups)
	Clinical significance: Diagnosis, treatment, and nursing care of adults with hypoglycemia and diabetes mellitus
Multiple-marker screening	Biocultural variations in blood levels for protein and hormones in pregnant women
	Alphafetoprotein (AFP), hCG, and estriol levels in Black and Asian women > Whites
	Clinical significance:
	High AFP levels signal that the woman is at increased risk for being delivered of an infant with spina bifida and neural tube defects, whereas low levels may signal Down syndrome; Down syndrome also is associated with low levels of estriol and high levels of hCG
	Black and Asian American women have higher average levels of AFP, hCG, and estriol than White counterparts
	Using a single median for women of all cultures:
	• Causes Black and Asian women to be falsely identified as being *at risk* for having infants with spina bifida and neural tube defects; by being classified as *high risk*, women are more likely to be subjected to invasive and expensive procedures such as amniocentesis; some may elect to abort the pregnancy based on screening test results
	• Inappropriately lowers the identified Down syndrome risk for Black and Asian women

TEST	REMARKS
Lecithin/ sphingomyelin ratio	Biocultural variations in amniotic fluid measures of fetal pulmonary maturity Blacks have higher ratios than Whites from 23 to 42 weeks gestation
	Clinical significance: The ratio is used to calculate the risk of respiratory distress in premature infants: lung maturity in Blacks is reached 1 week earlier than in Whites (34 vs. 35 weeks); racial differences should be considered in making decisions about inducing labor or delivering by caesarean section

Table based on data from:

Allanson, A., Michie, S., & Matreau, T. M. (1997). Presentation of screen negative results on serum screening for Down's Syndrome. *Journal of Medical Screening, 4*(1), 21–22.

Chapman, S. J., Brumfield, C. G., Wenstrom, K. D., & DuBard, M. B. (1997). Pregnancy outcomes following false-positive multiple marker screening test. *American Journal of Perinatology, 14*(8), 475–478.

O'Brien, J. E., Dvorin, E., Drugan, A., Johnson, M. P., Yaron, Y., & Evans, M. I. (1997). Race-ethnicity-specific variation in multiple-marker biochemical screening: Alpha-fetoprotein, hCG, and estriol. *Obstetrics and Gynecology, 89*(3), 355–358.

Overfield, T. (1995). *Biologic variation in health and illness: Race, age, and sex differences.* New York: CRC Press.

Although the reasons for these differences are unknown, genetic, environmental, dietary, socioeconomic, cultural, and lifestyle factors are being studied to determine the extent to which they contribute to the differences in test results. Table 3-8 identifies biocultural variations and their clinical significance for selected laboratory tests.

Clinical Decision Making and Nursing Actions

After you have completed a comprehensive cultural assessment, you are ready to analyze your subjective and objective data, set mutual goals with the client, develop a plan of care, make referrals as needed, and implement a plan of care, either alone or with others. Before **clinical decision making** or **nursing actions** can occur, you should identify the client's strengths and limitations, including his or her social support network: family, friends, clergy, and other visitors from the client's place of worship, ethnic or cultural organizations, or other sources that can be mobilized to assist the client. Next, you will want to determine whether there are client goals or needs for which professional nursing care is required.

Modes to Guide Nursing Judgments, Decisions, and Actions

Leininger (1991; Leininger & McFarland, 2002) suggests three major modalities to guide nursing judgments, decisions, and actions for the purpose of providing culturally congruent care that is beneficial, satisfying, and meaningful to the people served by nurses. The three modes are *cultural preservation or maintenance, cultural care accommodation or negotiation,* and *cultural care repatterning or restructuring.* Let us briefly examine each of these modes.

Cultural preservation or maintenance refers to "those professional actions and decisions that help people of a particular culture to retain and/or preserve relevant care values so that they can maintain their well-being, recover from illness, or face handicaps and/or death" (Leininger, 1991; Leininger & McFarland, 2002).

Cultural care accommodation or negotiation refers to professional actions and decisions that help people of a designated culture to adapt to or to negotiate with others for beneficial or satisfying health outcomes with professional care providers (Leininger, 1991; Leininger & McFarland, 2002).

Cultural care repatterning or restructuring refers to professional actions and decisions that help clients reorder, change, or greatly modify their lifeways for new, different, and beneficial health care patterns while respecting the clients' cultural values and beliefs and yet providing more beneficial or healthier lifeways than before the changes were coestablished with the clients (Leininger, 1991; Leininger & McFarland, 2002).

These modes are care-centered and based on the use of the client's care knowledge. The use of these modes of care increases understanding between the client and the nurse and promotes culturally congruent nursing care.

Evaluation

Evaluation of the effectiveness of clinical decisions and nursing actions should occur in collaboration with the client and his or her significant others—which may include members of the extended family, traditional healers, those with culturally determined nonfamilial relationships, and friends. A careful evaluation of each component of the transcultural nursing interaction should be undertaken in collaboration with the client. It may be necessary to gather further data, reinterpret existing findings, redefine mutual nurse–client goals, or renegotiate the roles and responsibilities of nurses, clients, and members of their support system.

The previous discussion has focused to a large extent on the individual during the period of hospitalization or while being cared for by nurses in the home or community environment. Next, we will look at the issue of evaluation after discharge. In the current managed care environment, there is growing emphasis on client *outcomes* and reported satisfaction with the care provided by nurses and other health care providers. You will need to participate in the establishment of *quality assurance, total quality management,* and/or *continuous quality improvement* initiatives aimed at gathering information from clients about their overall satisfaction with care. You also need to ensure that the process and instruments are culturally appropriate. For example, how are the needs of linguistically diverse clients met? Is translation or interpretation available? Are the questions asked in a culturally appropriate manner? It is imperative that nurses be included in all aspects of the evaluation and that they use this kind of feedback to improve their nursing care in the future.

SUMMARY

In this chapter we have examined transcultural perspectives on the health history and physical examination, key components of the cultural assessment. In the first section we provided an overview of the major data categories that nurses should consider if they are to demonstrate cultural competence in conducting the health history. In the second section we identified biocultural variations in the physical examination in health and illness. In the final section we examined cultural factors that influence clinical decision making, nursing actions, and evaluation.

REVIEW QUESTIONS

1. In your own words, describe the key components of cultural assessment.
2. Analyze the difference in body proportions, height, and weight among clients from diverse cultural backgrounds, and indicate the reasons for differences among the groups.
3. Compare and contrast your approach to the assessment of light- and dark-skinned clients for cyanosis, jaundice, pallor, erythema, and petechiae.
4. Review the biocultural variations in laboratory tests for hemoglobin, hematocrit, serum cholesterol, serum transferrin, multiple-marker screening, and amniotic fluid constituents.
5. Critically analyze the reasons for the current interest in ethnopharmacology by nurses, physicians, pharmacists, and other health care providers. How does knowledge of ethnopharmacology and cultural differences in response to medications facilitate your ability to provide culturally competent and congruent nursing care?

CRITICAL THINKING ACTIVITIES

1. Critically analyze the instrument, tool, or form used by nurses when conducting an initial patient or resident admission assessment at a hospital, extended care facility, or other health care agency in terms of its relevance to the health and nursing needs of persons from diverse cultures. From a transcultural nursing perspective, identify the strengths and limitations of the admission assessment instrument. What suggestions would you make to enhance the effectiveness of the instrument in assessing the cultural needs of newly admitted patients or residents? Be sure to consider the practical constraints that nurses face in the current managed care environment, such as time limitations, external forces that require us to care for increasingly large numbers of patients, and other constraints, before you suggest modifications.

2. Using the Andrews and Boyle Transcultural Nursing Assessment Guide for Individuals and Families (Appendix A), answer the questions in each data category as they apply to *yourself*. As you write your responses to the questions, critically reflect on your own health-related cultural values, attitudes, beliefs, and practices.

3. Using the Andrews and Boyle Transcultural Nursing Assessment Guide for Individuals and Families (Appendix A), interview someone from a cultural background different from your own to assess his or her health-related cultural values, attitudes, beliefs, and practices. After you have completed the interview, compare and contrast those responses with your own responses in Question 2. Identify the ways in which you are *alike*. Critically analyze the *differences* as potential sources of cross-cultural conflict, and explore ways in which they might influence the nurse–client interaction.

4. Conduct a head-to-toe physical examination of a person from a racial background different from your own. Summarize your findings in writing. In a constructively self-critical manner, reflect on what aspects of the exam were (a) easiest and (b) most difficult for you. Try to determine the reason(s) why some aspects were relatively easy or difficult for you. What further information or skill development would assist you in gaining confidence in your ability to conduct physical examinations on people from diverse racial backgrounds?

REFERENCES

Allanson, A., Michie, S., & Matreau, T. M. (1997). Presentation of screen negative results on serum screening for Down's syndrome. *Journal of Medical Screening, 4*(1), 21–22.

BCC Research. (2009). *Botanical and plant-derived drugs* [Report]. Retrieved February 10, 2010 from: http://www.piribo.com/publications/drug/_discovery/botanical_plantderived_drugs.html

Bloche, M. G. (2006). Race, money, and medicines. *The Journal of Law, Medicine, and Ethics, 34*(3), 555–558.

Chapman, S. J., Brumfield, C. G., Wenstrom, K. D., & DuBard, M. B. (1997). Pregnancy outcomes following false-positive multiple marker screening tests. *American Journal of Perinatology, 14*(8), 475–478.

Davies, S. (2006). Pharmacogenetics, pharmacogenomics and personalized medicine: Are we there yet? *Hematology, 2006*, 111–117.

Good, B. J., & Good, M. J. (1980). The meaning of symptoms: A cultural hermeneutic model for clinical practice. In: L. Eisenberg & A. Kleinman (Eds.). *The relevance of social science for medicine.* Boston: D. Reidel.

Harty, L., Johnson, K., & Power, A. (2006). Race and ethnicity in the era of emerging pharmacogenomics. *Journal of Clinical Pharmacology, 46*, 405–407.

Kleinman, A. (1980). *Patients and healers in the context of culture.* Berkeley, CA: University of California Press.

Leininger, M. M. (1991). *Culture care diversity and universality: A theory of nursing.* New York: NLN Press.

Leininger, M. M. (1995). *Transcultural nursing: Concepts, theories, research and practices.* New York: McGraw-Hill.

Leininger, M. M., & McFarland, M. R. (2002). *Transcultural nursing: Concepts, theories, research and practices.* New York: McGraw-Hill.

Levin, S. (1966). Effect of age, ethnic background and disease on sweat chloride. *Israeli Journal of Medical Science, 2*(3), 333–337.

Lin, K., Anderson, D., & Poland, R. (1995). Ethnicity and psychopharmacology: Bridging the gap. *Psychiatric Clinics of North America, 18*(3), 635–647.

Ma, J. K., Chikwamba, R., Sparrow, P., Fischer, R., Mahoney, R., & Twyman, R. M. (2005). Plant-derived pharmaceuticals—the road forward. *Trends in Plant Science, 10*(12), 580–585.

Mathis, A. S., & Knipp, G. T. (2002). Do sex and ethnicity influence drug pharmacokinetics in solid organ transplantation? *Graft, 5*(50), 294–302.

O'Brien, J. E., Dvorin, E., Drugan, A., Johnson, M. P., Yaron, Y., & Evans, M. I. (1997). Race-ethnicity-specific variation in multiple-marker biochemical screening: Alpha-fetoprotein, hCG, and estriol. *Obstretrics and Gynecology, 89*(3), 355–358.

Overfield, T. (1995). *Biologic variation in health and illness: Race, age and sex differences.* New York: CRC Press.

Schultz, J. (2003). FDA guidelines on race and ethnicity: Obstacle or remedy? *Journal of the National Cancer Institute, 95*(6), 425–426.

Wenger, A. F. (1993). Cultural meaning of symptoms. *Holistic Nursing Practice, 7*(2), 22–35.

Zhou, H. H., Sheller, J. R., Nu, H., Wood, M., & Wood, A. J. J. (1993). Ethnic differences in response to morphine. *Clinical Pharmacology and Therapeutics, 54*(3), 507–513.

The Influence of Cultural and Health Belief Systems on Health Care Practices

Margaret M. Andrews

KEY TERMS

Allopathic medicine
Alternative medicine
Complementary and alternative
    medicine (CAM)
Complementary medicine
Cultural belief systems
Folk healers
Folk healing system
Healing system
Health behavior
Health belief systems
Holistic paradigm
Hot/cold theory of disease
Illness behavior
Magico-religious paradigm
Metaphor
Paradigm
Professional care systems
Scientific paradigm
Self-care
Sick role behavior
Worldview
Yin and yang

LEARNING OBJECTIVES

1. Describe the major cultural belief systems of people from diverse cultures.
2. Compare and contrast professional and folk healing systems.
3. Identify the major complementary and alternative health care therapies.
4. Describe the influence of culture on symptoms and illness behaviors.
5. Critically analyze the efficacy of selected herbal remedies in the treatment of health problems.

In this chapter we shall examine the major cultural belief systems embraced by people from diverse cultures and explore the characteristics of three of the most prevalent worldviews, or paradigms, related to health–illness beliefs: the magico-religious, the scientific/biomedical, and the holistic health paradigms. We shall explore self-treatment, professional care systems, and folk (indigenous, traditional, generic) care systems and their respective healers. After analyzing the influence of culture on symptoms and sick role as well as illness behaviors, we shall examine selected complementary and alternative therapies used to treat physical and psychological diseases and illnesses.

Cultural Belief Systems

Cultural meanings and **cultural belief systems** develop from the shared experiences of a group in society and are expressed symbolically. The use of symbols to define, describe, and relate to the world around us is one of the basic characteristics of being human. One of the most common expressions of symbolism is the **metaphor**. In metaphor, one aspect of life is connected to another through a shared symbol. For example, the phrases "what a tangled web we weave" and "all the world's a stage" express metaphorically the relationship between two normally disparate concepts (such as human deception and a spider's web). People often use metaphors as a way of thinking about and explaining life's events.

Every group of people has found it necessary to explain the phenomena of nature. From the explanations developed emerges a common belief system. The explanations usually involve metaphoric imagery of magical, religious, natural/holistic, or biological form. The range of explanations is limited only by the human imagination.

The set of metaphoric explanations used by a group of people to explain life's events and to offer solutions to life's mysteries can be viewed as the group's **worldview**. A worldview can also be defined as a major paradigm. A **paradigm**, like any general perspective, is a way of viewing the world and the phenomena in it. A paradigm includes the assumptions, premises, and glue (linkages) that hold together a prevailing interpretation of reality. Paradigms are slow to change and do so only if and when their explanatory power has been exhausted.

The worldview developed reflects the group's total configuration of beliefs and practices and permeates every aspect of life within the culture of that group. Members of a culture share a worldview without necessarily recognizing it. Thinking itself is patterned on or derived from this worldview because the culture imparts a particular set of symbols to be used in thinking. Because these symbols are taken for granted, people do not normally question the cultural bias of their very thoughts. The use in the United States of the term *American* reflects such an unconscious cultural bias. This term is understood by citizens of the United States to refer only to themselves collectively; although in reality, it is a generic term referring to anyone in this hemisphere, including Canadians, Mexicans, Colombians, and so on.

Another example of symbolism and worldview can be seen in the way nurses use terms such as *nursing care*, *health promotion*, and *illness and disease*. Nurses often take for granted that all their clients define and relate to these concepts in the same way they do. This reflects an unconscious belief that the same cultural symbols are shared by all and therefore do not require reinterpretation in any given nurse–client context. Such an assumption accounts for many of the problems nurses face when they try to communicate with others who are not members of the health profession culture.

Health Belief Systems

Generally, theories of health and disease or illness causation are based on the prevailing worldview held by a group. These worldviews include a group's health-related attitudes, beliefs, and practices and frequently are referred to as health belief systems. People embrace three major **health belief systems** or worldviews: magico-religious, scientific, and holistic, each with its own corresponding system of health beliefs. In two of these worldviews, disease is thought of as an entity separate from self, caused by an agent that is external to the body but capable of "getting in" and causing damage. This causative agent has been attributed to a variety of natural and supernatural phenomena. Furthermore, many of us sometimes adhere to or believe in aspects of two or even three of the systems at any one time. For example, we may be ill and understand that our illness has an identified causative agent; at the same time we may pray to recover quickly and perhaps embark on a sacred journey to see a vortex specialist to unite our body, mind and spirit.

Magico-Religious Health Paradigm

In the **magico-religious paradigm**, the world is an arena in which supernatural forces dominate. The fate of the world and those in it, including humans, depends on the actions of God, or the gods, or other supernatural forces for good or evil. In some cases, the human individual is at the mercy of such forces regardless of behavior. In other cases, the gods punish humans for their transgressions. Many Latino, African American, and Middle Eastern cultures are grounded in the magico-religious paradigm. Magic involves the calling forth and control of supernatural forces for and against others. Some African and Caribbean cultures, for example, voodoo, have aspects of magic in their belief systems. In Western cultures there are examples of this paradigm in which metaphysical reality interrelates with human society. For instance, Christian Scientists believe that physical healing can be effected through prayer alone.

Ackerknecht (1971), in an article about the history of medicine, states that "magic or religion seems to satisfy better than any other device a certain eternal psychic or 'metaphysical' need of mankind, sick and healthy, for integration and harmony." Magic and religion are logical in their own way, but not on the basis of empiric premises; that is, they defy the demands of the physical world and the use of one's senses, particularly observation. In the magico-religious paradigm, disease is viewed as the action and result of supernatural forces that cause the intrusion of a disease-producing foreign body or the entrance of a health-damaging spirit.

Widespread throughout the world are five categories of events that are believed to be responsible for illness in the magico-religious paradigm. These categories, derived from the work of Clements (1932), are sorcery, breach of taboo, intrusion of a disease object, intrusion of a disease-causing spirit, and loss of soul. One of these belief categories, or any combination of them, may be offered to explain the origin of disease.

Native Alaskans, for example, refer to soul loss and breach of taboo (breaking a social norm, such as committing adultery). West Indians and some Africans and African Americans believe that the malevolence of sorcerers is the cause of many conditions. *Mal ojo*, or the evil eye, common in Latino and other cultures, can be viewed as the intrusion of a disease-causing spirit.

In the magico-religious paradigm, illness is initiated by a supernatural agent with or without justification, or by another person who practices sorcery or engages the services of sorcerers. The cause-and-effect relationship is not an organic one; rather, the cause of health or illness is mystical. Health is seen as a gift or reward given as a sign of God's blessing and goodwill. Illness may be seen as a sign of God's special favor insofar as it gives the affected person the opportunity to become resigned to God's will, or it may be seen as a sign of God's possession or as a punishment. For example, in many Christian religions, the faithful gather communally to pray to God to heal those who are ill or to practice healing rituals such as laying on of hands or anointing the sick with oil.

In addition, in this paradigm, health and illness are viewed as belonging first to the community and then to the individual. Therefore, one person's actions may directly or indirectly influence the health or illness of another person. This sense of community is virtually absent from the other paradigms.

Scientific or Biomedical Health Paradigm

The **scientific paradigm** is the newest and most removed from the interpersonal human arena of life. According to this worldview, life is controlled by a series of physical and biochemical processes that can be studied and manipulated by humans. Several specific forms of symbolic thought processes characterize the scientific paradigm. The first is determinism, which states that a cause-and-effect relationship exists for all natural phenomena. The second, mechanism, relates life to the structure and function of machines; according to mechanism, it is possible to control life processes through mechanical, genetic, and other engineered interventions. The third form is reductionism, according to which all life can be reduced or divided into smaller parts; study of the unique characteristics of these isolated parts is thought to reveal aspects or properties of the whole. One idea of reductionism is Cartesian dualism: the idea that the mind and the body can be separated into two distinct entities. The final thought process is objective materialism: What is real can be observed and measured. There is a further distinction between subjective and objective realities in this paradigm.

In general, the scientific paradigm disavows the metaphysical, though in recent years, there has been growing recognition that the positive and negative effects on health brought about by religious and holistic practices can be measured scientifically. When beneficial effects are identified, some who embrace the scientific paradigm include these practices in what is sometimes referred to as *integrative medicine*. The scientific paradigm usually ignores the holistic forces of the universe as well, unless explanations for such forces fit into the symbolic forms discussed previously. Members of most Western cultures, including the dominant cultural groups in the United States and Canada, espouse this paradigm. When the scientific paradigm is applied to matters of health, it is often referred to as the *biomedical model*.

Biomedical beliefs and concepts dominate medical thought in Western societies and must be understood to appreciate the practice of modern health care. In the biomedical model, all aspects of human health can be understood in physical and chemical terms. This fosters the belief that psychological processes can be reduced to the study of biochemical exchanges. Only the organic is real and worthy of study. Effective treatment consists of physical and chemical interventions, regardless of human relationships.

In this model, disease is viewed metaphorically as the breakdown of the human machine as a result of wear and tear (stress), external trauma (injury, accident), external invasion (pathogens), or internal damages (fluid and chemical imbalances or structural changes). Disease is held to cause illness, to have a more or less specific cause, and to have a predictable time course and set of treatment

requirements. This paradigm is similar to the magico-religious belief in external agents, having replaced supernatural forces with infectious agents.

Using the metaphor of the machine, Western medicine uses specialists to take care of the "parts"; "fixing" a part enables the machine to function. The computer is the analogy for the brain; engineering is a task for biomedical practitioners. The discovery of DNA and human genome research have led to the field of genetic engineering, an eloquent biomedical metaphor. The symbols used to discuss health and disease reflect the American cultural values of aggression and mastery: Microorganisms attack the body, war is raged against these invaders, money is donated for the campaign against cancer, and illness is a struggle in which the patient must put up a good defense. The biomedical model defines health as the absence of disease or the signs and symptoms of disease. To be healthy, one must be free of all disease.

Holistic Health Paradigm

In the **holistic paradigm**, the forces of nature itself must be kept in natural balance or *harmony*. Human life is only one aspect of nature and a part of the general order of the cosmos. Everything in the universe has a place and a role to perform according to natural laws that maintain order. Disturbing these laws creates imbalance, chaos, and disease. The holistic paradigm has existed for centuries in many parts of the world, particularly in Native American Indian cultures and Asian cultures. It is gaining increasing acceptance in the United States and Canada because it complements a growing awareness that the biomedical view fails to account fully for most diseases as they naturally occur.

The holistic paradigm seeks to maintain a sense of balance or harmony between humans and the larger universe. Explanations for health and disease are based not so much on external agents as on imbalance or disharmony among the human, geophysical, and metaphysical forces of the universe. For example, in the biomedical model, the cause of tuberculosis is clearly defined as the invasion of mycobacterium. In the holistic paradigm, whereby disease is the result of multiple environment–host interactions, tuberculosis is caused by the interrelationship of poverty, malnutrition, overcrowding, and mycobacterium.

The term *holistic*, coined in 1926 by Jan Christian Smuts, defines an attitude or mode of perception in which the whole person is viewed in the context of the total environment. Its Indo-European root word, *kailo*, means "whole, intact, or uninjured." From this root have come the words *hale, hail, hallow, holy, whole, heal*, and *health*. The essence of health and healing is the quality of wholeness we associate with healthy functioning and well-being.

In this paradigm, health is viewed as a positive process that encompasses more than the absence of signs and symptoms of disease. It is not restricted to biologic or somatic wellness but rather involves broader environmental, sociocultural, and behavioral determinants. In this model, diseases of civilization, such as unemployment, racial discrimination, ghettos, and suicide, are just as much illnesses as are biomedical diseases.

Metaphors used in this paradigm, such as the *healing power of nature, health foods*, and *Mother Earth*, reflect the connection of humans to the cosmos and nature. Voltaire's statement that an efficient physician is one who successfully bemuses the patient so that nature can affect a cure stems from this belief. The belief system of Florence Nightingale, who emphasized nursing's control of the environment so that patients could heal naturally, was also holistic.

A strong metaphor in the holistic paradigm is exemplified by the Chinese concept of **yin and yang**, in which the forces of nature are balanced to produce harmony. The *yin* force in the universe represents the female aspect of nature. It is characterized as the negative pole, encompassing darkness, cold, and emptiness. The *yang*, or male force, is characterized by fullness, light, and warmth. It represents the positive pole. An imbalance of forces creates illness.

Illness is the outward expression of disharmony. This disharmony may result from seasonal changes, emotional imbalances, or any other pattern of events. Illness is not perceived as an intruding agent but as a natural part of life's rhythmic course. Going in and out of balance is seen as a natural process that happens constantly throughout the life cycle. No sharp line is drawn between health and illness; both are seen as natural and as being part of a continuum. They are aspects of the same process, in which the individual organism changes continually in relation to the changing environment.

In the holistic health paradigm, because illness is inevitable, perfect health is not the goal. Rather, achieving the best possible adaptation to the environment by living according to society's rules and caring appropriately for one's body is the ultimate aim. This places a greater emphasis on preventive and maintenance measures than does Western biomedicine.

Another common metaphor for health and illness in the holistic paradigm is the **hot/cold theory of disease**. This is founded on the ancient Greek concept of the four body humors: yellow bile, black bile, phlegm, and blood. These humors are balanced in the healthy individual. The treatment of disease becomes the process of restoring the body's humoral balance through the addition or subtraction of substances that affect each of these humors. Foods, beverages, herbs, and other drugs are all classified as hot or cold depending on their effect, not their actual physical state. Disease conditions are also classified as either hot or cold. Imbalance or disharmony is thought to result in internal damage and altered physiologic functions. Medicine is directed at correcting the imbalance as well as restoring body functioning. Each cultural group defines what it believes to be hot and cold entities, and little agreement exists across cultures, although the concept of hot and cold is itself widespread, being found in Asian, Latino, Black, Arab, Muslim, and Caribbean societies.

Health and Illness Behaviors

The series of behaviors typifying the health-seeking process have been labeled *health and illness behaviors*. These behaviors are expressed in the roles people assume after identifying a symptom. Related to these behaviors are the roles individuals assign to others and the status given to the role players. People assume various types of behaviors once they have recognized a symptom. **Health behavior** is any activity undertaken by a person who believes himself or herself to be healthy for the purpose of preventing disease or detecting disease in an asymptomatic stage. **Illness behavior** is any activity undertaken by a person who feels ill for the purpose of defining the state of his health and of discovering a suitable remedy. **Sick role behavior** is any activity undertaken by a person who considers himself ill for the purpose of getting well or to deal with the illness.

Three sets of factors influence the course of behaviors and practices carried out to maintain health and prevent disease: (1) one's beliefs about health and illness; (2) personal factors such as age, education, knowledge, or experience with a given disease condition; and (3) cues to action, such as advertisements in the media, the illness of a relative, or the advice of friends.

A useful model of illness behavior has been proposed by Mechanic (1978), who outlines 10 determinants of illness behavior that are important in the help-seeking process (Table 4-1). Knowledge of these factors can help the nurse appreciate the client's behaviors and decisions about seeking and complying with health care. Awareness of these motivational factors can help nurses offer the appropriate assistance to clients as they work through the illness process.

Types of Healing Systems

The term *healing system* refers to the accumulated sciences, arts, and techniques of restoring and preserving health that are used by any cultural group. In complex societies in which several cultural traditions flourish, healers tend to compete with one another and/or to view their scopes of practice as separate from one another. In some instances, however, practitioners may

make referrals to different healing systems. For example, a nurse may contact a rabbi to assist a Jewish patient with spiritual needs, or a *curandero* may advise a Mexican-American patient to visit a physician or nurse practitioner for an antibiotic when traditional practices fail to heal a wound.

Self-Care

For common minor illnesses, an estimated 70% to 90% of all people initially try **self-care** with over-the-counter medicines, megavitamins, herbs, exercise, and/or foods that they believe have healing powers. Many self-care practices have been handed down from generation to generation, frequently by oral tradition. When self-treatment is ineffective, people are likely to turn to *professional* and/or *folk* (indigenous, generic, traditional) healing systems. Or perhaps it might be more accurate to say that professional health care procedures include those that supplement or substitute for self-care practices. Self-care is the largest component of the American health care system and accounts for billions of dollars in revenue annually (Vallerand, Fouladabakhsh, & Templin, 2004). The use of over-the-counter medications, or those medications that can be purchased by the consumer without a prescription from a physician are a popular form of self-care. Dietary supplements such as herbals, vitamins, minerals, or other substances are very popular and used extensively in the United States. Box 4-1 shows tips for making informed decisions and evaluating information about dietary supplements.

Professional Care Systems

According to Leininger (1991, 1997; Leininger & McFarland, 2002; Leininger & McFarland, 2005), **professional care systems** are formally taught, learned, and transmitted professional care, health, illness, wellness, and related knowledge and practice skills that prevail in professional institutions, usually with multidisciplinary personnel to serve consumers. Professional care

TABLE 4-1
Mechanic's Determinants of Illness Behavior

DETERMINANT	DESCRIPTION
Quality of symptom	The more frightening or visible the symptom, the greater is the likelihood that the individual will intervene.
Seriousness of symptom	The perceived threat of the symptom must be serious for action to be taken. Often others will step in if the person's behavior is considered dangerous (e.g., suicidal behavior) but will be unaware of potential problems if the person's behavior seems natural ("he always acts that way").
Disruption of daily activities	Behaviors that are very disruptive in work or other social situations are likely to be labeled as illness much sooner than the same behaviors in a family setting. An individual whose activities are disrupted by a symptom is likely to take that symptom seriously even if on another occasion he would consider the same symptom trivial (e.g., acne just before a date).
Rate and persistence of symptom	The frequency of a symptom is directly related to its importance; a symptom that persists is also likely to be taken seriously.
Tolerance of symptom	The extent to which others, especially family, tolerate the symptom before reacting varies; individuals also have different tolerance thresholds.
Sociocognitive status	A person's information about the symptom, knowledge base, and cultural values all influence that person's perception of illness.
Denial of symptom	Often, the individual or family members need to deny a symptom for personal or social reasons. The amount of fear and anxiety present can interfere with perception of a symptom.
Motivation	Competing needs may motivate a person to delay or enhance symptoms. A person who has no time or money to be sick will often not acknowledge the seriousness of symptoms.
Assigning of meaning	Once perceived, the symptom must be interpreted. Often people explain symptoms within normal parameters ("I'm just tired").
Treatment accessibility	The greater the barriers to treatment—whether psychologic, economic, physical, or social—the greater the likelihood that the symptom will not be interpreted as serious or that the person will seek an alternative form of care.

From Mechanic, D. (1978). *Medical sociology* (2nd ed). New York: The Free Press, a Division of Macmillan, Inc. Copyright © 1978 by David Mechanic. By permission.

is characterized by specialized education and knowledge, responsibility for care, and expectation of remuneration for services rendered. Nurses, physicians, physical therapists, and other licensed health care providers are examples of professionals who constitute professional care systems in the United States, Canada, and other parts of the world.

Folk Healing System

A **folk healing system** is a set of beliefs that has a shared social dimension and reflects what people actually do when they are ill versus what society says they ought to do according to a set of social standards (Wing, 1998). According to Leininger (1991; Leininger & McFarland, 2002), all cultures

---

BOX 4-1

Tips for Making Informed Decisions and Evaluating Information about Dietary Supplements

---

Basic Points to Consider

1. Do I need to think about my total diet?

   Yes, dietary supplements are intended to supplement your diet, not to replace the varieties of food that are important for your health

2. Should I check with my doctor or healthcare provider before using a supplement?

   Yes, this is a good idea. Dietary supplements are not always risk free.
   Always check with your health care provider if you are pregnant, nursing a baby, or if you have a chronic medical condition such as diabetes, hypertension. or heart disease.
   *Some supplements may interact with prescription and over-the-counter medicines.
   *Some supplements can have unwanted effects during surgery.
   *Adverse effects from the use of dietary supplements should be reported to the FDA by calling 1-800-FDA-1088.

3. Evaluate the websites as well as labels carefully as under the law, manufacturers of dietary supplements are responsible for making sure their products are safe before they are marketed.

   * Who operates the website?
   * What is the purpose of the website?
   * What is the source of the information on the site and does the site have references?
   * Is the information current?
   * How reliable is the internet or e-mail solicitations?

4. Ask yourself: Is it too good to be true? Don't believe everything you read.

5. Think twice about believing what you read. Here are some questionable assumptions.

   (1) *"Even if a product may not help me, it at least will not hurt me"*

   (2) *"When I see the term 'natural', it means that a product is healthful and safe"*

   (3) *"A product is safe when there is no cautionary information on the product label"*

   (4) *"a recall of a harmful product guarantees that all such harmful products will be immediately and completely removed from the marketplace"*

6. Contact the manufacturer for more information about the specific product that you are purchasing.

From: U.S. Food and Drug Administration, Center for Food Safety and Applied Nutrition (2009). Tips for the savvy supplement users: Making informed decisions and evaluating information http://www.fda.gov/Food/Dietary Supplements/ConsumerInformation/ucm110567.htm

---

of the world have had a lay health care system, which is sometimes referred to as indigenous or generic. Although the terms *complementary, alternative,* and *naturalistic healing* are sometimes used interchangeably with folk healing systems, the key consideration that defines folk systems is their history of tradition. Many folk healing systems have endured over time and rely on oral tradition for the transmission of beliefs and practices from one generation to the next. A folk healing system is a mixture of nonprofessional systems and uses healing practices that are learned informally. The folk healing system is often divided into secular and sacred components.

Most cultures have **folk healers** (sometimes referred to as traditional, lay, indigenous, or generic healers), most of whom speak the native tongue of the client, sometimes make house calls, and usually charge significantly less than healers practicing in the biomedical or scientific health care system (Leininger, 1997; Leininger & McFarland, 2002). In addition, many cultures have lay midwives (e.g., *parteras* for Hispanic women), *doulas* (support women for new mothers and babies), or other health care providers available for meeting the needs of clients. Table 4-2 identifies indigenous or folk healers for selected groups.

TABLE 4-2
Healers and Their Scope of Practice

CULTURE/FOLK PRACTITIONER	PREPARATION	SCOPE OF PRACTICE
Hispanic		
Family member	Possesses knowledge of folk medicine	Common illnesses of a mild nature that may or may not be recognized by modern medicine
Curandero	May receive training in an apprenticeship; may receive a "gift from God" that enables him or her to cure; knowledgeable in use of herbs, diet, massage, and rituals	Treats almost all of the traditional illnesses; some may not treat illness caused by witchcraft for fear of being accused of possessing evil powers; usually admired by members of the community
Espiritualista or spiritualist	Born with the special gifts of being able to analyze dreams and foretell future events; may serve apprenticeship with an older practitioner	Emphasis on prevention of illness or bewitchment through use of medals, prayers, amulets; may also be sought for cure of existing illness
Yerbero	No formal training. Knowledgeable in growing and prescribing herbs	Consulted for preventive and curative use of herbs for both traditional and Western illnesses
Sabador	Knowledgeable in massage and manipulation of bones and muscles	Treats many traditional illnesses, particularly those affecting the musculoskeletal system; may also treat nontraditional illnesses
Black		
"Old lady"	Usually an older woman who has successfully raised her own family; knowledgeable in child care and folk remedies	Consulted about common ailments and for advice on child care; found in rural and urban communities
Spiritualist	Called by God to help others; no formal training; usually associated with a fundamentalist Christian church	Assists with problems that are financial, personal, spiritual, or physical; predominantly found in urban communities
Voodoo priest and priestess or *Houngan* and *Mambo*	May be trained by other priests(esses). In the United States the eldest son of a priest becomes a priest; the daughter of a priest(ess) becomes a priestess if she is born with a veil (amniotic sac) over her face	Knowledgeable about properties of herbs; interpretation of signs and omens; able to cure illness caused by voodoo; uses communication techniques to establish a therapeutic milieu like a psychiatrist; treats Blacks, Mexican Americans, and Native Americans
Chinese		
Herbalist	Knowledgeable in diagnosis of illness and herbal remedies	Both diagnostic and therapeutic; diagnostic techniques include interviewing, inspection, auscultation, and assessment of pulses
Acupuncturist	3 1/2 to 4 1/2 years (1,500 to 1,800 hours) of courses on acupuncture, Western anatomy and physiology, Chinese herbs; usually requires a period of apprenticeship, learning from someone else who is licensed or certified	Diagnosis and treatment of yin/yang disorders by inserting needles into *meridians*, pathways through which life energy flows; when heat is applied to the acupuncture needle, the term *moxibustion* is used

(table continues on page 82)

TABLE 4-2
Healers and Their Scope of Practice *(continued)*

CULTURE/FOLK PRACTITIONER	PREPARATION	SCOPE OF PRACTICE
	Licensure required in the United States	May combine acupuncture with herbal remedies and/or dietary recommendations. Acupuncture is sometimes used as a surgical anesthetic
Amish		
Braucher or baruch-doktor	Apprenticeship	Men or women who use a combination of modalities including physical manipulation, massage, herbs, teas, reflexology, and *brauche*, folk-healing art with origins in 18th and 19th century Europe; especially effective in the treatment of bedwetting, nervousness, and women's health problems; may be generalist or specialist in practice; some set up treatment rooms; some see non-Amish as well as Amish patients
Lay midwives	Apprenticeship	Care for women before, during, and after delivery
Greek		
Magissa "magician"	Apprenticeship	Woman who cures *matiasma* or evil eye May be referred to as doctor
Bonesetters	Apprenticeship	Specialize in treating uncomplicated fractures
Priest (Orthodox)	Ordained clergy Formal theological study	May be called on for advice, blessings, exorcisms, or direct healing
Native Americans		
Shaman	Spiritually chosen Apprenticeship	Uses incantations, prayers, and herbs to cure a wide range of physical, psychologic, and spiritual illnesses
Crystal gazer, hand trembler (Navajo)	Spiritually chosen Apprenticeship	Diviner diagnostician who can identify the cause of a problem, either by using crystals or placing hand over the sick person; does not implement treatment

Adapted with permission from Hautman, M. A. (1979). Folk health and illness beliefs. *Nurse Practitioner,* *4*(4), 23, 26–27, 31.

If clients use folk healers, these healers should be an integral part of the health care team and should be included in as many aspects of the client's care as possible. For example, you might include the folk healer in obtaining a health history and in determining what treatments already have been used in an effort to bring about healing. In discussing traditional remedies, it is important to be respectful and to listen attentively to healers who effectively combine spiritual and herbal remedies and practices for a wide variety of illnesses, both physical and psychological in origin. Chapter 14 provides detailed information about the religious beliefs and spiritual healers in major religious groups.

Complementary and Alternative Medicine

Complementary and Alternative Medicine (CAM) is an umbrella term for hundreds of therapies based on health care systems of people from around the world. Some CAM therapies have ancient origins in Egyptian, Chinese, Greek, and Native North American cultures. Others, such as osteopathy and magnet therapy, have evolved in more recent times. *Western biomedicine*, or **allopathic medicine**, is the reference point, with all other therapies being considered complementary (in addition to) or alternative (instead of) to it. Coined by homeopathic physician Samuel Hahnemann in the 19th century, *allopathic medicine* is used most often to refer to conventional medical practice, which emphasizes killing bacteria and suppressing symptoms. Conventional medicine (or more accurately health care) is practiced by those who have earned either MD (medical doctor) or DO (doctor of osteopathy) degrees and by other related health professionals such as registered nurses, physical therapists, and psychologists. Some dietary supplements have been incorporated into conventional medicine. For example, research has demonstrated that folic acid prevents certain birth defects (Folic Acid and Pregnancy, n.d.), so folic acid is commonly prescribed for pregnant women.

The National Center for Complementary and Alternative Medicine (NCCAM), the U.S. Federal Government's lead agency for scientific research on CAM, has defined CAM as a group of diverse medical and health care systems, practices, and products that are not currently considered to be part of conventional or allopathic medicine. **Complementary medicine** is *used together* with conventional medicine. An example of a complementary therapy is using magnet therapy to help lessen a patient's discomfort following surgery. **Alternative medicine** is *used in place* of conventional medicine. An example of an alternative therapy is using a special diet to treat cancer instead of undergoing surgery, radiation, or chemotherapy that has been recommended by a conventional physician (NCCAM, 2007). NCCAM's mission is to examine complementary and alternative healing practices in the context of rigorous science, train CAM researchers, and disseminate authoritative information to the public and professionals. While some scientific evidence exists to support the safety and efficacy of selected CAM therapies, there needs to be a great deal more research on most of these therapies before their safety and efficacy can be documented for treating the diseases or medical conditions for which they are used (Ernst, Pittler, Stevinson, & White, 2001; Fontaine, 2000; Keegan, 2001; NCCAM, 2007). The list of what is considered to be CAM tends to change continually as those therapies that are proven to be safe and effective become adopted into conventional health care (Balneaves, 2006; Burke, Upchurch, Dye, & Chuy, 2005; Burrowes & Brommage, 2006; Chong, 2006; Foster, 1996; Fouladabakhsh, Stommel, Given, & Given, 2005; Grzywacz, 2006; Hsiao, Wong, Goldstein, Yu, Andersen, & Brown, 2006; Jagtenberg, 2006; Kuhn & Winston, 2000; Lenacher et al., 2006; Magin, 2006; Menzies, 2006; NCCAM, 2007; Taylor, 2006).

NCCAM classifies CAM therapies into five categories:

1. *Alternative medical systems* are built upon complete systems of theory and practice. Often these systems have evolved apart from and earlier than the conventional medical approach used in the United States or Canada. Examples of alternative medical systems that have developed in Western cultures include homeopathic medicine and naturopathic medicine. Examples of systems that have developed in non-Western cultures include traditional Chinese medicine and Ayurveda, which originated in India.

2. *Mind–body medicine* uses a variety of techniques designed to enhance the mind's capacity to affect bodily functions and symptoms. Some techniques that were considered CAM in the past have become mainstream (e.g., patient support groups and cognitive-behavioral therapy). Other mind–body techniques are still considered CAM, including meditation, prayer, mental healing, and therapies that use creative outlets such as art, music, or dance.

3. *Biologically based therapies* in CAM use substances found in nature, such as herbs, foods, and vitamins. Some examples include dietary supplements, herbal products, and the use of other so-called "natural" but as yet scientifically

unproven therapies (e.g., using shark cartilage to treat cancer).

4. *Manipulative and body-based methods* in CAM are based on manipulation and/or movement of one or more parts of the body. Some examples include chiropractic or osteopathic manipulation, and massage therapy.

5. *Energy therapies* involve the use of energy fields in two ways:

   a. *Biofield therapies* are intended to affect energy fields that purportedly surround and penetrate the human body. The existence of such fields has not yet been scientifically proven. Some forms of energy therapy manipulate biofields by applying pressure and/or manipulating the body by placing the hands in, or through, these fields. Examples include qigong, Reiki, and Therapeutic Touch.

   b. *Bioelectromagnetic-based therapies* involve the unconventional use of electromagnetic fields, such as pulsed fields, magnetic fields, or alternating-current or direct-current fields.

Box 4-2 identifies selected CAM therapies currently used by people in the United States and Canada to promote health and prevent and treat disease.

BOX 4-2

Selected Complementary and Alternative Therapies

Acupuncture ("AK-yoo-pungk-cher") refers to a family of procedures involving stimulation of anatomical points on the body by a variety of techniques. The acupuncture technique that has been most studied scientifically involves penetrating the skin with thin, solid, metallic needles that are manipulated by the hands or by electrical stimulation. When heat is applied to the needles, it is referred to as moxibustion ("mox-eh-BUST-chun").

Aromatherapy ("ah-roam-uh-THER-ah-py") involves the use of essential oils (extracts or essences) from flowers, herbs, and trees to promote health and well-being.

Ayurveda ("ah-yur-VAY-dah") includes diet and herbal remedies and emphasizes the use of body, mind, and spirit in disease prevention and treatment.

Chiropractic ("kie-roh-PRAC-tic") focuses on the relationship between bodily structure (primarily that of the spine) and function, and how that relationship affects the preservation and restoration of health. Chiropractors use manipulative therapy as an integral treatment tool.

Dietary supplements are products (other than tobacco) taken by mouth that contain a *dietary ingredient* intended to supplement the diet. *Dietary ingredients* may include vitamins, minerals, herbs or other botanicals, amino acids, and substances such as enzymes, organ tissues, and metabolites. *Dietary supplements* come in many forms, including extracts, concentrates, tablets, capsules, gelcaps, liquids, and powders. In the United States and Canada they have special requirements for labeling and are considered foods, not drugs.

Homeopathic ("home-ee-oh-PATH-ic") **medicine** is a CAM alternative medical system. In homeopathic medicine, there is a belief that "like cures like," meaning that small, highly diluted quantities of medicinal substances are given to cure symptoms, even though the same substances given at higher or more concentrated doses would actually cause those symptoms.

Massage ("muh-SAHJ") therapists manipulate muscle and connective tissue to enhance function of those tissues and promote relaxation and well-being.

Naturopathic ("nay-chur-o-PATH-ic") **medicine**, or naturopathy, is based on the premise that there is a healing power in the body that establishes, maintains, and restores health. Practitioners work with the patient with a goal of supporting this power through treatments such as nutrition and lifestyle counseling, dietary supplements, medicinal plants, exercise, homeopathy, and traditional Chinese medicine.

Osteopathic ("ahs-tee-oh-PATH-ic") **medicine** is a form of conventional medicine that, in part, emphasizes diseases arising in the musculoskeletal system. There is an underlying belief that all of the body's systems work together, and disturbances in one system may affect function elsewhere in the body.

BOX 4-2 (*continued*)

Some osteopathic physicians practice osteopathic manipulation, a full-body system of hands-on techniques to alleviate pain, restore function, and promote health and well-being.

Qigong ("chee-GUNG") is a component of traditional Chinese medicine that combines movement, meditation, and regulation of breathing to enhance the flow of qi (pronounced "chee" and meaning *vital energy*) in the body, improve blood circulation, and enhance immune function.

Reiki ("RAY-kee") is a Japanese word representing *Universal Life Energy*. Reiki is based on the belief that when spiritual energy is channeled through a Reiki practitioner, the patient's spirit is healed, which in turn heals the physical body.

Therapeutic Touch is based on the premise that it is the healing force of the therapist that affects the patient's recovery; healing is promoted when the body's energies are in balance, and by passing their hands over the patient, healers can identify energy imbalances.

Traditional Chinese medicine (TCM) is the current name for an ancient system of health care from China. TCM is based on a concept of balanced qi or *vital energy*, which is believed to flow throughout the body. Qi regulates a person's spiritual, emotional, mental, and physical balance and is influenced by the opposing forces of yin (negative energy) and yang (positive energy). Disease is proposed to result from the flow of qi being disrupted and yin and yang becoming imbalanced. Among the components of TCM are herbal and nutritional therapy, restorative physical exercises, meditation, acupuncture, and remedial massage.

SUMMARY

In this chapter we have examined the major cultural belief systems embraced by people of the world, including the top three: magico-religious, scientific, and holistic health paradigms or worldviews. We examined self-treatment, professional care systems, and folk (indigenous, traditional, or generic) care systems and the types of healers who practice in them. After analyzing the influence of culture on symptoms and sick role behavior, we explored CAM and healing modalities that are frequently used to treat physical and psychological conditions.

REVIEW QUESTIONS

1. In your own words, describe what is meant by the following terms: (a) cultural belief system, (b) worldview, and (c) paradigm.
2. What are the primary characteristics of the three major health belief systems: magico-religious, scientific, and holistic paradigms?
3. What are the differences between professional and folk care systems?
4. What is allopathic medicine?
5. What is the primary mission of the NCCAM?
6. Identify the seven major categories of CAM as defined by the NCCAM.

CRITICAL THINKING ACTIVITIES

1. Select a complementary or alternative practice that you would like to know more about, for example, acupuncture, chiropractic, or homeopathy. Search the Internet for information about this practice, and go to a library to conduct background research. After you have learned more about the practice, contact a healer who uses the type of practice that interests you and ask the following questions:

a. How did you prepare to be a practitioner of _____ ?

b. What do you believe are the major benefits of _____ to patients?

   c. What health-related conditions do you believe respond best to _____?

   d. Are there any risks to clients resulting from the use of _____?

2. According to the World Health Organization, 80% of the people in the world use CAM for the treatment of common illnesses. Select a common illness, such as upper respiratory infection, arthritis, or a similar condition, and identify the various complementary and alternative approaches to allopathic medicine that clients might use. What is the efficacy of each intervention that you have identified? How effective do you think the complementary and alternative practices are compared with allopathic medicine? Compare cost of each practice as well as efficacy.

3. The herb echinacea is frequently used for the prevention and treatment of the common cold. If a patient asked your opinion about the use of echinacea, how would you reply? Would you recommend that the patient use this herb for treatment of a cold? Explain why or why not.

4. Visit three of the following Web sites for further information about specific types of alternative and complementary medicine.

Acupressure and Massage

Acupressure Institute
http://www.acupressure.com
American Massage Therapy Association
http://www.amtamassage.org/

International Massage Association
http://www.imagroup.com
Rolf Institute of Structural Integration
http://www.rolf.org

Acupuncture and Chinese Medicine

American Association of Oriental Medicine (provides referrals to acupuncturists in local areas)
http://www.aaom.org

National Acupuncture and Oriental Medicine Alliance
http://www.acuall.org/

Aromatherapy

American Alliance of Aromatherapy
http://www.healthy.net/aromatherapy

National Association for Holistic Aromatherapy
http://www.naha.org/

Ayurvedic Medicine

Ayurvedic Institute

http://www.ayurveda.com

Biofeedback

Association for Applied Psychophysiology and Biofeedback

http://www.aapb.org

Chiropractic

American Chiropractic Association
http://www.amerchiro.org

International Chiropractors Association
http://www.chiropractic.org

Dietary Supplements

Office of Dietary Supplements, National Institutes of Health (NIH)

http://ods.od.nih.gov

International Bibliographic Information on Dietary Supplements (IBIDS) database

http://ods.od.nih.gov/Health_Information/IBIDS.aspx

U.S. Food and Drug Administration (FDA) Center for Food Safety and Applied Nutrition

http://www.cfsan.fda.gov/

Toll-free U.S. phone no.: 1-888-723-3366

Information includes *Tips for the Savvy Supplement User: Making Informed Decisions and Evaluating Information* (U.S. Food and Drug Administration, Center for Food Safety and Applied Nutrition, 2002) and updated safety information on supplements (www.cfsan.fda.gov/~dms/ds-warn.html). Adverse effects from a supplement can be reported to the FDA's MedWatch program, which collects and monitors such information (1-800-FDA-1088 or www.fda.gov/medwatch).

Environmental Medicine

American Academy of Environmental Medicine

http://www.aaem.com/

Guided Imagery

Academy for Guided Imagery

http://www.academyforguidedimagery.com/

Herbal Medicine

American Botanical Council

http://www.herbalgram.org

American Herbalist Guild

http://www.americanherbalistsguild.com/

Herb Research Foundation

http://www.herbs.org

Hypnosis

American Board of Hypnotherapy

http://www.abh-abnlp.com/

Mind/Body Medicine

Benson-Henry Institute for Mind Body Medicine

http://mindbody.harvard.edu/home/

Center for Mind/Body Medicine

http://www.cmbm.org/

Music Therapy

American Music Therapy Association

http://www.musictherapy.org

Naturopathic Medicine

American Association of Naturopathic Physicians

http://www.naturopathic.org

Qigong

The Qigong Institute

http://www.qigonginstitute.org/main_page/main_page.php

REFERENCES

Ackernecht, E. (1971). Natural diseases and rational treatment in primitive medicine. *Bulletin of the History of Medicine, 19*, 467–497.

Balneaves, L. G. (2006). Levels of commitment: Exploring complementary therapy use by women with breast cancer. *Journal of Alternative and Complementary Medicine, 12*(5), 459–466.

Burke, A., Upchurch, D. M., Dye, C., & Chuy, L. (2005). Acupuncture use in the United States: Findings from the National Health Interview Survey. *Journal of Alternative and Complementary Medicine, 12*(7), 639–648.

Burrowes, J. D., & Brommage, D. (2006). Issues in renal nutrition: Focus on nutritional care for nephrology patients. Herbs and dietary supplement use with stage 5 chronic kidney disease. *Nephrology Journal, 33*(1), 85–88.

Chong, O. (2006). An integrative approach to addressing clinical issues in complementary and alternative medicine in an outpatient oncology center. *Clinical Journal of Oncology Nursing, 10*(1), 83–92.

Clements, F. E. (1932). Primitive concepts of disease. *University of California Publications in Archeology and Ethnology, 32*(2), 185–252.

Ernst, E., Pittler, M. H., Stevinson, C., & White, A. (2001). *The desktop guide to complementary and alternative medicine: An evidence-based approach.* New York: Mosby.

Folic acid and pregnancy (n.d.) Retrieved February 16, 2010 from: http://kidshealth.org/parent/pregnancy_newborn/pregnancy/folic_acid.html.

Fontaine, K. L. (2000). *Healing practices: Alternative therapies for nursing.* Upper Saddle River, NJ: Prentice Hall.

Foster, S. (1996). *Herbs for your health.* Loveland, CO: Interweave Press.

Fouladabakhsh, J. M., Stommel, M., Given, B., & Given, C. (2005). Predictors of use of complementary and alternative therapies by cancer patients. *Oncology Nursing Forum, 32*(6), 115–123.

Grzywacz, J. G., (2006). Older adults' use of complementary and alternative medicine for mental health: Findings from the 2002 National Health Interview Survey. *Journal of Alternative and Complementary Medicine, 12*(5), 467–473.

Hautman, M. A. (1979). Folk health and illness beliefs. *Nurse Practitioner, 4*(4), 23–31.

Hsiao, A., Wong, M. D., Goldstein, M. S., Yu, H. J., Andersen, R. M., & Brown, E. R., et al. (2006). Variation in complementary and alternative medicine (CAM) use across racial/ethnic groups and the development of ethnic-specific measures of CAM use. *Journal of Alternative and Complementary Medicine, 12*(3), 281–290.

Jagtenberg, T. (2006). Evidence-based medicine and naturopathy. *Journal of Alternative and Complementary Medicine, 12*(3), 323–328.

Keegan, L. (2001). *Healing with complementary and alternative therapies.* Albany, NY: Delmar.

Kuhn, M. A., & Winston, D. (2000). *Herbal therapy and supplements: A scientific and traditional approach.* Philadelphia: Lippincott Williams & Wilkins.

Leininger, M. M. (1991). *Culture care diversity and universality: A theory of nursing.* New York: National League for Nursing Press.

Leininger, M. M. (1997). Founder's focus alternative to what? Generic vs. professional caring, treatments and healing modes. *Journal of Transcultural Nursing, 91*(1), 37.

Leininger, M. M., & McFarland, M. R. (2002). *Transcultural nursing: Concepts, theories, research and practices.* New York: McGraw-Hill.

Leininger, M. M. & McFarland, M. R. (2005). *Culture care diversity & universality: A worldwide nursing theory* (2nd ed.). Sudbury, MA: Jones & Bartlett, Publishers.

Lenacher, C. A., Bennett, M. P., Kip, K. E., Gonzalez, L., Jacobsen, P., & Cox, C. E. (2006). Relief of symptoms, side effects, and psychological distress through complementary and alternative medicine for women with breast cancer. *Oncology Nursing Forum, 33*(1), 97–104.

Magin, P. J. (2006). Complementary and alternative therapies in acne, psoriasis, and atopic dermatitis. *Journal of Alternative and Complementary Medicine, 12*(5), 451–457.

Mechanic, D. (1978). *Medical sociology* (2nd ed.). New York: Free Press.

Menzies, V. (2006). Effects of guided imagery on outcomes of pain, functional status, and self-efficacy in persons diagnosed with fibromyalgia. *Journal of Alternative and Complementary Medicine, 12*(1), 23–30.

Monte, T. (1997). *The complete guide to natural healing.* New York: Berkeley Publishing Group.

National Center for Complementary and Alternative Medicine (NCCAM) (2007). *What is CAM?* (NCCAM Publication No. D347). Retrieved February 16, 2010, from http://nccam.nih.gov/health/whatiscam/overview.htm.

Taylor, D. N. (2006). Health care industry shaping chiropractic's future. *Journal of the American Chiropractic Association, 43*(6), 19–23.

U.S. Food and Drug Administration, Center for Food Safety and Applied Nutrition. (2002). *Tips for the savvy supplement user: Making informed decisions and evaluating information.* Retrieved February 16, 2010 from http://www.cfsan.fda.gov/~dms/ds-savvy.html

Vallerand, A. H., Fouladbakhsh, J. M., & Templin, T. (2004). Use of complementary and alternative therapies in urban, suburban, and rural communities. *American Journal of Public Health, 93*(6), 923–925.

Wing, D. M. (1998). A comparison of traditional folk healing concepts with contemporary healing concepts. *Journal of Community Health Nursing, 15*(3), 143–154.

PART TWO

Transcultural Nursing: Across the Lifespan

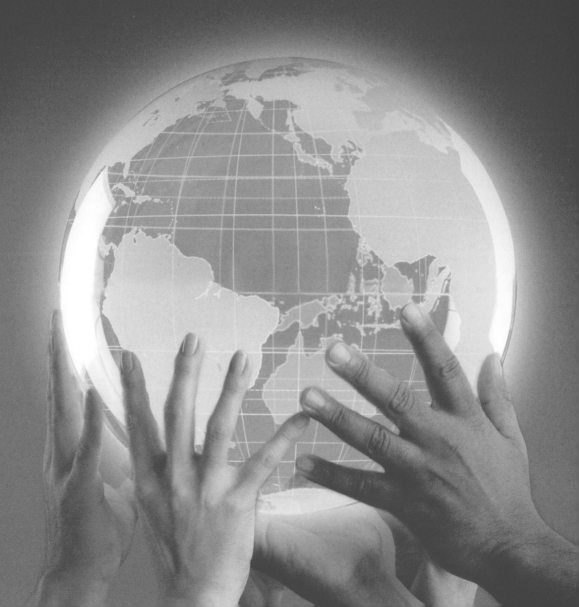

CHAPTER

5

Transcultural Perspectives in Childbearing

Jana Lauderdale

KEY TERMS

Abortion
Childbearing
Contraception
Culture
Domestic violence during pregnancy
Fertility controls
Hot/cold theories
Imbalance
Infant relinquishment
IUDs (intrauterine devices)
Maternal morbidity
Maternal mortality
Pregnancy
Prescriptive beliefs
Restrictive beliefs
Taboos

LEARNING OBJECTIVES

1. Analyze how culturally related issues influence the beliefs and behaviors of the childbearing woman and her family during pregnancy.
2. Explore one's own cultural values and norms toward members of vulnerable populations of childbearing women.
3. Understand the childbearing beliefs and practices of diverse cultures.
4. Examine the needs of women making alternative lifestyle choices regarding childbirth and child rearing.
5. Explore how the shared ideologies of vulnerable childbearing populations can influence pregnancy outcomes.

This chapter will discuss how **culture** influences the experience of **childbearing**. The experiences of the woman and those of her significant other during pregnancy, birth, and the postpartum period are examined. Recommendations for practice are provided in each section for nurses caring for childbearing women and their families. Also presented for the reader's consideration are discussions related to culturally specific circumstances and behaviors of the childbearing woman and her family.

Overview of Cultural Belief Systems and Practices Related to Childbearing

Childbearing is a time of transition and social celebration of central importance in any society, signaling a realignment of existing cultural roles and responsibilities, psychologic and biologic states, and social relationships. The different ways in which a particular society views this transitional period and manages childbirth are dependent on the culture's consensus about health, medical care, reproduction, and the role and status of women (Dickason, Silverman, & Schult, 1994).

Pregnancy and childbirth practices in contemporary Western society have seen dramatic changes over the past three decades. An increase in the number of women in the work force, advances in reproductive technology, self-care,

alternative therapies, the explosion of health information available to consumers on the Internet, and the influx of immigrants and refugees are but a few of the trends that require nurses to examine and rethink how we can better care for our clients (Tiedje, 2000). The dominant medical practices related to pregnancy and childbirth in the United States include the use of various state-of-the-art technologies such as fetal monitoring devices and sometimes cesarean sections. Medical care focuses on the pregnant woman and fetus; the father and other family members or significant others, if they are included at all, are relegated to observer rather than participant status. Although it is certainly much more common for a father to be present in the delivery room and to take a more active role in helping his wife or significant other during the laboring process, the dominant cultural practices or rituals in the United States and Canada include formal

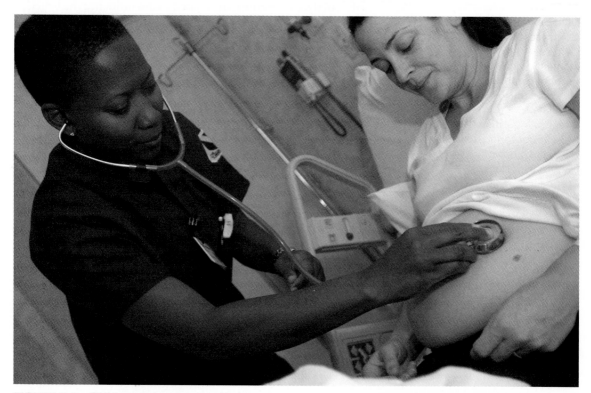

FIGURE 5-1 CNM assessing mom and baby.

prenatal care (including childbirth classes), ultrasonography to view the fetus, and hospital delivery. Figure 5-1 provides an example of monitoring fetal status, inducing labor, providing anesthesia for labor and delivery, and placing the woman in the lithotomy position, all of which are part of routine hospital care in modern health care facilities in the United States. A highly specialized group of nurses, obstetricians, perinatologists, and pediatricians actively monitors the mother's physiologic status, delivers the infant, and provides newborn care. However, because there is not total cultural agreement about the value of these practices, some health care providers elect to offer their pregnant

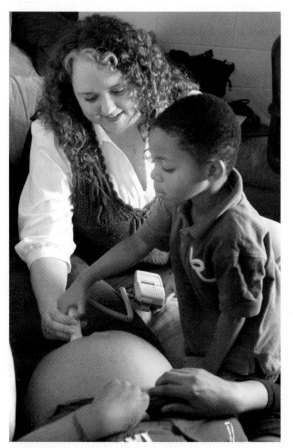

FIGURE 5-2 CNM offering family-oriented pregnancy care.

clients alternative health care services. As noted in Figure 5-2, these alternatives include in-hospital and freestanding birth centers and care by nurse practitioners and nurse midwives, who promote family-centered care and emphasize pregnancy as a normal process requiring minimal technologic intervention.

While advanced medical technology has become very common in childbirth, this has not necessarily led to healthy newborns and mothers. There has recently been great concern because maternal mortality ratios have increased from 6.6 deaths per 100,000 live births in 1987 to 13.3 deaths per 100,000 live births in 2006. The United States spends more than any other country on health care, and more on maternal health than any other type of hospital care. Despite this, women in the United States have a higher risk of dying of pregnancy-related complications than those in 40 other countries. In addition, the health disparities in the United States also play a role in increased **maternal morbidity** and **maternal mortality**, although it is unclear to what extent. For example, African American women are nearly four times more likely to die of pregnancy-related complications than white women. These rates and disparities have not improved in more than 20 years (Amnesty International, USA, 2010).

Subcultures within the United States have very different practices, values, and beliefs about childbirth and the roles of women, men, social support networks, and health care practitioners. They include proponents of the "back to nature" movement, who are often vegetarian, use lay midwives for home deliveries, and practice herbal or naturopathic medicine. Other groups that might have distinct cultural practices include African Americans, American Indians, Hispanics, Middle Eastern groups, Orthodox Jewish groups, Asians, and recent immigrants, among others. Additionally, religious background, regional variations, age, urban or rural background, sexual preference, and other individual characteristics all might contribute to cultural differences in the experience of childbirth.

Great variations exist in the social class, ethnic origin, family structure, and social support networks of women, men, and families in the United States. Despite these differences, many health care providers unfortunately assume that the changes in status and rites of passage associated with pregnancy and birth are experienced similarly by all people. In addition, many of the traditional cultural beliefs, values, and practices related to childbirth have been viewed by some professional nurses as "old-fashioned" or "old wives' tales." Although some of these customs are changing rapidly, many women and families are attempting to preserve their own valued patterns of experiencing childbirth. In recent years, nurses and other health professionals have attempted to understand the client's lifestyle, value system, and health and illness behaviors so that effective interventions can be implemented to reduce risks in a manner that is culturally congruent with community, group, and individual values.

Fertility Control and Culture

There is not much information in the professional literature about specific cultural beliefs and practices related to the control of fertility. A woman's fertility varies depending on several factors, including the likelihood of sterility as well as the probability of conceiving and of intrauterine mortality. In addition, the duration of a postpartum period, during which a woman is unlikely to ovulate or conceive, also influences fertility. These variables are further modified by cultural and social variables, including marriage and residence patterns, diet, religion, the availability of **abortion**, the incidence of venereal disease, and the regulation of birth intervals by cultural or artificial means. The focus in this section will be on those societal factors that influence reproductive rights and population control. These societal factors are highly influenced by our cultural values, norms, and traditions.

In 2001, approximately one-half of pregnancies in the United States were unintended (Finer,

2006), and the United States has set a national goal of decreasing unintended pregnancies to 30% by 2010. Unintended pregnancy has been cited as a critical factor in understanding the fertility of populations and the unmet need for contraception (Centers for Disease Control and Prevention [CDC], 2006). We have known for some time that unintended pregnancy can have numerous negative effects on the mother and the fetus, including a delay in prenatal care, continued or increased tobacco and alcohol and other drug use, as well as increased physical abuse during pregnancy, any of which can lead to preterm labor or low birth weight (LBW) infants (Santelli et al., 2003). Luker (1999) noted that the pattern of *when* unintended pregnancy occurs has changed from the end of the reproductive cycle (when family size is complete) to the start of the cycle (when to start a family). The author believes the result is caused by a change in social mores sanctioning motherhood outside of marriage, **contraception** availability including abortion, earlier sexual activity, and multiple partners. As mentioned above, one of the goals of Healthy People 2010 is to decrease unintended pregnancies from 49% to 30% by 2010 (U.S. Department of Health and Human Services, 2000) as of this printing; whether this goal has been reached is yet to be determined. Programs aimed at reducing or preventing unintended pregnancy must build on the cultural meaning of the problem and focus on the processes women and their partners use to make fertility decisions.

Commonly used methods of contraception in the United States include hormonal methods, **intrauterine devices (IUDs)**, permanent sterilization, and to a lesser degree, barrier and "natural" methods. Natural methods of family planning are based on the recognition of fertility through signs and symptoms and abstinence during periods of fertility. The religious beliefs of some cultural groups might affect their use of **fertility controls** such as abortion or artificial regulation of conception; for example, Roman Catholics might follow church edicts against artificial control of conception, and Mormon families might follow their church's teaching

BOX 5-1

CDC Refugee Reproductive Health Activities Goals

1. Initiate epidemiologic studies to evaluate the reproductive health status of women in refugee and IDP settings to better provide information to improve service, quality, and accessibility.

2. Design, implement, and evaluate reproductive health rapid assessment tools and behavioral and epidemiologic surveillance systems appropriate to refugee settings.

3. Design, recommend, and evaluate interventions and "best practices" identified through epidemiologic research, rapid assessment, and surveillance.

4. Strengthen the capacity of the refugee/IDP community, as well as the agencies providing health services, to collect and use data to improve reproductive health status and services.

5. Translate and communicate study findings and best practices to refugees and supporting agencies.

CDC, Division of Reproductive Health, National Center for Chronic Disease Prevention and Health Promotion, Atlanta, GA. (2006). Retrieved from http://www.cdc.gov.

regarding the spiritual responsibility to have large families and promote church growth (Andrews & Hanson, 2008). The ability to control fertility successfully also requires an understanding of the menstrual cycle and the times and conditions under which pregnancy is more or less likely to occur—in essence, an understanding of bodily functions. When these functions change, the woman might perceive the changes as abnormal or unhealthy. Because the use of artificial methods of fertility control might alter the body's usual cycles, women who use them might become anxious, consider themselves ill, and discontinue the method. American Indian women monitor their monthly bleeding cycles closely and believe in the importance of monthly menstruation for maintaining harmony and physical well-being. Contraceptives such as the IUD are generally better accepted than hormonal methods because of the normal or increased flow associated with the IUD. Because the mechanism of action of an IUD might include the expulsion of a fertilized ovum, some women oppose the use of the IUD for religious reasons.

At the beginning of 2006, there were estimated to be 20.8 million people uprooted and displaced from their homes due to war, ethnic and civil unrest, and political instability (UNHCR, 2006). Women and children account for approximately 80% of the world's refugees and displaced women are extremely vulnerable to poor reproductive illness and outcomes (CDC, Division of Reproductive Health, National Center for Chronic Disease Prevention and Health Promotion, 2006). The CDC has developed a refugee program with a focus on refugee reproductive health. The goals for the program are presented in Box 5-1. Women living in refugee situations encounter many barriers to contraceptive use.

Religious beliefs can also influence birth control choices. For example, the Hindu religion teaches that the right hand is clean and the left is dirty. The right hand is for holding religious books and eating utensils, and the left hand is used for dirty things, such as touching the genitals. This belief complicates the use of contraceptives requiring the use of both hands, such as a diaphragm (Bromwich & Parson, 1990).

Fertility practices among Arabs are swayed by their traditional Bedouin beliefs. In most cases, birth control is seen as an act of God. Purnell and Selekman (2008) describe Muslims believe abortion is "haram" unless the mother's life is in danger, consequently, unintended pregnancies are dealt with by praying a miscarriage will occur. Perhaps of greater significance to fertility in Muslim women, may be that sterility of a woman can be reason for abandonment or divorce. The authors go on to say that Islamic law forbids adoption and infertility treatment is limited to artificial insemination using the couple's own sperm and eggs.

Orthodox Jewish contraception and fertility beliefs are fairly straightforward. Infertility counseling and intervention such as sperm and egg donation (from the couple) meet with religious approval, with adoption viewed as a last resort (Washofsky, 2001). To the Orthodox, contraception beliefs vary. The use of condoms and birth control pills are acceptable with the barrier technique, random abortion and sterilization being the least supported birth control methods. However in cases where the mother's life is in jeopardy, abortion is not opposed (Kolatch, 2000).

In some African cultures, the beliefs and practices related to birth spacing has traditionally been a taboo in relation to postpartum sexual activity, with some women leaving their home for as long as 2 years to avoid pregnancy (Miller, 1992). The influence of religious beliefs on birth control choices obviously varies within and between groups and adherence to these beliefs may change over time. In the United States there has been great controversy over abortion and to some extent, the use of an IUD.

EVIDENCE-BASED PRACTICE 5-1

Reproductive Decisions for Women with HIV: Motherhood's Role in Envisioning a Future

Cultural influences more influence on HIV-positive women's reproductive choices than do HIV-related conditions. The authors conducted a grounded theory study on how women with HIV made reproductive decisions during a time of transition from when HIV was potentially fatal to mothers and newborns to its current status as a controllable chronic disease. Eighty HIV-positive women in Oakland, CA, Chicago, IL, and Rochester, NY were recruited to the study. The sample members were primarily women of color with a mean age of 35 years.

Women made their reproductive decisions based on the degree to which they could envision motherhood as part of their future. This judgment required women to weigh the negative hostile public opinion (You should not have a baby) to their equally strong personal reasons for seeking or continuing a pregnancy. Forces against choosing pregnancy were: public opinion, medical providers, family and other HIV women who discouraged a pregnancy. Reasons for choosing pregnancy were: (1) the social value of motherhood (2) "missed" motherhood as many of the women reported other babies had been "taken

away" from them because of substance abuse; and (3) Belief in God's protection. The results from this study support findings that cultural and personal influences are more relevant than HIV-related conditions to understanding women's reproductive choices.

Clinical Application

1. Encourage women-centered policies and services that are culturally-sensitive and considerable of the complexities of reproductive decisions for women with HIV.
2. Support programs that view motherhood as central to women's lives.
3. Recognize the complexities for women making reproductive decisions within competing and varied cultural influences.
4. Support counseling services that address the ambivalence that women might feel about their reproductive decisions and the uncertain future for themselves and their children.
5. Provide services to women with HIV in a non-coercive style with nonjudgmental attitudes.
6. Consider and reflect on your own attitudes and stereotypes about motherhood for women with HIV.

Reference: Barnes, D. B., & Murphy, S. (2009). Reproductive decisions for women with HIV: Motherhood's role in envisioning a future. *Qualitative Health Research, 19*(4), 481–491.

It is not uncommon for health professionals to identify many misconceptions about contraception and the prevention of pregnancy in our own culture as well as others. In a study by Otoide, Oronsaye, and Okonofua (2001), Nigerian adolescents participated in focus groups to explore their level of understanding regarding contraception. The researchers were aware that in this particular group there is a low level of contraceptive use but a high reliance on abortion. According to the results, the participants perceived that modern contraceptives would have a prolonged, adverse effect on future fertility, whereas abortion was seen as an immediate solution to unplanned pregnancy. This indicates a need to educate Nigerian adolescents regarding contraceptive action and side effects versus the use of unsafe abortion practices. Few cultural groups give unqualified social approval to abortion. In the United States and Canada, religious affiliation is the variable most closely associated with attitudes toward abortion. Women from traditional societies are questioning long-held beliefs related to fertility control.

Nurses providing family planning services must take care to be culturally sensitive so that women can be assisted in examining their own attitudes, beliefs, and sense of gynecologic well-being regarding fertility control. For example, Barnes and Murphy (2009) found that cultural influences are more important on HIV-positive women's reproductive choices than HIV-related conditions. This study is highlighted in Evidence-Based Practice 5-1.

Pregnancy and Culture

All cultures recognize **pregnancy** as a special transition period, and many have particular customs and beliefs that dictate activity and behavior during pregnancy. Recent reports of childbirth customs in the United States have focused on accounts of differing beliefs and practices relative to pregnancy among various ethnic and cultural groups. This section describes some of the biologic and cultural variations that might influence the provision of nursing care during pregnancy.

Biologic Variations

Knowledge of certain biologic variations resulting from genetic and environmental backgrounds is important for nurses who care for childbearing families. For example, pregnant women who have the sickle cell trait and are heterozygous for the sickle cell gene are at increased risk for asymptomatic bacteriuria and urinary tract infections such as pyelonephritis. Obviously, this places them at greater-than-normal risk for premature labor as well. Although heterozygotes are found most commonly among African Americans (8% to 14%), individuals living in the United States and Canada who are of Mediterranean ancestry, as well as of Germanic and Native North American descent, might occasionally carry the trait (Overfield, 1985; Perry, 2000). If both parents are heterozygous, there is a one-in-four chance that the infant will be born with sickle cell disease.

Another important biologic variation relative to pregnancy is diabetes mellitus. The incidence of non-insulin-dependent and gestational diabetes is much higher than normal among some Native American groups—a problem that increases maternal and infant morbidity. Illnesses that are common among European Americans might manifest themselves differently in Native American clients. For example, an American Indian woman might have a high blood sugar level but be asymptomatic for diabetes mellitus. It is important to be aware that the mortality rate in pregnant American Indian women with diabetes is higher than in White European American women. Diabetes during pregnancy, particularly with uncontrolled hyperglycemia, is associated with an increased risk of congenital anomalies, stillbirth, macrosomia, birth injury, cesarean section, neonatal hypoglycemia, and other problems.

Because long-term studies have been conducted among the Pima Indians of Arizona, we know that, for the last 40 years or so, they have a very high incidence of gestational diabetes and other health problems during pregnancy (Pettitt, Baird, Aleck, Bennett, & Knowler, 1983). Because some of the children born to Pima mothers after the studies began are now 28 to 30 years old, we can understand how a mother's diabetes can influence a child's health in adulthood. Researchers have found that the children of women with diabetes during pregnancy have a higher risk of becoming obese and getting diabetes earlier in life than those born to mothers who had normal blood sugar (Chamberlain, n.d.; The Pima Indians: Obesity and Diabetes, 2010).

Pregnant American Indians and Alaskan Native women with type 2 diabetes are at an increased risk of having babies born with birth defects. Gestational diabetes increases the baby's risk for problems such as macrosomia (large body size) and neonatal hypoglycaemia (low blood sugar). Although the blood glucoses of American Indian and Alaskan Native women usually return to normal after childbirth, these women have an increased risk of developing gestational diabetes in future pregnancies. In addition, studies show that many women with gestational diabetes will develop type 2 diabetes later in life (The Diabetes Monitor, 2005).

Cultural Variations Influencing Pregnancy Outcomes

Several cultural variations might influence pregnancy outcomes. Those highlighted in this chapter include alternative lifestyle choices, nontraditional support systems, cultural beliefs related to parental activity during pregnancy, and food taboos and cravings. Nurses must be able to differentiate among beliefs and practices that are harmful, benign, and health promoting. Few cultural customs related to pregnancy are dangerous; although they might cause a woman to limit her activity and her exposure to some aspects of life, they are rarely harmful to herself or her fetus.

Alternative Lifestyle Choices

Despite recent cultural changes that have made it more acceptable for women to have careers and pursue alternative lifestyles, the dominant cultural expectation for North American women remains motherhood within the context of the nuclear family. Changing cultural expectations have influenced many middle-class North American women and couples to delay childbearing until their late 20s and early 30s and to have small families. Many of today's women are very career-oriented and they may delay childbirth until they finish college and establish their career. Some women are making choices regarding childbearing that might not involve a marital relationship.

For another group of mothers who choose not to parent, the choices are not as clear. **Infant relinquishment** is in direct conflict with Western ideal cultural values, which suggest that all parents want a child. Nurses must examine their own cultural values when caring for women in this situation, making certain to avoid negatively stereotyping mothers who decide to relinquish their babies for adoption. The decision to relinquish is almost always difficult, and the birth mother does not forget the experience. Not all infant relinquishments result merely from the mother "not wanting the baby." For example, Native Americans living on reservations have been known to relinquish young and older children in the hope that their children will have "a better life off the reservation." Even with such good intentions, the relinquishment is difficult for all concerned. In one of the few studies on the experience of infant relinquishment by Lauderdale and Boyle (1994), the most common reasons given by birth mothers for relinquishment were strictly altruistic: The birth mothers wanted a better life for the baby than they believed they could offer, and they wanted the baby to have both a mother and a father. Box 5-2 lists considerations in the nursing care of relinquishing birth mothers who are making this difficult decision.

Lesbian couple childbearing occurs in another subculture of pregnant women with special needs. This group of women faces psychosocial dilemmas related to their lifestyle and social stigma. The most common fear reported by lesbian mothers is the fear of unsafe and inadequate care from the

BOX 5-2

Considerations in the Care of Relinquishing Birth Mothers

1. During pregnancy, be open to the discussions of single parenting or adoption; be supportive of the woman's decision.

2. Encourage early and appropriate prenatal care.

3. During hospitalization, acknowledge the adoption as a loss; discuss the grief and grieving process with the birth mother.

4. Accept the birth mother as a "real mother," encourage questions, discuss her hospital expectations.

5. Encourage the midwife and/or obstetrician and the pediatrician to provide follow-up care to the birth mother.

6. Include the birth mother in postpartum teaching as appropriate.

7. Assist with the creation of memories in the form of picture taking, saving locks of hair, making footprints, or other acts that have meaning to the birth mother.

8. If desired by the birth mother, allow a formal closure ceremony. Examples of closure could be a quiet "good-bye" between mother and infant or a prayer with family and clergy present. This is important because it facilitates the grief and grieving process.

9. After relinquishment, it might be helpful for the birth mother to link with other mothers who have successfully coped with a similar experience. Support groups can be located in association with hospitals, adoption agencies, and other interested community agencies.

10. Encourage postpartum follow-up so that the birth mother's physical and emotional recovery can be monitored.

Lauderdale, J., & Boyle, J. (1994). Infant relinquishment through adoption. *Image Journal of Nursing Scholarship, 26*(3), 213–217.

practitioner once the mother's sexual orientation is revealed (Spinks, Andrews, & Boyle, 2000). Reluctance to disclose sexual orientation to one's health care provider can act as a barrier to a woman's receiving appropriate services and referrals (Polek, Hardie, & Crowley, 2008). This situation requires health care providers to examine their own cultural value systems. Keep in mind that lesbian parents are dedicated to bringing a new life safely into the world to love and care for to the best of their abilities—the same hopes all parents have for their newborns. The findings from the study by McManus, Hunter, and Renn (2006) further support other research with lesbian health. There are four areas in their review of the literature that are significant in regards to lesbians considering parenting: (1) sexual orientation disclosure to providers and finding sensitive caregivers, (2) conception options, (3) assurance of partner involvement, and (4) how to legally protect both the parents and the child. Lesbian and heterosexual pregnancies have many similarities, and health care providers should not overlook the parallels. Issues of sexual activity, psychosocial changes related to attaining the traditionally defined maternal tasks of pregnancy (Rubin, 1984), and birth education all need to be addressed with lesbian couples. Special needs of the lesbian couple requiring assessment include social discrimination, family and social support networks, obstacles in becoming pregnant (i.e., coitus versus artificial insemination), lesbian maternal role development, legal issues of adoption by the partner, and coparenting roles.

Buchholz's (2000) qualitative study examined the childbirth experiences of lesbian couples. The researcher focused on the positive aspects of the experience and the reasons why they were positive for the mother. Preparation of the nursing staff before the couples' arrival in the delivery area was seen by the couples as helpful. This preparation assisted the staff with the execution of the couple's birth plan and helped identify, ahead of time, nurses who would prefer not to work with the couple. The nurses' inclusion of the mother's partner in the labor and delivery process, by acknowledging their approaching parenthood and allowing the partner to assist with newborn care after delivery, was seen as positive. The nursing staff conveyed support by using comforting gestures, checking with the couple frequently, answering questions, and just "being there" for them (Buchholz, 2000).

Buchholz's study identified two major concerns of lesbian couples. The first centered on legal issues such as power of attorney, visiting restrictions for the partner, and birth certificate information (father identification). Some of these concerns may be addressed in the 2010 ruling by President Obama that will make it easier for gay men and lesbians to make medical decisions on behalf of their partners (New York Times, 2010). The second concern described in Buchholz's study dealt with the couple's attention to nurses' behavioral cues and questioning whether "busyness" on the part of the nurses might somehow equate to discomfort with the situation. To further illustrate the issues surrounding nursing care and lesbian childbearing needs, a recent study by Renaud (2007) used critical ethnography to examine lesbians' personal experiences on becoming pregnant, giving birth, and becoming mothers and comothers. See Evidence-Based Practice 5-2.

To meet lesbian parents' special needs and provide sensitive and appropriate care, nurses must come to understand the lifestyle and culture of the lesbian couple and work with them in addressing both their physical and their psychosocial concerns. Equally important, nurses must understand their own cultural values and norms, being careful not to impose them on couples with special needs. Last, hospital policies and procedures might need to be adapted to reflect the changing times, lifestyles, attitudes, and needs of all our clients. Recent polls indicate that American attitudes toward gays and lesbians are changing with society as a whole becoming tolerant and supportive. For example, among younger Americans, there is support for legalization of gay marriage (U.S. News & World Report, 2010).

Maternal Role Attainment Alterations

Maternal role attainment is an attribute many times taken for granted in Western culture. If you give birth and become a mother, the assumption is you automatically become "maternal" and successfully care for and nurture your infant. However, many factors can affect maternal role attainment, including separation of mother and infant in cases such as illness,

---

EVIDENCE-BASED PRACTICE 5-2

We Are Mothers Too: Childbearing Experiences of Lesbian Families

Critical ethnography was used to describe lesbians' personal and health care experiences focusing on pregnancy and mothering within the context of potentially oppressive family, social, and political structures. The findings revealed seven themes: preparing the way: becoming ready; conception: you can't just fall into it; you can hear a heartbeat: pregnancy; birthing our babies; the work of mothers and mothers who work; families who sustain and families who oppose; and sources of support in everyday life.

Clinical Application

- Health care providers, policy makers, and the public need to keep in mind research findings and exercise increased sensitivity when providing care and establishing evidence-based practice standards and policies, in order to meet the needs of the expanding view of "family."
- Consider the special needs of lesbian couples during the childbearing process.

Reference: Renaud, M.T. (2007) We are mothers too: childbearing experiences of lesbian families. *Journal of Obstetric Gynecological Neonatal Nursing, 36*(2):190–199.

incarceration, or adoption, to name only a few. An example of successful maternal role attainment superimposed with a chronic illness is described in a phenomenological study that explored factors affecting maternal role attainment in Thai HIV-positive mothers selected for their successful adaptation to the maternal role. The results indicated six internal and external factors used to assist in attainment: (1) setting a purpose of raising their babies; (2) keeping their HIV status secret; (3) maintaining feelings of autonomy and optimism by living as if nothing were wrong, that is, normalization; (4) belief of quality versus quantity of support from husbands, mothers, or sisters; (5) hope for a cure; and (6) belief that their secret is safe with their health care providers. The study results indicated that while the diagnosis of HIV created challenges in attaining their mothering role, the women's feelings of shame of infection (seen as a disease of prostitutes in Thai culture) were buffered by their will to live, love for, and hope for a future with their children. The researcher notes in Thai society, women are the major agents of socialization in a child's life. As such, the knowledge gained by studying how HIV-positive Thai mothers manage the dual demands of survival and the attainment of the maternal role will help health care providers as they work to care for and provide support to women in these circumstances (Jirapaet, 2001). Obviously the decision to have a child is a complex one and while predominant ideas about social role obligations suggest that with HIV, women should not have children, the preponderance of research findings suggests that women's HIV serostatus and/or knowledge of their HIV transmission do not significantly influence their reproductive decisions (Barnes & Murphy, 2009).

Nontraditional Support Systems

A cultural variation that has important implications is a woman's perception of the need for formalized assistance from health care providers during the antepartum period. Western medicine is generally perceived as having a curative rather than a preventive focus. Indeed, many health care providers view pregnancy as a disaster waiting to happen, a physiologic state that at any moment will become pathologic. Because many cultural groups perceive pregnancy as a normal physiologic process, not seeing pregnant women as ill or in need of the curative services of a doctor, women in these diverse groups often delay seeking, or even neglect to seek, prenatal care.

Pregnant women and their partners are placing increased emphasis on the quality of pregnancy and childbirth, and many childbearing women rely on nontraditional support systems. For couples who are married, White, middle class, and infrequent users of their extended family for advice and support in childbirth-related matters, this kind of support might not be crucial. However, for other more traditional cultural groups, including African Americans, Hispanics, Filipinos, Asians, and Native Americans, the family and social network (especially the grandmother or other maternal relatives) may be of primary importance in advising and supporting the pregnant woman.

Childbearing practices for Filipino women are influenced by a number of factors including their cultural beliefs, socioeconomic factors, and in recent years, by Western medicine. Approximately 41% of Filipino births are supported by indigenous attendants called *hilots*. The attendants act as a consultant throughout the pregnancy. During the postpartum period the *hilot* performs a ritualistic sponge bath with oils and herbs, which is believed to have both physical and psychological benefits. The extended family is involved in the care of the baby, mother, and the household. Breast-feeding is encouraged and hot soups are encouraged to increase milk production (Pacquiao, 2008).

In Arab countries, labor and delivery is considered the business of women. Traditionally, *dayahs* and midwives presided over home deliveries. The *dayahs* provide support during the pregnancy and labor and are considered by traditional Arab women to be most knowledgeable due to their experience in caring for other pregnant women. Currently, hospital births are on the rise in most

Arab countries, decreasing the number of traditional home births (Purnell & Selekman, 2008). Kulwicki (2008) reports, following the traditional birth of an Arab newborn, the stomach is wrapped to prevent cold wind from entering the baby. This is done in an effort to decrease possible illnesses in the newborn.

It is essential that the nurse do a thorough cultural assessment to ascertain how much the pregnant woman uses nontraditional support systems and/or Western health care during her pregnancy. Once this assessment is complete and a trusting relationship has been established, the woman's pregnancy can be managed and consideration given to all the components that both she and the nurse believe are important for a successful outcome. We have known for some time that support during labor has positive effects, such as reduced labor pain, reduced stress, shorter duration of labor, less medication need, increased maternal satisfaction, and a positive attitude going into motherhood (Chalmers & Wolman, 1993; Gordon et al., , 1999). The decision for a supporter to be present during birth is a personal one

---

BOX 5-3

Cultural Beliefs Regarding Activity and Pregnancy

Prescriptive Beliefs

- Remain active during pregnancy to aid the baby's circulation (Crow Indian)
- Remain happy to bring the baby joy and good fortune (Pueblo and Navajo Indian, Mexican, Japanese)
- Sleep flat on your back to protect the baby (Mexican)
- Keep active during pregnancy to ensure a small baby and an easy delivery (Mexican and Cambodian Canadian)
- Continue sexual intercourse to lubricate the birth canal and prevent a dry labor (Haitian, Mexican)
- Continue daily baths and frequent shampoos during pregnancy to produce a clean baby (Filipino)

Restrictive Beliefs

- Avoid cold air during pregnancy (Mexican, Haitian, Asian)
- Do not reach over your head or the cord will wrap around the baby's neck (African American, Hispanic, White, Asian)
- Avoid weddings and funerals or you will bring bad fortune to the baby (Vietnamese)
- Do not continue sexual   intercourse or harm will come to you and baby (Vietnamese, Filipino, Samoan)

- Do not tie knots or braid or allow the baby's father to do so because it will cause difficult labor (Navajo Indian)
- Do not sew (Pueblo Indian, Asian)
- Avoid heavy physical work, eat rich and healthy foods, and get frequent rest (Iranian Canadian)

Taboos

- Avoid lunar eclipses and moonlight or the baby might be born with a deformity (Mexican)
- Do not walk on the streets at noon or 5 o'clock because this might make the spirits angry (Vietnamese)
- Do not join in traditional ceremonies like Yei or Squaw dances or spirits will harm the baby (Navajo Indian)
- Do not get involved with persons who cast spells or the baby will be eaten in the womb (Haitian)
- Do not say the baby's name before the naming ceremony or harm might come to the baby (Orthodox Jewish)
- Do not have your picture taken because it might cause stillbirth (African American)
- During the postpartum period, avoid visits from widows, women who have lost children, and people in mourning because they will bring bad fortune to the baby (South Asian Canadian)

From Waxler-Morrison, N., Andrews, J., & Richardson, E. (1990). *Cross-cultural caring: A handbook for health professionals in Western Canada.* Vancouver, BC: University of British Columbia Press.

and should be made individually by each couple in terms of their knowledge of one another and of the woman's coping style.

Cultural Beliefs Related to Activity During Pregnancy

Cultural variations also involve beliefs about activities during pregnancy. A belief is something held to be actual or true on the basis of a specific rationale or explanatory model. **Prescriptive beliefs**, which are phrased positively, describe what should be done to have a healthy baby; the more common restrictive beliefs, which are phrased negatively, limit choices and behaviors, and are practices/behaviors that the mother should not do in order to have a healthy baby. Taboo beliefs are practices believed to harm the baby or the mother. Many people believe that the activities of the mother—and to a lesser extent of the father—influence newborn outcome. Box 5-3 describes some traditional prescriptive and restrictive beliefs and taboos that provide cultural boundaries for parental activity during pregnancy. These beliefs are attempts to increase a sense of control over the outcome of pregnancy.

Positive or prescriptive beliefs might involve wearing special articles of clothing, such as the *muneco* worn by some traditional Hispanic women to ensure a safe delivery and prevent morning sickness. Other beliefs and practices involve ceremonies and recommendations about physical and sexual activity. One event in which a prescriptive belief might cause harm occurs when there is a poor neonatal outcome and the mother blames herself. For example, the mother whose fetus has died as a result of a cord accident, and who believed that hanging laundry caused the cord to encircle the baby's neck or body, might experience severe guilt. The nurse who is sensitive to the mother's anguish might say, "Many people say that if you reach over your head during pregnancy, it will cause the cord to wrap around the baby's neck. Have you heard this belief?" Once the woman responds, the nurse can explore her feelings about the practice. Do others in her family or social support network share her belief?

The nurse might share her own views by saying, "I have not read in any medical or nursing books that this practice is related to cord problems, although I know many people share your belief." The discussion can then continue focusing on the feelings and perceptions of the event as it is experienced by the woman and her family.

Negative or **restrictive beliefs** are widespread and numerous. They include activity, work, and sexual, emotional, and environmental prescriptions. **Taboos,** or restrictions with serious supernatural consequences, include the Orthodox Jewish avoidance of baby showers, divulgence of the infant's name before the infant's official naming ceremony, and laws, customs, and practices during labor and delivery (Bash, 1980; Noble, Newsome-Wicks, Engelhardt, & Woloski-Wruble, 2009). A Hispanic taboo involves the traditional belief that an early baby shower will invite bad luck, or *mal ojo*, the evil eye (Spector, 2008).

Food Taboos and Cravings

Among many cultures, a traditional belief was that the mother had little control over the outcome of pregnancy except through the avoidance of foods that are considered taboo. Another traditional belief in many cultures is that a pregnant woman must be given the food that she smells to eat, otherwise the fetus will move inside of her and a miscarriage will result (Spector, 2008). Spicy, cold, and sour foods are often believed to be the foods that a pregnant woman should avoid during pregnancy.

Some pregnant women experience pica: the craving for and ingestion of nonfood substances, such as clay, laundry starch, or cornstarch. Some Hispanic women prefer the solid milk of magnesia that can be purchased in Mexico, whereas other women eat the ice or frost that forms inside refrigerator units. The causes of pica are poorly understood, but there are some cultural implications because women from certain ethnic or cultural groups experience this disorder. In the United States, pica is common in African American women raised in the rural South and in women from lower socioeconomic levels. It is not uncommon to see small balls of clay in plastic bags and sold in country stores in the rural South. The phenomenon of pica has been described in Kenya, Uganda, and Saudi Arabia (Boyle & Mackey, 1999).

Cultural Issues Impacting Prenatal Care

Morgan's study (1996) is one of the few studies that explored African American women's beliefs, practices, and values related to prenatal care. The findings indicated that many of the women in urban areas lacked trust and were apprehensive about their current life circumstances. Establishing a good relationship and providing a safe environment increased attendance at prenatal clinics. Urban African American women indicated that they had less support than their contemporaries in the rural South. Nurses should be encouraged to set up peer social and educational groups for women who are similar to those in this study. In addition, the findings indicated that adherence to folk health care beliefs and practices were prevalent among study participants. Nurses must learn more about the practices of their clients and have a nonjudgmental attitude. Acceptance of alternative healers might even be therapeutic and helpful for many clients.

Using Leininger's Theory of Cultural Care Diversity and Universality, Berry's ethnonursing study (1999) focused on pregnant Mexican American women. The findings revealed the meanings and experiences attached to generic care (family and extended family pregnancy guidance) and professional care during pregnancy. Significant themes for generic culture care were identified as protection of the mother and fetus by elderly Mexican American women, who were affected by religious and family practices, and the value attached to the family providing care for the mother and being with her. Professional culture care themes included (1) respecting the family roles of caring for the mother in relation to age and gender, (2) expressing concern, knowledge, protection, and explanations and attending to the needs of the mother, (3) using the Spanish language while caring for the mother, and (4) believing that professional prenatal care was valued by the women even though access was in many cases problematic.

Incorporating the value of respect into the culture care of Mexican American pregnant women can be achieved on many levels and might be demonstrated by the following practices:

1. Supporting the religious or spiritual needs of clients by helping to locate religious advisors and providing time for prayer or quiet meditation when indicated.
2. Addressing clients by last name and conversing with clients about their families before the initiation of care.
3. Acknowledging elder generic guidance during pregnancy and, when appropriate, incorporating these practices into the client's care.
4. Respecting the family's beliefs in a male authority as the protector and final decision maker.
5. Encouraging a client to include her spouse in prenatal visits when decisions regarding care must be made, or making the information available for the client to take home for approval, especially when consents are required (Berry, 1999).

Both studies (Morgan, 1996; Berry, 1999) reported similar barriers to prenatal care access, including (1) lack of telephones for communicating with health care providers, (2) lack of transportation to the clinics, (3) legal issues surrounding immigration that affected access, (4) bureaucratic paperwork, and (5) inflexible clinic schedules. Nurses need to exercise creativity when solving these problems. For instance, they can explore the possibility that city or county governments will provide free transportation to health care sites for women in need of such assistance. Nurses can support the development of telephone health information systems in appropriate languages to explain access to health care, especially for newly immigrated clients. Lastly, nurses can rethink and restructure clinic schedules to include weekend and evening appointments as one way of easing the burden of access (Berry, 1999).

Traditional beliefs surrounding care during pregnancy when interfaced with Western medicine has, in some situations, forced an adjustment in the way Mexican American women engage in pregnancy care behaviors. Mexican American childbearing women seem to represent a healthy model for preventing low birth weight infants. However, acculturation to U.S. lifestyle may also put them at an increased risk for poor birth outcomes according to a study conducted by Martin et al. (2004). An ethnographic study in California examined the influence of acculturation on pregnancy beliefs and practices of Mexican American childbearing women. Lagana (2003) reported that "selective biculturalism" emerged as a protective approach to stress reduction and health promotion. The women interviewed indicated that regardless of the level of acculturation to U.S. culture, during pregnancy, they returned to traditional Mexican practices. Such practices include a low-fat, high-protein, natural diet (eat right—*come bien*); exercise for well-being (walk—*camina*); and avoidance of worry or stress, which could have a negative effect on the pregnancy outcome (don't worry—*no se preocupe*). The women described the family as a major support during pregnancy but also valued the economic and personal freedom available to women in the United States. The resulting conflicts lead to the adoption of a "selective bicultural perspective." This perspective allowed the women to maintain or reject cultural practices as needed. The fact that the women in this study lived in a largely Latino town might have limited their bicultural stress, whereas pregnant Mexican women living in a more heterogeneous environment might experience higher levels of stress related to cultural conflicts. The author suggests, "It is likely that some cultural traits protective of pregnancy are lost through the process of acculturation" (Lagana, 2003, p. 123). This statement indicates that health care providers need to consider not only the support from family and social support networks, but also explore the impact of stress from cultural conflicts on pregnancy outcomes. Some research has shown that preventive and health-promoting behaviors in pregnant minority women can be used to encourage healthy lifestyles and optimal utilization of health services and to obtain better outcomes of pregnancy (Feng, Zhang, & Owen, 2007).

Cultural Interpretation of Obstetric Testing

Many women do not understand the emphasis that Western prenatal care places on urinalysis, blood pressure readings, and abdominal measurements. For traditional Islamic women from the Middle East, the vaginal examination can be so intrusive and embarrassing that they avoid prenatal visits or request a female physician or midwife. For women of other cultural groups, common discomforts of pregnancy might be managed with folk, herbal, home, or over-the-counter remedies on the advice of a relative (generally the maternal grandmother) or friends (Spector, 2008). Health care providers can attempt to meet the needs of women from traditional cultures by explaining health regimens so that they have meaning within the cultural belief system. However, such explanations are only an initial step. Nursing visits can be made to the home, or group prenatal visits might be made based on self-care models instituted by nurses in local community centers. Additionally, nurses can incorporate significant others into the plan of care. During prenatal visits, nurses can provide information on normal fetal growth and development, and they can discuss how the health and behavior of the mother and those around her can influence fetal outcome.

Cultural Preparation for Childbirth

Preparation for childbirth can be developed through programs that allow for cultural variations, including classes during and after the usual clinic hours in busy urban settings, teen-only classes, single-mother classes, group classes combined with prenatal checkups at home, classes on rural reservations, and presentations that incorporate the older "wise women" of the community. In addition, nurses can organize classes in languages other than English and conduct these classes in community settings that are culturally appropriate and welcoming to women.

Birth and Culture

Beliefs and customs surrounding the experience of labor and delivery are influenced by the fact that the physiologic processes are basically the same in all cultures. Factors such as cultural attitudes toward the achievement of birth, methods of dealing with the pain of labor, recommended positions during delivery, the preferred location for the birth, the role of the father and the family, and expectations of the health care practitioner might vary according to the degree of acculturation to Western childbirth customs, geographic location, religious beliefs, and individual preference.

Traditionally, cultures have viewed the birth of a child in two very different ways; for example, the birth of the first son may be considered a great achievement worthy of celebration, or the birth may be viewed as a state of defilement or pollution requiring various purification ceremonies. In general North American culture, birth is often viewed as an achievement—unfortunately not always for the mother but rather for the medical staff. The obstetrician "manages" the labor and "delivers" the infant; for this active role, the doctor is often profusely thanked even before the mother is praised or congratulated. Gifts and celebrations are centered on the newborn rather than the mother. The recent consumer movement in childbirth and the upsurge of feminism has caused some redefinition of the cultural focus and has encouraged women and their partners to assume active roles in the management of their own health and birth experiences. Unfortunately, some women who have prepared themselves for a totally "natural" childbirth might feel disappointment and a sense of failure if they require analgesia or a cesarean section.

Traditional Home Birth

All cultures have an approach to birth rooted in a tradition in which childbirth occurs at home, within the province of women. For generations, traditions among the poor included the use of "granny" midwives by rural Appalachian Whites and southern African Americans and *parteras* by Mexican Americans. A dependence on self-management, a belief in the normality of labor and birth, and a tradition of delivery at home might influence some women to arrive at the hospital only in advanced labor. The need to travel a long distance to the closest hospital might also be a factor contributing to arrival during late labor or to out-of-hospital delivery for many American Indian women living on rural, isolated reservations.

Lori and Boyle (2011) examined beliefs and practices about maternal mortality and morbidity with women in Liberia. Liberian women are reluctant to share information about pregnancy and childbirth as these subjects are taboo to talk about with others. Husbands or male elders are the ones who make decisions about allowing a woman to seek care at a clinic or hospital when she is experiencing a difficult and arduous labor. Further complicating this situation, women are reluctant to seek professional health care at clinics or hospitals because they are more comfortable in their own homes with traditional (but untrained) birth attendants. These findings reinforce the notion that we need to understand the social and cultural context of childbirth and childbirth related practices before we can make an impact on the seemingly intractable problems of maternal morbidity and mortality.

This raises the question of how many informal systems are operating in the United States among rural/or traditional women with no access to mainstream health care, and how can they be identified and integrated in order to have the best of both worlds? One such example currently in existence involves Latinos in the United States, which are one of the most medically underserved populations (Center for American Progress Action Fund, 2010). Latino women have the highest birthrate among ethnic groups in the United States, but because of unaffordable insurance, program cuts, and limited access to appropriate prenatal care, this group of women and their unborn babies traditionally have been placed in a precarious situation (Martin et al., 2004). However, the Patient Protection and Affordable Care Act (PPACA) of 2010 makes important contributions toward addressing Hispanic/Latino Americans' health care needs. Expanding primary care, promoting community-based health services, and emphasizing culturally sensitive care will create a bridge between providers of care and the underserved and hard-to-reach populations they serve. It is possible to integrate the informal Hispanic care system with the mainstream in such a way as to ensure a complementary system. The Hispanic informal care system for pregnant women includes the use of lay midwives (*parteras*), labor and postpartum support persons (*doulas*), and health workers in the community (*promotoras*).

McEwen, Baird, Pasvogel, and Gallegos (2007) describe how community lay workers or *promotoras* can be used for outreach, including sharing information regarding availability of formal care, empowering women with cultural care knowledge and working with communities to preserve healthy Hispanic beliefs and practices that might otherwise be lost to acculturation. Of equal importance, *promotoras* provide a cultural and social support system that is beneficial to Hispanic or Mexican American women. Other U.S. health care facilities have taken this information to heart and have incorporated similar culturally sensitive innovations with great success.

The literature offers yet another example of the impact culture has on perinatal care practices. Walsh (2006) examined the beliefs and practices of an indigenous Guatemalan community's traditional birth attendants (TBAs) by using ethnographic methods, identifying the major themes as sacred calling (being called to service by God or a saint), sacred knowledge (skills learned through dreams or visions via communication with God), and sacred rituals (candles, incense, and other religious artifacts to create a sacred environment, along with prayer). The researcher found that commonly the birth attendant in Guatemala is the *comadrona*, a woman in the community who is trusted and has a calling for the role of a midwife. The women may or

may not have training, and because many lack formal training, they are often blamed for the high mortality rates. Currently, most health care practices in urban and rural areas in Guatemala use Western approaches; however, many traditional and isolated Guatemalan villages continue to use TBAs. The midwives in the Guatemalan highlands attend monthly meetings in which nurses and physicians provide education on obstetrical problems and emergencies. Walsh (2006) reported the *comadronas* are incorporating the information and skills learned in the monthly training sessions into their practices. These findings would indicate that as health care groups work to design programs to improve health outcomes, integrating cultural beliefs and rituals into health care training might ultimately improve health outcomes. As our immigration numbers continue to grow and diversity continues to increase, hopefully, so too will the number of health care institutions that strive to integrate these informal systems into their models for care.

Support During Childbirth

Despite the traditional emphasis on female support and guidance during labor, the inclusion of spouses and male partners in North American labor and birth rooms has been seen as positive by women of many cultures. Women from diverse cultures report a desire to have husbands or partners present for the birth. Unfortunately, some U.S. hospitals still enforce rules that limit the support person to the spouse or that prevent a husband from attending the birth unless he has attended a formal childbirth education program with his wife. Fortunately, this situation has changed a great deal in the past few years so that husbands or partners now make important contributions in supporting and helping pregnant women during labor. A description of the effects of Turkish fathers attendance in labor and delivery on the experience of childbirth is presented in Evidence-Based Practice 5-3.

Another source of conflict is the desire of many women to have the mother or some other female

EVIDENCE-BASED PRACTICE 5-3

Effects of Fathers' Attendance to Labor and Delivery on the Experience of Childbirth in Turkey

This study was planned to experimentally determine the effects of fathers' attendance to labor and delivery on the experience of childbirth. The concept of allowing partners attendance in labor and delivery did not become popular in Turkey because of cultural and religious reasons, hospital policies, and environmental conditions in delivery units. In recent years, this situation is beginning to change but the opportunity is still limited and only available in a few hospitals.

The study recruited 50 primigravidae low-risk women and their partners, assigned 25 women and their partners to an experimental group. The Perception of Birth Scale was used to measure women's attitudes about labor and delivery experience and the Father Interview Form was used to describe fathers' participation styles and their experience in labor and delivery. Women in the control group did not have their husbands in the labor and delivery rooms where they received routine care.

The fathers attending the birth indicated they were there "to support their wives." They assisted their wives with breathing, relaxation techniques, and emotional support. The fathers adopted active roles in coaching their wives; 44% of the fathers'-to-be chose to leave the delivery room at the moment of delivery, while the rest wanted to stay and continued supporting their wives. Wives whose husbands adopted an active support role reported more positive perceptions about their delivery experience and were more aware of events during the birth. The researchers concluded that fathers' presence and support have positive effects on all aspects of childbirth. This study supports other research that provides powerful evidence of improved outcomes such as shorter labors, less analgesia use, less operative vaginal delivery, or caesarean section when mothers are supported in labor.

Clinical Application

- Support childbirth education and preparation for both fathers and mothers when culturally acceptable and appropriate.
- Encourage and support fathers to adopt an active role in childbirth.
- Work to change hospital policies and cultural myths that exclude fathers' involvement in pregnancy, birth, and the postpartum period.

Reference: Gunger, I., & Beji, N. K. (2007). Effects of fathers' attendance to labor and delivery on the experience of childbirth in Turkey. *Western Journal of Nursing Research*, 29, 213–231.

relative or friend present during labor and birth. Because many hospitals have rules limiting the number of persons present, the mother-to-be might be forced to make a difficult choice among the persons close to her.

For an Orthodox Jewish woman in labor and for reasons of modesty, her choice of a labor support person may be a woman from the community (Lewis, 2003; Noble, Rom, Newsome-Wicks, Engelhardt, & Woloski-Wruble, 2009). The spouse may elect to stay in the labor room provided the mother's private parts are covered. Similar findings are reported from women of Islamic, Chinese, and Asian Indian backgrounds. Practices followed by these groups might include strict religious and cultural prohibitions against viewing the woman's body by *either* the husband or any other man. Labor practices are explicit for Orthodox Jewish women. Men are expected to not touch their wife or view their wife's genital area. They may offer verbal support and every effort should be made by the staff to cover or drape the woman appropriately. The husband should be given the opportunity to excuse himself during the delivery without fear of being viewed as being insensitive (Purnell & Selekman, 2008). It is always appropriate for the culturally sensitive nurse to raise these issues with clients and their spouses. Other noteworthy considerations when caring for laboring Orthodox Jewish couples include keeping the laboring mother's head covered at all times, perhaps by providing her with a surgical cap, and allowing an Orthodox man to pick up his newborn directly from the crib versus having a female nurse or physician hand him the newborn because practicing Orthodox men are not allowed contact with adult women other than their spouses (Lewis, 2003). Nurses must determine how much personal control and involvement are desired by a woman and her family during the birth experience. Again, due to a wide variation of customs and beliefs, it is always best for the nurse to ask patients directly about their beliefs and preferred cultural ways so that hospital practices can be aligned with individual needs.

For particular groups of women, religion or spirituality is central to their belief system and is the guiding factor in the childbirth experience. A study by Callister et al. (1999) of Orthodox Jewish and Mormon childbearing women investigated the meaning of culture and religion as they relate to childbirth. Five themes were identified that identified the importance of spirituality and God in the lives of the women and the significance and value placed on childbearing and childrearing in these cultures.

Cultural Expression of Labor Pain

Although the pain threshold is remarkably similar in all persons regardless of gender, social, ethnic, or cultural differences, these differences play a definite role in a woman's perception of labor pain. Pain is a highly personal experience, depending on cultural learning, the context of the situation, and other factors unique to the individual (Ludwig-Beymer, 2008). Because nurses

care for women and families from a variety of cultural backgrounds in labor and birth, it is imperative to understand the populations you care for to understand how culture mediates pain. In the past it was commonly believed that women from Asian and Native American cultures were stoic and did not feel pain in labor (Bachman, 2000). Such views are ethnocentric and should be avoided. Many factors interact to influence labor and the perception of pain. They include cultural attitudes toward the normalcy and conduct of birth, expectations of how a woman should act in labor, the role of significant others, and the physiologic processes involved.

Callister and Vega (1998) reported that Guatemalan women in labor tend to vocalize their pain. Coping strategies include moaning or breathing rhythmically and massaging the thighs and abdomen. Japanese, Chinese, Vietnamese, Laotian, and other women of Asian descent maintain that screaming or crying out during labor or birth is shameful; birth is believed to be painful but something to be endured (Bachman, 2000). Although many women from diverse cultures are deemed unprepared by some health professionals because they do not use formal breathing and relaxation techniques, women often use culturally appropriate ways of preparing for labor and delivery. These methods might include assisting with childbirth from the time of adolescence, listening to birth and baby stories told by respected elderly women, or following special dietary and activity prescriptions during the antepartal period. Most commonly in American culture, pregnant women and their significant others attend childbirth classes.

Birth Positions

Numerous anecdotal reports in the literature describe "typical" birth positions for women of diverse cultures, from the seated position in a birth chair favored by Mexican American women to the squatting position chosen by Laotian Hmong women. The nurse who cares for laboring women must realize, however, that the choice of positions is influenced by many factors other than culture and that the socialization that occurs when a woman arrives in a labor and delivery unit might prevent her from stating her preference.

Economically disadvantaged women from culturally diverse backgrounds have few birth options; most labor and give birth in large public hospitals. Routine patterns of care and decreased individualization are common in these institutions. These and other problems, such as language barriers, make the provision of culturally competent care during the birth process a challenge. However, any special provisions or attempts to understand the client from her perspective will be received with cooperation and gratitude. Recommendations for intrapartum nursing care of the culturally diverse pregnant woman are presented in Box 5-4.

BOX 5-4

Intrapartum Nursing Care for Culturally Diverse Women

1. If you are unable to speak the woman's language, make every effort to arrange for an interpreter.

2. If your nursing agency commonly cares for culturally diverse clients, find out whether other nurses have had experiences with similar clients. Share resources and your expertise with staff members.

3. Attempt to gain as much information as possible by completing a cultural assessment. See Appendix A for the Andrews/Boyle Transcultural Nursing Assessment Guide for Individuals and Families.

4. Elicit the mother's expectations about her labor and delivery experience.

5. Ask if she wants a support person with her? If so, have her identify that person.

6. Explore with her any cultural rituals she wants incorporated into her plan of care. If requests are manageable, honor them.

7. Be patient, draw pictures, gesture. Identify key words from family or the interpreter that you will need to be able to express yourself to her, for example, push, blow, pant, stop.

Cultural Meaning Attached to Infant Gender or Multiple Births

The meaning that parents attach to having a son, a daughter, or multiple births varies from culture to culture. Traditionally, the male gender is highly regarded, which places female infants in a position of "less than favorable" and in some cultures, places female infants at risk for infanticide. In certain Asian and Islamic cultures, it is believed that a male child is preferable to a female child. Twin births also carry a significance that varies from culture to culture. Twins may be viewed as something very special, while other cultural groups may view multiple births more negatively. In these situations, the nurse might find the best course of action is simply to point out all the positive attributes of the newborn(s).

Culture and the Postpartum Period

Western medicine considers pregnancy and birth the most dangerous and vulnerable time for the childbearing woman. However, other cultures place much more emphasis on the postpartum period. Many cultures have developed practices that balance and cushion this special time of vulnerability for the mother and the infant. Such strategies are thought to mobilize support for the new mother. Interestingly, support that comes from family and friends is usually considered "nontraditional" in approach by Western medicine. However, other cultural practices, particularly as they relate to restrictive dietary customs, activity levels, and certain taboos and rituals associated with purification and seclusion, might seem unusual to the nurse but have been noted to positively influence the mother's postpartum mental health, thus reducing the incidence of problems such as postpartum depression (PPD) (Stewart & Jambunathan, 1996).

Posmontier and Horowitz's (2004) review of the literature reports that PPD occurs in a wide variety of cultures worldwide. While it is apparent that the majority of PPD research has been conducted with Western cultures (Affonso, De, Horowitz, & Mayberry, 2000), identifying and reporting of the phenomenon in non-Western culture may be hindered by culturally unacceptable labeling of the disorder, variance of symptoms from group to group, or differences in diagnostic standards from culture to culture (Yoshida, Yamashita, Ueda, & Tashiro, 2001; Committee on Cultural Psychiatry, 2002; American Psychiatric Association, 2000).

Insights provided by the literature suggest nurses should assess all new mothers of diverse backgrounds for culture-specific signs of PPD. Women may express symptoms as somatic in nature, especially in cultures that have no name or definition for PPD, such as the Korean culture (Posmontier & Horowitz, 2004). In order to provide culturally competent nursing care for childbearing women and families from diverse backgrounds, nurses need to incorporate culturally sensitive assessments into their models of care in order to identify significant aspects that can be combined with Western approaches of care. Questions the nurse might ask as part of their assessment include: Have you felt alone or afraid when caring for your baby? Do you cry or feel sad when at home with your baby? How many times during the day do you feel this way? What do you do when you feel sad? What do you think about when you are alone with your baby?

Routine postpartum nursing care usually includes encouraging a healthy diet, adequate fluid intake, and self-care practices such as good hygiene practices, sitz baths, showering, bathing, ambulation, and exercise. However, these practices, common in North American obstetric care, might seem strange and even dangerous to women of other cultural groups. Nurses must take time not only to teach their clients, but to listen to them, making accommodations and being flexible when possible. In many cultures, the concept of postpartum vulnerability is based on one or more beliefs related to imbalance or "pollution." In one of the first transcultural research studies conducted, Horn (1981) examined

childbirth practices of the Muckelshoot Indians. She found that the Muckelshoot held unique ideas about the time surrounding childbirth. **Imbalance** was perceived to be the result of disharmony caused by the processes of pregnancy and birth, and pollution was believed to be caused by the "unclean" bleeding associated with birth and the postpartum period. Restitution of physical balance and purification occurred through many cultural practices, including dietary restrictions, ritual baths, seclusion, restriction of activity, and other ceremonial events.

Hot/Cold Theory

Central to the belief of perceived imbalance in the mother's physical state is adherence to the **hot/cold theories** of disease causation. Pregnancy is considered a "hot" state. Because a great deal of the heat of pregnancy is thought to be lost during the birth process, postpartum practices focus on restoring the balance between the hot/cold beliefs, or yin and yang. Common components of this theory focus on the avoidance of cold, in the form of either air or food. This real fear of the detrimental effects of cold air and water in the postpartum period can cause cultural conflict when the woman and infant are hospitalized. Nurses must assess the woman's beliefs regarding bathing and other self-care practices in a nonjudgmental manner.

Many women will pretend to follow the activities suggested by nurses, to the point of pretending to shower while in reality avoiding the nurses' prescriptions. The common use of perineal ice packs and sitz baths to promote healing can be replaced with the use of heat lamps, heat packs, and anesthetic or astringent topical agents for those who prefer to avoid cold influences. The routine distribution of ice water to all postpartum women is another aspect of care that can be modified to meet women's culturally diverse needs. Offering women a choice of water at room temperature, warm tea or coffee, broth, or another beverage should satisfy most women's needs for warmth, along with the offering of additional bed blankets. It is always appropriate to discuss cultural practices with the new mother to elicit her concerns, needs, and preferences.

Postpartum Dietary Prescriptions and Activity Levels

Dietary prescriptions are also common in this period. The nurse might note that a woman eats little "hospital" food and relies on family and friends to bring food to her while she is in the hospital. If there are no diet restrictions for health reasons, this practice should be respected. Indeed, the nurse should assess what types of food are being eaten by the woman and documenting them as appropriate.

Regulation of activity in relation to the concept of disharmony or imbalance includes the avoidance of air, cold, and evil spirits. Hispanic women are encouraged to stay indoors and avoid strenuous work. Obviously, if pregnancy and birth cause a "hot" state, the woman should avoid "hot" activities such as ironing. Fruits and vegetables and certainly cold drinks might be avoided because they are considered "cold" foods. Some women from traditional cultural groups view themselves as "sick" during the postpartal lochial flow. They might avoid heavy work, showering, bathing, or washing their hair during this vulnerable time. Cultural prescriptions vary regarding when women can return to full activity after childbirth, but many traditional cultures suggest that a woman can resume normal activities in as little as two weeks, and some take up to four months.

Postpartum Seclusion

The period of postpartum vulnerability and seclusion in most non-Western cultures varies between 7 and 40 days. Hispanic women, especially primigravidas, might follow a set of dietary and activity rules called *la dieta* (Spector, 2008). The Hispanic midwife or *partera* will frequently stay at the home of the mother for several hours after the delivery and may make a follow-up visit the next day.

Placental burial rituals are also part of the traditional Hmong culture, and with the continued growth in the number of Hmong Americans emigrating from California to different areas of the United States, cultural conflicts are common, especially in the areas of reproductive health (Clemings, 2001). In an effort to assimilate, many Hmong have continued to use animistic ceremonies and herbal remedies in addition to using Western medicine. Helsel and Mochel's (2002) study explored Hmong Americans' attitudes regarding placental disposition, cultural values affecting those attitudes, and perceptions of the willingness of Western providers to accommodate Hmong patients' wishes regarding placental disposal. The Hmong believe the placenta is the baby's "first clothing" and must be buried at the family's home, in a place where the soul can find the afterlife garment once the person is deceased. If the soul is unable to find the placental "jacket," it will not be able to reunite with its ancestors and will spend eternity wandering. Helsel and Mochel's study (2002) suggests that even though the Hmong have made giant leaps in transitioning from their traditional culture to that of Western culture, traditional Hmong beliefs in placental burial persist. Health care providers need to examine their own beliefs and institutional policy regarding the assumption that the placenta is medical waste and consider beliefs that regard the placenta as a necessary vehicle into the afterlife. This change in attitude and behavior by health care professionals would not only serve to accommodate the needs and wishes of traditional cultures, but it would indicate a commitment to provide culturally competent care.

In some cultures, women are considered to be in a state of impurity or pollution during the postpartum period. Consequently, ritual seclusion and elimination of activity might be practiced to reduce the risk of increasing personal vulnerability to the influence of spirits or of spreading evil and misfortune. In many cultures, this time of seclusion coincides with the period of lochial flow or postpartum bleeding. Common taboos include seclusion and avoidance of contact with others, avoidance of contact with certain food or objects, and avoidance of sexual relations.

Cultural Influences on Breast-Feeding and Weaning Practices

In an effort to increase the practice of breast-feeding, the World Health Organization and UNICEF (2004) recommend children worldwide be breast-fed for a minimum of two years, with no defined upper limit on the duration. Physiologically, children can be breast-fed over a period of several years. Only a few women in the United States participate in extended breast-feeding (longer than three years) for fear of disapproval; therefore, prolonged breast-feeding is usually concealed from family, friends, and health care providers. Dettwyler's work (2004) in this area reports segments of the country where relatively large groups of women nurse longer than three years. These areas include Seattle, WA; Salt Lake City, UT; College Station, TX; and Wilmington, DE. Culturally, breast-feeding and weaning can be affected by a variety of values and beliefs related to societal trends, religious beliefs, the mother's work activities, ethnic cultural beliefs, social support, access to information on breast-feeding, and the health care provider's personal beliefs and experiences regarding breast-feeding and/or weaning practices, to name a few.

For breast-feeding women from traditional backgrounds, it is important for nurses to be aware of factors that have been shown to affect the quality and duration of the breast-feeding experience, along with factors impacting weaning practices. McKee, Zayas, and Jankowski (2004) examined predictors of successful breast-feeding initiation and persistence in a sample of low-income African American and Hispanic women in the urban Northeast. The findings indicated that those women with a strong cultural identification and cultural social support, tended to initiate breast-feeding and continue with breast-feeding longer than those in the groups who did not have strong cultural identification. Adolescent African American and Latina mothers

in Chicago were interviewed to explore the teens' perceptions of breast-feeding and what influenced their infant-feeding decisions and practices. Reported influences included perceptions of breast-feeding benefits (bonding, baby's health), perceptions of the problems with breast-feeding (pain, embarrassment, no experience with the act of breast-feeding), and respected, influential people (Hannon, Willis, Bishop-Townsend, Martinez, & Scrimshaw, 2000). In a related study of the influence of grandmothers on breast-feeding, Almroth, Mohale, and Latham (2000) indicated maternal grandmothers to be positively influential in sharing information, advising new mothers, and providing hands-on and how-to suggestions. Conversely, Susin, Giugliani, and Kummer (2005) found that grandmothers in Brazil having daily contact with mothers were negatively impacting the duration of breast-feeding, citing that both maternal and paternal grandmothers encouraged the introduction of teas, water, and "other" milk. The study confirmed the need to include grandmothers in breast-feeding education so that they would exert a more positive influence on the new mother and baby.

There are few recent studies on cultural practices and breast-feeding, so it is worth reviewing studies of the past two decades as it is important for nurses to be aware of traditional practices that may or may not still be important to new mothers. In a qualitative study by Ingalsbe (1999) of U.S.-residing, Japanese- and Mexican-born mothers, several cultural practices were identified as influential in the type of infant feeding practiced. The Japanese mothers indicated a reluctance to ask questions of U.S. health providers (believe questioning to be inappropriate), which impacted the quality of information and direct teaching they received during the prenatal and postnatal periods. Many first-time moms in this study chose bottle-feeding as a result. The Mexican mothers described mixing Maizena, a cornstarch powder, with cow's milk, for use in weaning from breast- or bottle-feeding, citing its benefits as a thickening agent, keeping the stomach fuller for longer periods and thereby increasing times between breast- or bottle-feedings as solid foods were introduced. Reifsnider and Luck (2007) successfully increased the initiation and duration of breast-feeding to six months in a group of low-income Hispanic women though an intervention that included prenatal education and home-based postpartum support. The findings from this study demonstrate how important it is to have information and support for successful breast-feeding.

Cultural beliefs of women in Hong Kong indicate that even "Westernized" Chinese women hold fast to the basic teachings of Confucius, that is, the family's well-being is central, the father is the head of the family, and harmony with others is essential (Chen, 2001). If a Chinese breast-feeding mother is told by her spouse or family to wean her baby to maintain harmony, she will usually follow their advice (Fok, 1996).

Researchers have studied ethnicity, cultural beliefs or practices, and social mores as a way to understand the influences on infant-feeding practices. However, one group, in particular—the Native American population—has been studied less closely. Breast-feeding among indigenous populations (e.g., Aboriginal/Alaska Native and American Indian women) declined with the advent of infant formula availability. However, there has been a push from within Native American communities to a return to infant feeding "the natural way." Banks (2003) describes how breast-feeding is being successfully promoted among the Kanesatake, a rural Mohawk community in Quebec, Canada, using culturally competent community-based interventions. The promotion strategies include educating extended family on breast-feeding benefits; teaching the nutritional merits of breast-feeding, particularly to the maternal grandmother; addressing the social, emotional, and spiritual aspects of breast-feeding; using the oral tradition as a way to share information, setting the stage for cooperative and interactive learning; and creating teaching methods which avoid conventional courses, lectures, or written materials on infant-feeding practices, as native women are not attracted to or affected by these methods.

In the Kanesatake project, a respected elder volunteered to promote breast-feeding in her community. After completing a training session she chose to use subtle teaching encounters at banks, grocery stores, and social gatherings as a way to promote breast-feeding. Support groups or "talking circles" were organized for extended family and grandmothers of pregnant women where breast-feeding issues were discussed openly and freely, led by the elder. This approach is a good example of how community strengths, incorporation of culturally specific learning styles, and cultural sensitivity can be used as the foundation for successful program development.

Dodgson, Duckett, Garwick, and Graham (2002) examined breast-feeding practices among Ojibwe women. Incorporating family and elders into decision making about breast-feeding, weaning, and health-seeking behaviors was of great importance to Ojibwe mothers. They identified four "patterns of influence" on breast-feeding. They were: (1) mixed messages or conflicting information about breast-feeding; (2) life circumstances such as poverty, high crime, impoverished neighborhoods; (3) Nurturing and support of family members; and, (4) traditions that supported breast-feeding as the "natural" and preferred way to feed infants.

Prior to the industrialized age, women always breast-fed or if they were of "royal" blood or upper class, they used "wet nurses," women who had recently had a baby themselves and breast-fed other women's babies. Midwives attended births. They had a variety of names: aunties, medicine women, midwives, doulas, or grandmothers (grannies), but whatever their names, they were women that have and still are providing the support necessary for successful birthing and breast-feeding experiences. As immigrants continue to pour into the United States and American-born women adhering to their traditional cultural heritage attempt to make informed decisions regarding infant-feeding practices, it is imperative as nurses to examine specific cultural norms and practices that influence breast-feeding outcomes as we work to develop successful strategies.

Cultural Issues Related to Domestic Violence During Pregnancy

Domestic violence has emerged as one of the most significant health care threats for women and their unborn children. Numerous issues cross all cultural boundaries and influence the prevalence and response to domestic violence. These include a history of family violence, sexual abuse experienced as a child, alcohol and drug abuse by the mother or significant other, shame associated with abuse, fear of retaliation by the abuser, or fear of financial implications if the mother leaves the abuser, to cite a few. Outcomes of abuse shared by these women regardless of culture include stress (physical and emotional), poor lifestyle health practices, delayed prenatal care, and lack of support. Champion and Salazar (2008) studied health behavior in Mexican pregnant women with a history of violence and found that an experience of violence was associated with initiation of prenatal care, number of pregnancies, perception of barriers to care, and negative attitudes toward pregnancy.

A shocking study by Shadigian and Bauer (2005) identified homicide as a leading cause of pregnancy-associated death and suicide also as an important cause of death among pregnant and recently pregnant women. Health care providers must now acknowledge and understand that homicide is a leading cause of pregnancy-associated death, most commonly as a result of partner violence. Obviously, screening for both partner violence and suicidal ideation are essential components of comprehensive health and nursing care for women during and after pregnancy.

It has been documented for some time in the literature (Bewley & Gibbs, 1994) that physical abuse during pregnancy focuses on attack on the abdomen, breasts, and/or genitals, which puts not only the mother, but also the unborn child

at risk. Along with the physical abuse come the psychological consequences, including possible addiction to drugs and alcohol, stress, and depression. These factors not only affect the mother's health but can have a future effect on the newborn and later as the child develops. Many forms of abuse in the pregnant population warrant attention and discussion. However, this discussion will focus on three culturally different groups of women who may experience **domestic violence during pregnancy.** They are Hispanic, African American, and American Indian pregnant women. What links these groups of pregnant women are shared ideologies or characteristics that influence their behavior and have profound effects on their pregnancy outcomes. Ideologies of each group will be examined and recommendations identified for nurses working with these vulnerable pregnant women in these unique circumstances.

Information regarding women in abusive situations is scarce, partly because of underreporting. Important information we do know is that abused women are less likely to seek health care because their abuser limits access to resources and that battering occurs more frequently during pregnancy. This has implications for the pregnant woman and places her in double jeopardy, not only for herself, but also for her unborn baby as battering of pregnant women has long been associated with adverse pregnancy outcomes. In a National Violence Against Women study sponsored by the National Institute of Justice and the Centers for Disease Control and Prevention, it was estimated that 1.9 million women in the United States are assaulted annually (Tjadin & Thoennes, 1998; Rynerson, 2000). During pregnancy, 25 to 45% of women are beaten, and it is estimated that this percentage may be increasing (Rynerson, 2000).

An abused pregnant woman has a greater risk of delivering a LBW infant. One of the associations between abuse and LBW is delay in obtaining prenatal care. Indeed, findings from studies conducted during the past two decades have clearly shown that physical and sexual abuse predicts poor health during pregnancy and the postpartum period (Leserman, Stewart, & Dell, 1999). Taggert's and Mattson's 1996 study of the relationship between battering and prenatal care is still pertinent for nurses who care for pregnant women. Evidence-Based Practice 5-4 discusses this study and its importance in identifying delays in obtaining prenatal care as a result of battering.

The legacy of patriarchy, which is still deeply embedded in our culture, undoubtedly contributes to violence against women as do other factors, especially alcohol and drug abuse. Other issues associated with violence against women also influence pregnancy outcomes. These include exposure to physical harm or death, delayed prenatal care because of restricted access by the abuser, restricted support-seeking behaviors, and exposure to drugs and alcohol. Recommendations for health care providers will follow each discussion and will emphasize the importance of culturally competent care to these at-risk clients.

Hispanic Pregnant Women

Although there are many different Hispanic groups, they do share some important commonalities, for example, religion, customs, and language. As with any cultural group, differences do exist among the members. The incidence of spouse abuse among pregnant Hispanic women is not clear in the literature. However, we have known for a long time that, although violence during pregnancy is likely to be the most common form of family violence, it is also the least reported (Richwald & McClusky, 1985). Access to health care for pregnant Hispanic women is problematic. Barriers to prenatal health care include lack of health care insurance, language barriers, and low levels of education, all of which may encourage the use of traditional healers and remedies and might foster mistrust of health care professionals, leading to noncompliance. Hispanic women tend to be in low-paying jobs whose annual earnings are considerably less than those of non-Hispanic women. They also have less education than White women

---

EVIDENCE-BASED PRACTICE 5-4

Prenatal Care Delays Related to Battering

This study evaluated patterns of abuse during the pregnancies of 132 African American, 208 Hispanic, and 162 White American women from low-income clinics in large metropolitan cities in the West. The researchers found that the incidence of abuse did not vary significantly among ethnic groups and that the abused women from these groups sought prenatal care 6.5 weeks later than did the nonabused group. In this study, 1 in 4 women reported that they had been physically abused since their current pregnancy began, with African American women experiencing the most severe and most frequent abuse.

Clinical Application

- Include questions about abuse in every routine history taken during pregnancy in order to identify abused women.
- Offer information about abuse and available community resources. Women reporting abuse will need further screening with specific tools. Nurses should be aware of subtle signs of abuse. For example, psychosomatic complaints, injuries inconsistent with the explanation, failure to keep clinic appointments, and overprotective partners might be indications of abuse.
- Become familiar with community resources for referrals.

Reference: Taggart, L., & Mattson, S. (1996). Delay in prenatal care as a result of battering in pregnancy: Crosscultural implications. *Health Care for Women International, 17*, 25–34.

and live in large, extended households, often made up of several children and extended family members. The economic status of Hispanics, and therefore their health status, is closely tied to economic levels because economic status has determined access to care during the past decades (Suarez & Ramirez, 1999; Center for American Progress Action Fund, 2010). These many factors place Hispanic women at a distinct disadvantage when it comes to accessing prenatal care. Furthermore, these same factors tend to discourage the pregnant Hispanic woman from disclosing a situation of abuse and violence. Her choices are the same as those of other women in abusive situations: She can try to make the relationship work, or she can leave her abuser. If you are poor, have no friends or family members nearby, and have several little children who depend on you, leaving the family provider will be very difficult.

The Hispanic pregnant woman who chooses to leave her abuser must face the reality of language barriers, a poor economic situation, no insurance, and perhaps leaving her traditional family support network. These same factors inhibit the seeking of information regarding resources available to abused women. Even when faced with death, some abused women find it very difficult to expose their private situation to someone outside their cultural circle. Furthermore, certain groups of Hispanic women, such as migrants, are at higher risk because they are separated from family support systems in addition to confronting barriers related to poverty and language.

Nurses and other health practitioners in prenatal clinics are in an ideal position to facilitate a trusting relationship with an abused woman. Good assessment skills are crucial, because the first sign of abuse might not be an admission of abuse but physical findings of trauma. It is also helpful that the nurses have strong interpersonal skills and a genuine interest in Hispanic culture. In this situation, a Spanish-speaking health care provider might be able to form a trusting relationship more quickly, enabling the woman to share information about domestic violence. Recommendations for

assistance of abused pregnant Hispanic women include working with and mobilizing support, using the family and kinship structure, educating the abused woman regarding available resources for abused women, encouraging the woman's inner strength, and assisting in the development of skills necessary to mobilize resources.

African American Pregnant Women

Many cultural values of African Americans emphasize the larger Black society rather than focusing on individuals, making "all" collectively responsible for one another (Hine & Thompson, 1998). Therefore, many African American women exist in a social context supported by social connectedness versus that of autonomy. It is difficult to be specific about an assessment of factors related to domestic violence among African American women because of the lack of information. However, poor economic conditions might be a primary reason why violence occurs in African American families because often domestic violence is related to social and economic resources. The risk of wife abuse is thought to increase when the woman has a higher educational status than her partner or when the man is unemployed or has trouble keeping a job. This has long been identified as a familiar social situation in African American male–female relationships (Barnes, 1999).

One of the most difficult barriers confronting African American abused women who attempt to get help from police or from the legal system is the stereotypical view that violence among African Americans is normal. This view can lead to an unequal response to African American victims of violence. Since this behavior might be viewed as "normal," it could be dismissed or ignored.

Again, the nurse in the prenatal setting is in an ideal position to gather information and initiate a trusting relationship. As has been pointed out, the abused pregnant African American woman might not be willing to incriminate her spouse or significant other because she already sees him as a "victim of society." The nurse might need to rely heavily on her assessment and history-taking skills, being particularly alert to instances of trauma and to problems with past pregnancies. Education must stress that although the women see their men as "victims," women cannot and must not tolerate abuse. The nurse can identify shelter facilities in the woman's neighborhood and in other areas. If the woman feels uncomfortable going outside her neighborhood (and many do for fear they will not be understood outside their culture) the nurse can encourage her to go to members of her extended family, which might be more acceptable within African American culture. What is most important is that she has a plan of what to do, where to go, and who to call for help the next time she is afraid for her own safety. Last, the nurse must realize that in most instances, African American women believe that it is the responsibility of the woman to maintain the family, regardless of other factors. Therefore, African American women may be more likely to stay in an abusive relationship.

American Indian Pregnant Women

Violence within families has not always been part of American Indian society. Before contact with Europeans, American Indian society was based on harmony and respect for nature and all living things, sharing, and cooperation. Contributions from both sexes were valued, and many activities were shared, including the roles of warrior and hunter. As Indian communities strive to maintain cultural ties, the concepts of spirituality (balance, harmony, oneness), passive forbearance (humility, respect, circularity, connection, honor), and behaviors that promote harmonious living are reinforced in daily living (Nichols, 2004). Traditionally, cruelty to women and children resulted in public humiliation and loss of honor. Cultural disintegration, poverty, isolation, racism, and alcoholism are just a few of the problems that have fostered violence in American Indian cultures. Nevertheless, despite its prevalence, cruelty to women and children continues to be viewed by American Indians as a social disgrace (Green, 1996). In a recent study by Bohn (2002), the complicating factor of lifetime abuse events was shown to be a significant contributor to preterm birth and LBW infants. This means that the nurse

should not only assess for current abuse by the spouse or significant other, but also evaluate the other types of abuse inflicted over the lifetime of the mother, such as alcohol or drug abuse. Since the 1970s, American Indian tribes have made an effort to develop programs to meet the many needs of their communities. However, violence against women has not been addressed adequately because of the male-dominated leadership, other needs of the tribes, and the shame associated with abuse (Bohn, 1993). This trend is changing gradually as Indian communities have recognized that domestic abuse is a significant social problem and are taking measures to address it.

Recommendations for health care providers include identification of the abused person by direct questioning in a private setting, following the establishment of a trusting relationship with a health care provider; assessment of the woman's chart or medical record may provide an opening for discussion of abuse-related questions. A physical exam may identify signs of abuse, for example, injuries to the abdomen, breasts, or genitals, and a thorough history may identify signs of depression, alcohol and/or drug abuse, suicide attempts, eating disorders, miscarriages, and/or a history of complications of pregnancy.

In interviews with American Indian women, a sense of humor is most helpful because they view someone with whom they can laugh as easy to talk to. Open-ended questions are preferable. The nurse should also learn to become comfortable with periods of silence after questions. This does not mean that clients are not listening but rather just the opposite. These women think the question is worthy of thoughtful consideration before answering.

Once abuse has been identified, then the extent of abuse must be evaluated. The nurse must then intervene by providing information, discussing alternatives, and supporting the woman in her decision. Options should focus on Native American resources because such resources have usually been designed to be culturally sensitive. If only non-Indian resources are available, the nurse should follow through within these agencies. Variables to be considered in a discussion of options should include the woman's support system, her personal and cultural value system, and her financial status.

Abuse within Indian culture is traditionally handled within the family first. The abused woman might be reluctant to go outside for help because this might cause both families (hers and her spouse's or significant other's family members) to ostracize her. It is important to know that an American Indian woman considers it a virtue to stay with her mate no matter what the circumstance, especially if the marriage was performed or "blessed" by a traditional medicine man or woman. A woman who chooses to stay with her abuser might do so out of loyalty because he is Indian rather than because he is a man. It is essential to understand that when a woman attempts to leave an abusive relationship, she must know that her health care provider cares about her. Safety for the woman and her unborn baby is the priority. The woman will need phone numbers of shelters although transportation to a shelter may be a problem from the reservation. Like women in abusive situations elsewhere, having a plan to exit the situation is very important. Other resources are also necessary. Information related to drug and alcohol counseling, legal advise as well as information about job training and educational opportunities would be important to provide to the woman. It is important to focus on the woman's strengths, her sense of humor, and her skills and resources. She must be able to believe that both she and her abuser will heal.

SUMMARY

Culture, as it relates to pregnancy and childbirth, was discussed from many vantage points. Biologic and cultural variations that can affect childbearing outcomes were identified and analyzed. Women choosing alternative childbearing lifestyles were examined. The importance of nontraditional support systems to pregnant women, along with discussions of cultural beliefs and practices as they relate to pregnancy, birth, and the postpartum period, were presented with suggestions for care.

Vulnerable pregnant populations at risk for abuse were selected for discussion, including Hispanic, African American, and American Indian pregnant women. Culturally appropriate nursing care recommendations were offered for each cultural group.

Cultural beliefs and practices are continuously evolving, making it necessary for the nurse to acknowledge the various cultures and explore the meaning of childbearing with each family with whom she has contact. It is also important to remember that behavior must be evaluated from within each person's cultural context so that the care provided is not only knowledge based but meaningful. It is always important for the culturally competent nurse to demonstrate genuine concern, interest, and respect for clients' differing backgrounds. Only when these aspects are fully realized can we develop and provide culturally appropriate care for childbearing women and their families.

REVIEW QUESTIONS

1. List the biologic variations discussed and the implications for nursing care of the childbearing woman and her family.
2. Identify nursing interventions for women who relinquish infants during the postpartum period. Identify the typical cultural values in North American society about women who relinquish their infants.
3. Describe the special needs of lesbian couples during the childbearing process. What are common pejorative values about lesbian mothers?
4. Compare traditional Western medical support for pregnant women with nontraditional support, and describe why both might be critical for successful pregnancy outcomes in culturally diverse women.
5. Describe the differences between prescriptive and restrictive beliefs of a mother's behavior during pregnancy.
6. Describe two barriers that African American women face as they attempt to get help in abusive situations.
7. Describe the issues for consideration when developing a breast-feeding program for a traditional American Indian community.

CRITICAL THINKING ACTIVITIES

1. Critically analyze the culturally competent nursing interventions for a Hispanic woman after fetal demise from a cord accident.

2. Analyze the responses the culturally competent postpartum nurse should initiate when an African American woman refuses to get out of bed and shower?

3. Discuss and critically analyze how you would respond to your labor patient's request to allow her lesbian partner to participate in the birth of their child. What activities would you include in the plan of care? Why?

4. Describe and analyze how the nurse might offer culturally appropriate support to an Orthodox Jewish husband who has followed his cultural traditions and refuses to accept his newborn from a female nurse.

REFERENCES

Affonso, D., De, A., Horowitz, J., & Mayberry, L. (2000). An international study exploring levels of postpartum depressive symptomatology. *Journal of Psychosomatic Research, 49*, 207–216.

Almroth, S., Mohale, M., & Latham, M. C. (2000). Unnecessary water supplementation for babies: Grandmothers blame clinics. *Acta Paediatrican, 89,* 1408–1413.

American Psychiatric Association (2000). *Diagnostic and statistical manual of mental disorders* (4th ed., text revision). Washington, DC: Author.

Amnesty International, USA (2010). Deadly delivery: The maternal health care crises in the USA. AMR 51/007/2010.

Andrews, M. M., & Hanson, P. A. (2008). Religion, culture and nursing. In: M. M. Andrews, & J. S. Boyle (Eds.), *Transcultural concepts in nursing* (4th ed., pp. 432–502). Philadelphia: Lippincott, Williams & Wilkins.

Bachman, J. A. (2000). Management of discomfort. In: D. L. Lowdermilk, S. E. Perry, & I. M. Bobak (Eds.), *Maternity and women's health care* (7th ed., pp. 463–487). St. Louis, MO: Mosby.

Banks, J. W. (2003). Ka'nistenhsera Teiakotihsnie's: A native community rekindles the tradition of breastfeeding. *AWHONN Lifelines, 7*(4), 340–347.

Barnes, D. B., & Murphy S. (2009). Reproductive decisions for women with HIV: Motherhood's role in envisioning a future. *Qualitative Health Research, 19*(4), 481–491.

Barnes, S. Y. (1999). Theories of spouse abuse: Relevance to African Americans. *Issues in Mental Health Nursing, 20,* 357–371.

Bash, D. M. (1980). Jewish religious practices related to childbearing. *Journal of Nurse-Midwifery, 25*(5), 39–42.

Berry, A. B. (1999). Mexican American women's expressions of the meaning of culturally congruent prenatal care. *Journal of Transcultural Nursing, 10*(3), 203–212.

Bewley, C., & Gibbs, A. (1994). Coping with domestic violence in pregnancy. *Nursing Standard, 8*(50), 25–28.

Bohn, D. K. (1993). Nursing care of Native American battered women. *AWHONN's Clinical Issues in Perinatal and Women's Health Nursing,* 4(3), 424–436.

Bohn, D. K. (2002). Lifetime and current abuse, pregnancy risks, and outcomes among Native American women. *Journal of Health Care for the Poor and Underserved, 13*(2), 184–198.

Boyle, J. S., & Mackey, M. (1999). Pica: Sorting it out. *Journal of Transcultural Nursing, 10*(1), 65–68.

Bromwich, P., & Parsons, T. (1990). *Contraception: The facts* (2nd ed.). Oxford: Oxford University Press.

Buchholz, S. (2000). Experiences of lesbian couples during childbirth. *Nursing Outlook, 48*(6), 307–311.

CDC. *Unintended pregnancy prevention, home.* Retrieved January 5, 2007, from http://www.cdc.gov/reproductivehealth/UnintendedPregnancy/index.htm

CDC, Division of Reproductive Health and the National Center for Chronic Disease Prevention and Health Promotion. (2006). Retrieved January 5, 2007, from http://www.cdc.gov.

Callister, L. C., Semenic, S., & Foster, J. C. (1999). Cultural and spiritual meanings of childbirth: Orthodox Jewish and Mormon women. *Journal of Holistic Nursing, 17*(3), 280–295.

Callister, L. C., & Vega, R. (1998). Giving birth: Guatemalan women's voices. *Journal of Obstetric, Gynecologic, and Neonatal Nursing, 27,* 289–295.

Center for American Progress Action Fund (2010). Retrieved April 22, 2010 from http://www.amerianprogressaction.org/issues.2010/03/hispanic_health.html

Chalmers, B., & Wolman, W. (1993). Social support in labour—A selective review. *Journal of Psychosomatic Obstetrics Gynaecology, 14,* 1–15.

Chamberlain, J. (n.d.). *The Pima Indians: The vicious cycle.* Retrieved January 3, 2007, from National Institutes of Health, National Institute of Diabetes and Digestive and Kidney Diseases Web site: http://diabetes.niddk.nih.gov/dm/pubs/pima/vicious/vicious.htm

Champion, J. D., & Salazar, B. C. (2008). Health behaviour in Mexican pregnant women with a history of violence. *Western Journal of Nursing Research, 30*(8), 1005–1018.

Chen, Y. C. (2001). Chinese values, health and nursing. *Journal of Advanced Nursing, 36,* 270–273.

Clemings, R. (2001). Fresno's Hmong leave for new lives. *Fresno Bee*, pp. A1, A12.

Committee on Cultural Psychiatry (2002). *Cultural assessment in clinical psychiatry*. Washington, DC: American Psychiatric Publishing.

Dettwyler, K. A. (2004). When to wean: Biological versus cultural perspectives. *Clincial Obstetrics and Gynecology, 47*(3), 712–723.

Diabetes Monitor (2005). *Health Problems in American India/Alaska Native women: Diabetes*. Retrieved April 25, 2010 from http://www.diabetesmonitor.com/b350.htm.

Dickason, E. J., Silverman, B. L., & Schult, M. O. (1994). *Maternal infant nursing care* (2nd ed.). St. Louis, MO: Mosby.

Dodgson, J. E., Duckett, L., Garwick, A., & Graham, B. (2002). An ecological perspective of breastfeeding in an indigenous community. *Journal of Nursing Scholarship, 34*(3), 235–241.

Feng, D., Zhang, Y., & Owen, D. (2007). Health behaviors of low-income pregnant minority women. *Western Journal of Nursing Research, 29,* 284–300.

Finer, L. B. (2006). Disparities in rates of unintended pregnancy in the United States, 1994 and 2001. *Perspectives on Sexual Reproductive Health, 38,* 90–96.

Fok, D. (1996). Cross cultural practice and its influence on breastfeeding—The Chinese culture. *Breastfeeding Review, 4*(1), 13–18.

Green, K. (1996). *Family violence in aboriginal communities: An aboriginal perspective*. Ottawa, ON: National Clearing House on Family Violence.

Gordon, N. P., Walton, D., McAdam, E., Derman, J., Gallitero, G., & Garrett, L. (1999). Effects of providing hospital based doulas in health maintenance organization births. *Obstetrics and Gynecology, 98,* 756–764.

Gunger, I., & Beji, N. K. (2007). Effects of fathers' attendance to labor and delivery on the experience of childbirth in Turkey. *Western Journal of Nursing Research, 29,* 213–231.

Hannon, P. R., Willis, S. K., Bishop-Townsend, V., Martinez, I. M., & Scrimshaw, S. C. (2000). African-American and Latina adolescent mothers' infant feeding decisions and breastfeeding practices: A qualitative study. *Journal of Adolescent Health, 26*(6), 399–407.

Helsel, D., & Mochel, M. (2002). Afterbirths in the afterlife: Cultural meaning of placental disposal in a Hmong American community. *Journal of Transcultural Nursing, 13*(4), 282–286.

Hine, D. C., & Thompson, K. (1998). *A shining thread of hope*. New York: Broadway Books.

Horn, B. M. (1981). Cultural concepts and postpartal care. *Nursing and Health Care, 2*(9), 516–517.

Ingalsbe, K. S. (1999). *Infant feeding practices of Japanese and Mexican mothers who live in the United States*. Unpublished doctoral dissertation, Saint Louis University.

Jirapaet, V. (2001). Factors affecting maternal role attainment among low-income, Thai, HIV-positive mothers. *Journal of Transcultural Nursing, 12*(1), 25–33.

Kolatch, A. (2000). *The second Jewish book of why*. Middle Village, NY: Jonathan David.

Kulwicki, A. (2008). People of Arab heritage. In: L. Purnell, & B. Paulanka (Eds.). *Transcultural health care: A culturally competent approach* (3rd ed., pp. 113–128). Philadelphia: F.A. Davis Co.

Lagana, K. (2003). Come bien, camina y no se preocupe—Eat right, walk and do not worry: Selective biculturalism during pregnancy in a Mexican American Community. *Journal of Transcultural Nursing, 14*(2), 117–124.

Lauderdale, J., & Boyle, J. (1994). Infant relinquishment through adoption. *Image Journal of Nursing Scholarship, 26*(3), 213–217.

Leserman, J., Stewart, J., & Dell, D. (1999). Sexual and physical abuse predicts poor health in pregnancy and postpartum. *Psychosomatic Medicine, 61,* 92.

Lewis, J. A. (2003). Jewish perspectives on pregnancy and childbearing. *The American Journal of Maternal/Child Nursing, 28*(5), 306–312.

Lori, J. R., & Boyle, J. S. (2011). Cultural childbirth practices, beliefs, and traditions in post-conflict Liberia. *Health Care for Women International, 32*(6), 1–20.

Ludwig-Beymer, P. (2008). Transcultural aspects of pain. In: M.M. Andrews, & J.S. Boyle (Eds.), *Cultural aspects of nursing care* (pp. 329–354). Philadelphia: Wolters Kluwer Health/Lippincott Williams & Wilkins.

Luker, K. C. (1999). A reminder that human behavior frequently refuses to conform to models created by researchers. *Family Planning Perspectives, 31*(5), 248–249.

Martin, J. A., Hamilton, B. E., Sutton, P. D., Ventura, S. J., Menacker, F., & Munson, M. L. (2004). Births: Final date for 2002 [Data file]. *National Vital Statistics Reports, 52*(10). Available from CDC Web site, http://www.cdc.gov.

McEwen, M. M., Baird, M., Pasvogel, A., & Gallegos, G. (2007). Health–illness transition experiences among Mexican immigrant women with diabetes. *Family and Community Health, 30*(3), 201–212.

McKee, M. D., Zayas, L. H., & Jankowski, K. R. B. (2004). Breastfeeding intention and practice in an urban minority population: Relationship to maternal depressive symptoms and mother–infant closeness. *Journal of Reproductive and Infant Psychology, 22*(3), 167–181.

McManus, A. J., Hunter, L. P., & Renn, H. (2006). Lesbian experiences and needs during childbirth: Guidance for health care providers. *Journal of Obstetric, Gynecologic and Neonatal Nursing, 35*(1), 13–23.

Miller, M. A. (1992). Contraception outside North America: Options and popular choices. *NAACOG's Clinical Issues in Perinatal and Women's Health Nursing, 3*(2), 253–265.

Morgan, M. (1996). Prenatal care of African American women in selected USA urban and rural cultural contexts. *Journal of Transcultural Nursing, 7*(2), 3–9.

Nichols, L. A. (2004). The infant caring process among Cherokee mothers. *Journal of Holistic Nursing, 22*(3), 1–28.

Noble, A., Rom, M., Newsome-Wicks, M., Engelhardt, K., & Woloski-Wruble, A. (2009). Jewish laws, customs, and practice in labor, delivery and postpartum care. *Journal of Transcultural Nursing, 20,* 323–333.

Otoide, V. O., Oronsaye, F., & Okonofua, F. E. (2001). Why Nigerian adolescents seek abortion rather than contraception: Evidence from focus-group discussions. *International Family Planning Perspectives, 27*(2), 77–81.

Overfield, T. (1985). *Biologic variation in health and illness*. Menlo Park, CA: Addison-Wesley.

Pacquiao, D.F. (2008). People of Filipino heritage. In: L. Purnell, & B. Paulanka (Eds.), *Transcultural health care:*

A culturally competent approach (3rd ed., pp. 175–195). Philadelphia: F.A. Davis Co.

Perry, S. E. (2000). Medical-surgical problems in pregnancy. In: D. L. Lowdermilk, S. E. Perry, & I. M. Bobak (Eds.), *Maternity and women's health care* (7th ed., pp. 887–911). St. Louis, MO: Mosby.

Pettitt, D. J., Baird, H. R., Aleck, K. A., Bennett, P. H., & Knowler, W. C. (1983). *New England Journal of Medicine, 308,* 242–245.

Polek, C. A., Hardie, T. L., & Crowley, E. M. (2008). Lesbians' disclosure of sexual orientation and satisfaction with care. *Journal of Transcultural Nursing, 19,* 243–249.

Posmontier, B., & Horowitz, J. (2004). Postpartum practices and depression prevalences: Technocentric and ethnokinship cultural perspectives. *Journal of Transcultural Nursing, 15*(1), 34–43.

Purnell, L., & Selekman, J. (2008). People of Jewish heritage. In: L. Purnell, & B. Paulanka (Eds.). *Transcultural health care: A culturally competent approach* (3rd ed., pp. 278–292). Philadelphia: F.A. Davis Co.

Reifsnider, E. L., & Luck, J. F. (2007). Breast feeding by Hispanic women. Journal of *Gynecologic & Neonatal Nursing, 38*(2), 244–252.

Renaud, M.T. (2007). We are mothers too: Childbearing experiences of lesbian families. *Journal of Obstetric Gynecological Neonatal Nursing, 36*(2), 190–199.

Richwald, G. A., & McClusky, T. E. (1985). Family violence during pregnancy. In: D. B. Jeliffe, & E. F. T. Jeliffe (Eds.), *Advances in international maternal and child health* (pp. 87–96). New York: Oxford University Press.

Rubin, R. (1984). *Maternal identity and the maternal experience.* New York: Springer.

Rynerson, B. C. (2000). Violence against women. In: D. L. Lowdermilk, S. E. Perry, & I. M. Bobak (Eds.), *Maternity and women's health care* (7th ed., pp. 225–246). St. Louis, MO: Mosby.

Santelli, J., Rochat, R., Hatfield-Timajchy, K., Gilbert, B., Curtis, K., & Cabral, R. (2003). The measurement and meaning of unintended pregnancy. *Perspectives on Sexual and Reproductive Health, 35*(2), 94–101.

Shadigian, E. M., & Bauer, S. T. (2005). Pregnancy-associated death: A qualitative systematic review of homicide and suicide. *Obstetrical and Gynecological Survey, 60*(3), 183–190.

Spector, R. (2008). *Cultural diversity in health and illness* (7th ed.). Upper Saddle River, NJ: Prentice Hall Health.

Spinks, V. S., Andrews, J., & Boyle, J. S. (2000). Providing health care for lesbian clients. *Journal of Transcultural Nursing, 11,* 137–143.

Stewart, S., & Jambunathan, J. (1996). Hmong women and postpartum depression. *Health Care for Women International, 17,* 319–330.

Suarez, L., & Ramirez, A. G. (1999). Hispanic/Latino health and disease. In: R. M. Huff, & M. V. Kline (Eds.), *Promoting health in multicultural populations* (pp. 115–136). Thousand Oaks, CA: Sage.

Susin, L. R., Giugliani, E., & Kummer, S. (2005). Influence of grandmothers on breastfeeding practices. *Revista de Saúde Pública/Journal of Public Health, 39*(2), 1–6.

Taggart, L., & Mattson, S. (1996). Delay in prenatal care as a result of battering in pregnancy: Crosscultural implications. *Health Care for Women International, 17,* 25–34.

Tiedje, L. B. (2000). Returning to our roots: 25 years of maternal/child nursing in the community. *Maternal/Child Nursing, 25*(6), 315–317.

The Pima Indians: Obesity and Diabetes. Retrieved April 25, 2010, from http://diabetes.niddk.nih.gov/dm/pubs/pima/obesity.htm

The New York Times (2010). *Obama widens medical rights for gay partners.* Retrieved April 25, 2010 from http://www.nytimes.com/2010/04/16/us/politics/16webhosp.html

Tjadin, P., & Thoennes, N. (1998). Prevalence, incidence and consequences of violence against women: Findings from the national violence against women survey. *U.S. Department of Justice Research in Brief.* Washington, D.C.: U.S. Department of Justice.

UNHCR. (2006). *Refugees by numbers 2006 edition. Basic facts.* Retrieved April 22, 2010, from http://www.unhcr.org/basics/BASICS/3b028097c.html#NUMBERS.

U.S. Department of Health and Human Services. (2000). With understanding and improving health and objectives for improving health. *Healthy People 2010* (2nd ed.). Washington DC: U.S. Government Printing Office.

U.S. News, & World Report (2010). *CNN Poll: Most Americans oppose gay marriage, but those under 35 back it.* Retrieved from http://www.usnews.com/news.blogs/god-and-country/2009/05/05cnn-poll-most-americans

Walsh, L. (2006). Beliefs and rituals in traditional birth attendant practice in Guatemala. *Journal of Transcultural Nursing, 17*(2), 148–154.

Washofsky, M. (2000). *Jewish living: A guide to contemporary reform practice.* New York: UAHC (Union of American Hebrew Congregations) Press.

Waxler-Morrison, N., Andrews, J., & Richardson, E. (1990). *Cross-cultural caring: A handbook for health professionals in Western Canada.* Vancouver, BC: University of British Columbia Press.

World Health Organization and UNICEF. (2004). *Global strategy for infant and young child feeding.* Geneva: Switzerland World Health Organization.

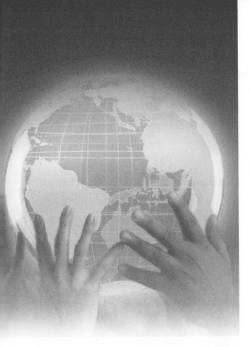

Transcultural Perspectives in the Nursing Care of Children

Barbara C. Woodring and
Margaret M. Andrews

KEY TERMS

Caida de la mollera (fallen fontanel)
Cosleeping
Cradleboard
Culture-bound syndromes
Curandero (male), *curandera* (female)
Empacho
Extended family
Ghost illness/possession
Infant attachment
Mal ojo
Nuclear family
Pandanus mat
Premasticate
Pujos
Susto

LEARNING OBJECTIVES

1. Analyze the impact of various cultural beliefs and practices on the development of children.
2. Examine the biocultural aspects of selected acute and chronic conditions affecting children.
3. Synthesize the transcultural concepts and evidence-based practices that support the delivery of culturally competent care for children and adolescents.

Children in a Culturally Diverse Society

Cultural survival depends on the transmission of values and customs from one generation to the next; this process relies on the presence of children for success. This interdependent nature of children and society reinforces the need for the greater society to nurture, care for, and socialize members of the next generation. In this chapter, the cultural influences on child growth, development, health, and illness will be examined. Figure 6-1—provides a visual representation of the interrelationship among culture, communication, and parental decisions/actions during child rearing. This schematic representation also serves as a model for understanding culturally significant decisions that affect the care of children and, therefore, will be evident throughout this chapter.

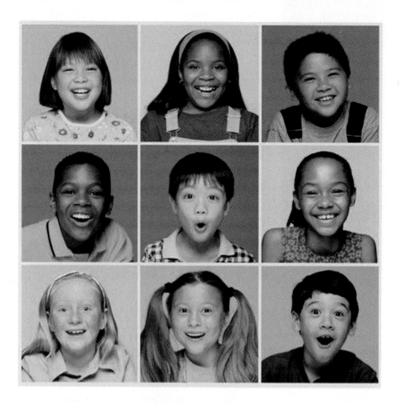

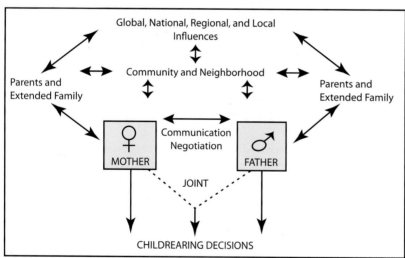

FIGURE 6-1   Model depicting the interrelation of culture, communication, and parental decisions about child-rearing practices.

Most children are cared for by their natural or adoptive parents. In this chapter the term parent refers to the primary care provider whether natural, adoptive, relational (grandparents, aunts, uncles, cousins), or those who are unrelated but who function as primary providers of care and/or parent surrogates for varying periods of time. In some cases, the primary provider of care looks after the infant, child, or adolescent for a brief time, perhaps for an hour or two, while the parents are unable to do so. In other cases, this person might function as a long-term or permanent parent substitute even though legal adoption has not occurred. For example, a grandparent might assume responsibility for a child in the event of parental death, illness, disability, or imprisonment. Health care providers should be aware that the same factors influencing the parents' cultural perspectives on child rearing also influence others who might assume the care of the child.

Children as a Population

Racial and Ethnic Composition

According to the U.S. Census Bureau (2009), there are 73.8 million people under the age of 18 who live in the United States; of these, 65% are White, 15% Hispanic (of any race), 13% Black, and 4% Asian/Pacific Islander/Native American/ Alaska Native. The number of Hispanic children has increased faster than that of any other group. It is estimated that by 2020, 40% of school-aged children in the United States will represent federal minority groups. More than 2 million children in the United States are foreign-born, and millions more are the children of recent immigrants. Many of these children constitute the more than 6 million school-age children who speak a language other than English at home. Approximately two-thirds of these children come from Spanish-speaking homes, and a large percentage of the remainder speak a variety of Asian languages. Many children of immigrants live in linguistic isolation in households where no member age 14 or older speaks English "very well," nationwide, 4% of children age 5 to 17 years live in such households (U.S. Census Bureau, 2009).

Although immigrants and their children are found throughout the United States and Canada, they tend to cluster in certain geographic areas. California, Texas, Illinois, and New York are homes for almost two-thirds of all foreign-born children. New Mexico, Arizona, New Jersey, and Florida also have relatively high numbers of children whose parents recently immigrated to the United States (U.S. Census Bureau, 2009). In Canada, most immigrants reside in one of the Canadian metropolitan areas. Toronto, Vancouver, and Montreal are home for the majority of children of recent immigrants (Statistics Canada, 2006).

Poverty

The impact of poverty on children's health is cumulative throughout the life cycle. The Life-Course Health Development framework (Halfron & Hochstein, 2002) indicates that disease in adulthood frequently is the result of early assaults to a child's health that becomes compounded over time. For example, when poverty leads to malnutrition during critical growth periods, either prenatally or during the first 2 years of life, the consequences can be catastrophic and irreversible, resulting in damage to the neurologic and musculoskeletal systems. If the brain fails to receive sufficient nutrients during critical growth periods, the child is likely to experience diminished cognitive development, leading to poor academic performance and later poorer job performance, lower pay, and thus perpetuation of the cycle of poverty and poor health.

Child poverty in the United States continues to grow even though 90% of poor children live in working families. In the United Stares one in six children (14 million) live in poverty, and a disproportionate number of these are from African American and Latino backgrounds. Children in mother-only families are five times as likely to be in poverty as those in married-couple families. Research links poverty to numerous risks and disadvantages for children, including increased abuse, neglect, lower reading scores, and overall less success in the classroom, failure, delinquency, malnutrition, and violence (Children's Defense Organization, 2009).

Children's Health Status

Indicators of child health status include birth weight, infant mortality, and immunization rates. In general, children from diverse cultural

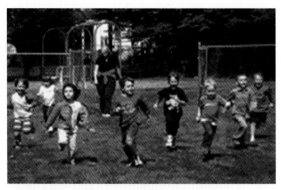

FIGURE 6-2 Children at play demonstrate common developmental milestones.

backgrounds have less favorable indicators of health status than their White counterparts. Health status is influenced by many factors, including access to health services. In 2009 the Children's Defense Fund reported 8.1 million children, one in ten, lived in working family households of U.S. citizens, but was uninsured and unable to attain appropriate health care. There are numerous barriers to quality health care services for children such as poverty, geography, lack of cultural competence by health care providers, racism, and other forms of prejudice. Families from diverse cultures (Figure 6-2) might experience difficulties in their interactions with nurses and other health care providers, and these difficulties might have an adverse impact on the delivery of health care. Because ethnic minorities are underrepresented among health care professionals, parents and children often have different cultural backgrounds from their health care providers (Goode & Jones, 2006; Goode, Hayewood, Wells, & Rhee, 2009).

Growth and Development

Although the growth and development of children are similar in all cultures, important racial, ethnic, and gender differences can be identified. From the moment of conception, the developmental processes of the human life cycle take place in the context of culture. Throughout life, culture exerts an all-pervasive influence on the developing infant, child, and adolescent. For example, there is cross-cultural similarity in the sequence, timing, and achievement of developmental milestones such as smiling, separation anxiety, and language acquisition. Developmental researchers who have worked in other cultures have become convinced that human functioning cannot be separated from the cultural and more immediate context in which children develop (Fleer, 2006). Figure 6-3 presents a model that summarizes the cultural factors that influence parental beliefs and practices related to child rearing.

Many developmental theories are based on observations of Western children and, therefore, may not have cross-cultural generalization. Investigations of the universality of the stages of development proposed by Piaget, the family role relations emphasized by Freud, and patterns of mother–infant interaction suggested by Bowlby to indicate security of attachment have resulted in modifications of the theories to reflect newer cross-cultural data.

Certain growth patterns appear across cultural boundaries. For example, regardless of culture, neuromuscular activities evolve from general-to-specific, from the center of the body to the extremities (proximal-to-distal development), and from the head to the toes (cephalocaudal development). Adult head size is reached by the age of 5 years, whereas the remainder of the body continues to grow through adolescence. Physiologic maturation of organ systems such as the renal, circulatory, and respiratory systems occurs early, whereas maturation of the central nervous system continues beyond childhood.

Other growth patterns seem to be specific to cultural groups. For example, in some cultures, the standard Western mobility pattern of sitting—creeping—crawling—standing—walking—squatting is not followed. The Balinese infant goes from sitting to squatting to standing. Hopi (Native American) children begin walking 1 to 2 months later than Anglo-American children. Tooth eruption occurs earlier in Asian and African American infants than in their White counterparts.

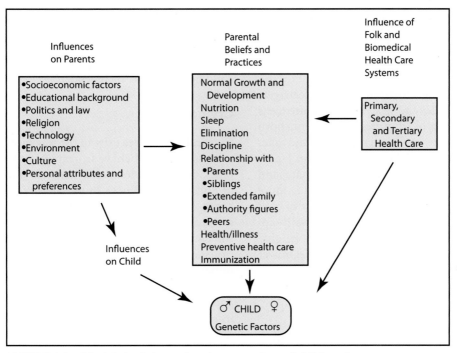

FIGURE 6-3   Model depicting cultural perspectives of child rearing.

Height and Weight

In the United States, African American and White children differ in mean birth weight, with African Americans being 181 to 240 grams lighter. This explains, in part, why low birth weight/prematurity (birth weight less than 2,500 g) appears twice as frequently in African Americans as it does in Whites. Chinese, Filipinos, Hawaiians, Japanese, and Puerto Ricans also have lower mean birth weights than Whites in the United States. Intertribal variation in the birth weights of Native American children also occurs; Hopi infant girls weigh about 400 grams less at birth than Cheyenne infant girls. Native North Americans from British Columbia and Northwestern Ontario have higher mean birth weights than non-Native Canadians. Overall, Native North Americans have a larger number of infants weighing 4,000 g or more at birth—a fact that is believed to be associated with the high incidence of diabetes in Native North Americans (Overfield, 1995).

Although it is difficult to separate nongenetic from genetic influences, some populations are shorter or taller than others during various periods of growth and in adulthood. African American infants are approximately three-fourths of an inch shorter at birth than Whites. In general, African American and White children are tallest, followed by Native Americans; Asian children are the shortest. Children of higher socioeconomic status are taller in all cultures. Data on African American and White children between 1 and 6 years old show that at age 6, African Americans are taller than Whites. Around age 9 or 10 years, White boys begin to catch up in height. White girls catch up with their African American counterparts around 14 or 15 years of age. African American children have longer legs in proportion to height than other groups (Overfield, 1995). During puberty, growth in African American children begins to slow down, and White children catch up so that the two races achieve similar heights in adulthood. The growth spurt of adolescence involves the skeletal and muscular systems, leading to significant changes in size and strength in both sexes but particularly in boys. White North American youths age 12 to 18 years are 22 to 33 pounds heavier and 6 inches taller than Filipino youths the same age. African American teenagers are somewhat taller and heavier than White teens up to age 15 years old. Japanese adolescents born in the United States or Canada are larger and taller than Japanese who are born and raised in Japan, primarily due to differences in diet, climate, and social milieu (Overfield, 1995). To provide more consistent comparisons of height/weight of children, the WHO has developed universally approved benchmarks for age-appropriate height/weight measures (deOnis et al., 2007; deOnis et al., 2009; WHO, 2009).

Infant Attachment

When **infant attachment** is examined, cross-cultural differences become apparent. Researchers have discovered that German and Anglo-American mothers expect early autonomy in the child and have fewer physical interventions as the child plays, thus encouraging exploration and independence. Japanese children are seldom separated from their mother and there is close physical interaction with the child. Similarly, Puerto Rican and Dominican mothers display close mother–child relationships with more verbal and physical expression of affection than European American parents (Reebye, Ross, & Jamison, 2009). Anglo-American mothers tend to give greater emphasis to qualities associated with the mainstream American ideal of individualism such as autonomy, self-control, and activity, whereas Puerto Rican mothers describe children in terms congruent with Puerto Rican culture; emphasis is placed on relatedness (e.g., affection, dignity, respectfulness, responsiveness to mother) and proximity seeking. Studies suggest that differences in infant attachment are linked to cultural variations in parenting behavior and life experiences. The development of African children is strongly related to the nutritional status of the child: those who tend to be malnourished have lessened attachment (DeWar, 2008). Parental socialization, values, beliefs, goals, and behaviors are determined in large measure by how culture defines good parenting and preferred child behaviors for each gender.

Crying

Cultural differences exist in the way mothers perceive, react, and behave in response to their infants' cues, behaviors, and demands. Knowledge of cultural differences in parental responses to crying is relevant for nurses as assessment of the severity of an infant's distress is often based on the parent's interpretation of the crying. The seriousness of a problem may be overestimated or underestimated because of cultural variations in perception of the infant's distress. The degree of parental concern toward an infant may be misinterpreted if one's cultural beliefs and practices differ from those of the parent (DeWar, 2009). For example, in Asian and Latino cultures the male child is expected to maintain strong control over their emotions, and not cry in the presence of others; therefore, a child crying in pain may be interpreted one way by a nurse and dismissed as inappropriate by a parent.

Culture-Universal and Culture-Specific Child Rearing

The values, attitudes, beliefs, and practices of one's culture affect the way parents and other providers of care relate to a child during various developmental stages. In all cultures, infants and children are valued and nurtured because they represent the promise of future generations. From the moment of birth, differentiation between the sexes is recognized. The early differentiation of gender roles is manifested in gender-specific tasks, play, and dress (Figure 6-4). Throughout infancy, childhood, and adolescence, girls and boys undergo a process of socialization aimed at preparing them to assume adult roles in the larger society into which they

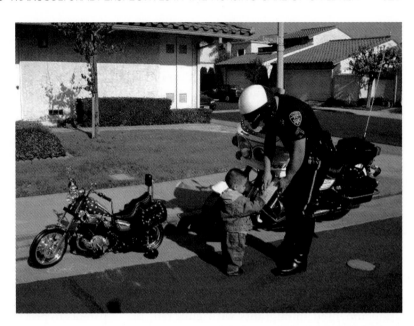

FIGURE 6-4 There is an early differentiation of gender-specific tasks, play, and dress.

have been born or to which they have migrated. As children grow and develop, their communications/interactions occur within a cultural context. That which is considered acceptable is strongly influenced by parental education, social expectation, religious background, and cultural ties. However, all parents want to be treated respectfully by their children and want their children to show respect toward others, thus becoming a source of pride and honor to their family and cultural heritage.

There are many universal child-rearing practices, but most research has focused on specific cultural differences rather than on similarities. It is important to distinguish between cultural practices and those that reflect the economic well-being of the family, for example, the stereotypes that suggest that teenage pregnancy is more common and more acceptable among African Americans than among counterparts in other cultures. When socioeconomic factors are considered, the myth is shattered. Although African American adolescents from the lower socioeconomic groups have higher rates of teen pregnancy, this is not true for middle- and upper-income African Americans.

Although not an exhaustive review of child-rearing customs, the following discussion will focus on clinically significant child-rearing behaviors among families from diverse cultures. Special consideration will be given to nutrition, sleep, elimination, parent–child relationships, and discipline.

Nutrition: Feeding and Eating Behaviors

In many cultures, breast-feeding is traditionally practiced for varying lengths of time ranging from several weeks to several years. The growing availability and convenience of extensively marketed prepared formula have resulted in a decrease in the number of women who attempt to breast-feed.

Some cultural feeding practices might result in threats to the infant's health. The practice of propping a bottle filled with milk, juice, or carbonated beverages to quiet a child or lull them to sleep is known to result in dental caries; this practice should be discouraged. In some cultures, mothers **premasticate**, or chew, food for young children in the belief that this will facilitate digestion. This practice, most frequently reported among Black and Hispanic mothers, is of questionable benefit and may transmit infection from the mother's mouth to the baby.

Health status is dependent in part on nutritional intake, thus integrally linking the child's nutritional status and wellness. Although the United States is the world's greatest food-producing nation, nutritional status has not been a priority for many people in this country. An estimated 1 million children in the United States experience malnutrition. Malnutrition is described as undernutrition (not enough essential nutrients or nutrients excreted too rapidly) or overnutrition (eating too much of the wrong food or not excreting enough food) (WHO, 2009). Malnutrition may be serious enough to interfere with neuro- and musculoskeletal development. Some parents of refugee children, undocumented immigrants with children, or parents of children living below poverty level may be unable to provide their children with an adequate and/or appropriate food intake. However, malnutrition is not exclusive to children from poor, lower socioeconomic groups. By definition many middle- and upper-income families have obese children who are also malnourished. Obesity frequently begins during infancy, when mothers succumb to cultural pressures to overfeed. For example, among many who identify themselves as Filipino, Vietnamese, and Mexican, to name a few cultures, fat babies generally are considered healthy babies. In most African tribes, fat babies are considered healthy, and mild to moderate obesity is considered a sign of affluence and health later in life.

The popularity of fast-food restaurants and "junk" foods has resulted in a high-calorie, high-fat, high-cholesterol, and high-carbohydrate diet for many children. Parents are frequently involved in numerous activities outside the house and have little time for traditional tasks such as cooking or seating the family together for a meal. Because fast foods have some intrinsic nutritional value, their benefit should be evaluated on the basis of age-specific requirements. Poverty forces many parents to provide inexpensive substitutes for the expensive, often unavailable, essential nutrients. These lower nutrient, high fat, high calorie foods are referred to as "empty calories" and have led to the recently documented epidemic of childhood obesity. As exhibited in Figure 6-5, the prevalence of childhood obesity among various cultural and ethnic groups within the United States was described by Anderson and Whitaker (2009) and Harbaugh

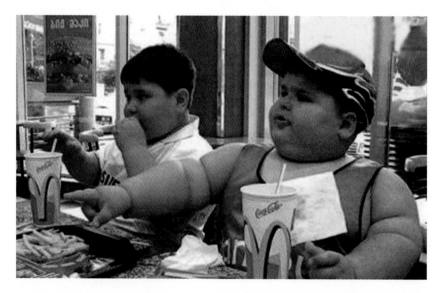

FIGURE 6-5 Childhood obesity is often initiated or reinforced through diets of "fast foods."

and Jordan (2009). The reported weight-for-age imbalance among preschool, school-age, and adolescent African American children was especially disturbing and purports serious complications of hypertension, diabetes, and cardiovascular disease for young Black adults.

The extent to which families retain their cultural practices at mealtime varies widely; an example of this can be found in Evidence-Based Practice 6-1. Because a hospitalized child's recovery might be enhanced by familiar foods, nurses need to assess the influence of culture on eating habits. For hospitalized children, you should foster an environment that closely simulates the home (e.g., use of chopsticks rather than silverware). Family members can be encouraged to visit during mealtime; depending upon the child's condition, food may be brought from home and/or the family encouraged to eat with the child if this is appropriate. For example, most Asian parents believe that children should be fed separately from adults and that they should acquire "good table manners" by the time they are 5 years old; these practices can be supported during hospitalization.

In many cultures illness is viewed as a punishment for an evil act, while fasting (abstaining from solid food and sometimes liquids) is viewed as penance for evil. A situation may become dangerous, and even deadly, should a parent view the child's illness as an "evil" event and consequently withhold food and/or water. Dehydration rapidly occurs and malnutrition may quickly follow. These dangerous issues may require legal intervention to protect the child and may produce difficult, culturally insensitive outcomes. Nurses

---

EVIDENCE-BASED PRACTICE 6-1

Best Practices for Preventing Overweight and Obesity in Children from Diverse Cultures

Obesity leads to chronic disease and poor health. Childhood obesity has risen to epidemic proportions in Western industrialized nations. Experts agree that prevention is the best method of curbing the obesity in children. Promoting and protecting the health of children and adolescents in the wake of the growing obesity epidemic requires a comprehensive and carefully constructed plan that draws on past and present research in the area of obesity management. The investigator conducted a meta-analysis of research garnered from experts in the areas of child health, immigrant health care, public health, psychology, nutrition, exercise, and health policy on the best ways to prevent and treat obesity in children.

Clinical Application

- Childhood obesity programs in clinics and schools are helpful in reducing chronic disease risk factor levels (blood fat/cholesterol, blood pressure), reducing body fat, and improving fitness.
- Participating in culturally appropriate physical activities, away from TV and technology, is an important factor in reducing and preventing obesity.
- Involving program participants in the development of activities is important to building acceptance by children, families, and communities.
- Successful programs used multiple strategies such as health education, physical activity, family support, behavior modification, improvement of access to healthy food choices, and exercise in schools, accompanied by culturally appropriate and meaningful rewards or incentives.

Reference: Flynn, M. (2004). Best practices for the prevention of overweight and obesity in children: A focus on immigrants new to industrialized countries. Calgary Health Region. Project No. 6795-15-2002/5440004. Retrieved March 4, 2007, from http://www.hc-sc.gc.ca/sr-sr/finance/hprp-prpms/results-resultats/2004-flynn_e.html

must be vigilant to support cultural eating habits, but be prepared to educate parents and children about the prevention and intervention into malnutrition and dehydration.

One cannot discuss nutrition and hydration without mentioning the problem of safe drinking water. Children die daily from water-borne diseases that could be prevented with a few drops of bleach and a safe water supply. Contaminated water is found in all countries at some time and in some countries at all times. Weather-related disasters, earthquakes, famine, and war typically escalate the water crises. In cases of vomiting, diarrhea, and dehydration contaminated water supplies should always be investigated as the source.

Sleep

Although the amount of sleep required at various ages is similar across cultures, differences in sleep patterns and bedtime rituals exist. The sleep practices in a family household reflect some of the deepest moral ideals of a cultural community. Nurses working with families of young children in both community and inpatient settings frequently encounter cultural differences in family sleeping behaviors.

Community health, psychiatric, and pediatric nurses who work with young children and their families often assess the family's sleep and rest patterns. On the issue of family cosleeping, nurses traditionally have taken a rigid approach that excludes this common cultural practice. Although some degree of **cosleeping**—the practice of parents and children sleeping together for all or part of the night—is common in families with young children, there are marked cultural differences in the proportion that regularly implement this practice (Ball, 2002; McCoy, Hunt, & Lesko, 2004).

Research has found that the majority of parents bring their children into bed with them at some time. Some parents allow the child into their bed only occasionally, after a nightmare or if the child is upset, whereas others routinely have children in bed with them. A few parents, especially mothers who breast-feed, indicated that

they sleep with their children all the time (McKenna, 2000; McKenna & McDade, 2005).

Cosleeping is more acceptable, and occurs most frequently among African American families. Most White middle-class North American and European families believe that infants and children should sleep alone because it fosters autonomy, privacy, and independence, while other cultures place a high value on protection of the vulnerable child and believe that cosleeping is especially helpful to those children who feel insecure. It has, however, been documented that children who cosleep are more likely to wake at night or to have trouble falling asleep alone at bedtime (Worthman & Brown, 2007).

For the hospitalized child, caregivers need to identify the child's usual bedtime routines. Bedtime routines and preparation for sleep might include a snack, prayers, and/or a favorite toy or story. Common bedtime routines should be continued in the hospital as much as possible.

The type of bed in which a child sleeps might vary considerably. In a traditional American Samoan home, infants sleep on a **pandanus mat** covered with a blanket, and sometimes a pillow is used. The **cradleboard** has been used by several Native American nations. Constructed by a family member, a cradleboard is made of wood and might be decorated in various ways depending on the affluence of the family and tribal customs (see Figure 6-6). The cradleboard helps the infant feel secure and is easily moved while the family engages in work, travel, or other activities. Although cradleboards have been blamed for exacerbating hip dysplasias in Native American infants, diapering counterbalances this by causing a slight abduction of the hips.

In the United States and Canada, the common developmental milestone of sleeping for 8 uninterrupted hours by age 4 to 5 months is regarded as a sign of neurologic maturity. In many other cultures, however, the infant sleeps with the mother and is allowed to breast-feed on demand with minimal disturbance of adult sleep. In such an arrangement, there is less parental motivation to enforce "sleeping through the night," and

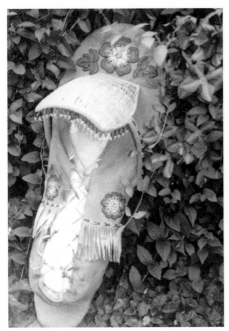

FIGURE 6-6 The cradleboard, created many centuries before the car seat, helps to promote infant mobility and safety and its use is still prevalent among Native Americans.

infants continue to wake up every 4 hours during the night to be fed. Thus, it appears that this developmental milestone, in addition to its biologic basis, is a function of context.

A common transition from sleeping in a crib to a bed without side rails is a developmental marker that is important to the child. This transition usually occurs during preschool years depending upon the physical space in the home, the parental attitude toward the child's independence, and the child's neuromuscular development/coordination. Once a child has gained the independence of leaving a crib, it may be emotionally traumatic for them to be placed into a hospital bed with side rails of any kind. Health care providers need to be sensitive to this situation and reassure both child and parent that any regressive behavior that occurs as a result of reverting to a bed with side rails will be short-lived.

Homelessness presents many problems, one of which is the lack of a consistent place for a child to sleep. Although nomadic tribes have for cen-

turies moved their habitat on a daily basis, even they generally had a consistent tent or covering. Today millions of children are haunted by nightmares and daily face the issues of not having a permanent, safe or secure place in which to lay their head. Whether by poverty, disease, war, or disaster, children with or without families nightly wander without a safe place to sleep. The toll of the massive number of homeless children that are the result of recent Haitian earthquakes, Samolian devastations, and mid-Eastern wars has yet to be estimated. Lack of a safe place to sleep is only one of many issues to be considered (Figure 6-7).

Elimination

Elimination refers to ridding the body of wastes. It is a function that is accomplished by the combined work of the gastrointestinal, genitourinary, respiratory, and integumentary systems of the body. Of primary concern to parents of toddlers and preschoolers is bowel and bladder control. Toilet training is a major developmental milestone, perhaps more for the parents than for the child, and is taught through a variety of cultural patterns.

Most children are capable of achieving dryness by 2½ to 3 years of age. Bowel training is more easily accomplished than bladder training. Daytime (diurnal) dryness is more easily attained than nighttime (nocturnal) dryness. Some cultures start toilet training a child before his or her first birthday and consider the child a "failure" if dryness is not achieved by 18 months. Often there is significant shaming, blaming, and embarrassment of the child who has not achieved dryness by the culturally acceptable timetable. The nurse should remember that due to spinal cord/nerve development, maintenance of dryness is not physiologically possible until the child is able to walk without assistance. In some cultures, children are not expected to be dry until 5 years of age and boys have a more difficult time achieving bladder control than girls. Constipation in a child is a persistent concern among parents who expect a ritualistic daily pattern of bowel movements. In some cultures, infants are given herbs aimed at purging them when they are a few days, weeks, or months

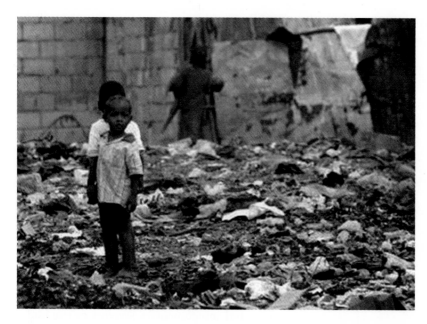

FIGURE 6-7 A Haitian child stand amidst earthquake rubble without clean water, food, or a place to sleep.

old to remove evil spirits from the body. Parents should be advised against using purgatives in infants because fluid and electrolyte imbalance occurs, and dehydration can ensue rapidly.

The role of the nurse is to acknowledge that toilet training can be taught through a variety of cultural patterns but that physical and psychosocial health are promoted by accepting, flexible approaches. A previously toilet-trained child might become incontinent as a result of the stress of hospitalization but generally will regain control quickly when returned to the familiar home environment. Parents should be reassured that regression of bowel and bladder control frequently occurs when a child is hospitalized; this is normal and is expected to be a short-term occurrence.

Menstruation

Ethnicity is the strongest determinant of the duration and character of menstrual flow. The roles of diet, exercise, and stress are known to influence menstruation in women of all ages. In the United States, African American girls have menses that are longer in duration and heavier in nature.

Attitudes toward menstruation are often culturally based, and the adolescent girl might be taught many folk beliefs. For example, in traditional Mexican American families, girls and women are not permitted to walk barefooted, wash their hair, or take showers or baths during menses. In encouraging hygienic practices, respect cultural directives by encouraging sponge bathing, frequent changing of sanitary pads or tampons, and other interventions that promote cleanliness (Lee, 2006). Some Mexican Americans believe that sour or iced foods cause the menstrual flow to thicken, and some Puerto Rican teenagers have been taught that drinking lemon or pineapple juice will increase menstrual cramping. The nurse should be aware of these beliefs and should respect personal preferences concerning beverages. The teenager has probably been taught the folk practices by her mother or by another woman in her family who might be watchful during the girl's menstrual periods. If menstruation coincides with hospitalization, you need to respect the teenager's preferences and might need to reassure the mother or significant other that cultural practices will be respected.

Many cultural groups treat menstrual cramping with herbs and a variety of home remedies. Be certain to ask the adolescent whether she takes anything special during menstruation or in the absence of menstrual flow. Verify the amount and type of home remedies used to determine possible interactive effect with prescribed medications.

Adolescent girls of Islamic religious backgrounds have cultural and/or religious prohibitions and duties during and after menstruation. In Islamic law, blood is considered unclean. The blood of menstruation, as well as blood lost during childbirth, is believed to render the female impure. Because one must be in a pure state to pray, menstruating girls and women are forbidden to perform certain acts of worship such as touching the Koran, entering a mosque, praying, and participating in the feast of Ramadan. During the menstrual period, sexual intercourse is forbidden for both men and women. When the menstrual flow stops, the girl or woman performs a special washing to purify herself. In Islam, sexual pollution applies equally to men and women. For men, sexual intercourse and the discharge of semen is an act that renders a man impure and requires a ritual washing before being able to perform the prayer. Buddist and Hindu women do not enter the kitchen and may sleep in separate/special rooms during menses (Figure 6-8) (New World Encyclopedia, 2008).

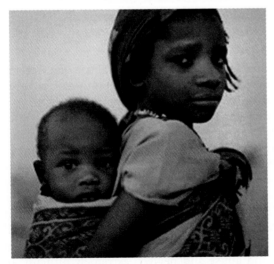

FIGURE 6-8 Menarche sets the developmental stage for girls to become mothers: children parenting children.

Parent–Child Relationships and Discipline

In some cultures, both parents assume responsibility for the care of children, whereas in other cultures, the relationship with the mother is primary and the father remains somewhat distant (Figure 6-9). With the approach of adolescence, the gender-related aspects of the **parent–child relationship** might be modified to conform with cultural expectations.

Some cultures encourage children to participate in family decision making and to discuss or even argue points with their parents. Some African American families, for example, encourage children to express opinions verbally and to take an active role in all family activities. Many Asian parents value respectful, deferential behavior toward adults, who are considered experienced and wise; therefore, children are discouraged from making decisions independently. The witty, fast reply that is viewed in some European cultures as a sign of intelligence and cleverness might be punished in some non-Western circles as a sign of rudeness and disrespect.

The use of physical acts, such as spanking, various restraining and other actions bordering on physical abuse, are connected with discipline in many groups. Physical punishment of Native North American children is rare. Instead of using loud scolding and reprimands, Native North American parents generally discipline with a quiet voice, telling the child what is expected. During breast-feeding and toilet training, Native North American children are typically permitted to set their own pace. Parents tend to be permissive and nondemanding. African American parents tend to point out negative behaviors of a child in loud, demanding tones; spanking and physical punishment is also used in an attempt to quickly gain the child's attention and rapidly attain adherent behaviors.

With the approach of adolescence, parental relationships and discipline generally change. Teens are usually given increasing amounts of freedom and are encouraged to try out adult roles but in a supervised way that enables parents to retain

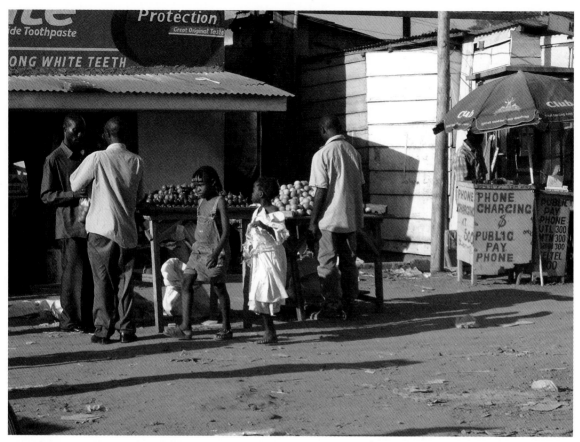

FIGURE 6-9   African fathers frequently take daughters food shopping in neighborhood markets.

considerable control. In many cultures, adolescent boys are permitted more freedom than girls of the same age. Among some religious groups, such as the American Amish, adolescents are given a period of time (a month to a year) of more independent lifestyle prior to commitment to specific religious life rules.

Child Abuse Versus Folk Healing

Child abuse and neglect have been documented throughout human history and are known across cultures. International attention to child maltreatment emerged in the late 1970s, and the International Society for the Prevention of Child Abuse and Neglect (ISPCAN) held an international congress to explore physical abuse and neglect, molestation, child prostitution, nutritional deprivation, and emotional maltreatment from a cross-national perspective. This congress led to the formation of a multicountry study of child maltreatment/abuse and the recently released United Nations–WHO joint publication "Enhancing the Rights of Adolescent Girls" (WHO, 2010).

Cross-cultural variability in child-rearing beliefs and practices has created a dilemma that makes the establishment of a universal standard for optimal child care, as well as definitions of child abuse and neglect, extremely difficult. In defining child maltreatment across cultures, the WHO and UNICEF have included Korbin's (1991) classic characteristics: (1) cultural differences in child-rearing practices and beliefs, (2) departure from one's culturally acceptable behavior, and (3) harm to children (Korbin, 1991).

Practices that are acceptable in the culture in which they occur may be considered abusive or neglectful by outsiders; some examples follow. In many Middle Eastern cultures, despite warm temperatures, infants are covered with multiple layers of clothing and might be observed to sweat profusely because parents believe that young children become chilled easily and die of exposure to the cold. Many African nations continue to practice rites of initiation for boys and girls, usually at the time of puberty. In some cases, ritual circumcision—of both boys and girls—is performed without anesthesia, and the ability to endure the associated pain is considered to be a manifestation of the maturity expected of an adult. In the United States and Canada, the African American parental use of physical forms of discipline might present controversial and ethical dilemmas for the nurse. The same is true for some Southeast Asian folk healing practices such as coining, pinching, and burning that produce marks on the body and are used for treatment of pain and various illnesses.

In some Middle Eastern and Mexican societies, fondling of the genitals of infants and young children is used to soothe them or encourage sleep; however, such fondling of older children or for the sexual gratification of adults would fall outside of acceptable cultural behaviors.

Although African American children are three times more likely than White children to die of child abuse, there is considerable disagreement about whether race differences exist in the prevalence of child abuse independent from socioeconomic factors such as income, education, and employment status. Health care providers need to become knowledgeable about folk beliefs, child-rearing practices, and cultural variability in defining child maltreatment.

Gender Differences

Physiologically, adult men differ from adult women in both primary and secondary sex characteristics.

On average, men have a higher oxygen-carrying capacity in the blood, a higher muscle-to-fat ratio, more body hair, a larger skeleton, and greater height. Behaviorally, there are also differences between the two sexes, especially in the division of labor.

For children, gender differences can be identified cross-culturally in six classes of behavior: nurturance, responsibility, obedience, self-reliance, achievement, and independence (Barry, Bacon, & Child, 1967). Differences between boys and girls appear early in life and form the basis for adult roles within a culture. Normal newborn boys are larger, more active, and have more muscle development than newborn girls. Normal newborn girls react more positively to comforting than do newborn boys.

Variability in sex-role behavior is common. Most people in a society adopt common behaviors defined as appropriate to their biologic sex, but there are many exceptions. Sex roles are themselves highly variable by age, social class, religious orientation, and sexual preference. The stringency of expectations also varies: girls and women in the United States and Canada can violate sex-role norms with fewer explicit sanctions than their Middle Eastern counterparts.

Health and Health Promotion

The concept of health varies widely across cultures. Regardless of culture, most parents desire health for their children and engage in activities that they believe to be health promoting. Because health-related beliefs and practices are such an integral part of culture, parents might persist with culturally based beliefs and practices even when scientific evidence refutes them, or they might modify them to be more congruent with contemporary knowledge of health and illness.

Illness

The family is the primary health care provider for infants, children, and adolescents. It is the family that determines when a child is ill and decides to seek help in managing an illness. The family determines the acceptability of illness and sick-role behaviors for children and adolescents. Societal and economic trends influence the cultural beliefs that are passed from generation to generation. Health, illness, and treatment (care/cure) are part of every child's cultural heritage. Every society has an organized response to defined health problems. Certain people are designated as being responsible for deciding who is sick, what kind of sickness the person has, and what kind of treatment is required to restore the person to health.

Research has consistently demonstrated that African American and Hispanic children are less likely to have seen a physician than are Whites (Figure 6-10). They also have a lower average number of ambulatory visits than their White counterparts. Even when children are hospitalized, minorities receive fewer services than do Whites (Federal Interagency Forum on Child and Family Statistics, 2006; Children's Defense Organization, 2009).

Health Belief Systems and Culture-Bound Syndromes

Among many cultural groups, traditional health beliefs coexist with Western medical beliefs. Members of a cultural group choose the components of traditional (Western) medicine, Eastern medicine, or folk beliefs that seem appropriate to them. A Mexican American family, for example, might take a child to a physician and/or a traditional

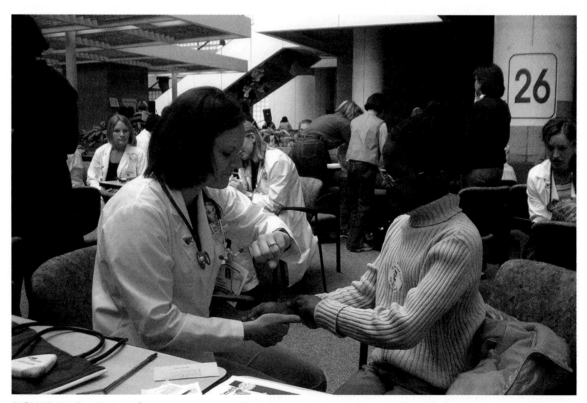

FIGURE 6-10 Fewer African American children receive preventative health care than their white counterparts. This child is taking advantage of a health fair in a local shopping mall to learn about her health status.

healer (curandero). After visiting the physician and the *curandero*, the mother might consult with her own mother and then give her sick child the antibiotics prescribed by the physician and the herbal tea prescribed by the traditional healer. If the problem is viral in origin, the child will recover because of his or her own innate immunologic defenses, independent of either treatment. Thus, both the herbal tea of the *curandero* and the penicillin prescribed by the physician might be viewed as folk remedies; neither intervention is responsible for the child's recovery.

Belief systems about specific symptoms are culturally unique. These are referred to as **culture-bound syndromes**. In Hispanic culture, *susto* is caused by a frightening experience and is recognized by nervousness, loss of appetite, and loss of sleep. Mexican American babies must be protected from these experiences. *Pujos* (grunting) is an illness manifested by grunting sounds and protrusion of the umbilicus. It is believed to be caused by contact with a woman who is menstruating or by the infant's own mother if she menstruated sooner than 60 days after delivery.

The evil eye, *mal ojo*, is an affliction feared throughout much of the world. The condition is said to be caused by an individual who voluntarily or involuntarily injures a child by looking at or admiring him or her. The individual has a desire to hold the child, but the wish is frustrated, either by the parent of the infant or by the reserve of the individual. Several hours later, the child might become listless, cry, experience fever, vomiting, and/or diarrhea. The most serious threat to the infant with *mal ojo* is dehydration; the nurse encountering this problem in the community setting needs to assess the severity of the dehydration and plan for immediate fluid and electrolyte replacement. Parents should be taught the warning signs and the potential seriousness of dehydration. A simple explanation of the causes and treatment of dehydration should be provided. If the parents adhere strongly to traditional beliefs, you should respect their desire for the *curandera* to participate in the care. Parents or grandparents might wish to place an

amulet, talisman, or religious object such as a crucifix or rosary on the child or near the bed.

For the Mexican American family, a variety of causes is attributed to *Caida de la mollera*, or **fallen fontanel**, which arises from a number of causes such as failure of the midwife to press preventively on the palate after delivery, falling on the head, abruptly removing the nipple from the infant's mouth, and failing to place a cap on the infant's head. The signs of this condition include crying, fever, vomiting, and diarrhea. Given that health care providers frequently note the correspondence of these symptoms with those of dehydration, many parents see *deshidratacion* (dehydration) or *carencia de agua* (lack of water) as synonymous with *caida de la mollera*. Although regional differences exist, parental treatment usually is directed at rehydration, thus, raising the fontanel.

Empacho is a digestive condition believed by Mexicans to be caused by the adherence of undigested food to some part of the gastrointestinal tract. This condition causes an "internal fever," which cannot be observed but which betrays its presence by excessive thirst and abdominal swelling believed to be caused by drinking water to quench the thirst. Children who are prone to swallowing chewing gum are believed to experience *empacho*, but it can affect persons of any age.

Among some Hindus from northern India, there is a strong belief in **ghost illness** and **ghost possession**. These culture-bound syndromes, or folk illnesses, are based on the belief that a ghost enters its victim and tries to seize the soul. If the ghost is successful, it causes death. Illness and the supernatural world are linked by the concepts of fever and the ghost, which is a supernatural being discussed in Hindu sacred scriptures.

One sign of ghost illness is a voice speaking through a delirious victim; this may occur in children and adults. Other signs are convulsions and body movements, indicating pain and discomfort, and choking or difficulty breathing. In the case of an infant, incessant crying is a sign. The psychologic state of the parents is often involved in the diagnosis, and some believe that ghosts might be cultural scapegoats for the illness and death of children. When an infant or small child becomes ill and dies, a mother or father might be relieved of psychic tension from feelings of personal guilt by transferring the blame for the death to a ghost.

Biocultural Influences on Childhood Disorders

Children may be born with a genetic constitution inherited from their biologic parents, who have inherited their own genetic compositions. The child's genetic makeup affects his or her likelihood of both contracting and inheriting specific conditions. In both children and adults, genetic composition has been demonstrated to affect the individual's susceptibility to specific diseases and disorders. It is often difficult to separate genetic influences from socioeconomic factors such as poverty, lack of proper nutrition, poor hygiene, and such environmental conditions as lack of ventilation, sanitary facilities, heat during cold weather, and clothing that is insufficient to provide protection during the various seasons. Other factors responsible for differing susceptibilities to specific conditions are variations in natural and acquired immunity, intermarriage, geographic and climatic conditions, ethnic background, race, and religious practices. Some studies have attempted to explain differences in susceptibility solely on the basis of cultural heritage, but they have not succeeded in doing so. This section examines some common conditions in which genetic constitution seems to be a factor influencing child health.

Immunity

Perhaps one of the most frequently cited examples of the connection between immunity and race is that of malaria and the sickle cell trait in Africans. Black Africans possessing the sickle cell trait are known to have increased immunity to malaria, a serious endemic disease found in warm, moist climates. Thus, Blacks with the sickle cell trait survived malarial attacks and reproduced offspring who also possessed the sickle cell trait. As dictated by Mendelian probability, the sickle cell anemia disease eventually developed and continues to be genetically transmitted. The transfer of immunity to many contagious diseases via injection/ingestion of live or attenuated viruses has been a major factor in decreasing childhood deaths. However, there is no evidence of culture-bound positive or negative effects where vaccines are available. Some religious groups refuse immunizations and often experience outbreaks of preventable communicable diseases within their community. Other parents refuse immunizations based on the belief of a connection between childhood autism and vaccines; the clinical research to support this opinion has not yet been found.

Intermarriage

Intermarriage among certain cultural groups has led to a wide variety of childhood disorders. For example, there is an increased incidence of ventricular septal defects (VSDs) among the Amish, amyloidosis among Indiana/Swiss and Maryland/German families, and mental retardation in several other groups (GeneReview, 2009). In the extreme, intermarriage among groups having few members can lead to total extinction; the number of Samaritans in Israel, for example, has dwindled to a handful of surviving, aging members.

Ethnicity

Although the role of socioeconomic factors in tuberculosis—such as overcrowding and poor nutrition—cannot be disregarded, ethnicity also appears to be a factor in this disease. Groups with a relatively high incidence of tuberculosis are Native North Americans living in the Southwest United States and in northern and prairie regions of Canada, Mexican Americans, and Africans and refugees from third world countries. Ethnicity is also linked to several noncommunicable conditions such as Tay-Sachs disease, a neurologic condition affecting Ashkenazic Jews of northeastern European descent, and phenylketonuria (PKU), a metabolic disorder primarily affecting Scandinavians.

Race

Race has been linked to the incidence of a variety of disorders of childhood. For example, the endocrine disorder cystic fibrosis primarily affects White children, whereas sickle cell anemia has its primary influence among Blacks and those of Mediterranean descent. Black children are known to be at risk for inherited blood disorders, such as thalassemia, G-6-PD deficiency, and hemoglobin C disease. In addition, an estimated 70% to 90% of Black children have an enzyme deficiency that results in difficulty with the digestion and metabolism of milk.

Hereditary Predisposition to Illness

The predisposition to certain disorders also has been linked to cultural influences. For example, the incidences of obesity, hypertension, and diabetes are especially high among Blacks, and those of dysentery, alcoholism, and suicide are high among Native North American children and adolescents. Mexican American children are known to succumb to pneumonia more frequently than Anglo North American children of similar socioeconomic status.

Chronic Illness and Disability in Children

Chronic illnesses and disabilities have become the dominant health care problem in North America and are the leading causes of morbidity and mortality.

Beliefs Regarding the Cause of Chronic Illnesses and Disabilities

Illness is viewed by many cultures as a form of punishment. The child and/or family with a chronic illness or disability might be perceived to be cursed by a supreme being, to have sinned, or to have violated a taboo. In some cultural groups, the affected child is seen as tangible evidence of divine displeasure, and its arrival is accompanied throughout the community by prolonged private and public discussions about what wrongs the family might have committed.

Inherited disorders and illnesses are frequently envisioned as being caused by a family curse that is passed along from one generation to the next through blood. Within such families, the nurse's desire to determine who is the carrier for a particular gene might be interpreted as an attempt to discover who is at fault and might be met with family resistance.

Folk beliefs mingled with eugenics have resulted in the notion that many chronic conditions, particularly mental retardation, are the products of intermarriage among close relatives. The belief that a chronically ill or disabled child might be the product of an incestuous relationship can further complicate attempts to encourage parents to seek assistance.

Among those who believe that chronic illness and disability are caused by an imbalance of hot and cold or yin and yang, the burden of responsibility for life care lies with the affected individual. For many individuals from Latino or Southeast Asian cultures, the cause and potential cure lie within the individual. He or she must try to reestablish equilibrium through regaining balance. Unfortunately for those with permanent disabilities who cannot be fully healed within this conceptual system, society might perceive them as living in a continually impure or diseased state.

Traditional beliefs are tenacious and tend to remain even after genetic inheritance or physiologic patterns of chronic disease progression are explained to the family. Often new information is quickly integrated into the traditional system of folk beliefs, as is evidenced by the addition of currently prescribed medications to the hot/cold classification system embraced by many Hispanic families. An explanation of the genetic transmission of disease might be given to a family, but this does not guarantee that the older belief in a curse or "bad blood" will disappear.

When disability is seen as a divine punishment, an inherited evil, or the result of a personal state of impurity, the very presence of a child with a disability might be something about which the family is deeply ashamed or with which they are unable to cope (Figure 6-11). In addition to suffering from public disgrace, some parents or families, especially immigrant groups from Eastern Europe and Southeast Asia, also fear that disabled

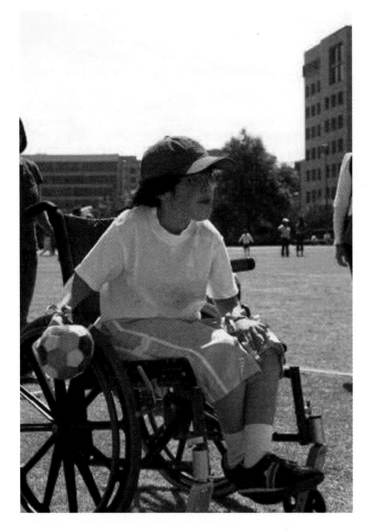

FIGURE 6-11 Children with physical disabilities are viewed in some cultures as a reflection of family evil and in others as a special blessing later in life.

children will be taken away and institutionalized against their will.

It must be emphasized that some cultural explanations of the cause of chronic disease or disability are quite positive. For example, some Mexican American parents of chronically ill children believed that a certain number of ill and disabled children would always be born into the world. Many Mexican American parents who embrace Roman Catholicism believe that God has singled them out for the role because of their past kindnesses to a relative or neighbor who was disabled and view the birth of the disabled infant as God's will.

The number of chronically ill children in developed nations has increased markedly over the past decade. This increase is primarily due to dramatic changes in available treatments the delivery of health care. This is particularly evident in the delivery of neonatal care where, in the United States, no expense is spared to save the life of very low birth weight infants. The lifesaving efforts often leave a child with multiple chronic illnesses, in contrast to countries with fewer medical resources, such as Uganda and Haiti, where these same very low birth weight babies will not survive infancy (Figure 6-12).

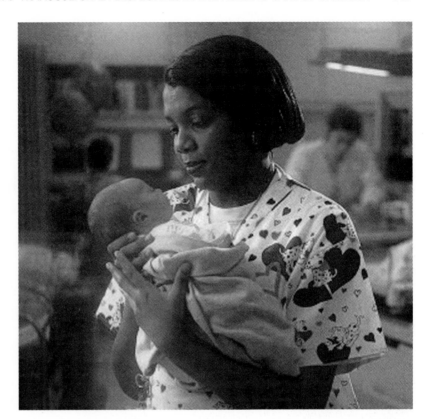

FIGURE 6-12 Many low birth weight infants are "saved" by the availability of high tech-health care only to experience multiple chronic illnesses.

Special Considerations for Adolescents

Culture and Adolescent Development

Adolescence is a developmental passage to adulthood marked by major physical, emotional, and social changes. In many ways, adolescents from different cultural backgrounds grow and develop in similar ways and experience common physical, emotional, and social changes. It is believed that all adolescents show concerns over changes occurring during puberty, such as self-identity, self-image, gender identity, increased autonomy, relationships with peers of the opposite sex, and career aspirations. Cultural forces, however, influence the manner in which adolescents respond to these developmental changes.

Many believe the major task of adolescence is the achievement of self-identity. Havighurst's classic work on adolescent development (1974) identified eight tasks that adolescents must complete before entering adulthood: (1) develop relationships with peers, (2) accept a sex role, (3) accept one's physical appearance, (4) become emotionally independent from parents, (5) prepare for marriage and family life, (6) prepare for economic independence, (7) acquire an ideology and value system, and (8) achieve and accept socially responsible behavior. Havighurst indicated that the tasks are both historically and culturally relative and acknowledged that variations exist in the type and timing of the tasks faced by adolescents raised in different cultural settings.

From a cultural and developmental task perspective, competent development occurs with successful completion of the tasks that confront

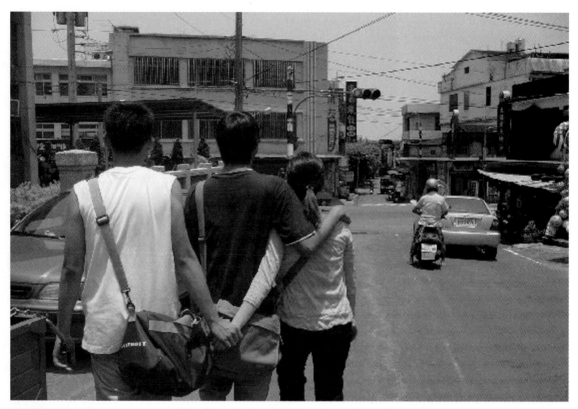

FIGURE 6-13 As teens grow and explore their world, they make friends from many different cultures.

the individual at different points in the life course and concomitant development of the social and cognitive skills required by the task and permitted by the culture. Adolescents from a wide range of cultural backgrounds are believed to face different tasks at different points in their lives (Figure 6-13).

As children grow older, they are likely to encounter more people from other cultures and, therefore, to become increasingly influenced by factors external to their family. By making comparisons between themselves and members of other cultures, adolescents develop a better awareness of their own culture and might begin to select values, behaviors, or attitudes from cultural groups outside the family. The increased sensitivity to cultural differences experienced by adolescents is largely the result of four factors: (1) increased mobility and independence, which permits greater exposure to the world outside the home; (2) growing cognitive ability, which permits greater awareness and understanding of cultural issues; (3) widening social networks in which diversity manifests itself, and (4) available technology that transmits culturally diverse music, values, and social imperatives into personal devices (earphones, headsets, iPods) and social media.

Adolescents who identify with minority groups, especially those that are gang related, are frequently faced with choices about maintaining separateness or going through the process of assimilation or acculturation to the group. In traditional assimilation, adolescents take on the values, beliefs, and behaviors of the majority culture and abandon their original ethnic traditions. In acculturation, they accept both their own culture and other cultures, adapting elements of each. Acculturated teenagers demonstrate flexibility in adapting their behavior

EVIDENCE-BASED PRACTICE 6-2

Predictors of Unprotected Intercourse of Adolescents Girls

In recent years, the United States has had the highest rate of adolescent pregnancies in the developed world. In addition to pregnancy, sexually transmitted diseases are an end result of unprotected sex creating major long-term repercussions. The purpose of this study was to identify predictors of unprotected sex in adolescent women. Aruda surveyed a convenience sample of adolescents who sought pregnancy testing in an ambulatory clinic. The participants were 15 to 21 years of age and based upon the laws of the state (MA), reproductive confidentiality was assured during the health visit.

The Interaction Model of Client Health Behaviors (IMCHB), abroad-based multifactor model developed by an advance practice nurse formed the basis for the study. From the model items related to the individual's contextual background were developed. A questionnaire was developed that focused on the teens previous health care experiences, social influences, and environmental resource. Several tools were used to collect data, including the Index of Reproductive and Contraceptive Knowledge, a resiliency scale and open response questions related to self-reported use of condoms.

Results

A multiracial group of 305 adolescents participated in this study they identified themselves as: Black (50%), Other (22%), White (17%), American Indian (4%), Asian (0.3%); in a separate questions 36% self-identified as Hispanic. The mean age of the participants was 18 years and their partners were 21 years of age, most couples had dated over a years. Eighteen percent some type of reported sexual assault. Most participants (41%) lived in a female-headed households. Although condoms were reported as the major method of contraception used, 52% indicated they were not used consistently. Ten percent of the participants indicated they did not use any contraceptives.

Although only a few of the study results are reported here, of interest was that 51% of the participants expressed "fertility fears," fear about their ability to become pregnant. This is especially interesting as 45% reported prior pregnancies. The variables found to directly influence unprotected sexual activity (condom use) were age of partner, fertility fears, age of menarche, knowledge about pregnancy, motivation, and duration of dating.

Implications

Use of the IMCHB model focuses on research findings into interventions that are tailored for the unique client. Since the age of menarche and "fertility fears" significantly influence the use of condoms and, thus, the resultant pregnancy and STDs, these two factors should be addressed through education. During each health care encounter the nurses should ask direct specific questions to the teen to assess her knowledge of pregnancy and contraception, what she believes constitutes responsible sexual behavior, and what resources she needs to prevent unprotected sex. In addition, the possibility and/or practice of initiating sexual activity in early teen years to prove that one can should be discussed. Fears of the future can be clarified by assuring the teen that early sexual intercourse does not positively influence her ability to become pregnant later, but instead could lead to STDs and unplanned pregnancy that would effect later life. Age-appropriate educational materials should be made available in the schools, Boys & Girls Clubs, local discount stores, and other locations frequented by teens. Nurses should encourage use of newer social networks devices such as text messaging and Twitter, to educate teens on pregnancy/prevention and condom use.

Reference: Aruda, M. (in press). Predictors of unprotected intercourse for female adolescents measured at their request for as pregnancy test. *Journal of Pediatric Nursing.*

White, E., Rosengard, C., Weitzen, S., Meers, A., & Phipps, M. (2006). Fear of inability to conceive in pregnant adolescents. *Obstetrics & Gynecology,* 108, 1411–1416.

to multiple cultures and are sometimes referred to as having bicultural or multicultural competence. An example of such acculturation is the appearance of body tattoos. A teen may want to have a body tattoo because it is in vogue with the peer group, but it is unacceptable to the majority culture (namely the parent), so they obtain a tattoo on a body part that is not revealed when wearing clothing (e.g., breast, thigh, or buttocks). This action may then become acceptable to both cultures.

Special Health Care Needs of Adolescents

There are approximately 22 million adolescents in the United States and Canada. Teenagers are in a process of evolving from childhood to adulthood, and they belong not only to the cultural groups that have formed the basis for their values, attitudes, and beliefs, but also to the subculture of adolescents. This subculture links the adolescent with other adolescents through a system of socially transmitted behaviors and belongings, such as brand-named clothing, music, and technostatus symbols. The adolescent subculture has its own set of values, beliefs, and practices that may or may not be in harmony with those of the cultural group that previously guided their behaviors.

The adolescent subculture is vaguely structured and lacks formal written laws or codes. Conformity with the peer group behavior is expected. One of the most outstanding characteristics of the adolescent subculture is preoccupation with clothing, hairstyles, and grooming. Clothing mirrors the personal feelings of the adolescent and facilitates identity with the peer group.

In the hospital setting, gowns might stifle the individual's sense of identity, so the adolescent should be permitted to wear familiar clothing whenever the style does not interfere with safety, comfort, or hygiene. Whether or not one personally approves, there is no harm in allowing a reasonable amount of makeup, jewelry, or other items of apparel that might be important to the adolescent. Body piercing, prominent in some

culture for years, has become widely accepted to the adolescent subculture worldwide. The nurse must assess the placement of the piercing to determine whether it may safely remain in place or must be removed. Piercing of the tongue may prove a hygienic issue and must be discussed with the teen before requiring removal.

Some young men and women prefer to dress in traditional clothing. It is important for the nurse to determine what the adolescent finds most comfortable to wear during hospitalization and accommodate as much as possible as long as safe standards are upheld.

There is a relationship between some diseases and socioeconomic status; consequently, low-income teenagers may have a wide range of diagnosed and undiagnosed diseases. During the transition from dependent children to independent adults, some disorders might interfere with their development of a positive body image, sexual and personal identity, and value system. The entrance of HIV/AIDS as a global health issue has caused adolescents to seriously evaluate their sexual behavior. The U.S. AID in collaboration with the World Bank has embarked upon a 13-nation study of adolescent health in Asia and the Near East. The key educational tool is teaching the ABCs of sex: **A**bstinence, **B**e Faithful, and use **C**ondoms (Utomo, 2003). Unfortunately, condoms are not always used and unplanned pregnancies and/or unwanted disease often follow. Evidence-Based Practice 6-2 describes some factors that predict the causes of unprotected sexual activity in adolescents.

Culturally Competent Nursing Care for Children and Adolescents

A few principles of care for specific cultural groups have been provided to illustrate the practical ways in which culturally competent nursing care should be provided. The examples are intended to be illustrative, not exhaustive.

Nursing Assessment of the Family

Cultural Background

Culture, like language, is acquired early in life, and cultural understanding is typically established by age 5. Every interaction, sound, touch, odor, and experience has a cultural component that is absorbed by the child even when it is not taught directly. Lessons learned at such early ages become an integral part of thinking and behavior. Table manners, the proper behavior when interacting with adults, sick role behaviors, and the rules of acceptable emotional response are anchored in culture. Many beliefs and behaviors learned at an early age persist into adulthood.

Over time, culture has influenced family functioning in many ways, including marriage forms and ceremonies; choice of mates; postmarital residence; family kinship system; rules governing inheritance, household, and family structure; family obligations; family–community dynamics and alternative family formations. These traditions have given families a sense of stability and support from which members draw comfort, guidance, and a means of coping with the problems of life, including physical and mental illness, handicaps, disabilities, dying, and death.

Each family modifies the culture of the larger group in ways that are uniquely its own. Some beliefs, practices, and customs are maintained, whereas others are altered or abandoned. Although it is helpful for you to have a basic knowledge of children's cultural backgrounds, it is also necessary to view each family on an individual basis. Assumptions or biased expectations cannot be allowed to replace accurate assessment. It is essential for you to remember that not all members of a cultural group behave in a stereotypical fashion. For example, although many Chinese North American children behave in the manner congruent with the stereotype—showing respect for authority, polite social behavior, and a moderate-to-soft voice—some are disrespectful, impolite, and boisterous and illness only exaggerates the differences. Evidence-Based Practice 6-3 exemplifies this difficulty as it reviews the situation of a Chinese family with a chronically ill child in the American health care system. Individual differences, changing norms over time, the degree of acculturation, the length of time the family has lived in a country, and other factors account for variations from the stereotype.

Family Belief Systems

The behavior of children and adolescents is influenced by child-rearing practices, parental beliefs about involvement with children, and the type and frequency of disciplinary measures. Although both parents exert an influence on the child's orientation to health, research indicates that a wide cultural variability exists, with the mother being the most influential parent in most cultural groups; this is easily verified in most single-parent households, and also very visible in matriarchal societies of African and African American families. Thus, identifying the attitudes, values, and beliefs about health and illness held by the parents and other providers of child care is an important part of the cultural assessment of the family.

Mothers' attitudes toward health and illnesses are related to their educational level. Mothers with little formal education tend to be more fatalistic about illness and less concerned with detecting clinical manifestations of disease in their children than are well-educated mothers. The former are also less likely to follow up on precautionary measures suggested by health care providers. A mother who believes that people have no control over whether they become sick is more likely to seek care in an emergency facility and less likely to have a preventive approach to health. She is also less likely to seek preventative education and might not comply with recommended immunization schedules. Nursing interventions with a mother who believes that there is much a person can do to keep from becoming ill will be different with regard to the nature of health education and counseling provided.

With assessment data related to the belief system(s) of the family, you have facts from which to choose approaches and priorities. For a

EVIDENCE-BASED PRACTICE 6-3

When Health Care Provider Decisions Clash with Parental Preference

Each year health care research unravels the mystery of previously unknown diseases and conditions; recently, expanded knowledge about Proteus syndrome has been revealed. This rare congenital and progressive disorder causes soft tissue overgrowth (nonmalignant tumors), resulting in swelling that compresses nerves, vessels, and organs. Asymmetrical growth of skeletal and soft tissue also produces spinal deformities and respiratory compromise. It was a 12-year-old with Proteus syndrome who attracted the attention of the health care team. Turner (2010) provides unique insight into two years in the life of this child. These two years reflected a situation in which the care perceived necessary for the longevity of the child was in direct conflict with the traditional cultural beliefs of a Chinese family who immigrated to the United States. Over several years the child deteriorated from attending school regularly to a nonverbal, agitated child exhibiting self-injurious behavior (head banging, scratching, and banging of extremities); she was hospitalized seven times. The mother had difficulty physically managing the child; the family had limited financial resources, lived in a small apartment that could not accommodate needed care equipment, was unable to communicate in English, and had no extended-family available; the parents voluntarily placed the child in medical foster care.

Over nearly two years in foster care the child improved significantly. Consistent pain management helped to eliminate the self-injurious behavior; mobility improved; she demonstrated the understanding of simple words and began smiling. Since the course/progression of Proteus syndrome is unknown and hospitalizations were becoming more frequent, the primary medical team requested a palliative care consultation.

To determine the outcome of the ethical dilemma the health care team utilized a four-quadrant ethical decision-making tool taking into consideration: medical indications (principles of beneficence and nonmalfeasance), patient preference (respect for autonomy), quality of life (principles of beneficence, nonmalfeasance, and autonomy), and contextual features (loyalty and fairness). When the decisions were made and presented to the parents, they determined it was their familial duty to take the child out of foster care and back to their home to provide a dignified death. The health care team was severely divided about this decision: some felt, for the child's well-being, she should return to the foster care home where she was showing emotional improvement, others believed it was a parental decision related to the care of a minor child. This dilemma was taken to the hospital ethics committee for decision. The committee determined that the rights of the parents superseded the other factors and the child was discharged to the parental home with a home care and pain management plan.

This was clearly a difficult decision; however, the solution has ended being a correct one. Once again in her home environment the child began to thrive, smile, make eye contact with her family, and even walk as few feet. She has been at home for two years and her parents seemed quite comfortable with the results: supported by strong cultural ties her mother never stops smiling.

Reference: Turner, H. N. (2010). Parental preference or child well-being: An ethical dilemma. *Journal of Pediatric Nursing, 25*(1), 58–63.

mother who is not oriented to prevention of illness or maintenance of health, focusing energies on teaching might not be productive; it might be more useful to spend time designing family follow-up care or establishing an interpersonal relationship that invites the parent to follow recommended immunization schedules, well-child care, and other aspects of health promotion.

Extended Family

Early in the nurse–parent relationship, it is necessary to identify members of the nuclear and/or **extended family** who play a significant role in the care of the child. Among families worldwide, the **nuclear family** is a rarity. In only 6% of the world's societies are families as isolated and nuclear as in the United States and Canada. The extended family is far more universally the norm. Kin residence sharing, for example, has long been acknowledged as characteristic of many African American, Chinese American, Mexican American, Amish, Mormon, and other groups.

In societies where the extended family is the norm, parents—particularly those who married at a young age—might be considered too inexperienced to make major decisions on behalf of their child. In these groups, key decisions are frequently made in consultation with more mature relatives such as grandparents, uncles, aunts, cousins, or other kin. Sometimes nonkin are considered to be part of the extended family. In many religions, the members of one's church, synagogue, temple, or mosque are viewed as extended family members who might be relied on for various types of support, including child care. Not coincidentally, members of some congregations refer to one another as brothers and sisters. The Amish family pattern is referred to as *friendscraft*, or three-generational family structure. Amish parents know that they can rely on the support of their entire church community. For example, a young Amish couple might turn to that community for assistance with decision making, finances, and emotional and spiritual support when a child is ill. You should ask the parents if anyone else will be participating in the decision making that affects their child. Once that information is known, you should include the person(s) identified by the parents in the child's plan of care.

The influence of the extended family or the social support network on the child's development becomes particularly important when the number of single-parent families in some culturally diverse groups is considered. According to an update of the U.S. 2000 Census (2009), the percentage of children living with two parents varied by race and origin. Eighty-five percent of Asian children lived with two parents, as did 78% of White non-Hispanic children, 70% of Hispanic children, and 38% of Black children. Five percent of U.S. children live in a household with neither parent present (U.S. Census Bureau, 2009).

The nuclear family is the unit for which most health care programs are designed. Consider the implicit message about the family when you note the number of chairs for visitors typically placed in hospital rooms, physician or nurse practitioner offices, and other health care settings. Although a handful of rural hospitals make special accommodations for the extended and church family of patients, few provide a place for the Amish to hitch their horses and buggies adjacent to the facility. With the advent of Family Centered Care in the United States, all children's hospitals provide more flexible visiting hours and extend visiting privileges to include siblings, extended family and friends; however, no hitching post could be found.

Nursing Interventions

Physical Care of the Child or Adolescent

Care of the hospitalized child's body is the primary domain of the nurse. Despite its importance, hair care is sometimes omitted for Black children because White, Hispanic, Asian, and Native American nurses might be unfamiliar with proper care. The hair of Black children varies widely in texture and is usually fragile. Hair might be long and straight or short, thick, and kinky. The hair and scalp have a natural tendency to be dry and to require daily combing, gentle brushing, and application to the scalp of a light oil such as Vaseline or mineral oil. The hair might be rolled on curlers, braided, or left loose according to personal preference. Bobby pins or combs might be used to keep the hair in place. If an individual has cornrow braids or shaved, sculptured hair, the scalp might be massaged, oiled, and shampooed without unbraiding the hair.

Some Blacks prefer straightened hair, which might be obtained chemically or thermally. Hair that has been straightened with a pressing comb will return to its naturally kinky state when exposed to moisture or humidity or when hair growth occurs. Children of Asian descent tend to have straight hair that does not require the same amount of care as the hair of most African Americans or Whites.

Textural variations also are found in the facial hair of culturally diverse boys and men during adolescence and adulthood. Many Asian teenage boys have light facial hair and require infrequent shaving, whereas African American boys and men tend to have a heavy growth of facial hair requiring regular attention. Some Black teenage boys have tightly curled facial hair, which when shaved curls back upon itself and penetrates the skin. This may result in a local foreign-body reaction on the face that can lead to the formation of papules, pustules, and multiple small keloids. Some African American teens and men might prefer to grow beards rather than shave, particularly when they are ill. Before shaving a teen determine his usual method of facial grooming and attempt to shave or apply depilatories (agents that remove hair) in a similar manner. When using depilatories, you should protect the skin from irritation by keeping the chemical from contacting the client's nose, mouth, eyes, and ears. Straight and safety razors are contraindicated when depilatories are used because they can cause local irritation to the skin.

Principles related to personal hygiene apply to children of all racial and ethnic backgrounds, but the specific manner in which care is given might vary widely. When in doubt, you should ask the child's parent or extended family member how hair care is carried out at home. Children might feel more secure if a parent or close family member actually provides the care. If you determine that the child would benefit from care by a familiar caregiver from home, the rationale for requesting family intervention should be explained. Comments that the nursing staff is too busy or uninterested in providing hair care should be avoided; rather, the benefit to the child's security and sense of well-being should be emphasized.

When bathing a client, you should remember that the washcloth removes some parts of the outermost skin layer. Such sloughed skin, which will be evident on the washcloth and in the bathwater, will vary in color depending on the ethnic group of the person being bathed. The sloughed skin of a darkly pigmented child, for example, will be a brownish black color. This does not mean that the child was dirty; the normal sloughing of skin is simply more evident in darkly pigmented people when compared with lightly pigmented groups. The more melanin that is present, the darker the skin color will be. Because dryness is more evident on darkly pigmented skin, Vaseline, baby oil, lanolin cream, and lotions can be applied after the bath to give the skin a shiny, healthy appearance.

Communicating with the Hospitalized Child and Family

Communicating with the child and the family are key components in a successful hospitalization and recovery. Verbal communication is especially difficult when the child–family–health care provider do not speak the same language. The natural response would be to obtain the services of an interpreter. The nurse should be aware of gender- and age-related customs before doing so. For instance, an adolescent girl might be uncomfortable with an older male interpreter, and an older boy might prefer a friend to translate rather than an interpreter connected to the health agency. Attention should also be paid to the correct national origin of the child before seeking an interpreter; for example, an individual from Southeast Asia may speak Vietnamese, Cambodian, or Laotian—vastly different languages. Approximately 15% of migrant/immigrant families speak English in the home; this factor should be included in the nursing assessment. Most children and adolescent involved in the American school system learn English quickly and may serve as interpreters for family members. Even in families who have mastered English as a second language, the stress of illness and hospitalization may cause them to regress to their primary language. The use of a formal or informal interpreter is still recommended.

Nonverbal expressions are not to be overlooked as powerful communication tools. Nurses should take their cues from observing the family interactions. Some Italian parents/families are very demonstrative with facial expressions and arm/hand gestures—while the children may remain quiet. On the other hand, Asian parents and children both remain quiet and often wear "masked faces" showing very little emotional expression. Nurses must be aware of their own nonverbal expressions of acceptance of appearance or actions as they are often interpreted as disrespect or dislike of the individual rather than a situation.

Evaluation of the Nursing Care Plan

Obtaining a thorough cultural assessment, including use of folk remedies, during the initial encounter with the child/adolescent and parents is essential. It is upon this basis that the plan of care is developed, negotiated, and evaluated. To evaluate the effectiveness of the nursing care plan in providing culturally competent care, first you should ask a few probing questions to determine whether the plan was successful in achieving the desired outcomes, including the mutual goals established with the child and parents. Second, if the goals were not met, you should ask a few probing questions to determine the reasons for failure. Were the child and parents included in the planning and implementation of the nursing care? Were extended family members included in the plan? Did the true decision maker in the family participate in the care plan? For example, the grandparent, uncle, aunt, or other extended family member—not the biologic mother or father—is

the family decision maker. Third, if the goals were met, the reasons for their success should be evaluated and communicated to other members of the health care team for future reference.

Application of Cultural Concepts to Nursing Care

Two case studies are presented here to demonstrate the application of transcultural nursing concepts, theories, and research findings to clinical nursing practice. The first, Case Study 6-1, focuses on a very young child from an American Amish family, and the second, Case Study 6-2, on a dying child from a Buddhist family. Each case exemplifies the need for involvement of extended families of varying types. Each also reflects how the response of the nursing team affected the end result of the child's care. In addition a specific, individualized plan of care for the Amish family is presented. As shown, the nursing issues in each case are complex and multifaceted. The interconnectedness of the various components of the child's situation with the larger system is often minimized or disregarded. The values and beliefs of both the nurses within the health care delivery system and the family's extended social network must be considered. For the purpose of analysis, some fundamental conflicts in values and beliefs have been identified. Similarities and differences also have been indicated in the nursing plan of care.

In the case involving the Amish child, the young nurse was clearly advocating for a patient, in a situation requiring change in hospital practice, if not policy. It is assumed that this facility had not yet implemented principles of family-centered care, which are common practice in most agencies that care for children. Given the negative response of the nursing supervisor, it would seem she needs to reassess her approach to the problem. She would be wise to first gather data from her colleagues to help her understand the immediate, inflexible response of the supervisor, and then determine whether there are possible compromises that would be acceptable to both family

CASE STUDY 6-1

Presence of Immediate and Extended Family

A rural Amish community is located about 50 miles from an urban medical center, the only facility available for care of an acutely ill child. An enthusiastic new RN emphatically presents her case to allow the presence of family/extended family of a 6-month-old Amish child who has been admitted for the repair of a cardiac VSD. The nurse is passionate about the issue, rational in her approach, and assured that she can prevail to change existing visitation policies.

The problem of overnight accommodation for the extended community family has become a topic of debate among the nursing staff. Sensitive to the cultural practices and beliefs of the Amish child and his family, the new RN begins stating her position on behalf of the family's right to adhere to Amish cultural practices to her supervisor. The supervisor listens impatiently and quickly interrupts with her decision. "These people are such a nuisance. The child wouldn't even have the VSD if they didn't insist on intermarriage within their own community.

Then they come here in droves and think we have to give them a place to sleep. This isn't a hotel. They can just go back to their horses and buggies and old-fashioned ways. The answer is NO! The natural, biologic mother and father may spend the night. Everyone else is to go home. And that's final."

The nurse leaves the discussion with her supervisor feeling dejected; however, she completes her data collection. Using Leininger's transcultural model (1991), she examines the underlying attitudes, values, and beliefs among the Amish parents and those of the health care providers and then develops an individualized, culturally congruent, plan of care. Prior to discharge, the nurse, in collaboration with the parents and other significant members of the extended family, evaluates the effectiveness of the nursing care from a transcultural nursing perspective. The young nurse must also review the process in which change can be accomplished within the agency. She needs to determine what parts of the system can/should be manipulated to bring about desired change and who are the formal and informal leaders who can effect change.

and supervisor. She will need to present the risk versus benefits of having the extended family remain with the child: consider factors from agency perspective, the legal perspective, perspective of other patients, and the child/family perspective (Box 6-1). A review of the literature will reveal significant data that support involvement of extended family in hastening recovery of the child by supporting the entire family.

Outcome: There are no definitive solutions or answers for this dilemma. The case study is intended to demonstrate the complexity of the

---

BOX 6-1

Nursing Plan of Care: Hospitalization of an Amish Child: Conflicting Cultural Values (Related to Case Study 6-1 Above)

Goal: Child's recovery and ultimate discharge from the hospital (return to parents) in an optimal state of health. This is a mutual goal of the Amish child's parents and of the health care providers within the health care system. In order to plan care for this child, the nurse needs to examine the underlying attitudes, values, and beliefs of the two groups that are in conflict. Points on which there is agreement must be identified as well.

Amish–rural, agricultural lifestyle	Urban health care providers
Family	
Large families, extended sociocultural–religious network of community members who assist the natural parents.	Small family units, urban lifestyle, nuclear family.
Cooperation and support among extended family, especially in stressful "crisis" times such as hospitalization of a child.	Individual responsibility by members of a nuclear family; mother and father primarily responsible.

BOX 6-1 (*continued*)

Child generally not left alone when away from community; therefore, someone from the community visits or stays in absence of parents.

Concept of family includes "nonblood relatives."

Visiting by grandparents and siblings accepted but only two at any given time and only parents can remain over night.

Concept of family includes only biologically related persons.

Parental Obligations

Children are a part of a larger cultural group; adult members of the larger community have various relationships and obligations to the children and parents even though they are not biologically related.

Mother and father are responsible for children; only they may stay with the child overnight. Physical size of hospital facilities do not allow for a large number of visitors, who clutter rooms, violate fire safety rules by blocking doorways, and hindering delivery of care. Responding to requests for information from every visitor is time consuming and violates HIPAA policies

Economic Considerations

Communal sharing of resources; hospital bill is paid from a common fund; entire bill is paid in cash upon discharge.

Rely on private or state subsidized health insurance coverage for payment of all costs related to patient care, Sense of anonymity and impersonal involvement.

Traditional and Religious Values

Religious values permeate all aspects of daily living; time set aside daily for prayer and reading of scripture.

Religion is important and adherence to practices often vary based on severity of illness; worship usually limited to a single day of the week, such as Saturday or Sunday.

Belief that illness afflicts both the "just" and the less righteous and is to be endured with patience and faith.

Illness is part of a cause–effect relationship; science and technology will one day conquer illness.

Protestant work ethic (in an agricultural, rural sense).

Protestant work ethic (in an urban sense).

Dress is according to 19th-century traditions; specific colors and styles indicate marital status.

Fashions occur in trends; wide range of "acceptable" dress.

Married men wear beards; single men are clean-shaven.

Whether a man shaves is a matter of personal preference.

Simple, rural lifestyle; family-oriented living. For religious reasons, avoid "modern" conveniences such as electricity; use candles/kerosene lights, outdoor sanitary facilities.

Use high-tech electronic equipment, electricity and nuclear energy. Indoor plumbing is the norm; auto-flush toilets and water that runs with the wave of a hand are "ordinary."

cross-cultural issues and to emphasize the necessity for thoughtful analysis of various facets of the problem. The ability to synthesize information from previous learning—psychology, anthropology, religion and theology, history, economics, sociology, principles of leadership, and others—to the nursing care of children from culturally diverse backgrounds is invaluable.

The cultural assessment is the foundation of excellent transcultural care and cannot be overlooked even in the face of major obstacles of attitudes of others or limited time. A cultural assessment must become an integral part of the admission assessment of all children and adolescents, thus enabling excellent, individualized, family-centered care.

CASE STUDY 6-2

End-of-Life Care for a Buddhist Adolescent

Ving, 16 years of age, was born in Vietnam and immigrated to Australia with her family 15 years ago. She is a devout Buddhist. Ving was born hepatitis B positive, which is now complicated by advanced liver cancer. Over the past few weeks, Ving's pain has become unmanageable at home and her family has her admitted to the hospital for better pain management. Her family is concerned that appropriate preparations be made for her death.

In collaboration with Buddhists monks, the nurses of the inpatient unit agreed that Ving would be cared for through the final hours of her life with minimal noise and minimal activity in her room; this was to ensure that her soul was as untroubled as possible. Her family remained with Ving around the clock and agreed to notify the nurses when she died, the health care team agreed not to touch the body until the family agreed it was appropriate.

Outcome:

On the day of her death, family, close friends, and spiritual advisors were present to oversee the process. Eight hours after her death it was deemed that Ving consciousness had departed, she was then examined and the time of death documented.

This case study was adapted from: Clark, K., & Philips, J. (2010). End of life care: The importance of culture and ethnicity. *Australian Family Physician, 39*(4), 212.

SUMMARY

Culture exerts an all-pervasive influence on infants, children, and adolescents and determines the nursing interventions appropriate for the individual child, parents, and extended family members. Knowledge of the cultural background of the child and family is necessary for the provision of excellent transcultural nursing care. Your **cross-cultural communication** must convey genuine interest and allow for expression of expectations, concerns, and questions.

Culture influences the child's physical and psychosocial growth and development. Basic physiologic needs such as nutrition, sleep, and elimination have aspects that are culturally determined. Parent–child relationships vary significantly among families of different cultures, and individual differences among those with the same background add to the complexity. Cultural beliefs and values related to health and illness influence health-seeking behaviors by parents and determine the nature of care and cure expected.

Regardless of the cultural background of an adolescent, the transition from childhood to adulthood must be accomplished. This can be complicated when the adolescent's values, beliefs, and practices conflict with traditional cultural values or with those of the dominant culture in which the teenager lives. Acculturation of an adolescent presents multiple issues for the family as well as for the teen.

REVIEW QUESTIONS

1. Compare and contrast the child-rearing practices of three cultural groups; also
   a. Discuss the role of extended family members in raising children for each of the three groups.
   b. Describe the ways in which extended family members can assist parents during a child's illness.
2. Critically examine the perceived causes of chronic illness and disability in children from diverse cultures. Describe how the parental philosophic and religious beliefs affect their reaction to/explanations for the child's chronic illness and/or disability?
3. Describe the term and identify nursing interventions for the following Hispanic culture-bound syndromes as they affect children:
   a. *Pujos* (grunting)
   b. *Mal ojo* (evil eye)
   c. *Caida de la mollera* (fallen fontanel)
   d. *Empacho* (a digestive disorder)

4. Critically explore the impact of various cultural attitudes on teen pregnancy.

5. Compare and contrast cultural beliefs about contraceptive use by adolescents.

CRITICAL THINKING ACTIVITIES

1. Determine your own level of cultural sensitivity and competence by completing the self-assessment checklist developed by the Georgetown University's Center for Child and Human Development. Go to: http://www.nasponline.org/resources/culturalcompetence/checklist.aspx

2. Arrange for an observational experience in a classroom at a school known to have children from various cultures. Compare and contrast the behaviors observed. Does the student–teacher interaction vary according to cultural background? What culturally based attitudes, values, and beliefs are reflected in the children's behaviors? The teacher's attitude? Ask the teacher(s) to describe the cultural similarities and differences in the classroom.

3. When caring for a child from a cultural background different from your own, spend time talking with the child's parents or primary provider of care and discuss the child-rearing beliefs and practices specifically related to discipline, respect, and educational expectations for the child. Compare and contrast the parental responses with your own beliefs and practices.

4. When assigned to the pediatric unit, observe the number and relationship of visitors for children from various cultures. Who visits the child? If nonrelated visitors come, describe how they interact with the child? With the parent(s)?

5. When caring for a child from a cultural background different from your own, ask the parent(s) or primary provider(s) of care to tell you what they believe causes the child to be healthy and unhealthy. To what cause(s) do they attribute the current illness or hospitalization? What interventions do they believe will help the child to recover? Are there any healers outside of the professional health care system (e.g., folk, indigenous, or traditional healers) whom they believe could help the child return to health?

REFERENCES

Anderson, S., & Whitaker, R. (2009). Prevalence of obesity among U.S. preschool children in different racial and ethnic groups. *Arch Pediatr Adolesc Med. 163*(4), 344–348.

Aruda, M. (in press). Predictors of unprotected intercourse for female adolescents measured at their request for as pregnancy test. *Journal of Pediatric Nursing.*

Ball, H. (2002). Reasons for bedsharing: Why parents sleep with their infants. *Journal of Reproductive and Infant Psychology, 20,* 207–222.

Barry, H., Bacon, M. K., & Child, I. L. (1967). Definitions, ratings, and bibliographic sources of child-training practices of 110 cultures. In C. S. Ford (Ed.). *Cross-cultural approaches* (pp. 293–331). New Haven: HRAF Press.

Children's Defense Organization. (2009). *Children in poverty.* Retrieved February 11, 2007, from http:cdf.childrensdefense.org/site/PageServer?pagename=priorities_endchildpoverty

Clark, K., & Philips, J. (2010). End of life care: The importance of culture and ethnicity. *Australian Family Physician, 39*(4), 210–213.

deOnis, M., Onyango, A., Borghi, E., Siyam, A., Nishida, C., & Siekmann A. (2007). Development of a WHO growth reference for school age children and adolescents. *Bulletin of The WHO, 85,* 660–667.

DeWar, G. (2008). The science of attachment parenting. Retrieved March 1, 2010 from http://www.parentingscience.com/attachment-parenting.html

DeWar, G. (2009). Infant crying, fussing and colic: An anthropological perspective on the role of parenting.

Retrieved on March 1, 2010, from http://www. Parentingscience.com/infantcrying.hlml

Federal Interagency Forum on Child and Family Statistics (2006). America's children in brief: Key national indicators of well-being, 2006. Retrieved March 5, 2007, from http://www.childstats.gov/americaschildren

Fleer, M. (2006). The cultural construction of child development: Creating institutional and cultural intersubjectivity. *International Journal of Early Year Education, 14*(2), 127–140.

Flynn, M. (2004). *Best practices for the prevention of overweight and obesity in children: A focus on immigrants new to industrialized countries.* Calgary Health Region. Project No. 6795-15-2002/5440004. Retrieved March 4, 2007, from http://www.hc-sc.gc.ca/sr-sr/finance/hprp-prpms/results-resultats/2004-flynn_e.html

GeneReview (2009). Familial transthyretin amyloidosis. Retrieved March 1, 2010, from http://www.ncbin.nlm.nih.gov/pubmed/20301373

Goode, T., & Jones, W. (2006). *Definition of linguistic competence.* Washington, DC: National Center for Cultural Competence, Georgetown University Center for Child and Human Development.

Goode, T., Hayewood, S., Wells, N., & Rhee, K. (2009). Family-centered, culturally and linguistically competent care: Essential components of the medical home. *Pediatric Annals, 38*(9), 505–512.

Halfron, N., & Hochstein, M. (2002). Life course health development: An integrated framework for developing health policy and research. *Milbank Quarterly, 80*(3), 433–479.

Harbaugh, L., & Jordon-Welch, M. (2009). End the epidemic of childhood obesity...one family at a time. *American Nurse Today.* Retrieved March 1, 2010 from http://nursingworld.org/mods/mod461

Havighurst, R. J. (1974). *Developmental tasks and education.* New York: David McKay.

Korbin, J. E. (1991). Cross-cultural perspectives and research directions for the 21st century. *Child Abuse and Neglect, 15*(Suppl. 1), 67–77.

Lee, J. (2006). *Exposing longstanding taboos about menstruation: A cross-cultural study of the women's hygiene project.* Oral presentation at 2006 International Communication Association Conference, Dresden, Germany. Retrieved February 28, 2010, from http://www.allacademic.com//meta_mla_apa.reserach_citation.

Leininger, M. M. (1991). *Culture care delivery and universality: A theory of nursing.* New York: National League for Nursing Press.

McCoy, R., Hunt, C., & Lesko, S. (2006). Frequency of bed sharing and it's relationship to breasdtfeeding. *Developmental and Behavioral Pediatrics, 25*, 141–149.

McKenna, J. (2000). Cultural influences on infant and childhood sleep biology: Toward a more inclusive paradigm. In Loughlin, J., Carroll, J., Marcus, C. (Eds.). *Sleep and breathing in children.* I (pp. 199–230). Notre Dame, IN: Notre Dame Press.

McKenna, J., & McDade, T. (2005). Why babies should never sleep alone: A review of the co-sleeping controversy in relation to SIDS, bed sharing and breastfeeding. *Pediatric Respiratory Reviews, 6*, 134–162.

New World Encyclopedia. (2008). *Menstruation.* Retrieved March 20, 2010, from http://www.newworldencyclopedias.org/entry/menstrurastion

Overfield, T. (1995). *Biologic variation in health and illness: Race, age and sex differences* (2nd ed.). New York: CRC Press.

Reebye, P., Ross, S., & Jamieson, K. (2009). A literature review of child-parent/caregiver attachment theory and cross-cultural practices influencing attachment. Retrieved March 19, 2010, from http://www.attachmentacrosscultures.prg/reserch/html#12

Short, M., & Rosenthal, S. (2008). Psychosocial development and puberty. In C. Gordon (Ed.). *The menstrual cycle and adolescent health* (Chapter 4). Wiley-Blackwell.

Statistics Canada. (2006). *Census tract profiles.* Ottawa, ON. Retrieved March 1, 2010, from http://www12.statcan.gc.ca/census-recentement/2006/rt-td/as-eng.cfn

Turner, H. N. (2010). Parental preference or child well being: An ethical dilemma. *Journal of Pediatric Nursing, 25*(1), 58–63.

U.S. Census Bureau. (2009). Resident population and net change. Retrieved March 1, 2010, from http://quickfacts.census.gov/qfd/sdtates/00000.html

Utomo, I. D. (2005). Women's lives: Fifty years of change and continuity. In: Hull, T. H. (Ed.). *People, Population and Policy of Indonesia.* (pp. 71–124). Jakarta Equinox Publishing & Institute of Southeaster Asian Studies.

White, E., Rosengard, C., Weitzen, S., Meers, A., & Phipps, M. (2006). Fear of inability to conceive in pregnant adolescents. *Obstetrics & Gynecology, 108*, 1411–1416.

World Health Organization. (2009). Child growth standards. Retrieved March 1, 2010, from http://www.who.int/childgrowth/en

World Health Organization. (2010). *Enhancing the rights of adolescent girls.* Geneva: WHO.

Worthman, C., & Brown, R. (2007). Companionable sleep: Social regulation of sleep and cosleeping in Egyptian families. *Journal of Family Psychology, 21*, 124–135.

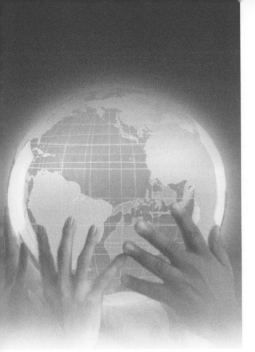

Transcultural Perspectives in the Nursing Care of Adults

Joyceen S. Boyle

KEY TERMS

Adulthood
Caregiving
Developmental crises
Developmental tasks
Developmental transitions
Generativity
"High blood"
HIV/AIDS
Middle adult
Midlife crisis
"Nerves" ("bad nerves")
Physiologic development
Psychosocial development
Sandwich generation
Situational crises
Situational transitions
Social age
Social roles
Stroke belt
"The virus"
Transitions of adulthood
Young adult

LEARNING OBJECTIVES

1. Understand how culture influences adult development.
2. Explore how health-related situational transitions might influence adult development.
3. Analyze the influences of culture on caregiving in the African American culture.
4. Analyze the influences of culture on women's development in the African American family.
5. Evaluate cultural influences in adulthood that assist individuals and families to manage during health-related crises.
6. Assess the ways in which gender, religious views, and culture influence health–illness and/or situational transitions in adult development.

This chapter discusses transcultural perspectives of health and nursing care associated with developmental events in the adult years. Chapter 8 of the text discusses transcultural nursing care of older adults; therefore, this chapter will focus primarily on young and middle adulthood. The first section presents an overview of cultural influences on adulthood, with an emphasis on how **transitions of adulthood** might be influenced by cultural variations. The second section gives an example of problems faced by a middle-aged African American woman who is experiencing a situational crisis, as well as personal health problems. The situational crisis or transition begins when her daughter is diagnosed with HIV/AIDS and returns home to live with her mother. The influences of culture on individual and family responses to health problems, caregiving, and situational transitions are described. In this chapter, we will discuss developmental tasks, those transitions that occur in a normal successful adulthood. We will also refer to specific transitions, those points in life that indicate change or turmoil as individuals struggle to cope with various life events.

Overview of Cultural Influences on Adulthood

Developmental processes and how they relate to health during adulthood are of interest as development stages often influence responses to illness. In addition, adult development structures how individuals respond to health promotion and wellness by shaping lifestyles, including eating habits, exercise, work, and leisure activities.

The middle years are a time of physical and psychosocial change. These changes are usually gradual and reflect the processes of normal aging. **Physiologic development** is evident in the hormonal changes that take place in midlife in both men and women, whereas **psychosocial development** may be more subtle, but equally important. These changes, both physiologic and psychosocial, are influenced by cultural values and norms.

Physiologic Development During Adulthood

Women undergo menopause, a gradual decrease in ovarian function with subsequent depletion of progesterone and estrogen. While these physiologic changes occur, self-image and self-concept change also. The influence of culture is relevant because women learn to respond to menopause within the context of their families and culture. The *perception* of menopause and *aspects* of the experience of menopausal symptoms seem to

vary across cultures. It has sometimes been assumed that non-Western women do not experience the menopausal problems seen in Western society because their status increases as they age; however, this assumption has been challenged. Certainly the treatment of menopause differs, as Western medicine has tended to treat the symptoms of menopause with hormone replacement therapy. This too is changing as we become aware that adult aging is a complex phenomenon and there are often unanticipated repercussions to medical interventions. Although there are not many studies on the perimenopausal transition across cultural groups, there seem to be cultural differences in the reporting of symptoms associated with menopause such as bodily pain and in the use of health care services, as well as prescribed treatments for menopausal symptoms. This reinforces an earlier statement that women (as well as others) learn to respond to menopause within the context of their families and culture. Recent studies have also shown that such factors as length of stay in the United States and social–economic status were significant predictors of number and severity of menopausal symptoms among immigrant women (Bokim, Im, & Chee, in press).

Men also have physical and emotional changes from the decreased levels of hormones. Loss of muscle mass and strength and a possible loss of sexual potency occur slowly. However, developmental differences among both men and women have not been examined cross-culturally, and most existing theoretical and conceptual models of adult health do not provide insight into cultural variations. Recognition of the cultural belief that aging, however gradual, is a normal process and not a cause for medical and/or surgical intervention may be more culturally appropriate for persons of diverse cultural groups.

Psychosocial Development During Adulthood

Development in adulthood was termed the "empty middle" by Bronfenbrenner (1977). A noted developmental psychologist, he implied that this term was an indication of Western culture's lack of interest in the adult years. Traditionally, these years were viewed as one long plateau that separates childhood from old age. It was assumed that decisions affecting marriage and career were made in the late teens and that drastic changes in developmental processes seldom occurred afterward. For many years, most developmental theorists saw adulthood as a period to adapt to and come to terms with aging and one's own mortality. Our thinking has changed considerably since Bronfenbrenner's observations. We now conceptualize middle age as a vigorous and changing stage of life involving challenges and transformations.

Sociocultural factors in our society have precipitated tremendous changes, producing crises, changes, and other unanticipated events in adult lives. Divorce, remarriage, career change, increased mobility, the sexual revolution, and the women's movement have had a profound impact on the adult years. Many middle-aged adults may be caught in the **sandwich generation**—still concerned with older children (and sometimes grandchildren) but increasingly concerned with the care of aging parents. Middle life can be a time of reassessment, turmoil, and change. Society acknowledges this with common terms such as *midlife crisis* or even *empty nest syndrome*, along with other terms that imply stress, dissatisfaction, and unrest. However, adulthood is not always a tumultuous, crisis-oriented state; many middle-aged persons welcome the space, time, and independence that middle age often brings. Midlife can be a time of challenge, enjoyment, and satisfaction for many persons. We now tend to view a "midlife crises" as a time of transition that can be a positive experience including the mastery of new skills and behaviors that helps an individual to change and grow in response to a new environment (Meleis, Sawyer, Im, Hilfinger Messias, & Schumacher, 2000).

Chronologic Standards for Appropriate Adult Behavior

Much of the work on adult development was done in the 1960s and 1970s by developmental psychologists such as Bronfenbrenner (1977),

Neugarten (1968), and Havighurst (1974), all of whom proposed different theories about adult development. We still rely on some of this early work as we attempt to understand the complexities of adult development. Neugarten (1968) observed that each culture has specific chronologic standards for appropriate adult behavior and that these cultural standards prescribe the ideal ages at which to leave the protection of one's parents, choose a vocation, marry, have children, and in general, get on with life. The events associated with these standards do not necessarily precipitate crises or change. What is more important is the timing of these events. As a result of each culture's sense of social time, individuals tend to measure their accomplishments and adjust their behavior according to a kind of social clock. Awareness of the social timetable is frequently reinforced by the judgments and urging of friends and family, who say, "It's time for you to . . ." or "You are getting too old to . . ." or "Act your age." Problems often arise when social timetables change for unpredictable reasons. An example is the recent trend of adult children, frequently divorced or unemployed or both, returning to live with their parents, often bringing along their own children. Grandparents caring for grandchildren are now a common phenomenon in our society. Being widowed in young adulthood or losing one's job at age 50 due to an economic downturn are examples of events that are likely to cause stress and conflict because they occur outside of our notions of social order.

Culture exerts important influences on human development in that it provides a means for recognizing stages in the continuum of individual development throughout the life span. It is culture that defines **social age**, or what is judged appropriate behavior in stages of the life cycle. In nearly all societies, adult role expectations are placed on young people when they reach a certain age. Several cultures have defined rites of passage that mark the line between youth and adulthood; in the United States, we tend to view the legal age to obtain a driver's license or to drink alcohol as markers of beginning adulthood.

Menarche is a milestone in women's development and a psychologically significant event, providing a rather dramatic demarcation between girlhood and womanhood. However, this is not an event that is celebrated openly in U.S. culture as most girls are too embarrassed to talk openly about it with anyone but their mothers or close friends. There are no definitive boundaries that mark adulthood for either young girls or young boys, although legal sanctions confer some rights and responsibilities at the ages of 18 and 21 years. Examples are the age requirements for obtaining a driver's license, for voting, and for purchasing alcohol and tobacco. Although the age of 21 years is often cited, there is no single criterion for the determination of when young adulthood begins, given that different individuals experience and cope with growth and development differently and at different chronologic ages. A young boy who joins the military forces at age 18 and serves in Iraq or Afghanistan may "grow up" more quickly than the young boy who lives with his parents, has a part-time job, and attends a local community college.

Adulthood as such is usually divided into young adulthood (late teens, 20s, and 30s) and middle adulthood (40s and 50s), but the age lines can be fuzzy. Generally, a **young adult** in his or her late teens and early 20s struggles with independence and issues related to intimacy and relationships outside the family. Role changes occur while the young adult is pursuing an education, experiencing marriage, and starting a family while establishing a career. A **middle adult** most often concentrates on career and family matters. However, as previously mentioned, adulthood is not necessarily an orderly or predictable plateau. Experiences at work have a direct bearing on the middle-aged adult's development through exposure to job-related stress, levels of physical and intellectual activity, and social relations formed with coworkers. "Re-careering" or changing careers during middle adulthood is also becoming more common and can be a source of change. At home, family life can be chaotic, with role changes and other transitions occurring with dizzying frequency. Often adults are faced with the realization that they are getting older and feel like they have made the wrong choices or have left many things still undone. This realization can lead to **developmental crises** and/or **situational crises**. How well individuals cope with and manage the challenges and transitions required in adulthood are influenced by their cultural values, traditions, and background.

Developmental Tasks

Throughout life, each individual is confronted with **developmental tasks**: responses to life situations encountered by all persons experiencing physiologic, psychologic, spiritual, and sociologic changes. Although the developmental tasks of childhood are widely known and have long been studied, the critical experiences of adulthood are less familiar to most nurses.

Several theorists have studied and defined the developmental or *midlife* tasks of adulthood. Many personality theorists, for example, Freud, Erikson, and Fromm, cite maturity as the major criterion of adulthood. These various theories have implications for how we define "development," "maturity," and "wisdom". According to Erikson (1963), the developmental task of middle adulthood is the attainment of generativity versus stagnation. **Generativity** is accomplished through parenting, working in one's career, participating in community activities, or working cooperatively with peers, spouse, family members, and others to reach mutually determined goals. Mature adults have a well-developed philosophy of life that serves as a basis for stability in their lives. Individuals in adulthood assume numerous **social roles**, such as spouse, parent, child of aging parent, worker, friend, organization member, and citizen. Each of these social roles involves expected behaviors established by the values and norms of society. Through the process of socialization, the individual is expected to learn the behaviors appropriate to the new role. It is important to note that many developmental theories have connotations of stability and blandness associated with adulthood, although this probably is not the case.

In many ways, the early theorists' views of what occurs in adulthood are the biases of "White" middle-class values and experiences. This constellation of characteristics has been attributed to predominantly White, Anglo-Saxon, Protestant (WASP) views and behaviors. For many cultural groups in Western society, the mastery of mainstream developmental tasks is not easily managed, and in some cases, it may even be undesirable. For some groups, developmental tasks may be accomplished through culturally defined patterns that are different from or outside of the norm of what is expected in the dominant culture. In Evidence-Based Practice 7-1,

we learn how an observant Jewish woman, and her family, in labor, delivery, and postpartum needs nursing care that allows her to abide by Jewish laws, customs, and practices that influence everyday life as well as those that pertain to childbearing. Childbearing is a special time for most cultures and there are cultural prescriptions to ensure the well-being of both the mother and the child. The nurse and/or midwife can assist the traditionally, religious and observant Jewish couple to maintain their religious laws, customs, and practices. These laws, customs, and practices frame their lives and parenthood with meaning and richness. The discussion

EVIDENCE-BASED PRACTICE 7-1

Jewish Laws, Customs, and Practice in Labor, Delivery, and Postpartum Care

This article provides a comprehensive and thorough guide to specific laws, customs, and practices of traditionally, religious observant Jews that assist the transcultural nurse or midwife to provide culturally congruent and sensitive care during labor, delivery, and the postpartum period. Providing culturally congruent care includes cultural knowledge, in this case, the nurse or midwife needs to understand the Jewish laws, customs, and practices that guide everyday life as well as those that pertain to childbearing. These cultural issues include adherence to the laws of intimacy issues between husband and wife or niddah, dietary laws or kashrut, and observance of the Sabbath. Detailed tables are provided that list: (1) observant Jewish customs, laws, and practices during labor, delivery and postpartum; (2) annual Jewish holidays and fast days; (3) a cultural assessment for Jewish clients in labor, delivery, and postpartum. Case studies are presented that describe cultural competence challenges for nurses who want to learn about the Jewish culture and how to provide culturally

competent care to Jewish women during childbirth.

Clinical Application

1. Recognize that observant Jewish couples are committed to maintaining their religious laws, customs, and practices as much as possible throughout the labor, delivery, and postpartum periods.
2. Acknowledge that childbirth is a time that is highly influenced by cultural values and beliefs.
3. The religious laws, customs, and practices that will be most apparent during labor, delivery, and postpartum will pertain to prayer, communication between husband and wife, dietary laws, the Sabbath, modesty issues, and labor and birth customs.
4. The culturally competent nurse follows the cues of the religious family, tailoring his or her health and nursing care in a manner that allows the family to practice their traditions in their specific designed manner while employing professionalism and creativity in providing quality patient care.

Reference: Noble, A., Rom, M., Newsome-Wicks, M., Englehardt, K., & Woloski-Wruble, A. (2009). Jewish laws, customs, and practice in labor, delivery and postpartum care. *Journal of Transcultural Nursing, 20*, 323–333.

includes intimacy issues between husband and wife, dietary laws, Sabbath observance, as well as those practices concerning prayer, modesty issues, and labor and birth customs. This childbearing time that occurs in young and middle adulthood is a prime example of the interface between culture, religion, childbearing practices, and transcultural nursing care.

During the last few decades, new studies have focused on the developmental experiences of women and have led several authors (Belenky, McVicker, Clinchy, Goldberger, & Tarule, 1997) to suggest that developmental stages and the associated developmental tasks of adulthood have been derived primarily from studies of men. These authors suggest that women experience adult development differently. Women's traditional location of responsibility was in the home, nurturing children and husbands as well as parents. This view is changing, prompted by societal changes and informed by scholars who are addressing women's psychosocial development in new ways. Some of these differences are described in the next section.

Adulthood has been conceptualized as step-by-step phases of development, but more recent theories (Demick & Andreoletti, 2003; McCrae & Costa, 2003) suggest that development is an evolutionary expanse involving different eras and transitions. These life transitions have triumphs, costs, and disruptions. Within nursing, Meleis et al. (2000) proposed a framework to study life transitions. They suggest that transitions can be developmental, situational, health–illness, and/or organizational. The next section discusses several important adult life transitions and examines how culture and life events influence adult growth and change during these transitions. These life transitions or successful progression through a developmental task occur slowly over many years, but they are important in terms of quality of life and life satisfaction. Culture influences these transitions, and it is important that nurses be able to evaluate their adult clients and to help them adjust and change in culturally appropriate ways.

Culture and Adult Transitions

Developmental Transition: Achieving Success in One's Career

Some Americans define a "successful career" as financial success, while others may see it as a way to provide service or make a contribution to the lives of their fellow citizens. It is important to recognize that women as well as men now achieve success in their chosen careers. Other "new" Americans may find that the goal of a successful career is not possible for them. The United States, as other countries in the world, has experienced a tremendous influx of immigrants and refugees from Southeast Asia, Latin America, Eastern Europe, Africa, and other areas. Although immigrants and refugees may aspire to a good job, that may be a difficult goal to attain. They may have difficulty with the language, with the skills and educational level required, and other factors necessary to holding a good job in the United States. Furthermore, many more women, including immigrants and refugees, are working outside of the home, and there may be a different division of time of energy for both spouses.

In many immigrant and refugee families, role conflict and stress occur within the family as gender roles begin to change during contact with American culture. For example, sometimes the male head of household is unable to find employment; if he was a professional in his former country, he may be reluctant to accept the menial jobs that are traditionally filled by immigrants or refugees when they first come to this country. Frequently, low-status jobs are more available to immigrant women, yet their traditional roles are closely tied to the home and family. When an immigrant or refugee woman begins to work outside of the home, her role changes and alters the traditional power structure and the roles within the family. The lack of adequate social supports, such as affordable day care and adequate compensation for work, and the additional physical and emotional stress result in an unacknowledged toll on immigrant and refugee families. Box 7-1 lists some characteristics of immigrant and refugee families.

BOX 7-1

Some Characteristics of Immigrant and Refugee Families

1. Traditional family values are evident; for example, roles of men and women are differentiated. Women's role is in the home, with the family. Men are heads of the household and family providers.

2. Families tend to be extended; if members do not actually live in the same household, they visit and contact each other frequently. Immigrants and refugees tend to keep in fairly close contact with family members in the home country.

3. Many immigrants come to the United States because they already have family members here.

4. Most immigrants and refugees are poor and struggle to earn an adequate income. Often men in refugee communities have been professionals in their home country but are unable to be employed in the same capacity in their new host country. Women are often more easily employed outside of the home and they often find employment as domestic or service workers. For many refugee or immigrant women, working outside of the home is a new experience for them. To earn a salary is very empowering for these women.

5. Refugees may be fleeing war and political persecution. Many may experience symptoms of posttraumatic stress syndrome.

6. Traditional health and illness beliefs may influence behavior. Immigrant and refugee families may combine traditional health practices with modern Western health care. The use of traditional practices is fairly common in some groups.

7. Language is a significant barrier for the first few years that immigrants and refugees live in the United States and Canada. Children tend to learn English and become acculturated faster than their parents.

At present, to expect members of certain groups, such as poor or ethnic minorities, newly arrived immigrants or refugees, the homeless, the mentally ill, or the unemployed, to achieve satisfaction from jobs that interest them or from status derived from succeeding in a career is unrealistic and indicates a lack of sensitivity to the problems faced by these groups. Thus, although the work role is valued in American society, the attainment of a successful career may not be realistic for some minority groups, immigrants, or even certain individuals within the majority culture, some of whom are returning to school in the hope of preparing for a second career.

Developmental Transition: Achieving Social and Civic Responsibility

Social and civic responsibilities are in part culturally defined. Although members of the dominant North American culture may value achieving an elected office in the local Parent Teacher Association (PTA) or Rotary Club, other cultures may find these goals baffling and emphasize other activities within the cultural group. For example, in some groups, religious obligations may be given priority over civic responsibilities. Usually, traditional religious groups have not encouraged the emergence of women in leadership roles within the church structure or the wider society, although this is being challenged by women within several religious groups.

Sometimes within traditional cultures, women who seek roles outside the family are criticized because recognition and acknowledgment outside the family group may conflict with the traditional role of women. Some religious and ethnic or cultural groups believe that a woman's place is in the home, and women who attempt to succeed in a career or in activities outside the home or group are frowned on by other members of the group. Civic responsibilities that relate to children or domestic matters may be viewed as appropriate for women to assume, whereas civic activities may be viewed as more within the province of men. Middle Eastern and Southeast Asian cultures emphasize responsibilities and contributions to the extended family or clan rather than to the wider society. Numerous researchers (Baird, 2009; Lipson & Miller, 1994) have reported that refugee women in the United States continue to socialize almost exclusively with other refugee women, often extended family/clan or tribe members.

During the past three decades, the majority (65%) of the refugees relocated to the United States are women (Gozdziak & Long, 2005), many of these are unmarried or widowed with children. Women, whose husbands are killed or stay behind to fight in various conflicts, are often forced to flee with children and/or elderly family members alone. Women refugees carry a substantial burden during the migration process and are considered an essential component in the adaption of the family. Coping with life in the United States becomes the focus of their daily lives. Finding a job, getting children into school, learning English, and other resettlement activities become challenging transitions for them. Refugee women experience stress as they undergo these transitions. It is not unusual for refugee women to associate their own health and well-being with that of their family members (Guruge & Khanlou, 2004). African refugees from Sudan, Somalia, Eritrea, and Ethiopia have identified informal social support networks, such as having family and friends nearby and religion as being important for the well-being of their families and themselves (Tilbury & Rapley, 2004). The social and civic responsibilities that we have associated with adulthood in White, middle-class America may not be appropriate for many other cultural groups. Clearly we need to rethink adult development and transitions in the lives of refugee and immigrants. Concepts such as social connectedness and integration, resilience and strength might help us better understand adult development and transitions in refugee and immigrant populations.

Developmental Transition: Marriage and Raising Children to Adulthood

The age at which young persons marry and become independent varies by custom or cultural norm as well as by socioeconomic status. Generally speaking, adults of lower socioeconomic status leave school, begin work, marry, and become parents and grandparents at earlier ages than middle-class or upper-class adults. It is relatively common in North American society for an 18-year-old, for example, to marry and move away from home or to leave home to pursue higher education or find employment. Indeed, many American families encourage early independence, or "leaving home," although this trend decreases when the economy declines. Other cultural groups, such as those from the Middle East and Latin America, place more emphasis on maintaining the extended family. Even after marriage, a son and his new wife may choose to live very close to both families and to visit relatives several times each day. Families from some cultural groups, such as Hispanics, or traditional religious groups, such as the Hutterites or the Amish, may be reluctant to allow their young daughters to leave home until they marry. In many Muslim families, girls do not leave home until they are married.

Increased mobility in American society has impacted family life as many young families now live far away from grandparents, and the traditional influences of grandparents on young grandchildren is decreasing. Sometimes because of geographical distance, grandparents barely know their grandchildren, although digital photos via home computers, cell phones, and other technological devices are helping to keep grandparents up-to-date with the growth and activities of their grandchildren.

Caring for and launching their own children and caring for their own aging parents place some middle-age adults between the demands of caregiving from parents and those from children. Primarily, caregivers have been women, and the stress resulting from the demands of caregiving places them at increased risk of health problems (Teel & Leenerts, 2005). In cultures that value and maintain extended family networks, the responsibilities of caring for both children and older parents can be shared. Many American families still maintain very close and extended family networks (Figure 7-1).

Adjusting to aging parents and associated responsibilities, as well as finding appropriate solutions to problems created by aging parents, are challenges created by situational, developmental, and even health–illness transitions. Placing an aged mother or father in a nursing home may be a decision made with reluctance and only when all other alternatives have been exhausted. Such actions may be totally unacceptable to some members of other cultural groups, in which family and community networks would facilitate the complex care required by an aged ill person. Such

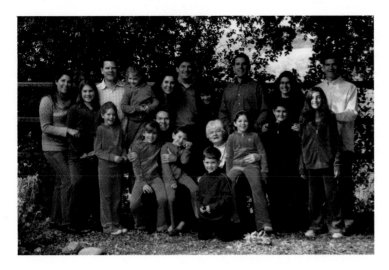

FIGURE 7-1 American families, such as the extended family of Teresa and Neil Cooper of Carlsbad, California, are multiethnic in each generation, yet maintaining close family ties is a priority. This emphasis on family has continued through three generations. The children look forward to seeing each other. Their parents and grandparents believe that this is the beginning of the fourth generation of close family ties.

cultural norms would exert a great deal of social pressure on an adult son (or especially a daughter) who failed in this obligation.

Developmental Transition: Changing Roles and Relationships

The relationship between a wife and husband is often enhanced in middle adulthood, although divorce at this time is not infrequent in the United States. The frequent need for both spouses to work may conflict with traditional roles and cause feelings of guilt on the part of both the husband and wife. Some women continue to assume all responsibility for domestic chores while working outside the home, and they experience considerable stress and fatigue as a result of multiple role demands. If either or both spouses are working in low-paying jobs and still struggling to make ends meet, or if the job holder is laid off or loses his or her job, adulthood may not be a time of enjoyment and leisure activities.

An emphasis on an emotionally close interpersonal relationship between a husband and wife may be a culturally defined value. In some Hispanic cultures, women develop more intense relationships or affective bonds with their children or relatives than with their husbands. Latin men, in turn, may form close bonds with siblings or friends—ties that meet the needs for companionship, emotional support, and caring that might

otherwise be expected from their wives. Touch between men (walking arm in arm) and between women is acceptable in many societies. Gender roles and how men and women go about establishing personal ties with either sex are heavily influenced by culture. In North American society, women are more likely to have intimate, self-disclosing friendships with other women than men have with other men. A man's male friends are likely to be working, drinking, or playing "buddies." In southern Europe and the Middle East, men are allowed to express their friendship with each other with words and embraces. Such expressions of affection between men are uncommon in North American culture and might be attributed to homosexuality.

Affiliation and friendship needs in adulthood and the satisfaction of these needs are facilitated or hindered by cultural expectations. Social support, family ties, and friendship needs can be met through the extended family and kinship system or through other culturally prescribed groups such as churches, singles bars, work, and civic associations. Something new for many single adults are the various Internet sites where one can meet others who are single and interested in starting new relationships. An individual's health may be affected by these social ties: persons who have a reliable set of close friends and an extensive network of acquaintances are usually healthier—both emotionally and physically—than persons without supportive networks and close friends.

Changing cultural values also influence professional health care roles and relationships. How individuals are approached and greeted as well as the kind and type of relationship established may be closely tied to cultural expectations and norms. A casual, first-name basis has become the norm in many health care situations, with medical receptionists (and often other health professionals as well) calling patients by their first names. This can be inappropriate in many instances. Health care professionals should inquire about the appropriate manner to use in approaching clients and their family members. Table 7-1 provides some suggestions and guidelines to use in approaching clients and using their names in professional relationships.

TABLE 7-1
Guidelines for Names

Arab	Both male and female children are given a first name. The father's first name is used as the middle name; the last name is the family name. Usually, a person is called formally by the first name, such as Mr. Mohammed or Dr. Anwar.
Chinese	The family name is stated or written first and then the given name, just opposite of European and North American tradition. Only very close friends use the given name. Politeness and formality are stressed; always use the whole name or family name. Use only the family name to address men, for example, if the family name is Chin and the man's given name is Wei-jing, address the man as Chin. Many Asians take an English name that they use in their North American host country. Use the title Mr. or Mrs. preceding the English name because the use of only the first name is considered rude. Some Asians switch the order of their names to be like Western names, and this can be very confusing to outsiders.
	Women in China do not use their husband's name after marriage. If the woman has lived in Hong Kong, Taiwan, or a Western country for a long time, her name may be the same as her husband's name.
Latin American	The use of surnames may differ by country. Many Latin Americans use two surnames, representing the mother's and father's sides of the family. "Maria Cordoba Lopez" indicates that her father's name is Cordoba and her mother's surname is Lopez. When Maria marries, she will retain her father's name and add the last name of her husband. Thus, Maria becomes Maria Cordoba de Recinos. Many Latin Americans drop their mother's surnames after they immigrate to the United States. In approaching clients of traditional Latin cultures, it is appropriate to use the Spanish terms *Señor* or *Señora*, followed by the primary surname (the husband's), if the nurse is comfortable with those terms.
Native North American	Native North American names differ by tribal affiliation. Many tend to follow the dominant cultural norms. In the Navajo culture, a health care provider may call an older Navajo client "grandfather" or "grandmother" as a sign of respect. In the past, some tribes have tended to convert traditional names into English surnames. Thus, there are names like Joe Calf Looking and Phyllis Greywolf.

The above-mentioned examples are very general. If in doubt, always ask because it can be embarrassing for the nurse and the client if the nurse uses a name in an inappropriate manner. Members of cultures that adhere to traditional values might be confused by our current practice of using Ms. as a designation for women. Generally speaking, it is *always best and most appropriate* to be formal and to use the surname with the appropriate title of Mr. or Mrs. preceding the name.

Adapted from Purnell, L. D., & Paulanka, B. J. (2008). *Transcultural health care: A culturally competent approach* (3rd ed.). Philadelphia: F.A. Davis.

Health-Related Situational Crises

The preceding section described developmental tasks, transitions, and some cultural variations influencing adulthood. This section contains an in-depth case study of a middle-aged African American woman who is experiencing health–illness **situational transitions** and **developmental transitions**. Transitions often occur because of a serious illness in middle age. Leading causes of death in the United States are heart disease, cancer, cerebrovascular disease, respiratory disease, accidents, and diabetes (Centers for Disease Control and Prevention [CDC], National Center for Health Statistics, 2009). These conditions affect individuals, but they also occur within a family system and affect children, spouses, aging parents, and other close relatives. Because middle-aged adults may be responsible for aging parents or ill adult children as well as for grandchildren, the illness of any one individual must be evaluated carefully for the myriad of ways in which it affects all members of the family.

Health care professionals need a better understanding of how families influence the health-related behavior of their members because definitions of health and illness and reactions to them form during childhood within the family context. Yet, there are many gaps in our knowledge. Cultural beliefs and values influence health promotion, disease prevention, and the treatment of illness. When the illness has social and/or cultural connotations, or involves shame and/or stigma, the issues become more complex. Medical treatment and nursing care must take into account the cultural history, values, beliefs, and practices that influence the client's and family's ability to cope with the illness, as well as assessing whether the interventions are congruent with their culture.

Caregiving and African American Women

African American women, like all women, receive and provide health care in the context of their families in which they perform multiple caregiving roles: as wives, mothers, daughters, widows, single women, and so on. Women's assumption of the caregiving role is in line with traditional expectations of women's domestic role, and the majority of caregivers are women; therefore, it is not surprising that the caregiving roles of women often predispose them to interrupted employment and limited access to health care insurance as well as pension and retirement plans. Shambley-Ebron and Boyle (2006a, 2006b) have documented that these general problems and characteristics of caregivers are compounded for African American women by the special circumstances of their lives and the lives of the men and children for whom they care. In the case of African American caregivers, prejudice, discrimination, and poverty often all interact to increase stress and pose challenges that frequently result in poor health.

Caregiving, as used in this chapter, implies the provision of long-term help to an impaired family member or close friend. Caregiving usually is labor intensive, time consuming, and stressful, although the exact effects on the physical and emotional health of caregivers are still being documented. Although positive outcomes, such as feelings of reward and satisfaction, do occur for caregivers, they still experience negative psychologic, emotional, social, and physical outcomes (Vitaliano, Shang, & Scanlan, 2003). When caregiving for other family members takes place during middle adulthood, the roles for both the caregiver and the recipient may change as new challenges emerge. In addition, culture and ethnicity influence beliefs, attitudes, and perceptions of what is normal and what is sickness, as well as what caregiving actions should be taken. Culture and ethnicity may influence how often individuals engage in self-care versus seeking formal health services, how many medications they take, how often they rest and exercise, and what types of foods they consume when ill. Caregiver research has been based predominantly on White subjects, and ethnic differences have been rarely analyzed. It has been only recently that nurse researchers and others have focused on specific cultural groups to study caregiving (Escandon, 2006) and the ethnocultural factors that are so important in planning support for caregivers (Crist, Kim, Pasvogel, & Velazquez, 2009; Gallagher-Thompson et al., 1997).

Studies of African American caregivers have found that they tend to use religious beliefs to help them cope with the stress of caregiving. Boyle, Hodnicki, and Ferrell (1999) described Black caregivers' belief in a personal God and their intense relationship with Him provided them with support during the illness of a family member and helped them cope with death and loss. Poindexter, Linsk, and Warner (1999) also found that a major source of support for Black caregivers was their personal relationships with "Jesus," "God," or "the Lord." These authors suggest that spirituality is both personal and empowering for some African Americans and is related to the deepest motivations in life. Spirituality is often expressed in the context of the daily life of Black caregivers, not necessarily by formal attendance at religious events. Holt and McClure (2006) noted that the specific nature of the religion–health connection among African Americans is of great interest to health professionals as it holds promise for integrating church-based health interventions.

African American women also face a special situation in relationship to **HIV/AIDS**. African American women are especially hard hit by HIV/AIDS. In 2006, African American women comprised only 12% of the female population in the United States, yet they accounted for 64% of women with HIV/AIDS (National Alliance of State & Territorial AIDS Directors [NASTAD], 2008). Three-fourths of the HIV/AIDS cases in African American women were caused by high-risk heterosexual contact (CDC, Fact Sheet: HIV/AIDS among African Americans, 2008). The rate of AIDS diagnosis for African American women was 20 times the rate of White women by the end of 2006 (NASTAD, 2008) and is the third leading cause of death for African American females, ages 25 to 34, in 2006 (WISQARS, CDC, 2006). Shambley-Ebron and Boyle (2006b) studied African American women who were diagnosed with HIV/AIDS and caring for children who were also HIV positive. These mother–caregivers relied on spiritual traditions and religious practices to help deal with the pressures of living and mothering with HIV/AIDS.

Although several studies show positive results of caregiving in African American caregivers, many caregivers pay a high emotional and physical price for their care. There is also some indication that African American caregivers may solve problems of caregiving differently and that these differences may result from social and cultural factors. For example, African American mothers whose adult children are living with HIV/AIDS may not always exhibit a proactive, problem-solving approach to effects of the disease (Boyle, Bunting, Hodnicki, & Ferrell, 2001). This is not because African American caregivers are uninterested in their adult children's health or cannot understand the complexity of medical regimens. Such behavior may be related more to the racial discrimination and racism that have remained significant factors in the health care of African Americans over time. In addition, there may be cultural influences that shape human behavior in such a way that problems arising from illness and caregiving are solved by different approaches.

The Context of HIV/AIDS and the African American Community

HIV/AIDS disproportionately affects African Americans and has had a devastating effect on African American communities. The CDC points out that at every stage—from HIV diagnosis through the death of persons with AIDS—the hardest-hit racial or ethnic group is African Americans. Even though African Americans make up only approximately 13% of the U.S. population, one-half of the estimated new cases of HIV/AIDS diagnoses in the United States in 2004 were for African Americans (CDC, HIV/AIDS Surveillance Report, 2008).

Prevention Challenges

From a public health standpoint, preventive education about HIV/AIDS has been hindered by an unwillingness to talk frankly about behaviors surrounding sex and drug use and this has been a substantial barrier in effective HIV preventive programs. In essence, the AIDS epidemic has forced society to examine and attempt to alter cultural behaviors and values that were largely ignored in the past. And, as a society, we have not always been comfortable with this frankness. In Evidence-Based Practice 7-2, we read about a culture- and-gender-based approach to HIV/AIDS prevention entitled *My Sister, Myself*. This age-appropriate intervention targeted preadolescent girls as sexual activity is often initiated in early adolescence. The intervention was an eight week program with a weekly session lasting 2.5 hours. Community input was solicited in the development of the intervention. Topics included Africana womanist values, discussions about female reproductive health, stress management skills, and healthy relationships between young men and women. This program suggested that as young African American girls learn to access their cultural and gender strengths, healthier women, families, and communities will develop.

Over the past 2 decades in the United States, the practice of high-risk HIV behaviors has changed from selected populations of White homosexual men with no history of drug use to heterosexuals having multiple sex partners and/or using drugs. HIV/AIDS disproportionately affects selected groups, especially Blacks and Hispanics, and risk patterns are different for men and women. *African American women*, a term that includes both adolescents and adults, are especially at risk. More than three-fourths of the HIV/AIDS cases diagnosed for African American women from 2001 to 2004 were caused by heterosexual contact. Injection drug use accounted for almost one-fifth of all

EVIDENCE-BASED PRACTICE 7-2

My Sister, Myself: A Culture- and Gender-Based Approach to HIV/AIDS Prevention

This article describes the development and implementation of a culture- and gender-based HIV prevention intervention entitled *My Sister, Myself*. African American women are bearing an excess burden of HIV/AIDS, becoming infected at a rate 25 times that of White American women. This places African American girls at the highest possible risk of becoming infected with HIV/AIDS. Age-appropriate interventions that target preadolescent girls have the potential to reach this high-risk group during the critical developmental stages of preadolescence and early adolescence, when sexual activity is often initiated. Cultural appropriateness is essential to the development of effective interventions and may be an important way to interrupt the growing rates of HIV/AIDS in African American women. Community action participatory research was used to involve the community in the development of the intervention. The intervention was an 8-week culture- and gender-based program, conducted in weekly sessions each lasting 2.5 hours. Eight girls participated in the intervention. The themes and content for each session were developed in conjunction with the community members. The sessions used guest educators, group leaders, and storytellers. Activities included studying the lives of successful African American women, Africentric and Africana womanist values and discussions about female reproductive health, stress management skills, and healthy relationships between young men and women. Data were gathered through a series of focus groups from the participants to evaluate cultural and gender awareness, sexual health knowledge, and future plans. All of the girls recognized that they knew very little about their body and sexual health and needed to have information to make appropriate choices. Girls also believed that they had traditionally centered resources to help them arrive at

(Evidence-Based Practice continues on page 170)

EVIDENCE-BASED PRACTICE 7-2

My Sister, Myself: A Culture- and Gender-Based Approach to HIV/AIDS Prevention (*continued*)

adulthood successfully. These methods included inner strength, female supportive networks, and spirituality. As young African American girls learn to embrace and access their cultural and gender strengths, healthier women, families, and communities are certain to follow.

Clinical Application

- Culture and gender are unique and distinct aspects of the lives of young African American girls and must be included in preventive interventions for health and well-being.
- Nursing interventions that focus on future aspirations of young African American girls can be useful in helping them direct their energies toward meeting these goals, while foregoing roadblocks such as early sexual activity.

- As many young girls (regardless of their cultural heritage) are reluctant to talk with their mothers about issues related to sexuality, it is important to provide avenues for girls to talk with knowledgeable adult women who are culturally similar for answers to questions about sexuality.
- Supportive networks for young African American girls can be broadened and strengthened by involving teachers, nurses, and women from their churches as support persons to help them achieve their goals in relation to age-appropriate relationships and sexual behaviors.
- The use of spirituality and religiosity appears consistently in the literature as a way to help young African American girls deal with life experiences.

Reference: Shambley-Ebron, D. Z. (2009). My sister, myself: A culture- and gender-based approach to HIV/AIDS prevention. *Journal of Transcultural Nursing, 20,* 28–36.

---

cases. By the end of 2006, the rate of AIDS diagnoses for African American women was 20 times the rate for White women (NASTAD, May, 2008). Although high-risk heterosexual behavior and drug use are important factors influencing HIV infection rates among African American women, other factors also contribute to circumstances that can lead to HIV transmission. Among these factors are biological vulnerabilities; unique characteristics and nuances of heterosexual relationships in African American communities. Structural influences also impacting HIV transmission and that are of concern to African American communities are poverty, employment, and education and incarceration (NASTAD, May 2008). Implementing intervention programs has proven extremely difficult. The CDC points out that the African American community faces numerous barriers that impact HIV prevention efforts.

Barriers to HIV Preventive Efforts in African American Communities

Influences on HIV/AIDS Status of African Americans

Poverty

African Americans, generally speaking, often have lower incomes than other Americans. Nearly one in four African Americans are living in poverty (U.S. Census Bureau, 1999) and studies have found an association between higher AIDS incidence and lower income (Diaz et al., 1994). Accessing health care services is a problem if an individual does not have health insurance. In addition, for many African Americans, day-to-day living activities often take precedence over whether an individual has access to educational information about HIV and AIDS. Poverty or lack of money and health insurance influence access to

HIV testing and state-of-the art treatment if an individual is diagnosed with HIV.

Denial

Many African Americans still believe that HIV/AIDS is a problem in Newark or New York, or even in Florida, but not in rural Georgia or Alabama. Homosexuality is a very sensitive topic in many African American communities as is drug use; therefore, talking about HIV/AIDS may be met with disapproval or disdain. Talking frankly about sexual behavior with new partners and insisting on the use of condoms may be very difficult for African American women. They may be afraid to ask a male partner about his sexual history or his use of or experience with drugs for fear of abruptly ending their relationship. Denial about HIV might be a reason why many African Americans who are HIV infected do not get tested and do not know they are HIV positive. Persons who do not know that they are HIV infected are more likely than those with a diagnosis to engage in risky behavior and to unintentionally transmit HIV to others (CDC, Heightened Response to HIV/AIDS, 2007)

Drug Use

Injecting drugs is the second leading cause of HIV infection for African American women and the third leading cause of HIV infection for African American men. In addition to the danger from contaminated needles, syringes, and other works, persons who use drugs are more likely to take other risks, such as unprotected sex, while under the influence of drugs (CDC, Fact Sheet: HIV/AIDS among African Americans, August, 2008). A recent study of HIV-infected women found that women who used drugs, compared with women who did not, were less likely to take their antiretroviral medicines exactly as prescribed (Sharpe, Lee, Nakashima, Elam-Evans, & Fleming, 2004).

Homophobia and Concealment of Homosexual Behavior

Homophobia and stigma can cause some homosexual African American men to identify themselves as heterosexual or not to disclose their sexual orientation and this presents challenges to prevention programs (Millett, Peterson, Wolitski, & Stall, 2006). It is extremely important to involve African American community stakeholders in developing and implementing programs that achieve significant reductions in HIV/AIDS and ultimately to end this epidemic among African Americans. Involving community stakeholders will mobilize African American communities to become more aware of the need to develop strategies that address broader social and cultural factors such as homophobia, stigma, and denial (CDC, Heightened Response to HIV/AIDS, 2007).

Culturally Competent Nursing Care of an African American Woman Experiencing a Situational Crisis

In the past decade or so, the nature of HIV/AIDS caregiving has changed because new antiretroviral medications have dramatically altered the course of HIV/AIDS. During the first part of the AIDS epidemic, caregivers to persons with AIDS often were men; however, mothers and other family members became more involved as the incidence of HIV disease changed from White homosexual men to the heterosexual population. Many African Americans living in the rural South first learned about HIV/AIDS from television programs, and many used to think of AIDS as a disease that was common in large cities; few thought it was something that could happen in small Southern towns or to a member of their own family. Unfortunately, many persons have become rather complacent because they now think that HIV/AIDS can be treated with new medications, and therefore, there is nothing to worry about any more. Although the new antiretroviral medications are effective, African Americans continue to be at risk, not only to contacting HIV/AIDS but in terms of accessing and following through with state-of-the-art treatment programs.

HIV/AIDS still carries a tremendous stigma in African American communities. Many African Americans, especially younger adults or teenagers refer to HIV/AIDS as **"the virus."** Case Study 7-1 provides an example of a middle-aged African American woman who provides care to her developmentally delayed sister, Ethel, and to her 26-year-old daughter, Tywanda, who has HIV/AIDS. Culturally appropriate ways in which the nurse might implement nursing care are suggested. The use of traditional family and religious systems is encouraged because these ties are of particular significance in rural African American culture.

CASE STUDY 7-1

Mrs. Ernestine Pollard, a 57-year-old Black woman, lives in a small town in rural Georgia. Mrs. Pollard cares for her older sister, Ethel, who is now 65 years old. Mrs. Pollard explains that her sister "can't talk, and her mind's not good." Mrs. Pollard says that even as a little girl, she knew that Ethel would be her special responsibility and when she (Mrs. Pollard) married, Ethel cane to live with her and her new husband. Mr. Pollard died a few years ago following a stroke. Recently Ethel's health has been deteriorating because of a series of what Mrs. Pollard calls "little strokes." Then, just a few months ago, Mrs. Pollard's 26-year-old daughter, Tywanda, returned home to live with her. Tywanda was living and working in New Jersey, where she had became ill. She was taken by friends to the emergency room and then admitted to the hospital. During this hospitalization, the results of a test for HIV disease were positive. After discharge from the hospital, Tywanda decided to return home to live with her mother. Tywanda has been a great worry to her mother for a number of years as Mrs. Pollard has known that Tywanda was occasionally using drugs. Although Mrs. Pollard welcomed Tywanda home again, she worried about her past high-risk behaviors and hoped they would not continue.

Despite successes in HIV/AIDS treatment and marked declines in HIV infection rates in other risk groups, HIV disease was still the third leading cause of death for African American females, ages 35 to 44 in 2006 (WISQARS, 10 Leading causes of death for Black females, August, 2006). While high-risk heterosexual sexual behavior and drug use are important factors influencing HIV

infection rates among African American women, other factors also contribute to the context of HIV/AIDS. NASTAD states that programs targeting African American women must recognize the complexities of HIV risk among African American women and address the complex web of social and cultural issues that place them at the crossroads of the HIV epidemic in the United States (NASTAD, May 2008). Issues such as poverty, employment, education and incarceration, as well as the unique characteristics and nuances of heterosexual relationships in African American communities must be taken into consideration.

Mrs. Pollard explains that sometimes with the stress of caregiving for Ethel and worrying about Tywanda, her "pressure goes sky high." She has had "high blood" for several years. Her physician prescribed medication for her blood pressure, and she tries to take it on a regular basis, but sometimes she forgets. Other times, she decides that she just does not have the money for medication. Lately, as Tywanda has been staying away from home and acting secretively, Mrs. Pollard is not sleeping well and she is worried that Tywanda may be taking drugs again. She told her doctor that she has "bad nerves" and explained that she is unable to sleep at night. The physician prescribed sleeping pills for her, but Mrs. Pollard is unwilling to take them because she fears that she will not hear Ethel if she gets up doing the night. In addition to her worry about Tywanda, she is concerned about her sister's health as Ethel seems to be getting more confused and disoriented, especially at night. Mrs. Pollard's other grown children, two daughters, live in Atlanta, several hours drive from the small town where Mrs. Pollard lives.

Health Promotion Strategies and Nursing Interventions

African American women are at high risk for cardiovascular diseases, particularly hypertension and stroke. Mrs. Pollard lives in that area of the South known as the **stroke belt** because morbidity and mortality from cardiovascular diseases (especially among African Americans) are so prevalent in this region (WISQARS, 10 Leading Causes of Death, United States, 1999–2006). The nursing management priorities for Mrs. Pollard will be to support her caregiving role and provide health promotion strategies to control her blood pressure and help reduce the stress she is currently experiencing. In terms of blood pressure management, a nurse might advise Mrs. Pollard to lose weight and incorporate changes in eating habits and regular exercise into her lifestyle. However, social and cultural factors as well as the caregiving situation may compromise these health goals. Nurses can become more culturally sensitive to cultural norms and values of clients like Mrs. Pollard by listening carefully, being empathetic, recognizing the client's self-interest and needs of her family members, being flexible, having a sense of timing, appropriately using the client's and family's resources, and giving relevant information at the appropriate time.

Although Mrs. Pollard does have a private physician and tries to seek care when appropriate, she considers Ethel's and Tywanda's needs before her own. Mrs. Pollard does not have health insurance and therefore access to care is compromised. Tywanda attends an infectious disease clinic about 50 miles from where her mother lives. Her medications are provided through Ryan White HIV/AIDS Program, a federal program focused exclusively on HIV/AIDS care. The program is for those who do not have sufficient health care coverage or financial resources for coping with HIV disease (U.S. Department of Health and Human Services, HIV/AIDS Bureau, n.d.). Mrs. Pollard does not accompany Tywanda when she visits the clinic because first of all, Tywanda acts as if she does not want her mother to go with her and secondly, Mrs. Pollard does not wish to leave her sister alone. The nurses at the clinic wonder if anyone in Tywanda's family really cares about her because she always comes alone to the clinic appointments. However, Tywanda does not always attend the clinic but she does not tell her mother when she misses an appointment. Mrs. Pollard does not know about the medications that Tywanda takes for HIV/AIDS. Tywanda does not readily disclose information and Mrs. Pollard tries to be sensitive to her daughter's wishes.

Mrs. Pollard is concerned about Ethel's appetite because she believes that the proper food will promote and enhance her health. Like many other adults, Mrs. Pollard has fairly definite preferences about food and the way it is prepared and served. The Pollard family frequently eats foods that are high in fat; for example, they enjoy servings of bacon or fatback for breakfast once or twice during the week. Breakfast is an important meal for them. They prefer their vegetables cooked with bacon or ham for flavoring. Symbolism is attached to food in every culture, and Mrs. Pollard believes that both Ethel and Tywanda's health will improve by eating what Mrs. Pollard considers "healthy" foods. In her concern for Tywanda and the time she spends with her sister, she neglects her own diet or eats whatever is convenient, often "fast foods" or those high in carbohydrates and sodium. Mrs. Pollard needs to be gently reminded by the nurse that it is important for her to pay some attention to her own nutrition also. The nurse could initiate a discussion about the kinds of nutritious foods that would be appropriate for the three of them.

Young-Mason (2009) suggested that understanding the art and culture of food of those we seek to help is paramount to being and becoming an astute and learned nurse. Clark (2003) observed that food could have many meanings as well as being nourishing. For example, food can serve as a means of enhancing interpersonal relationships or as a means of communicating love and caring. Being able to prepare food that her daughter and sister will eat and enjoy is a source of satisfaction for Mrs. Pollard and a reinforcement of her successful role as caregiver. It is an act of caring and love for her to prepare a meal for her family. At the same time, she must maintain her own health to continue to provide care for Tywanda and her sister. A priority is that she take her medication on a regular basis to control her blood pressure. Taking her medication regularly, resting as often as she can, and avoiding foods that are high in fat and/or sodium or eating them only in small or moderate amounts may be realistic goals for Mrs. Pollard.

Nurses providing care to clients like Mrs. Pollard will need to consider other cultural factors that ultimately influence the nursing goals. Rural African Americans often have cultural ways to view health and illness. **"High blood"** is an illness condition that is associated with African American culture in the rural South. Many health care professionals make the wrong assumption that "high blood" is the same as high blood pressure, and although there are similarities, the cultural explanation of "high blood" is different from the biomedical explanation of high blood pressure. "High blood" is conceptualized in terms of blood volume, blood thickness, or even elevations of the blood in the body (e.g., "blood rushes to your head").

"High blood" is believed to be caused primarily by factors that "run blood up," such as salt, fat, meats, and sweets. This condition results in an increased "pressure" or high blood pressure. Sometimes "high blood" leads to a feeling of faintness that may cause the afflicted person "to fall out" or faint. Other causal factors that result in "high blood" are emotional upsets or prolonged stress. Sometimes it is thought to be caused by a falling out with God or by eternal forces such as enemies putting a "hex" on someone. Many older African American clients believe that eating slightly acidic foods, such as greens with vinegar or dill pickles, will lower "high blood." Thus, although there are similarities between "high blood" and high blood pressure, the explanations and treatments are not always the same in the cultural prescriptions as in the biomedical model. Mrs. Pollard tries to be conscientious about taking her blood pressure medication, but she sometimes forgets to take it and sometimes does not get around to promptly renewing the prescription, so she might go without her medication for several days or a couple of weeks. The nurse should acknowledge Mrs. Pollard's active involvement in her own health promotion, encourage her to take her blood pressure medication as prescribed, and remind her to renew it promptly before she is completely out of medication.

"Nerves" or even **"bad nerves,"** while not unique to the rural South, are commonly described by many Southerners. "Bad nerves" are often equated with anxiety and worry but may refer to something as serious as a "mental breakdown" or severe emotional disorder. Mrs. Pollard uses the term to refer to her worry, concern, and anxiety about Tywanda and Ethel. Sometimes she has "crying spells" that she describes as "just crying and crying, and not being able to stop." She gets up several times at night to answer her sister's call or to check on Tywanda and make certain that they are all right. Lack of sleep and continued worry and anxiety accelerate her psychologic distress. Again, recognition and acknowledgment from the nurse that she is providing excellent care for her sister and her daughter will be reassuring for her. She should be encouraged to rest and should be assured that crying and feeling sad are normal reactions to her sister's deteriorating condition and Tywanda's HIV/AIDS.

Because of a lack of economic resources, African American midlife women are likely to be subjected to many stressful life events, such as job and marital instability, lack of male companions as heads of households, erratic income, and frequent changes and relocations. Because she has worked for self-employed businesses most of her life, Mrs. Pollard lacks health insurance. She has experienced many life stresses that were related to the lack of economic resources. Mrs. Pollard was working as a clerk in a local dry cleaning establishment when Tywanda returned home and told her mother that she had HIV/AIDS. However, as Ethel's health deteriorated and Tywanda's behaviors became more obvious and problematic, Mrs. Pollard decided to stop working for a while. She thought that if she stayed home, she could provide closer supervision and care to Ethel and be available to Tywanda when she needed her mother. Mrs. Pollard faces numerous situational crises: Tywanda's illness and high-risk behaviors, the poor health and aging of her sister, and economic hardship because she is the family provider and is not working at the present time.

Stress and anxiety are normal reactions in the lives of middle-aged adults like Mrs. Pollard. However, limited resources, lack of access to high-quality health care, and discrimination during an illness of a family member compound the stress and complicate a situational crisis. Mrs. Pollard's physician prescribed sleeping medication for her, assuming that would take care of her inability to sleep. Unfortunately, this reaction is fairly common: Physicians sometimes tend to prescribe medications for the symptoms reported by clients rather than probing more deeply into the situation. The nurse can reinforce Mrs. Pollard's decision not to take this medication and explore with her how to set aside time during the day when she might be able to take a nap. In addition, Mrs. Pollard's anxiety and inability to sleep well are directly related to the stress of caregiving. This can be dealt with in a more culturally acceptable manner than the routine prescription of sleeping medication. Some ways to support and help Mrs. Pollard deal with stress and anxiety may be family support, participation in religious activities, and coping through traditional spirituality. The nurse might suggest that Mrs. Pollard set aside some time during the day to quietly read the Bible and listen to religious music.

Close family and spiritual ties within the African American family and community support the caregiving role. Extended and nuclear family members willingly care for sick persons and assume these roles without hesitation. Mrs. Pollard's two daughters try to help their mother and Tywanda as much as possible, but they live several hours drive away. They try to visit one weekend each month and bring their children with them. Tywanda enjoys the company of her sisters and Mrs. Pollard notices that on weekends when one of the sisters is expected, Tywanda's mood seems improved as she obviously looks forward to the visit.

Many individuals with HIV disease and their close family members are reluctant to disclose the diagnosis to others outside the family because the stigma of disclosure in a small community can affect all members of the family. Shambley-Ebron and Boyle (2006b) report that in spite of its prevalence in African American communities, HIV/AIDS continues to be a highly stigmatized condition. Mrs. Pollard's minister is aware of Tywanda's condition, as are a few members of Mrs. Pollard's "church family." One of the

primary stressors of women during the midlife years is the loss of relationships and friendship networks, often because of competing demands on time. Caregivers have very little time for their own needs. It is extremely important for Mrs. Pollard's health and coping abilities that she continue to participate in church activities and to maintain those friendships and networks.

Spiritual beliefs form a foundation for Mrs. Pollard's daily life. Like other African Americans who live in the same rural community, Mrs. Pollard attends a small Protestant church whose membership is exclusively African American. Many, but not all, African Americans strongly believe in the use of prayer for all situations they may encounter. They use prayer as a means of dealing with everyday problems and concerns. Mrs. Pollard relies a great deal on prayer, and her religious beliefs and practices provide her with support and strength in her caregiving role. Encouraging Mrs. Pollard to take even 15 minutes each day to read familiar biblical verses might be one of the most helpful interventions the nurse could suggest.

Mrs. Pollard has a lifetime of experience with her church; she attended church services as a child and has continued this pattern in her adult years. The role of the church in the African American community has always been important; the church was the center of activities for African Americans for decades (Poindexter et al., 1999). Mrs. Pollard's religious beliefs are integrated into her daily life as a caregiver, and her belief in God enhances her ability to care for Ethel and Tywanda. She, like many other African Americans, has a personal relationship with God and is able to share her worries and concerns through prayer. Her traditional spirituality and church support provide a foundation for an active approach to coping with problems. Evidence-Based Practice 7-3 describes a group of African American women and their church leaders who discussed cultural health beliefs about creating healing lifeways. In particular, the women reported that prayer was the best action that they could take if they were ill. Prayer was a healing force for these African American women. The women talked

EVIDENCE-BASED PRACTICE 7-3

Faith and Feminism: How African American Women from a Storefront Church Resist Oppression in Health Care

It is well documented within the health profession that racism and discrimination negatively affect health care. These factors impede access to and acceptance of care by poor African American women. Unfortunately, a historical pattern of dehumanization of Black people is mirrored in contemporary experiences with the medical profession and health care system. However, women of color are not unknowingly victims, and over the years they have developed ways of combating racism and discriminatory objectification that they encounter in health care.

This article describes a group of African American women and their church leaders, who attended the Morning Sun Missionary Baptist Church (a pseudonym), a small storefront church in the Pacific Northwest. The church's pastor defines a storefront church as a building that was originally meant for another purpose; in this case, the church had once been a small white-frame house in a residential area of the city. Through interviews and life histories, the women described how they interpreted their day-to-day experiences in clinical encounters as well as health beliefs about how to survive and create healing lifeways. The women related that through their experiences, the best action anyone could take when ill was to pray. Prayer was a healing force in the women's lives and brought about an altered consciousness that occurred in times of intensely spiritual moments

and through the social action that was engendered as a result of the power of prayer. The women employed multiple strategies in preparing themselves to take control of the health interactions. They learned to be prepared, to take the initiative, and to ask questions. The women also made a point of taking the most assertive family member with them, especially if there was any procedure planned. They supported one another with discussions during church social times and reinforced the notion that they could redefine the dominant views of their experiences. Placing their trust in the Lord, believing that prayer had the power to change things, they were able to resist the dominant ideology of the health care system.

Clinical Application

- Read some of the sources cited in this article about Black feminism as they are enlightening about both institutional and individual racism in health care.
- Acknowledge the support and assistance that African Americans receive from their participation in religious activities.
- Incorporate the spiritual beliefs that strengthen and sustain African American women in your nursing care.
- Encourage the development of church-based and community-based educational efforts and support services for HIV-affected individuals and their family members.

Reference: Abrums, M. (2004). Faith and feminism: How African American women from a storefront church resist oppression in healthcare. *Advances in Nursing Science, 27*(3), 187–201.

about how they could take control of health situations, such as visiting a physician. The support, care, and social action of this group of women helped them employ multiple strategies to be assertive in health interactions.

A Situational Crises and Nursing Interventions

An important priority of nursing care for Mrs. Pollard and her family is to help them understand and adjust to the impact of HIV disease. The diagnosis of HIV/AIDS precipitated a situational crisis for the Pollard family. Such a situation can best be resolved by the provision of culturally relevant health-promotion and risk-reduction strategies. The health teaching and nursing interventions provided to the Pollard family should focus on wellness and health promotion. The nurse can continue this emphasis by helping Mrs. Pollard successfully manage the situational crises as well as the developmental transitions she is facing that are common to adulthood. The nurse can tell Mrs. Pollard about the social services available for patients who have HIV/AIDS and their family members. Mrs. Pollard may want to talk to a mental health counselor about the fears and concerns she has about Tywanda and drug use. In addition, the nurse can encourage Tywanda to keep clinic appointments and to see appropriate counseling and follow-up.

An important American cultural value is success in one's career, and over the past several decades, this has become as important to women as it has traditionally been for men. Mrs. Pollard has worked outside the home most of her adult life; yet, rural African American culture does not place the kind of emphasis on work and career that the wider American society does. Mrs. Pollard's ties of love and affection to Tywanda and to her sister, Ethel, are reinforced by African American cultural values. Family ties and the lifelong attachments, as well as the extension of the maternal role to an adult child, are highly valued in African American culture (Boyle et al., 1999). These values are emphasized over women's careers outside the home. In a historical study of African American women in America, Hine and Thompson (1998) suggested that Black women have always been the financial providers in Black families and that women's work roles have been culturally viewed as an inherent part of Black motherhood, not as individual careers. Mrs. Pollard has always been proud that she was able to take care of her family and that she could "make do" with very little. These values are important to family integrity and they can be positively reinforced by the nurse.

Many African American women of Mrs. Pollard's generation obtain meaning in their lives by caring for family members. Their feelings, behaviors, and attitudes go beyond a simple sentiment of affection or of family ties. In explaining why she cares for her older retarded sister, Mrs. Pollard says, "We were little girls together. I always knew that I was going to take care of her." In many societies, women disproportionally provide caregiving services and social policies, and home-based programs are organized around the assumption of women's availability and willingness to provide care. At the same time, it is important to understand that Mrs. Pollard values the traditional caregiving role, and she needs support and assistance in providing the care she believes her family members need.

It is important for the nurse to acknowledge that Mrs. Pollard is valued, recognized, and respected for her competence and expertise as a caregiver. The nurse could begin by including Mrs. Pollard, Tywanda, and her sisters in developing mutual goals for Tywanda's progress and care. At the same time, they can discuss Ethel's deteriorating condition and realistic expectations for her future. Mrs. Pollard should be encouraged in her role of providing help and care to family members and in promoting the health of her daughter and others. It is also important that her attention be directed toward her own needs on occasion, considering she tends to focus on meeting the needs of Tywanda and Ethel before her own. Of particular concern is the timing of Tywanda's illness. A serious health condition in a young, previously healthy adult child will cause unique trauma and conflict because of society's expectations that young adults will outlive their older parents. In addition, as a person diagnosed with HIV/AIDS, Tywanda has a condition that often generates shame and stigma.

It is important that these issues be acknowledged by both Mrs. Pollard and Tywanda.

Social and civic responsibilities among rural, older African Americans in the South are met almost entirely at the level of the extended family and the African American church. These ties and associations are very strong, are often complex, and are not readily understood by outsiders. African American pastors are key players in the lives of their congregations and in their communities. Mrs. Pollard should be encouraged to attend church services and to seek the help and support available to her through this important cultural resource. Mrs. Pollard sings in the church choir and tries to attend choir practice every Wednesday evening. Tywanda has agreed to stay home with her Aunt Ethel on Wednesday evenings while Mrs. Pollard is away for the evening. The Black church has been a traditional source of support, and congregations are frequently made up of middle-aged or older adults. Coping strategies such as prayer or reading the Bible and resources such as family and church support may help mediate Mrs. Pollard's reaction to stressful situations. A culturally competent nurse understands that spirituality is a traditional cultural value that can be supportive to African Americans during a health crisis.

Mrs. Pollard's life revolves around her family and church. The nurse must understand the importance of cultural ties with kin and others. The support provided by these ties is crucial when an illness develops and is necessary to successful health promotion and maintenance in caregiving activities. Although social support is very important in situations like Mrs. Pollard's, some researchers have found that many African American caregivers of persons with HIV illness have not disclosed the presence of HIV in the family to anyone outside the immediate family, including church members and ministers (Poindexter et al., 1999). When asked where they obtained help and support, these caregivers answered, "Jesus," "God," or "the Lord." It is not uncommon for older African Americans to cope without the amount of social support that would usually be expected in such a crisis, relying instead on internal spiritual resources (Poindexter et al., 1999, p. 231). Mrs. Pollard's Atlanta-based daughters are crucial to support and assistance during this stressful time. The nurse should encourage them and acknowledge their contributions. In addition, they should be involved in planning care for Tywanda and Ethel as they are instrumental in the support of their mother.

The nurse can continue to encourage Mrs. Pollard to attend church services because her social life is derived from her participation in the activities of her church. Providing positive enforcement for Tywanda's decision to stay with her aunt Ethel while Mrs. Pollard attends church services and choir practice would be appropriate. It will be the church family who will be instrumental in providing emotional support and help as Ethel's condition continues to decline. If Ethel should die, the church will offer spiritual support as well as the opportunity for Mrs. Pollard to find meaning and to cope with her loss and grief. If Tywanda continues risky drug and sexual behavior, Mrs. Pollard will need continued support and counseling from health care professionals to continue her caregiving role. Nursing interventions at the individual and family level are extremely important in maintaining and extending quality of life. Preventive interventions at the community level are essential to interrupt the trend of growing rates of HIV/AIDS in African American women.

SUMMARY

All individuals are confronted with life transitions or changes that we term *developmental tasks*. All cultures have acceptable and defined ways of responding to these life situations. There is a need to create new paradigms of adult development that reflect a more holistic picture of adult life. A situational crisis or transition was presented: an African American woman, Mrs. Pollard, who cared for her developmentally delayed sister, Ethel, and her 26-year-old daughter who had HIV/AIDS. Mrs. Pollard's own health problems were exacerbated by this situational transition, and her normal development through adulthood was disrupted. How nurses can understand such situations and provide culturally appropriate care was described.

REVIEW QUESTIONS

1. List and describe the types of transitions proposed by Meleis et al. (2000) and discussed in this chapter. Can you describe examples of these kinds of transitions in your family members and friends? Do you think it is helpful to think of "transitions" as opposed to "developmental tasks"? Why?

2. How does culture influence transitions or developmental tasks of adulthood? For example, explain how a woman from a traditional culture such as those in the Middle East might experience adulthood differently.

3. Discuss how gender might influence adult development in White "mainstream" North American culture.

4. Describe how social factors such as mobility, increased education, and changes in the economy have influenced adult development in mainstream North American culture.

5. How might caregiving for a family member bring about a situational transition for a middle-aged adult? Would this differ for cultural groups such as Chinese Americans or Mexican Americans? How?

6. Describe how culture influences the role of the caregiver in some African American cultures. What can you find in the literature about caregiving in other cultural groups?

CRITICAL THINKING ACTIVITIES

1. Interview a middle-aged colleague, a client, or a person from another cultural group. Ask about family adult roles and how they are depicted. How are these role descriptions typical of traditional roles that are described in the literature? If not, how are they different? What are some of the reasons why they have changed?

2. Interview a middle-aged client from another cultural group. Ask about the client's experiences within the health care system. What were the differences the client noted in health beliefs and practices? Ask the client about his or her health needs during middle age.

3. Using the cultural assessment guidelines provided in Appendix A, conduct a cultural assessment of a middle-aged client of another cultural group. Critically analyze how the client's culture affects the client's role within the family and the timing of developmental transitions. How might the assessment data differ if the client were older? Younger?

4. Review the literature on Mexican American culture. Describe the traditional Mexican American family. What are the cultural characteristics of Mexican Americans to consider in assessing the developmental tasks of adulthood in this group?

5. You are assigned a new patient, a 24-year-old man from El Salvador named Jose Calderon. At morning report you learn that he has been a gang member in El Salvador, and because he wanted to stop all gang-related activities, his life was threatened. He fled to the United States and has been granted political asylum. You are told that he has extensive tattoos on his body. What do you know about gang membership in Central America? In the United States? How does membership in a gang address the needs of adolescents? What are the cultural factors that are important to consider when you are planning nursing care for a patient like Jose? For example, how does our culture view body tattoos? What are the issues related to political asylum, immigration, and the like? How might you assist Jose to meet his developmental needs? What might be the problems he will encounter in U.S. society or in our health care system?

REFERENCES

Abrums, M. (2004). Faith and feminism: How African American women from a storefront church resist oppression in healthcare. *Advances in Nursing Science, 27*(3), 187–201.

Baird, M. B., (2009). *Resettlement transition experiences among Sudanese refugee women.* PhD dissertation, The University of Arizona, United States, Tucson, Arizona. Retrieved September 11, 2009, from Dissertations & Theses @ University of Arizona. (Publication No. AAT 3352364).

Belenky, M. F., McVicker, B., Clinchy, B. M., Goldberger, N. R., & Tarule, J. M. (1997). *Women's ways of knowing: The development of self, voice, and mind.* New York: Basic Books.

Bokim, L., Im, E. O., & Chee, W. (in press). Acculturation and menopausal symptoms among ethnic minority midlife women. *Journal of Transcultural Nursing.*

Boyle, J. S., Bunting, S. M., Hodnicki, D. R., & Ferrell, J. A. (2001). Critical thinking in African American mothers caring for adult children with HIV/AIDS. *Journal of Transcultural Nursing, 12*(3), 193–202.

Boyle, J. S., Hodnicki, D. R., & Ferrell, J. A. (1999). Patterns of resistance: African American mothers and adult children with HIV illness. *Scholarly Inquiry for Nursing Practice, 13,* 111–133.

Bronfenbrenner, U. (1977). Toward an experimental ecology of human development. *American Psychologist, 32,* 513–531.

Centers for Disease Control and Prevention. (2007). *A heightened national response to the HIV/AIDS crises among African Americans.* U.S. Department of Health and Human Services. Retrieved September 10, 2009, from http://www.cdc.gov/hiv/topics/aa/resources/reports/heightenedresponse.htm

Centers for Disease Control and Prevention. (August 2008). In *Fact Sheet: HIV/AIDS among African Americans.* U.S. Department of Health and Human Services. Retrieved September 9, 2009, from http://www.cdc.gov/hiv/topics/aa/resources/factsheets/aa.htm

Centers for Disease Control and Prevention. (2008). *HIV/AIDS surveillance report, 2008* (Vol. 18, pp. 1–54). Atlanta, GA: US Department of Health and Human Services. Retrieved September 8, 2009, from http://www.cdc.gov/hiv/topics/surveillance/resources/report/pdf/2006SurveillanceReport.pdf

Centers for Disease Control and Prevention, National Center for Health Statistics. (2009). In *Leading causes of death.* Retrieved August 15, 2009, from http://cdc.gov/nchs/fastats/lcod.htm

Clark, M. J. (Ed.). (2003). The cultural context. In M. J. Clark (Ed.), *Community health nursing: Caring for populations* (pp. 101–139). Upper Saddle River, NJ: Prentice Hall.

Crist, J. D., Kim, S., Pasvogel, A., & Velazquez, J. H. (2009). Mexican American elders' use of home care services. *Applied Nursing Research, 22*(1), 26–34.

Demick, J., & Andreoletti, C. (Eds.). (2003). *Handbook of adult development.* New York: Kluwer Academic/Plenum.

Diaz, T., Chu, S. Y., Buehler, J. W., Boyd, D., Checko, P. J., Conti, L. et al. (1994). Socioeconomic differences among people with AIDS: Results from a multistate surveillance project. *American Journal of Preventive Medicine, 10,* 217–222.

Erikson, E. (1963). *Childhood and society* (2nd ed.). New York: Norton.

Escandon, S. (2006). Mexican American intergenerational caregiving model. *Western Journal of Nursing Research, 28,* 564–585.

Gallagher-Thompson, D., Leary, M., Ossinalde, C., Romero, J., Wald, M. J., & Gernanadez-Gamarra, E. (1997). Hispanic caregivers of older adults with dementia: Cultural issues in outreach and intervention. *Group, 21,* 211–232.

Gozdziak, E., & Long, K. C. (2005). *Suffering and resiliency of refugee women: An annotated bibliography 1980-2005.* Washington, DC: Institute for the Study of International Migration: Georgetown University. Retrieved November 15, 2005, from http://www.georgetown.edu/sfs/programs/isim/

Guruge, S., & Khanlou, N. (2004). Intersectionalities of influence: Researching the health of immigrant and refugee women. *Canadian Journal of Nursing Research, 36*(3), 32–47.

Havighurst, R. J. (1974). *Developmental tasks and education.* New York: David McKay.

Hine, D. C., & Thompson, K. (1998). *A shining thread of hope: The history of Black women in America.* New York: Broadway Books.

Holt, C. L., & McClure, S. M. (2006). Perceptions of the religion-health connection among African American church members. *Qualitative Health Research, 16,* 268–281.

Lipson, J. G., & Miller, S. (1994). Changing roles of Afghan refugee women in the United States. *Health Care for Women International, 15,* 171–180.

McCrae, R. R., & Costa, P. T. (2003). *Personality in adulthood: A five-factor theory perspective* (2nd ed.). New York: Guilford Press.

Meleis, A. I., Sawyer, L. M., Im, E. O., Hilfinger Messias, D. K., & Schumacher, K. (2000). Experiencing transitions: An emerging middle-range theory. *Advances in Nursing Science, 23*(1), 12–28.

Millett, G. A., Peterson, J. L., Wolitski, R. J., & Stall, R. (2006). Great risk for HIV infection of black men who have sex with men: A critical literature review. *American Journal of Public Health, 96,* 1007–1019.

National Alliance of State & Territorial AIDS Directors. (May 2008). *The landscape of HIV/AIDS among African American women in the United States.* African American Women, Issue Brief No. 1, 444 North Capital Street, NW, Suite 339 Washington, DC.

Neugarten, B. (1968). *Middle age and aging: A reader in social psychology.* Chicago: University of Chicago Press.

Noble, A., Rom, M., Newsome-Wicks, M., Englehardt, K., & Woloski-Wruble, A. (2009). Jewish laws, customs, and practice in labor, delivery, and postpartum care. *Journal of Transcultural Nursing, 20,* 323–333.

Poindexter, C. C., Linsk, N. L., & Warner, R. S. (1999). "He listens. . .and never gossips:" Spiritual coping without church support among older, predominantly African-American caregivers of persons with HIV. *Review of Religious Research, 40,* 231–243.

Purnell, L. D., & Paulanka, B. J. (2003). *Transcultural health care: A culturally competent approach* (2nd ed.). Philadelphia: F.A. Davis.

Shambley-Ebron, D. (2009). My sister, myself: A culture- and gender-based approach to HIV/AIDS prevention. *Journal of Transcultural Nursing 20*, 28–36.

Shambley-Ebron, D., & Boyle, J. S. (2006a). In our grand-mothers' footsteps: Perceptions of being strong in African American women with HIV/AIDS. *Advances in Nursing Science, 29*(3), 195–206.

Shambley-Ebron, D., & Boyle, J. S. (2006b). Self-care and the cultural meaning of mothering in African American women with HIV/AIDS. *Western Journal of Nursing Research, 28*, 42–60.

Sharpe, T. T., Lee, L. M., Nakashima, A. K. Elam-Evans, L. D., & Fleming, P. (2004). Crack cocaine use and adherence to antiretroviral treatment among HIV-infected black women. *Journal of Community Health, 29*, 117–127.

Teel, C. S., & Leenerts, M. H. (2005). Developing and testing a self-care intervention for older adults in caregiving roles. *Nursing Research, 54*, 193–201.

Tilbury, F., & Rapley, M. (2004). 'There are orphans in Africa still looking for my hands': African women refugees and the sources of emotional distress. *Health Sociology Review, 13*, 54–64.

U.S. Census Bureau. Poverty (1999). *Census 2000 brief.* Retrieved September 9, 2009, from http://www.census.gov/prod/2003pubs/c2kbr-19, pdf

U.S. Department of Health and Human Services, HIV/AIDS Bureau. (n.d.). *The HIV/AIDS Program: Legislation.* Retrieved August 28, 2009, from http://hab.hrsa.gov/law/leg.htm

Vitaliano, P. P., Zhang, J., & Scanlan, J. M. (2003). Is caregiving hazardous to one's physical health? A meta-analysis. *Psychological Bulletin, 129*, 946–972.

WISQARS Leading Causes of Death Reports (1999–2006). Retrieved August 18, 2009, from http://webappa.cdc.gov/sasweb/ncipc/leadcaus10.html

WISQARS, National Center for Health Statistics (2006). *10 Leading causes of death, United States 2006, Black females.* Retrieved August 28, 2009, from http://webappa.cdc.gov/cgi-bin/broker.exe

Young-Mason, J. (2009). Understanding culture: The art of food from the Annuals of the Caliph's Kitchens. *Clinical Nurse Specialist, 23*, 175–176.

Transcultural Perspectives in the **Nursing Care** of **Older Adults**

Margaret A. McKenna

KEY TERMS

Formal support
Illness behavior
Informal social support
Long-term care
Traditional medicine or practices

LEARNING OBJECTIVES

1. Demonstrate knowledge of socioeconomic factors and community resources that influence the experiences of older adults in the health care system.
2. Apply concepts of cultural variation, life experiences, and acculturation to plan and implement nursing care for the older adults in community and institutional settings.
3. Integrate concepts of informal and formal support systems, patterns of caregiving, and available resources to plan appropriate nursing care of the older adult.
4. Develop nursing interventions for older adults in a variety of caregiving contexts that will be perceived as culturally acceptable.

Nurses and other health professionals will be caring for more older adults within 10 years when the population of people over 65 years of age will exceed the number of children under five for the first time in human history (U.S. Census Bureau, 2008). The number of Americans over 65 will increase from 40 million in 2010 to 55 million in 2020 (Administration on Aging, 2009). Older adults are a heterogeneous sector of our population and will have a range of strengths as well as various needs that require different levels of health care, assistance, and social support. The continuum of older adults' care needs will be met through a range of services that are provided in home-based care in community settings, retirement communities, congregate care facilities, assisted living centers, as well as acute and long-term care facilities. Nurses plan and implement care that facilitates the older adults' independence and promotes quality of life and well-being through the older adult clients' progression from self-care to extended care settings. Nurses in their many roles also care for hospitalized older adults showing consistent and sustained patient contact as well as coordination of acute care and extended care resources (Chang, Hancock, Hickman, Glasson, & Davidson 2007; Kim, Capezuti, Boltz, & Fairchild, 2009).

Culture influences how individuals view aging; thus, groups of older clients vary in their adjustments to aging and in their health- and illness-related behaviors and practices. Culture is not the sole determinant of behavior but is a critical dimension in understanding the interactions of older clients in their families and in an encompassing societal context. When nurses give attention to the older client's cultural background, they will implement care that is more individualized to the strengths and needs of each client and most appropriate to each individual's circumstances.

The available resources in the community as well as institutions, long-term care funding, and interventions at a societal level will affect any older client's options for care and the individual's movement on a continuum of care. Understanding that the older adult is a participant in the culturally influenced patterns of care within a family, the nurse may consider the family as one resource for care. The older clients' cultural traditions and values will influence their preferences for their residence, lifestyles, and caregivers. Social and economic factors, including acculturation, influence the retention of traditional cultural values and practices. In assessing older adults, nurses must consider individuals in the contexts of society, of their cultural upbringing, and of their families who have varying strengths, resources, and capacities for care of aging family members.

To develop culturally appropriate care for older adults, nurses will first want to consider that the context for delivering care to clients is set by how available and affordable national, state, and local health care resources are for older adults. States, and even rural and urban locations, differ in the range of information and referral sources, acute and extended care facilities, and community-based services that are available to older adults to support their quality of life. See Box 8-1 for highlights of multiple factors that will interact and shape the context for older adult clients who seek care or use health care services.

BOX 8-1

Factors that Influence Older Adults' Responses in Seeking Health Care

At the Societal Level

- Social and economic factors affect eligibility or limit older adults in receiving preventive care, acute care, or health care maintenance in the health care system.
- Interventions to control Medicare expenditures force shorter hospital stays.
- Gaps in health care services put greater burdens on older patients for home and community-based care.

Cultural Variation Within a Societal Context

- Different cultural traditions have values that influence patterns in caring for older adult family members as they age and come to require more assistance.
- Younger family members become acculturated and change traditional behaviors that may differ from older adults' expectations to be cared for at home.

At the Individual Level

- Female family members who were considered primary caregivers for older family members are entering the work force and may not be available as caregivers.
- Families' economic situations, proximity to the older adult, and sources of formal support in the community will determine options for residence and care needs of the older adult.

This chapter is organized in three sections that emphasize the dimensions that nurses will find relevant in planning care for older adults: (1) the encompassing social and economic factors that influence the older adult's help-seeking behavior and plans for long-term care, (2) the factors at the community level that include cultural values, practices, patterns of caregiving, and resources including informal and formal sources of help that are available to older clients, and (3) the interaction of needs and resources that impact older adults and their families who cope with illness and make decisions in a continuum of care and services.

The Older Adult in Contemporary Society: Factors Impacting Health Care

This section addresses the encompassing context that surrounds and influences older adult clients: demographic factors of the aging population, economic factors, and social theories of aging that shape how older adults in Western society perceive growing older.

Changing Demographics

One of every eight Americans was over 65 years old in 2009 and the number of people aged 85 and older will triple in the next 40 years (Administration on Aging, 2009). In 2008 nearly 20% of older adults over 65 were minorities, 8.3% were African Americans, nearly 7% had Hispanic ethnicity (who could be of any race), 3% were Asian or Pacific Islander, and less than 1% were American Indian or Native Alaskan. By 2030 the older minority population is expected to increase 217% compared to 81% for the older White population. An estimated 2 to 4 million Americans aged 60 or older are lesbian, gay, bisexual, or transgender, and research suggests they will experience discrimination based on their sexual orientation as well as their age. Improved living conditions, increasing life expectancies, and decreasing fertility rates are contributing to an increase in the proportion of older adults in the population of the United States and Canada, as well as in other developed countries.

Increased longevity may mean declining health and losses that increase isolation and loneliness for some older adults, different trajectories of relatively good health with a slow decline for some, or good health with recovery from illness episodes for others. One of three older persons reported some type of disability such as difficulty in hearing, seeing, or self-care but some of these were minor difficulties and 16% reported they needed assistance as a result of a disability (Administration on Aging, 2009). However, chronic illnesses affect a sector of older adults disproportionately and contribute to varying degrees of disability with 50% of older adults having at least two chronic conditions. The care and management of chronic conditions becomes more problematic and costly with advancing age. A subgroup of the older adult population will experience significant aspects of physical decline or functional disability that requires extended use of hospital, community, or home-based personal health services. The health care systems in the United States, Canada, and other developed countries must face expanded demands of some older clients that include care for multiple chronic conditions. Over 1.3 million older adults are in nursing homes and half of these residents are 85 years or older and typically have severe impairments including cognitive impairments or dementia.

Evidence indicates that older members of some racial and ethnic groups of color experience higher rates of several health conditions than do White populations. Cardiovascular disease (CVD) affects Black adults much more consistently than other racial groups, despite differences in socioeconomic status (Rooks et al., 2008). Health care reduced this disparity slightly, but race still holds a significant association with CVD (Rooks et al., 2008). Hospitalization for congestive heart failure was higher in African Americans, Hispanics, and American Indians/Alaska Natives than in non-Hispanic Whites (American Heart Association, 2007). Older adults who are African American, Hispanic (non-White), and American Indian/Alaska Native suffer a higher prevalence of CVD and diabetes than do White (non-Hispanic) populations (American Heart Association, 2007). The rate of diabetes for American Indians/Alaska Natives is more than twice that for Whites. Similarly, Mexican-born individuals report higher rates of diabetes and related chronic illness, which directly affects higher rates of disability, than individuals in the non-Hispanic elderly population (Markides, Eschbach, Ray, & Peek, 2007). These disparities exist for interrelated reasons, including lower-income levels, lack of insurance including supplemental insurance to Medicare, barriers in access to care, and lower quality of care for some health conditions even when the individual is insured and care is received (Angel, Angel, & Hill, 2008).

Both ethnicity and income level affect the older adults' health status and need for care. Older White males with the highest incomes can generally expect to live more than 3 years longer than those in the lowest income levels. Low-income seniors are significantly more likely to encounter these health risk exposures: losing a loved one or close friend, overwhelming caregiving demands for someone else, social isolation, and poor quality housing (Evans, Wethington, Coleman, Worms, & Frongillo, 2008). These multiple risk exposures largely accounted for the link between poverty and ill health (Evans et al., 2008). Elderly African Americans often suffer functional declines at earlier ages than White Americans. Older African American women have a much higher proportion of disabling conditions than older African American men and older White adults. Thus, there is no simple correlation between the need for care and increased age because care needs and health status are affected by many dimensions in an older person's life, including socioeconomic level, ethnicity, and lifestyle (e.g., dietary habits).

To serve the growing proportion of older clients and their complex demands, nurses should consider that social and economic factors, cultural variation, and available support interact and impact the **illness behavior** and related help-seeking responses of older clients. As nurses prepare to care for older clients, they must assess the heterogeneity of the population as ethnicity, cultural traditions, social and economic situations, living arrangements, employment status, and migration history of older adults are as varied as they are for younger adults. These background factors contribute to older adults' varied responses to the illness that brings them to the health care system.

Economic Factors

The cost of **long-term care** for older adults in the United States has contributed to growing Medicare expenditures for individuals aged 65 years and older as costs have shifted to management of chronic illness and not solely acute care episodes. Given that the numbers of older adults who may require long-term community-based or institutional care is likely to rise, financial burdens for health care at national, state, and local systems can only increase. The health care needs of older Americans, especially those who are 85 years or older and are referred to as the "old old," will place more burden on our health care system. These elderly Americans may have set aside resources for retirement, but they may not be sufficient to keep pace with their longer life spans. As the number of elderly who are 65 years or older increases, the elderly also continue to have the highest poverty level of adult Americans. Older adults who retire usually live on a fixed income, have increased health-related expenses, and may cope with the death of a spouse or life partner.

Among ethnic older adults, including Hispanics and African Americans, 40% have no private savings for their retirement and will look to state and federal reimbursement programs for health and social service needs. More than 20% of older Hispanics have incomes below the poverty level, compared to less than 10% of Anglo elderly. Poverty among a sector of the Mexican American elderly may be attributed to occupational history of low wage jobs, periods of unemployment, and lower educational levels as the proportion of Hispanic elderly with no formal education is eight times the rate for Anglo elderly. The reality is that many ethnic elderly of color have accumulated fewer financial assets; that is, they have a lower household income and have less income from private pensions than do elderly Whites. More ethnic elderly of color rely on Supplemental Security Income (SSI) as the primary source of income after age 65, whereas a much smaller number of elderly White clients (1 out of 20) relies on this source. One of the major problems that many ethnic older adults and their families face is that limited tangible assets and lower equity in their homes may limit possible care options because families cannot afford costly long-term care or community-based care of the older adult family member.

Community-based services may include homemakers, adult day care, transportation, personal care, and short-term institutional care. Combinations of these services offer promising results for frail elderly who meet eligibility criteria and who are carefully assessed that are provided at a cost savings from nursing home care. This evidence may lead to broader implementation of similar services that will enable more elderly to reside longer in their preferred community residences.

The majority of older adults prefer to "age in place," that is, to stay in their homes and in their neighborhoods as long as possible. The level of support and supervision needed by many older adults leads to their placement in assisted living communities. Assisted living combines long-term care with maximizing opportunities for autonomy and privacy in a home-like setting. Therefore, there is a wide variety of assisted living programs in terms of size, structure, sponsorship, amenities, cost, and service availability. Care of the elderly at home may require comprehensive services from a multidisciplinary team of providers along a continuum of care, and services provided at home in place of institutionalization may or may not be less costly and must include a broad spectrum of services, often using formal and informal networks of caregivers. Nurses who provide primary care have a vital role to assess the older adults' physical, mental, and social well-being within the contexts of family, culture, and community. Providing community-based

care has some limitations as frail older adults in very rural areas may have to enter nursing homes as a safe housing option when there are too few community-based support services or assisted living centers to sustain the frail adult.

Nurses may be case managers for older adult clients in active retirement communities or other settings, including community-based care. An example from the caseload of a nurse who provides preventive health care and assessments in a low-income housing complex for older adults illustrates that individuals have different experiences using health care services and Medicare. An 82-year-old woman who worked as a housekeeper did not seek health care until she had a stroke related to untreated hypertension four years ago. She had limited contributions to Social Security owing to an episodic work history, and her illness depleted any savings. She received Medicare-funded services and continues to receive home health care through Medicaid, which is state-funded health care coverage for individuals with low income. This situation is representative of the experiences of many older adults who have lower socioeconomic status and are affected by the societal interventions, including Medicare, that provide health care coverage for older clients.

As a home health nurse, you may realize that older patients on your caseload would benefit from nursing assessments and medication monitoring, but you are informed that the patient's insurance and Medicare will not cover such services. Medicare pays only a small portion of home health care services, and the patient must be medically eligible to qualify. Older adults who have other insurance may have some coverage for additional home health services for a limited period of time.

The care that older adults may receive will be influenced and determined by economic necessity as well as environmental situations such as resources for nursing services and homemaker resources; rural and urban locations will affect resource availability. Older adults' needs for care, their requests for assistance, and the sources of caregivers are also dimensions that are culturally influenced. Within the United States, nurses and health care professionals see numerous variations in community caregiving support resources, both formal and informal, that are provided for older adults.

In addition to the demographic and economic factors that affect the older population, several theoretical assumptions underlie how people feel about aging adults and shape how resources are made available to care for older adults in communities.

Social Theories of Aging

How older adults are viewed as members of society varies, and these perceptions influence the experiences of older adults. The older adult clients' requests for services and the reactions of others to older adults are shaped in part by the prevailing social theories of aging:

- *Disengagement theory* focuses on the withdrawal of older adults who are forced into retirement or who incur disabilities.
- *Activity theory* supports the selective substitution of activities by retired individuals.
- *Continuity theory* focuses on the adaptation or continuation of patterns and behaviors from younger adulthood.

There are other cultural theories of aging, and these are Western theories that provide a framework for assessing how older clients respond to growing older and make decisions about living arrangements and anticipated care needs. The theoretical frameworks are useful in working with older adults who were raised with Western values. In American society, the values of independence, self-reliance, and productivity contributed to the attitude that the aged, who no longer contribute to society as workers, had less self-worth. Research has shown that older adults who have persistently low feelings of usefulness may be vulnerable to increased risks for poor health outcomes as they age (Gruenewald, Karlamangla, Greendale, Singer, & Seeman, 2009). Traditionally, in mainstream American culture, retirement for many older individuals led to the loss of their occupations and status and to their disengagement from social interaction. However, researchers who study aging tend to promote a

more current "active aging" paradigm. Active aging reflects the realities that industrialized nations have older populations who may remain engaged in economically and socially productive activities. Older adults are recognized not for imposing a financial burden, but for being involved in socially important activities: volunteering, providing household and child-care help, giving care to the disabled elderly, and supporting social service organizations. Under the newer active aging paradigm, industrialized societies are promoting social and economic integration of older people with respect for individuals' choices. The active aging paradigm and other theoretical perspectives are summarized in Box 8-2.

BOX 8-2

Nonbiologic or Social Theories of Reactions to Aging

Disengagement Theory

- Proponents of this theory say a pattern of withdrawal is usually considered desirable by the older person.
- Time is allocated for reflection and leisure activities. Critics of this theory say that reclusive adults naturally tend to become disengaged in their older years.

Activity Theory

- Older adults who substitute activities for the tasks, such as employment, that are regulated and have been withdrawn from the worker will be more satisfied.

Selectivity Theory

- Some people become less engaged in some aspects of their lives such as work but become more active in other domains that provide them with personal satisfaction.

Continuity Theory

- Advocates for this theory say that older adults continue lifelong activities that contribute to their well-being.
- Individuals find meaning in adapting behaviors from younger adulthood.

Accommodating Cultural Diversity at the Community Level: Older Adults in Different Ethnic and Cultural Contexts

This section describes intergroup and intragroup differences in how older adults' life experiences will shape their responses in seeking health care. Some older adults experienced living through the Depression, seeing the invention of television, computers, and video teleconferences, migrating to find employment, and fighting in an international conflict. European Americans in their 90s may have been young adults fleeing Poland or Germany before World War II. Older Southeast Asian adults in their 60s may have fled Cambodia, Laos, or Vietnam when conflict and political unrest enclosed around them. Political refugees from countries in East Africa and immigrants from Eastern bloc nations who have lived through civil wars and political revolution could well have depleted their coping mechanisms as younger adults fleeing their homeland. As a newer wave of older adult immigrants, they may experience adjustment problems that warrant care in the health and mental health care system, but at the same time they may distrust the system or have no previous experience in seeking health care.

Nurses who are providing care to clients whose background differs from their own are usually sensitive to assessing the client's culture. Individuals who have immigrated from the same country or region will differ in their needs and in the ways that their cultural background influences their health- and illness-related actions. These differences are based on a number of factors:

- Regional or religious identity,
- Situation in their homeland that may have prompted them to emigrate,
- Length of time they have spent in the United States including degree of acculturation,
- Proximity to immediate family or extended family members,

- Network of friends and social support from their homeland, and/or
- Link with ethnic, social, and health-related institutions.

In the total Hispanic American population, persons of Mexican descent are most numerous (54%), Cubans represent 14%, Puerto Ricans 9%, and other Spanish-speaking countries represent 24%. Patterns of immigration and repatriation vary among these Hispanic groups and lead to substantial differences in the proportion of elderly Hispanic Americans. Many educated and professionally well-established Cubans immigrated to the United States in the 1960s and have remained here and are now retired. In contrast, families leaving from Mexico have been younger, some older Mexican immigrants returned to their homeland, and older Mexican Americans do not have as long a life expectancy as their Cuban American peers.

More attention should be given to understanding the diversity among Asian American, Native Hawaiian, and other Pacific Islanders as there are more than 40 distinct ethnic groups. Of the immigrant groups that have been represented in the United States for several generations (Chinese, Japanese, and Filipinos), the Chinese and Filipino elderly are the most numerous. Newer immigrants include Koreans and Thais, and among the refugees, the Vietnamese elderly are more numerous than Cambodians, Laotians, and Hmong.

Culture influences how individuals view aging, define health, manage interpersonal crises, and face alterations in health that accompany aging. Nurses should consider that for older adults, health has multiple dimensions: physical functioning, social and emotional well-being, plus quality-of-life measures, including life satisfaction and happiness. Older adults differ in their perceptions of health but generally regard their physical activity and psychologic well-being as indicators of health. Only 7% of older White Americans typically regarded their health as poor, whereas some older individuals from Latin American cultures were more inclined to state they had poor health

(Jang, Chiriboga, Herrera, & Branch, 2009). Poor health refers to self-reported problems with physical functioning or a need for assistance to complete daily activities.

Older adults are inclined to seek health information and to make behavioral changes to maintain their independence into old age. Older adults who use self-help strategies to maintain their health generally report better psychologic well-being and physical functioning than older adults who do not use these approaches. Older adults who decide to adopt positive health behaviors such as stopping smoking or starting exercise go through phases in making their decisions. Nurses typically provide information about the risks of not exercising as well as the benefits of increasing activity or stopping smoking or adopting healthy eating habits. Nurses may also ask older clients about the circumstances that lead to a lack of exercise and then help clients to take small steps such as seeing how others fit exercise in their lives. Nurses aware of cultural variations can appreciate that older individuals will have different value orientations underlying their decisions to adopt healthy behavior over at-risk behaviors. Older adults who have peer support, anticipate a possible setback in changing a behavior and plan how to get past a challenge, and use incentives through self-talk and rewards will be more likely to make positive health changes.

Practitioners should seek to understand the difficulties and different approaches that affect individual case management (Tanner, 2007). Interventions should take into account older adults' cognitive ways of coping and practical strategies, and support these strategies (Tanner, 2007). For example, the matriarch of an extended family who has always valued the social benefits that come from sharing meals with family members may be reluctant to stop that practice and substitute exercise and low-fat meals. Older adults will also have learned responses in their help-seeking behavior to cope with chronic illness and to assess new illness symptoms. Some older African Americans have been more resourceful in their problem solving, planning, and coping that may be due in

part to the lack of access to health care that they may experienced over time.

Culture will influence the older person's expectations of what constitutes illness and will also influence whether the older adult maintains the use of traditional sources of health care in place of or in addition to the use of biomedical sources of care. Some older clients will prefer the use of traditional medicine from their native country or practices that they recall from their childhood. Researchers have described the simultaneous use of Western medicine and traditional Chinese health practices that focus on restoring harmony and balance in the body and spirit among some groups of Chinese immigrants (Lai & Surood, 2009; Miltiades & Wu, 2008). The use of traditional sources of health care concurrently with or in place of the biomedical health care system is not limited to members of recently migrated cultural groups but is common to nearly all individuals. Several chronic conditions that often accompany age including osteoarthritis or diabetes increase the likelihood that older adults will use traditional sources or self-care to treat their symptoms. The older adult may resort to an over-the-counter medication and may use other popular remedies before, during, or after the use of prescribed sources of care. Nurses can show an interest in the client and ask them about any actions they take to treat their conditions, in order to assess the older client's concurrent use of traditional practices, folk medicine, or popular medicine. Case Study 8-1 illustrates that assessing the client's use of alternative sources of treatment is useful in developing a care plan that the client will accept.

Older adult clients may also use **traditional medicine or practices** from their family of origin as a means to prevent illness. Preventive measures may combine a magical or religious element, such as burning a candle, offering cornmeal to the spirits, wearing an amulet, or reciting a prayer. To assess the older adult's cultural beliefs and practices, the nurse can demonstrate a nonjudgmental attitude and ask questions similar to the ETHNIC or LEARN tool in Box 8-3.

CASE STUDY 8-1

Mr. S.L. was a 78-year-old retired machinist who had degenerative joint disease that caused recurring pain in his elbows and knees. He referred to his condition as "arthritis" and attributed his pain to the wear and tear of his long career working around machinery, hauling parts, handling equipment, and standing for long intervals. He was raised in West Virginia and recalled that his mother used rubbing liniment and kerosene to relieve aching joints. He lived outside a major Northwest city when he was interviewed by a nurse researcher about his use of alternative sources of treatment for his joint pain. He said that in addition to over-the-counter pain medication, he regularly rubbed kerosene and sheep liniment on his affected joints. He explained that his joints were not well lubricated and that they felt like gears that were clashing. An oil-based rubbing compound penetrated the joints and relieved his discomfort.

Clinical Application

The nurse assessed that the use of the rubbing compound did not interfere with the prescribed medications. The patient's belief that rubbing compound improved his condition and decreased his pain allowed him to participate in a prescribed exercise program. The nurse would continue to assess the treatment to determine whether the use of an alternative source of treatment would interfere with the prescribed care plan.

BOX 8-3

Two Tools for Interviewing an Older Adult Client—ETHNIC or LEARN

Explanation: Explore the patient's perceptions of why the patient thinks he or she has the symptoms

Treatment: Ask what home remedies or treatment the patient has used and what treatment the patient expects

Healers: Inquire if the patient has conferred with healers, ministers

Negotiate: Discuss how to include some of the patient's beliefs to reach a mutually agreed upon plan of care

Intervention: State the plan including diet, exercise, or other therapies.

Collaborate: Discuss how to work together with the family and community resources.

A very similar tool uses a LEARN mneumonic:
Listen to the client's explanation of the illness
Elicit what the client does to make the condition better
Ask the client what else he or she does to help alleviate symptoms
Respond with information about the biomedical model and recommended care plan for the illness
Negotiate with the patient a plan that integrates the client's culturally influenced explanatory model with biomedical model toward a goal accepted by the patient

Source for ETHNIC tool: Kobylarz, Heath, and Like (2002).

Older clients may use alternative sources of care and decide not to follow prescribed treatment plans. They do so based on their beliefs about the causes of their illness and their expectations for treatment. Older clients may blend some biomedical beliefs about the cause of illness with some traditional and popular notions about illness, so it follows that clients may adhere to some traditional practices and some biomedical treatments.

In a study of African American and White patients who had osteoarthritis the African American patients were more likely to use topical treatments for their symptoms, to report activity limitations based on severity and to use diet supplements than were the White patients (Silverman, Nutini,

Musa, King, & Albert, 2008). Among a multiethnic sample of older adult clients that had diabetes, the Mexican American older adults were twice as likely to use an unconventional therapy than were White, Black, or Native American clients. But among this sample of low-income older adults the overall resort to alternative medical strategies such as herbal remedies was very low (Schoenberg, Traywick, Jacobs-Lawson, & Kart, 2008).

In planning nursing care, nurses should consider that older adults from different backgrounds might share experiences of migration, changing social and family structures, structural forces or institutional racism that include discrimination, and historical events that include political conflict. The hardships that older clients have endured may increase their striving for autonomy in later years and push the client toward self-reliance. The older client may need time to reflect on decisions and may tend to regard health care cautiously. Some older clients will be fatalistic about many losses in life and weigh options about health care in relation to their fatalistic views. Support groups for older adults who have had age-related sensory losses or chronic illness have been found to have a positive effect on the quality of life for these patients. Similarly, in research with older Whites and African Americans, the older adults who had health challenges but also had positive perceptions of vitality and well-being maintained or enhanced their mental health. Because an overall sense of well-being affects the influence of physical health on mental health, interventions may succeed by targeting the individual's sense of vitality and well-being (Jang, Chiriboga, Borenstein, Small, & Mortimer, 2009). Nurses may implement educational or support programs focused on promoting positive perceptions of personal health and increased vitality that may help protect older adults from negative emotional consequences stemming from physical health conditions (Jang, Chiriboga, Borenstein, Small, & Mortimer, 2009).

Older clients may preserve their traditional values that connect them to their origins and give meaning to their lives. Nurses can provide culturally sensitive care when they identify that older clients retain traditional values or blend traditional values and practices with biomedical beliefs and practices. Many older clients could have grown up with limited preventive care and associate health care only with emergent conditions, so nurses should assess the older client's previous experiences in the health care system. Several examples of health care studies of older adults are highlighted in Table 8-1.

Understanding Culture Change in Older Adults

Some older adults have relocated to different regions of the country or have made a significant transition in their late adult years to be close to younger family members. Older clients may have the common experience of relocating or migrating, but the length of time that they have resided in one area may vary. A study of older Hispanic immigrants in Miami found that a more positive neighborhood social environment was associated with better mental health for these urban residents (Brown et al., 2009).

Older immigrants may have lost their social positions and may be clinging to family roles in light of the stress of acculturation that reduces their status. A study of Central American immigrants to a metropolitan area in the United States indicated that their perceived stress was correlated with their psychologic health (Dunn & O'Brien, 2009). The psychologic stress related to cultural change is more intense for older refugees. Elderly ethnic Vietnamese, Chinese Vietnamese, and Laotians who resided with immediate family members had a higher sense of social adjustment compared to older refugees who shared a living space with many extended family members and non-kin. The older refugee has sometimes left behind a career and a status associated with that career.

Some examples will illustrate these factors. Mai Bliatout fled from Laos in the late 1970s and settled in the Pacific Northwest. She and her husband had three daughters while they lived in Laos, and they had a fourth daughter in the United States. Mai and her family are Catholic as her family had been friends with missionaries, but some people from Laos follow Buddhism or animism. Since her husband's death, Mai has lived with her oldest daughter, son-in-law, and two granddaughters in an urban neighborhood where there are other Laotian families, Vietnamese, and some Korean families. The other three daughters live within two hours of Mai and visit her at least once a week. Mai travels with one of her daughters to a church that is in another part of the city to hear the mass in her native language, rather than hearing a native English speaker. She lives where she can shop in an international market and buy noodles similar to what she used to have at home. She has contact with immigrants

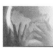

TABLE 8-1

Highlights of Selected Nursing Studies Related to Older Adults 2008–2010

STUDY (AUTHOR, DATE) AND TOPIC OR GROUP STUDIED	CULTURAL CONCEPTS RELEVANT IN CARE OF OLDER ADULT CLIENT	IMPLICATIONS FOR NURSING CARE
Fleming and Gilibrand (2009); Meta-synthesis of 11 studies of diabetes management in the context of South Asian groups (Pakistani, Gujarati, Bangladeshi)	The challenges that diverse groups of participants reported in managing their diabetes could not be attributed solely to cultural beliefs or practices.	Individuals from different cultural groups integrated culture along with personal beliefs and lifestyle choices into diabetes self-management decisions. An individual approach is called for in planning appropriate nursing care.
Phillips and Crist (2008); Mexican American and non-Hispanic White caregivers for elderly family members	The stereotypical assumptions that Mexican American families' supportive networks were extensive and that families required less formal intervention were explored and clarified.	Nurses should not assume that Mexican American families need less intervention, or that Mexican American families have more social support, or that Mexican American families' networks will be more stable over time.
Wan, Yu, and Kolanowski (2008) Chinese elders and their family members experiencing less available family care and diminishing social support	Family support of older adults is the first and foremost responsibility of family members who are expected to provide physical, emotional, social, and psychologic support for older Chinese.	Lessons learned from the United States on community nursing models and gerontological nursing curricula may be relevant for addressing China's unprecedented challenges in caring for its elderly population.
Warren-Findlow and Issel (2010); African American women with chronic heart disease who lived in a large Midwestern city in the United States	Some African American stress-coping strategies are identified as cultural responses in the form of collective coping, spiritual centered coping and ritual centered coping.	The women believed stress and family history caused their illness. They relied on God and their inner strength to reduce and mange stress. Health care providers should frame health behaviors as activities to reduce stress.

whose experience is similar to hers. Although Mai has lived in the United States for 30 years, she always preferred to speak her native language while at home with her husband. Mai and her husband are representative of approximately 85% of older Southeast Asian refugees who have traditional expectations of living with and receiving support from their children. In Case Study 8-2, an older immigrant parent assumes a new role and acquires a new source of status in the family.

Under the current immigration policies, some recent immigrants do have a financial responsibility to their older family members. The older adult usually does not have an option to work, nor is public assistance an option, so the family must provide for the older adult members. Older family members may reciprocate services for younger family members. Nurses have described that in approximately one-third of Hispanic families; older clients provided child care to younger family members and actively assisted in family decisions. As part of a nursing assessment, the nurse notes if older adults are primary care providers for grandchildren or other family members and if an illness episode in the older adult disrupts the family.

Many immigrants who have migrated after the age of 50 years experience more depression associated in part with their increased dependence.

CASE STUDY 8-2

Mrs. D.R. is a 79-year-old native of the Philippines. She moved to an urban area in California to be near her four children, who live in the same state. She had lived in the same town in the Philippines for her entire adult life and had stayed there to care for her husband and her sister, who both required care for chronic conditions. She is representative of Filipinos who migrate at a later age to join family members in North America. Although she was a much needed and highly esteemed member of her household in the Philippines, she, like many other immigrants, experienced role reversal when she lost the once dominant position within the family and became financially dependent on adult children during relocation. Mrs. D.R. was also like other older Filipino adults who had a more active social network before relocation. She also spoke a dialect and did not speak Tagalog, the language spoken by many younger residents of the Philippines. After her relocation to the United States, her communication and interaction became restricted to her extended family because she did not feel confident using her limited English and did not find other speakers of her dialect. Mrs. D.R. found increasing comfort through prayer and attendance at the Roman Catholic Church to buffer the disequilibrium she felt as a result of her migration.

An older Filipino adult's status changes if he or she assumes child care or other duties within an adult child's home. Doing so maintains the older member's respect within the family, and this reciprocal relationship may lead to the perception of filial obligation between the generations of family members. After Mrs. D.R. assumed the care of her two daughters' children, her self-esteem, personal dignity, and pride in her family increased. The nurse who treated Mrs. D.R. in the emergency department after she fractured her wrist in a fall assessed that Mrs. D.R.'s injury would place a strain on the family because they would temporarily be without their child-care provider. The nurse was able to involve her family members in the discharge plan for Mrs. D.R. so her recovery could be ensured, she would not lose respect, and she would not feel responsible to assume her usual duties until she felt better.

Clinical Application

The nurse caring for Mrs. D.R. assessed the following areas, which are relevant concerns for any older adult client:

- Interaction of the older client within the family—what role does the older adult have with a spouse, partner, adult children, grandchildren
- Environment to which the older client will return
- Adherence of the client and the family to traditional values
- Linguistic or social isolation of the older client

Depressed older adults are more likely to have lower self-rated health and may have more functional impairment, which suggests that nurses should assess the quality of the older adult's relationships as well as their functioning status.

For many Mexican American older adults, low socioeconomic status could be a barrier to health care, especially for early diagnosis and treatment of chronic conditions. However, for many years, deaths from heart disease were found to be somewhat lower in Mexican Americans than in non-Hispanic White people. This is suggestive of protective aspects of traditional Mexican American culture that may include older adults' integration in the extended family and their care at home that contributes to a slightly better-than-expected health status. However, recent research found that heart disease deaths in Mexican Americans were as high as in non-Hispanic White people. The protective aspects of Mexican American culture may diminish over time among families as they become more acculturated. Older Mexican Americans and other older Hispanics may have chronic conditions that could respond to positive lifestyle changes if the messages to develop healthy habits are delivered in culturally appropriate programs.

Membership in a cultural group or the shared experience of immigrating from the same country does not imply that older adults are similar. The life experiences of the individuals, including their occupations and education, and their acculturation will affect their needs and expectations for care in their advancing years.

There are three cultural values—respect for the aging, intergenerational duty, and the primacy of family bonds—that are similarly held among many of the cultural groups that compose the large group that is referred to as Asian Americans. In each group, the majority of individuals would likely expect and find that care for older adult family members is assumed by younger family members. Traditional Japanese culture offers us an example of the shared culturally influenced expectation that daughters and daughters-in-law would care for older family members as they face declines in personal health. However, although some families who are Japanese American may continue to uphold traditional values, there are increasing signs of conflicting traditional values and popular culture values.

Although traditional values among Asian American and Pacific Islander families may be desirable, other factors, including increasing education and career opportunities for women as well as economic necessity to enter the labor force, may influence the behavior of female family members to work outside the home and not to be full-time caregivers. There are other patterns that include the suburbanization of Japanese Americans and more varied geographic locations that reduce the relevance of traditional values in the lives of the Nisei (second-generation) Japanese Americans, which may impact lowered status and reduced authority for the Issei (first-generation) Japanese American elderly. Nurses may need to assess what could be disparities in what the older client expects for care and what the younger family members can realistically provide.

Caregiving of Older Adults by Family Members

Involving the family in the care of the older adult member is important because family members are participants in **informal social support** networks that often nurture and maintain older adults in their preferred community residences. It is also vital to consider the preferences of the older person and his or her family members, as well as the capacities of the older adult for self-care and the willingness and capabilities of the families to offer support and assistance with care. The type and duration of support that can be provided by family members must be considered in relation to sources of **formal support** that could be used to sustain the family care.

There are many contexts for formal support and health care for the older adults. The image of care for older adults in skilled nursing facilities has given way to a continuum of services that includes self-care, supported self-care, assisted living communities, and skilled care. The roles that family members take in each of these levels of care vary according to cultural, socioeconomic, and demographic characteristics. We hear of adults who are "sandwiched between the layers" in the care of their own children and care of aging parents. Although intergenerational caregiving is becoming increasingly common for families across the United States, families in other countries have values more consistent with caring for aging parents in extended families. All families have culturally influenced patterns of responsibility to care for older family members, but these patterns vary across cultures.

Culture definitely influences the role that the family members will take in the care of older family members. Nurses and health care professionals must be increasingly aware of how social and economic factors may alter families' retention of traditional values that affect caring for older family members. Nurses working with older adults should be sensitive to the evolving needs of family caregivers that will be influenced by the caregivers' acculturation and their time since immigration, two factors that place the caregiver between value systems. Although some Asian American women have a commitment to family caregiving, the increasing cultural diversity in North America calls for nurses to give more attention to assessing and understanding the cultural variations among individuals of Chinese, Japanese, Vietnamese, Hmong, or Cambodian heritage who may be expected to be caregivers.

The economic necessity that two adults in many households must work to provide adequate household income has contributed to a decline in the former taken-for-granted availability of adult female children as caregivers to parents and grandparents. The participation of women in the work place and the decline in the numbers of adult children in many families have contributed to families that are not available to provide personal care to the older adult family members. Adult children and other family members may be available to provide episodic assistance, emotional support through short visits, or some financial assistance to purchase in-home services. It is not possible to talk about older adults or their families as if they were a homogeneous group, in similar life situations. Rather it is necessary to consider that cultural diversity and lifestyle choices may actually influence and determine many different options for care of the older adult. Nurses working in acute, community, and long-term care settings will be asked to support family members who are involved and contributing to the care of older family members in different ways: tangible support, emotional support, financial assistance, personal caregivers, and relief caregivers.

In caring for older adults, community nurses may have to coordinate how families caring for older adult members can access and use formal support services (visiting nurse services, chore services, adult day care) and informal support services (family members, neighborhood volunteers, meal delivery). Nurses are giving increasing attention to assessing the caregiver's capacities, needs, and resources in planning for extended care of an older adult at home. A nurse needs to assess the caregiver's health and well-being as well as that of the older adult client, considering a caregiver may be a working mother sandwiched in the care of an older parent and adolescent children, or a caregiver may be a retired worker in her 60s with a chronic illness.

Nurses need to be increasingly aware of the growing cultural diversity and the increasing numbers of older adults who may require home care. Not only are clients more diverse, but their potential family caregivers vary widely in socioeconomic status, educational levels, and acculturation patterns. These factors will influence whether the caregivers, who are usually wives, daughters, or other close relatives will be expected to care for older family members. In a study of caregiving among Mexican American and non-Latino White elders, there were fewer Mexican American elders than non-Latino White elders who preferred to relay on professional help. A greater proportion of the Mexican American older adults turned to informal caregivers when recovering from a hip fracture (Min & Barrio, 2009).

Dimensions of Social Support

Social support assumes special relevance for the older client, but in contrast there are many older clients who sustain social deprivation from several sources:

- Separation from immediate family members because of geographic mobility
- Age-related segregation caused by increased nuclear families in neighborhoods
- Loss of spouse or partner because of death or illness
- Loss of leisure pursuits or entertainment due to illness or loss of income

It is especially important for many older adults to have social, emotional, and physical sources of support to assist them to remain as independent as possible. Understanding the patterns of support that older adults might need and assessing the cultural variations in these patterns of support is good preparation for nurses who may be working in acute, extended-care, or community settings. Social support has been delineated in three ways: affective support that refers to expressions of respect, love; affirmational support referring to having endorsement for one's behavior and perceptions; and tangible support that refers to receiving some kind of aid or physical assistance such as accompanying a person to an appointment.

One implication is to identify the importance that an older adult places on types of social support. Nurses may assess what the older client identifies as his or her sources of affective, affirmational, and tangible supports. Sources of social support are described in Table 8-2.

To understand that culture may influence the types of social support family members offer to older clients, nurses may assess the concept that the structure of families affects how informal support is provided. Some families, including the Yankee Americans, German Americans, and families of English heritage often have a linear structure. The expectation is that adult children will assume care

responsibilities for aging parents, and grandchildren will assume caregiving for aging parents and grandparents when needed. Another family structure is collateral when the perceived bonds are more diffuse. Parents, aunts, uncles, grandparents, and family friends may be part of the collateral bonds of families. Among families with a collateral structure are some Irish, Polish, and African American families, who expect to receive and to provide informal support among all collateral contacts. The expectation for care among many Irish families is that relatives must assist each other when needed. Many Irish and Irish American families would agree with the assumption that their relatives are obliged to enter into generalized reciprocity.

Although most studies have looked at family support, a recent study identified that older adults may also rely on support from friends. This study of visually impaired Chinese older adults showed that a friendship network correlated more than a

TABLE 8-2
Social Networks Common to Older Clients in Community Settings

NETWORK	PARTICIPANTS IN NETWORK	CHARACTERISTICS OF NETWORK
Integrated support network with local support	Family members living nearby, friends, neighbors	Based on long-term local residence of the older adult, frequent contact with available kin, usually a large network; older client remains involved in community. Friends may offer tangible assistance, affirmational support. Family offers affective support.
Community-based support network	Family members do not live in proximity, friends may be available, neighbors more accessible	Family members accessible by phone for affective support, friends may not be in good health to help, younger neighbors who are available help as they can for tangible support.
Family-dependent network	Adult children, other relatives, minimal or no contact with friends, contact with neighbors for emergencies or occasional relief support	Adult children and other relatives provide most sources of support. Network may depend on a primary caregiver with planned relief. Would benefit from some formal source of support: homemaker, aide.
Restricted support network	Spouse or adult children of the older client are primary caregivers; friends do not maintain contact or are not available because of their own illness or distance	Older client may be out of touch with peers. Older client may live in the adult child's home. Usually frailer older adult. Network may fall apart if the one primary caregiver becomes ill or loses touch with peers. Older adult unable to provide support. Usually needs formal source of support to be maintained.

family network with health-related quality-of-life measures (Wang, Chan, Ho, & Xiong, 2008).

Socially isolated older adults may have more self-reported health problems but may "do without" health care services due to their income status and lack of social support. When these older adults do seek care, they tend to be sicker and need more extensive care. Therefore, keeping older adults engaged in community life and seeking to understand what social constructs and/or personal circumstances may affect their health care may help defray long-term medical costs (Kobayashi, Cloutier-Fisher, & Roth, 2009). Access to needed services in a timely manner could help older adults address health conditions and promote well-being in the short term (Kobayashi et al., 2009).

In addition to cultural variation in patterns of giving help and support, it is not surprising that socioeconomic status will influence the amount and level of assistance that family members provide to older adult family members. It is important to identify the relative influence of two types of factors on patterns of family members providing support to their older members. These are (1) demographic factors such as family size, migration patterns, rural/urban residence, and (2) socioeconomic factors, including income level and educational level. Both of these sets of factors may determine the availability of family members to offer assistance and may influence the type of support that is offered. Thus, nurses must assess the influence of these factors on the older adult's social support network and identify that demographic and socioeconomic factors may be blended with culturally influenced patterns of behavior.

There are sectors of the Native American elderly population who have lived in urban areas and have generally assimilated more than their rural peers who live on reservations. Elder Native Americans tend to socialize less outside of their extended families and expect that the needs of clan members and extended family members will come before those of the individual. Native American values support the care of older family

members in the home, but the pool of available caregivers is diminishing because of declining fertility and employment mobility. Elder Native Americans living in multigenerational households are more likely than White peers to have significant disabilities. A pattern that has been seen in some Native American families is that each adult child, in birth order, assumes the burden of responsibility and cost of care for the aging parent, that may exhaust the son's or daughter's personal limited financial resources.

It is more likely that an older Mexican American or Chinese American in a traditional or immigrant family will live with an adult child and receive help from an adult child than an older European American. This suggests that economic necessity or the presence of larger families may lead to the observed pattern of residence and assistance for some families. Nurses and other health care professionals must also be cautious to identify the variations within groups and not just between groups. Nurses and health care professionals should certainly move beyond generalizations and toward appreciating the cultural differences among groups of older adults who may indicate on the census or on required forms that they are "Hispanic" or "Asian." We should not assume that all Hispanic families are familistic, nor should we assume that this is a characteristic among only Hispanic families. We would find that other groups are just as familistic in their attention to older adults and that some Hispanic families are not demonstrating that characteristic to any greater extent than are other families.

Variations Among Members of Cultural Groups

Among the groups referred to as *Hispanic,* there are differences in patterns of older adults regarding daily contacts, church attendance, and socialization with friends. Older Cuban Americans are more likely than Mexican Americans and older Puerto Ricans to get together often with friends. Older Mexican Americans are more likely than either Cuban Americans or Puerto Ricans to attend church and to have daily contact with their children. There are also significant variations in other groups of older Asian Americans and Pacific Islanders. Older Korean Americans may have immigrated with their highly educated adult children, but a higher proportion of the older clients wish to live independently from the adult children. The Korean American elderly may socialize with their peers through Korean churches but are more likely to be lonely and isolated than Chinese, Japanese, and Filipino elderly.

The nurse may look for ways to support an older adult in making ties to his or her home country to enhance self-esteem and feelings of belonging. Nurses may ask if an older adult can talk to a group of children at an ethnic community center, such as the Ukrainian Community Center, El Centro, or the Polish Association. The older adult can also tell the history of his or her immigration to adolescents who may be tracing their cultural heritage for an oral history project. Senior adults may also be connected to school-age children by walking them to and from school or tutoring them through an after-school project. Nurses who are working with ethnic elderly clients may want to look for resources in the local community to do outreach to these community members and to involve them in their care.

The Individual Level: Integrating Social and Cultural Factors in the Care of Older Adults

The purpose of this section is to identify that older adults will experience the interaction of socioeconomic factors at a societal level with their culturally determined values and practices. Social and cultural factors influence most older clients' progress in meeting the developmental tasks of aging. The developmental tasks that older adults achieve include the satisfaction of basic needs, such as safety, security and dignity, and the fulfillment of integrity and self-actualization. For the majority of older adults, these needs are intertwined with the lifestyle and the residence of the older adult. For that reason, this section focuses on the options that older adults have for community or institutional care as these options provide older clients with safety, security, and an opportunity to possess dignity and autonomy. The older adult also usually exerts some control over planning where he or she will live and exercises self-determination and self-esteem. Usually in conjunction with the community or institutional residence of the older client, the individual may find an outlet for individual or group activity, volunteer efforts, artistic activity, or socialization that are sources of self-esteem, give meaning to one's life, and contribute to positive fulfillment of the developmental tasks of aging.

Nurses are especially well prepared to work with older clients as they demonstrate a professional understanding that in all cultural groups aging is a developmental experience for individuals who are in a stage of reflecting on life experiences and finding meaning in their lives. Older adults may have many transitions that are chosen or are inevitable with growing older. In mainstream American society, these include retirement, grandchildren, changed living arrangements, family mobility, declining health, and deaths of family members including spouse, siblings, or children. Older adults may assume new roles, and nurses who work with older adults in community settings can reinforce changing roles as opportunities for positive growth. Nurses often view the strengths and residual abilities that older clients possess rather than dwelling on the losses, and in doing so, the nurse promotes optimal functioning when the older adult may be experiencing unavoidable dependency.

Cultural factors, including the cultural group history, and life experiences, including immigration, will interact and determine the older client's efforts to achieve security, autonomy, and integrity. In achieving integrity, the older client has a need to bring closure to life and acceptance of eventual death. A nurse may assess this need in a client's family and be a sensitive listener when the client works through the steps of achieving integrity.

Older clients need time for a purposeful life review. The older adult may relinquish some aspects such as paying bills to an adult child, so the older person is free to reflect on life successes and failures.

Faith and Spirituality in the Lives of Older Adults

The importance of religion, faith, and spirituality for older adults has been described in nursing and social work. Religion may be a source of instrumental or emotional support, a psychosocial resource, or a coping mechanism for older adults who experience challenging health conditions. Older adults who experience chronic pain may turn to their spiritual beliefs to help them cope. Evidence-Based Practice 8-1 highlights pain management in older adults.

Previous studies found that there were no significant differences in the use of religion that were related to gender or to race; rather, the members of all groups identified that religion had been a stable influence in their lives when there were

---

EVIDENCE-BASED PRACTICE 8-1

Pain Management in Older Adults: Accommodating for Cultural Variation

There are several established guidelines for pain management in older adults such as that of the University of Iowa Geriatric Nursing Interventions Research Center Acute Pain Management in Older Adults that are based on scientific evidence. All though the guidelines exist they are not consistently followed and there are reports of under-treatment of pain among older adults in nursing homes, hospice and hospitals. At a meeting of the American Pain Society study data were presented that only one of two patients receiving hospice care had their pain assessment adequately documented. Nursing home residents who had chronic pain had described "being constantly pained" as a feature of their life experience. They also elaborated on themes of the certainty and uncertainty of their pain and of "being old and worn out" and of "taking punishment." The themes stated by those study subjects suggest that nurses could help to reduce the patients' subjective experience of pain through assessing how the patient describes pain and then individualizing a care plan to include patient-requested pain-reduction measures. Assessment could include using a behavioral pain scale or observation of pain indicators for patients who cannot self-report pain.

Clinical Application

Nurses working in acute care settings, extended care settings, and in the community will be in roles to interact with patients and their caregivers to negotiate an acceptable pain management plan. Nurses should assess for the patient's tolerance for pain, past and present experience with pain, effect of pain on quality of life, and the meaning attached to pain that are all factors that can be influenced by the patient's cultural background and the patient's life experiences. The nurse who is striving to be culturally competent will assess the patient's culturally influenced explanatory model about the cause of the pain and the patient's expectations of treatments to relieve the pain. Behavioral therapies may include meditation, music, imagery, and aromatherapy. The nurse may assist in integrating the patient's preferences to use traditional and popular remedies including cold packs, herbal remedies, heat applications or other therapies along with the Western prescribed medicines when the traditional or alternative sources would not harm the patient.

Reference: Higgins, I. (2005).

numerous changes in living conditions, housing, and employment. Among older adults in rural areas, which included areas in the Southern United States, some Native American, European American, and African American elders had integrated their religious beliefs in their health-related practices. Groups of rural African American older adults presented complex health belief systems with religion being one of the interrelated dimensions and God sometimes personalized as a "divine other." As many older adults possess religious or spiritual beliefs, all older clients require culturally sensitive communication and intervention that is specific to their backgrounds.

Decisions on a Continuum of Care

Many older adults will require three types of care that can be summarized as (1) intensive personal health service, depending on the presence of acute and chronic conditions; (2) health maintenance and restorative care, depending on chronic conditions; and (3) coordinated nursing, social services, and ancillary services that may be provided on an episodic basis for older clients in the community. Depending on the level of disability that an older person suffers, he or she may be faced with a decision to continue to live in one's home with assistance, with family members, in an assisted living residence, or in a skilled nursing facility. Nurses will observe that older clients express different attitudes that range from resignation to acceptance when they must change residences. The nurse can assess that the older client's attitudes about community or facility residence have been influenced by social and peer groups, and the nurse can be sensitive to the older client's reactions.

Researchers have found that the most consistent factor in determining the placement of the older person into a skilled nursing facility is the lack of an adequate informal network. Nurses who provide care to older clients and families from different cultural backgrounds will notice that families vary in their capacities to provide care for the older relative who declines in functional abilities. Culture can influence the extent that functional disabilities will be perceived as disabling or merely annoying, and it will influence the extent that individuals seek help for their disabilities.

Families have often developed culturally influenced patterns of caregiving and social support. The nurse may assess the following: Does the family modify the environment and assist in home care so that the older adult remains at home? Do children and grandchildren share tasks, provide meals, and run errands so the grandparents can live alone? Do family members have a plan to have relatives share responsibility to provide support and supervision for an older family member? Does the older family member have caregivers and alternates who can provide care as needed if the older adult wishes to remain at home?

Some differences have been noted in the patterns of living arrangements according to ethnic background. Even when single older African Americans lost functional abilities, they were less likely than Whites with similar losses to enter skilled nursing facilities. That finding indicates that some older African Americans may be able to reside in the community with family assistance and informal and formal social support for a longer duration than White clients. In one study of Puerto Ricans in skilled nursing facilities in New York City, the residents had higher levels of disability than did a comparison group of other facility residents. This finding suggested that Puerto Rican family members might have been more inclined to care for family members with declining health status and for a period of time longer than other families. Older individuals with adequate support systems may maintain their health and remain in a community-based setting for a longer period of time before institutional care becomes necessary. Mexican American institutionalized elderly were more physically and functionally impaired than their non-Latino peers, which lends support to the theories that informal networks provided help with activities of daily living, transportation, nutrition, respite care, and social support that deferred the necessity of nursing home placement. Older Mexican Americans interacted more frequently with younger family members than their non-Latino counterparts, owing in part to closer geographic proximity. Nurses must also assess that the values of independence and self-reliance may be very strong for some older clients, and they may refuse any assistance from family members, so the nurse should evaluate clients' behaviors relative to underlying values.

Nursing facility admissions show that while 6% of Whites over the age of 65 years may reside in a nursing facility on a typical day, the percentage of Hispanics older than 65 residing in a nursing home is half of that, or 3%. The census category subsumes many different cultural groups under a broad category of Asian Americans, and only 3% of those older than the age of 65 years would reside in a nursing facility on a representative day. White elderly clients aged 85 years and older make up 23% of the nursing home residents in the United States. Hispanic and Asian/Pacific Islander older adult clients make up 10% of the nursing home population aged 85 years or older.

Historically, a higher proportion of older adults from diverse ethnic and racial groups have been cared for in home environments than have elders who are White. The interaction of other factors including the availability, acceptability, and affordability of a skilled nursing facility that is in proximity to the ethnic populations also definitely impacts the overall residence patterns by members of cultural and ethnic groups.

Older foreign-born Chinese American residents were asked about the desired residence for older adults with diminishing capacities for self-care, and the respondents indicated that a nursing home was a good choice for the older person to become healthy but was not preferred for the incapacitated person who would relinquish personal control in that setting. The elders' expectation was that adult children would care for them. In contrast, nearly one-third of elderly Korean respondents indicated that a nursing home was the best living arrangement for a chronically ill or disabled person. Although more elderly Korean respondents still preferred to remain in their own homes, they also expressed less willingness to be a burden to their adult children if they became incapacitated.

Older adults who for the majority, if not all, of their lifetime have spoken their native language and surrounded themselves with friends who also shared their customs could find it enormously difficult to enter a skilled nursing facility that would appear quite different in its practices. Much of the professionals' actions and behavior that occurs in health care facilities is the result of acculturation in the biomedical culture. Nurses and other health care professionals are not always aware that their behavior, such as an insistence on schedules, order, and cleanliness, would not be valued equally by older adults from different cultural groups. Thus, ethnic elders may feel especially uncomfortable if they do not understand why they are awakened at a certain time, required to be dressed, and asked to participate in group socialization. The ethnic elder may find the skilled nursing facility to be hostile and unfriendly.

Some older adults who have immigrated to North America from other nations may have negative perceptions of acute care facilities as well as skilled nursing facilities based on their experiences in their native countries. Nurses can do much to ease the entry of ethnic elders into health care facilities when they assess each resident's cultural background, food preferences, choices for daily care and personal schedule, and interaction with family members. The individual's life experiences and personality will certainly shape the reaction to being in a care facility. A nurse may ask questions on topics that were meaningful to the older client, for example, what was most important for them to maintain in their daily routines and what would they like to do so they could be as independent as possible. Older clients in long-term care facilities for care of their debilitating physical conditions have expressed their desires to maintain their quality of life by controlling personal care and making decisions about their personal affairs whenever possible.

Community-Based Services for Older Adults

The skilled nursing facility represents only one option for extended care of the older adult. The current nursing facility resident is regarded by experts in the field as an individual who has generally exhausted the opportunities for care in the community. This individual usually only enters a facility after home care and levels of assisted living have been implemented. Long-term care nursing consultants and nurses working in ambulatory care settings often are asked to assess older clients to help determine the best care option. Criteria that the nurse often considers to recommend the level of care or residential placement that would be most appropriate for an older client include mental orientation, physical mobility restrictions (use of assistive devices and ability to walk unaided), degree of assistance needed to complete activities of daily living, frequency of incontinence, and level of risk for accident or injury if living independently.

Nurses can assess social and cultural factors that influence the care that older adults will need, the resources to meet those needs, and the locations for residence and care that are most acceptable to the client. Nurses must assess the physiologic status of the older adult and consider the safety of the client in a residential setting. The nurse must also consider medication management of the older client, and there are physiologic changes in aging that must be considered for every client. Additionally, a nurse should reduce potential misunderstandings caused by language differences in a care plan for any older client. The nurse should assess for the older clients' understanding of medication directions as the client's eyesight may be failing and should clarify directions, which may be open to multiple interpretations. Other factors to assess include cultural values that affect the older adult's expectations for family member care. The cultural values held by the older client and his or her family will influence the available resources, including informal sources of support such as children and grandchildren who are called upon to provide personal care, assistance with activities of daily living, and financial support.

Nurses and health care professionals who are aware of the older adult client's preferences for in-home care or for residence in skilled nursing facilities realize that the client's economic resources may affect preferred care options. For the poor elderly person, purchasing part-time personal health care services or attendant care that would enable him or her to remain at home may not be an option, so the older adult manages in less-than-desirable or potentially unsafe living situations. Nurses who are working with individual clients and those who are assigned a caseload of groups of older adults in community settings, such as apartment complexes and assisted living centers, will assess the client's needs, available sources of support from the family, and formal sources of support that are affordable to the client in a total plan of care for each client. Local programs through the Division of Aging, Aging Services, or a comparable agency may leverage available state or federal funds in innovative programs to reduce rental costs to assist elderly clients so they can remain in the community.

Local or church affiliated agencies that recruit and train volunteer visitors and caregivers to the elderly may be used in conjunction with the aging agency programs to enable the fragile older adult to function at home with formal sources of support. These organized sources of support that may include a weekly visitor or a person to do chores for the elderly client may supplement the care and support that family members may provide. Nearly all older adults indicate their preferences for remaining in the community and in their homes rather than in institutional care. The desire to be independent is a cultural value that is highly regarded by many older adults who proudly proclaim how they have supported and cared for themselves for years. For the majority of older American adults, the long-held value to be independent is so strong that the person would rather live alone even in poor health than be a burden to his or her family.

Older individuals who are independent or self-sufficient in the previously mentioned areas are the most likely candidates for what are termed *continuing care retirement communities*. These are common residential locations that offer the older adult a comfortable apartment, a range of levels of assistance with activities of daily living, meals, social activities, and supervised exercise programs. Some residential communities have an attached facility for the skilled nursing care. Many of these communities have accommodations to move the client to higher and lower levels of care based on the older client's needs, which may change over time. Factors that could cause changes in the older client's condition that would warrant transfers from one level of care to another would include acute exacerbations of chronic illness, new illness episodes, surgical care, and declines in functional abilities associated with falls or accidents.

These continuing care retirement communities offer many older adults the security to summon health care assistance if needed, the opportunity to interact with peers, and the option to remain in a community setting with an increased likelihood of participating in community resources, including cultural events, shopping trips, or entertainment provided by younger adults or school children. But some older adults would feel stigmatized by residence in such a facility and would prefer to live in an independent location in the community. Other perspective residents might prefer the stimulation of intergenerational contact outside of an age-related residence and would prefer living on their own with other means of informal and formal support.

The challenge that the majority of older individuals will face is the high cost of paying for levels of care in residential communities or in skilled nursing facilities. Many older clients and their families assume that Medicare will be the means for paying for such care. However, Medicare is limited to reimbursement for posthospital acute nursing facility stays and does not cover what is termed custodial or maintenance care of the older client. Older individuals and their families may exhaust their personal resources to cover extended care needs and custodial care. Nurses working in ambulatory care are finding many new work experiences in caring for older adult clients for short-term posthospital care or for assessment of clients who need extended care.

There has been an increase in the development of day programs in communities that provide nursing assessment, physical or occupational therapy, group socialization, and nutrition to older adults. These programs may supplement the affective support and tangible assistance that families give, and the programs provide settings that affirm the older clients' dignity. The range of these services provided at each site varies according to the support of the local community, including volunteers and professional staff. Some sites provide group socialization and nutrition for a lunchtime meal. The older adults are usually ambulatory or able to be independent with assistive devices, so they may be transported to the sites by public or private transportation. In some Asian American communities, adult day centers offer programs and services for older adults who may be caregivers for their grandchildren. The grandparent may bring the grandchild for well-child examinations and also access a health care provider for himself or herself, so two generations access health care at the same site.

The options are expanding for the older client to continue to reside in the community and to participate in an adult day program. On Lok Senior Health Services is an adult day-care program pioneered in Chinatown, San Francisco, which hires a multidisciplinary team to provide comprehensive services to the very frail elderly who would be at risk for nursing home placement. The Cherokee Nation of Oklahoma is adapting a culturally specific approach to provide a Program of All-Inclusive Care for the Elderly (PACE) for the frail elderly in rural Oklahoma communities that have a high Cherokee population. Salud Para Su Corazon has been a comprehensive outreach program using a culturally acceptable *promotora* model to teach heart healthy behavior for the Hispanic elderly, their families, and their communities. Elderwise is a senior enrichment program in Seattle, Washington, with activities that include art, exercise, and discussion topics, so adults review events in their personal histories and they are validated as authorities on their lives and for their abilities (see Figures 8-1 and 8-2).

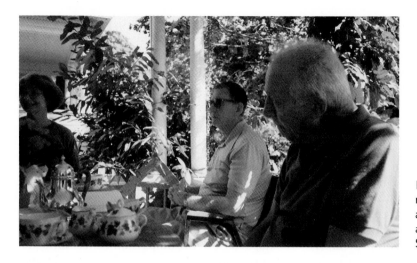

FIGURE 8-1 Opportunities to recall and share life experiences affirm the older client's identity and self-esteem (Elderwise in Seattle, Washington).

Nurses may want to assess the availability of enrichment programs in local settings and encourage attendance at such a program for older adult clients. Many mutual assistance associations or cultural affiliations, for example, the Khmer Community, Asian Counseling Services, Croatian Cultural Center, or the Eritrean Center may provide programs for older adults to interact with young people and to share cultural traditions. These cultural center programs and similar church-affiliated programs provide a means for older clients to receive affirmational peer support and to reinforce their cultural identity in a way that restores self-esteem and dignity.

Other intergenerational programs support older adults becoming involved within the community and the educational system. These types of program include the Older American Volunteer Program, the Retired Senior Volunteer Program, and the Foster Grandparents Program. There are also intergenerational child-care centers that are demonstrating that older volunteers are resources in the community, and the children and older adults benefit. Evaluations of multigenerational programs found that the older volunteers had a high level of life satisfaction, including psychosocial adjustment and self-esteem. Older adult volunteers experienced high life satisfaction prior to volunteering, so they appear to be successfully demonstrating the active aging theory.

Evaluating Services to Improve Delivery of Care

The nurse manager who evaluates the use of services by older clients can assess the cultural appropriateness and acceptability of services. Clients may be reluctant to use services for various reasons that include internal barriers such as not perceiving a need for care, contextual barriers

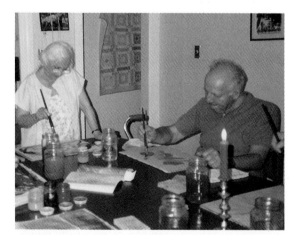

FIGURE 8-2 Creative expression stimulates discussion among participants in an older adult enrichment program (Elderwise in Seattle, Washington).

such as prior negative experiences in health care settings, and service barriers such as lack of health care insurance.

To overcome the barriers that are perceived by older clients, nurses can assume several approaches to interact effectively with older adults from diverse groups:

- Be sensitive to the life experiences and previous health care experiences of the older clients.
- Listen attentively to the older client's complaints, recollections, and strengths.
- Listen to related conversations to assess for underlying depression.
- Elicit information about the older client's preferences for care, including diet and use of self-care remedies, and include them when appropriate.
- Identify available sources of informal support and confirm availability.

SUMMARY

A cultural approach to the older client recognizes that individuals are the products of, as well as the participants in, an encompassing societal framework. Within the societal framework, the cultural backgrounds of the older clients will influence their variations in their perceptions, behavior, and practices. Culture serves as a guide to the older client to determine what choices and actions are appropriate and acceptable. Within cultural groups, individual variation is evident in response to the physiologic signs and the psychosocial demands of increasing age. Examples of older immigrant clients demonstrate that the clients' views and perceptions may differ from those of family members and from the views of the nurse. The different attitudes, practices, and behaviors among older clients result from their heritage, experiences, education acculturation, and socioeconomic status. Nursing care is not acceptable if it is based on assumptions that members of cultural groups are all the same. Instead, nursing care must be based on the assessment of individual differences in the variables that influence responses to illness and help-seeking behaviors.

Nurses who are providing care in acute care settings or in the community often ask several questions as part of the nursing assessment:

1. Is the older adult isolated from culturally relevant supportive people, or is the older client enmeshed in a caring network of relatives and friends?
2. Has a culturally appropriate network replaced family members in performing some tasks for the older adult client?
3. Does the older adult expect family members to provide care, including nurturance and emotional support, which family members are unable to provide?
4. Does language create a barrier in the older client's receipt of services from formal resources?

Older adult clients have often developed their own systems including informal support for coping with illness and with changes associated with age. Nurses who are working with older clients in a variety of settings will want to assess who provides affirmation and tangible support that maintains the older client in an optimal level of functioning. Formal resources may be used to sustain the informal support systems to promote the lifestyle preferred by the older client. It is increasingly important for nurses to recognize the expanded roles that the older client may have in his or her family as a caretaker of young grandchildren or another family member. Nurses caring for older adult clients should give attention to the client's family and social roles and develop care plans that maintain and restore the individual to his or her usual roles and patterns of activity. In the future, nurses will assess and work with more older clients as they progress along a continuum of services and through more than one type of residence in the community. By assessing the client's cultural background and available support resources, nurses will plan appropriate care that will help older clients to optimize their self-esteem and dignity based on the client's functional abilities, affective support, and affirmational support.

REVIEW QUESTIONS

1. What resources, needs, and limitations should the nurse assess to develop a care plan for a recently discharged 82-year-old chronically ill man who is returning to a single-room occupancy hotel in a crowded inner-city location?

2. As the nurse who does health assessments for frail older adults who attend a community comprehensive day program, what information should the nurse assess to identify culturally appropriate care plans or service delivery plans for older Filipino and Chinese American clients?

3. The short-term subacute unit where you are the nurse manager serves a multinational group of older clients who are admitted for orthopedic surgery. What cultural assessments do you teach the staff to use in identifying the needs of clients and their families?

CRITICAL THINKING ACTIVITIES

1. Many local communities offer adult day care for older adults with chronic health care problems who are residing alone or with family members. Services usually include health screening by a nurse as well as occupational health and/or physical activity sessions for these community-based older adults. Request permission to attend an activity as an observer and attentive listener. Through observation and, if possible, conversation with a participant, try to assess the levels of self-care that session participants possess and identify the types of assistance that these clients require to remain in the community.

2. If you are a case manager for a managed care organization, you receive many authorization requests for in-home nursing services to assist older adults who have been discharged home following hospitalization for acute illnesses or surgery. List the factors that you will consider and the types of data that you need to make an informed decision about the nursing and health-related services and the duration of services that the older client should receive while at home.

3. In many communities, nurses provide hospice services to residents in long-term care facilities or to older adults living in other settings. Contact a community-based hospice nurse to request information about how the services meet older adults' needs for love and belongingness, as well as reflection and recollection that are expressed late in life.

4. With your awareness that cultural traditions and life experiences influence many older adults to prefer independent living, prepare a letter as a home health nurse to the appropriate official to request government-funded home health services for older adults.

REFERENCES

Administration on Aging. (2009). *A profile of older Americans: 2009*. U.S. Department of Health and Human Services.

American Heart Association. (2007). *Statistical fact sheets*. Available from http://www.americanheart.org/presenter.jhtml?identifier=2007

Angel, R. J., Angel, J. L., & Hill, T. D. (2008). A comparison of the health of older Hispanics in the United States and Mexico. *Journal of Aging and Health, 20*(1), 3–31.

Brown, S. C., Mason, C. A., Spokane, A. R., Cruza-Guet, M. C., Lopez, B., & Szapocznik, J. (2009). The relationship of neighborhood climate to perceived social support and mental health in older Hispanic immigrants in Miami, Florida. *Journal of Aging and Health, 21*(3), 431–459.

Chang, E., Hancock, K., Hickman, L., Glasson, J., & Davidson, P. (2007). Outcomes of acutely ill older hospitalized patients following implementation of tailored models of care: A repeated measure (pre- and post-intervention) design. *International Journal of Nursing Standards, 44*(7), 1072–1092.

Dunn, M. G., & O'Brien, K. M. (2009). Psychological health and meaning in life: Stress, social support, and religious coping in Latina/Latino immigrants. *Hispanic Journal of Behavioral Sciences, 31*(2), 204–227.

Evans, G. W., Wethington, E., Coleman, M., Worms, M., & Frongillo, E. A. (2008). Income health inequalities among older persons: The mediating role of multiple risk exposures. *Journal of Aging and Health, 20*(1), 107–125.

Fleming, E., & Gillibrand, W. (2009). An exploration of culture, diabetes, and nursing in the South Asian community: A meta-synthesis of qualitative studies. *Journal of Transcultural Nursing, 20*(2), 146–155.

Gruenewald, T. L., Karlamangla, A. S., Greendale, G. A., Singer, B. H., & Seeman, T. E. (2009). Increased mortality risk in older adults with persistently low or declining feelings of usefulness to others. *Journal of Aging and Health, 21*(2), 398–425.

Higgins, I. (2005). The experience of chronic pain in elderly nursing home residents. *Journal of Research in Nursing, 10*(4), 369–382.

Jang, Y., Chiriboga, D. A., Borenstein, A. R., Small, B. J., & Mortimer, J. A. (2009). Health-related quality of life in community-dwelling older Whites and African Americans. *Journal of Aging and Health, 21*(2), 336–349.

Jang, Y., Chiriboga, D. A., Herrera, J. R., & Branch, L. G. (2009) Self-rating of poor health: A comparison of Cuban elders in Havana and Miami. *Journal of Cross Cultural Gerontology, 24*(2), 181–191.

Kim, H., Capezuti, E., Boltz, M., & Fairchild, S. (2009). The nursing practice environment and nurse-perceived quality of geriatric care in hospitals. Western *Journal of Nursing Research, 31*(4), 480–495.

Kobayashi, K. M., Cloutier-Fisher, D., & Roth, M. (2009). Making meaningful connections: A profile of social isolation and health among older adults in small town and small city, British Columbia. *Journal of Aging and Health, 21*(2), 374–397.

Kobylarz, F. A., Heath, J. M., & Like, R. C., (2002). The ETHNIC(S) mneumonic a clinical tool for ethnogeriatric education. *Journal of the American Geriatric Society, 50,* 1582–1589.

Lai, D. W. L., & Surood, S. (2009). Chinese health beliefs of older Chinese in Canada. *Journal of Aging and Health, 21*(1), 38–62.

Markides, K. S., Eschbach, K., Ray, L., & Peek, K. (2007). Census disability rates among older people by race/ethnicity and type of Hispanic origin. In J. L. Angel & K. E. Whitfield (Eds.). *The health of aging Hispanics: The Mexican-origin population* (pp. 26–39). New York: Springer.

Miltiades, H. B., & Wu, B. (2008). Factors affecting physician visits in Chinese and Chinese immigrant samples. *Social Science & Medicine, 66,* 704–714.

Min, J., & Barrio, C. (2009). Cultural values and caregiver preference for Mexican-American and non-Latino White elders. *Journal of Cross-Cultural Gerontology, 25*(3), 225–239.

Phillips, L. R., & Crist, J. (2008). Social relationships among family caregivers: A cross-cultural comparison between Mexican Americans and non-Hispanic White caregivers. *Journal of Transcultural Nursing, 19*(4), 326–337.

Rooks, R. N., Simonsick, E. M., Klesges, L. M., Newman, A. B., Ayonayon, H. N., & Harris, T. B. (2008). Racial disparities in health care access and cardiovascular disease indicators in Black and White older adults in the health ABC study. *Journal of Aging and Health, 20*(6), 599–614.

Schoenberg, N. E., Traywick, L. S., Jacobs-Lawson, J., & Kart, C. S. (2008). Diabetes self-care among a multiethnic sample of older adults. *Journal of Cross Cultural Gerontology, 23*(4), 361–376.

Silverman, M., Nutini, J., Musa, D., King, J., & Albert, S. (2008). Daily temporal self-care responses to osteoarthritis symptoms by older African American and Whites. *Journal of Cross Cultural Gerontology, 23*(4), 319–337.

Tanner, D. (2007). Starting with lives: Supporting older people's strategies and ways of coping. *Journal of Social Work, 7*(1), 7–30.

U.S. Census Bureau. (2008). An Aging World: 2008. Accessed online www.csnus.gov/prod/2009pubs/p95-09-1.pdf

Wan, H., Yu, F., & Kolanowski, A. (2008). Caring for aging Chinese: Lessons learned from the United States. *Journal of Transcultural Nursing, 19*(2), 114–120.

Wang, C., Chan, C. L. W., Ho, A. H. Y., & Xiong, Z. (2008). Social networks and health-related quality of life among Chinese older adults with vision impairments. *Journal of Aging and Health, 20*(7), 804–823.

Warren-Findlow, J., & Issel, L. M. (2010). Stress and coping in African American women with chronic heart disease: A cultural cognitive coping model. *Journal of Transcultural Nursing, 21*(1), 45–54.

PART THREE

Nursing in Multicultural Health Care Settings

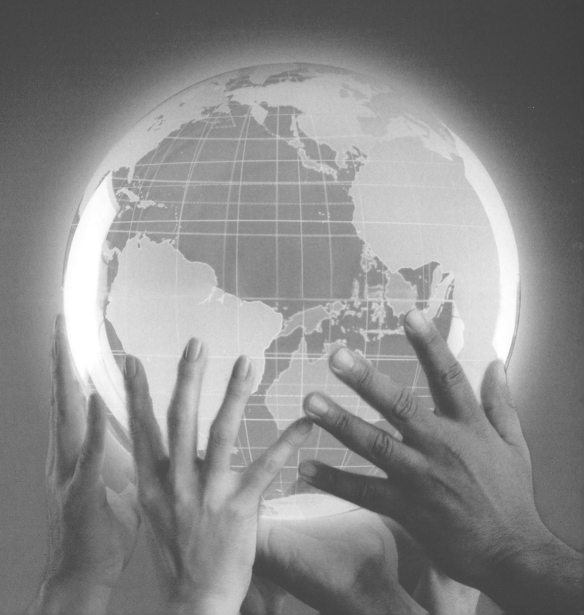

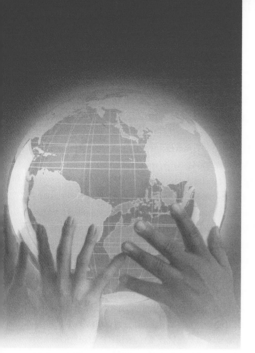

Creating Culturally Competent Organizations

Patti Ludwig-Beymer

KEY TERMS

CLAS Standards (Culturally and
    Linguistically Appropriate
    Services)
Community-based participatory
    research
Corporate culture
Cultural competence
Culturally competent organizations
Diversity
Dynamic hospital
Formal hospital
Health disparities
Healthy communities
Human resource frame
Institutional racism
Interpreter
Leininger's Culture Care Model
Limited English proficiency (LEP)
Magnet designation
Organizational culture
Participatory action research
Personal hospital
Political frame
Production-oriented hospital
Structural frame
Symbolic frame
Transcultural nursing administration

LEARNING OBJECTIVES

1. Describe how organizations can develop cultural competency.
2. Identify how health disparities can be decreased or eliminated.
3. Examine how organizations resolve conflict.
4. Evaluate organizational cultures.
5. Assess culturally competent initiatives designed and implemented by health care organizations.

An individual's culture affects access to care and health-seeking behaviors, as well as perceived quality of care. In addition to understanding the culture of patients or clients, however, it is also essential to examine the culture of providers and organizations. The interplay of client, provider, and **organizational cultures** may create barriers, cause cultural conflicts, lead to a client's lack of trust or reluctance to access services, and may ultimately result in health care inequities.

Leininger (1996) defines **transcultural nursing administration** as "a creative and knowledgeable process of assessing, planning, and making decisions and policies that will facilitate the provision of educational and clinical services that take into account the cultural caring values, beliefs, symbols, references and lifeways of people of diverse and similar cultures for beneficial or satisfying outcomes" (1996, p. 30). One very important role of nurse administrators is to ensure that organizational policies are culturally sensitive and appropriate and that they recognize the rights of individuals and families. Such policies should incorporate Leininger's (1991) decisions and actions of culture care preservation/maintenance, culture care accommodation/negotiation, and culture care repatterning/restructuring. According to the American Nurses Association Council on Cultural Diversity in Nursing Practice (1991), "[n]urse administrators must foster a climate in which nurses and other health care providers understand that provider-patient encounters include the interaction of three cultural systems." These three systems are the culture of the health care providers, the culture of the client, and the culture of the organizational setting.

Nurse leaders recognize the importance of transculturally based administrative practices in health care settings. The American Organization of Nurse Executives (AONE, 2005) has identified nurse executive competencies related to **diversity** as summarized in Box 9-1.

Malone (1997) describes several strategies for improving organizational cultural competence. First, health care organizations must implement training that helps **corporate culture** to value and manage cultural diversity. Second, nursing administration must reward practice that values differences and is culturally appropriate and collaborative. Third, nursing should seek members who are culturally competent. Finally, nursing should recruit and hire members who are culturally diverse, to better reflect the demographics of the country. Literature suggests that culturally diverse organizations outperform more homogenous organizations (Cox, 1994; Dreachslin, 1996).

This chapter serves to augment the current dialogue on creating **culturally competent organizations**. It defines a culturally competent organization, explains the need for culturally competent organizations, describes organizational culture, and provides a mechanism for assessing an organization's culture. Both the physical environment of care and the community context are considered. Finally, strategies for developing culturally competent initiatives and the role of health care providers in creating culturally competent organizations are described.

BOX 9-1

American Organization of Nurse Execuitves (AONE) Nurse Executive Competencies Related to Diversity

- Create an environment that recognizes and values differences in staff, physicians, patients, and communities.
- Assess current environment and establish indicators of progress toward cultural competency.
- Define diversity in terms of gender, race, religion, ethnicity, sexual orientation, age, and the like.
- Analyze population data to identify cultural clusters.
- Define cultural competency and permeate principles throughout the organization.
- Confront inappropriate behaviors and attitudes toward diverse groups.
- Develop processes to incorporate cultural beliefs into care.

Source: American Organization of Nurse Executives. (February 2005). AONE nurse executive competencies. *Nurse Leader,* 50–56.

Defining a Culturally Competent Organization

Culturally competent health care, broadly defined as services that are respectful of and responsive to the cultural and linguistic needs of patients, is increasingly viewed as essential in reducing racial and ethnic disparities, improving health care quality, and controlling costs. The U.S. government considers cultural competence as a method of increasing access to quality care for all patients. The aim should be to develop systems more responsive to diverse populations. Managed care organizations view cultural competence as driving both quality and business. By embedding cultural competence strategies into quality improvement initiatives to make care more efficient and effective, clinical outcomes are improved while costs are controlled. Those in academic settings agree that cultural competency education is crucial for preparing future health care workers, although appropriate education on the topic is provided in only half of the medical schools in the United States (Betancourt, Green, Carrillo, & Park, 2005).

According to the Office of Minority Health, **cultural competence** refers to the ability of health care providers and organizations to understand and respond effectively to the cultural and linguistic needs of patients (Office of Minority Health, 2001). Cultural competence encompasses a wide range of activities and considerations. It includes providing respectful care that is consistent with cultural health beliefs of the clients and family members.

Competent interpreter services and programs to promote staff diversity are other ways in which health care organizations can increase cultural competence (Clancy & Stryer, 2001). Because communication is a cornerstone of patient safety and quality care, every patient has the right to receive information in a manner he or she understands. Effective communication allows patients to participate more fully in their care. Communicating effectively with patients is also critical to the informed consent process and helps practitioners and hospitals give the best possible care. For communication to be effective, the information provided must be complete, accurate, timely, unambiguous, and understood by the patient. Many patients of varying circumstances require alternative communication methods: patients who speak and/or read languages other than English; patients who have limited literacy in any language; patients who have visual or hearing impairments; patients on ventilators; patients with cognitive impairments; and children. The hospital has many options available to assist in communication with these individuals, such as **interpreters**, translated written materials, pen and paper, communication boards, and speech therapy. It is up to the hospital to determine which method is the best for each

patient. Various laws, regulations, and guidelines are relevant to the use of interpreters. These include Title VI of the Civil Rights Act, 1964; Executive Order 13166; policy guidance from the Office of Civil Rights regarding compliance with Title VI, 2004; Title III of the Americans with Disabilities Act, 1990; state laws; and the American Medical Association Office Guide to **Limited English Proficiency** (LEP) Patient Care (Joint Commission Resources, 2010).

In the United States, a variety of organizations have addressed the need for culturally competent organizations. For example, The Joint Commission has set standards, outlined in Box 9-2, to ensure that patients receive care that respects their cultural, psychosocial, and spiritual values (Joint Commission Resources, 2010). As outlined in Box 9-3, the American Nurses Association (2001) and American Nurses Credentialing Center (2008) have also addressed the need for culturally competent care.

The United States government has also addressed culturally appropriate health care systems. For example, the Institute of Medicine (IOM) report "Health Professions Education: A Bridge to Quality" (Greiner & Knebel, 2003) identifies five core competencies for all health professionals: provide patient-centered care, work in interdisciplinary teams, employ evidence-based practice, apply quality improvement, and utilize informatics. Providing patient-centered care includes sharing power and responsibility with patients and caregivers; communicating with patients in a shared and fully open manner; taking into account patients' individuality, emotional needs, values, and life issues; implementing strategies for reaching those who do not present for care on their own, including care strategies that support the broader community; and enhancing prevention and health promotion. In order to accomplish the goal of meeting patients' individuality, emotional needs, values and life issues, the IOM report further indicates that clinicians must provide care in the context of the culture, heath status, and health needs of the patient.

BOX 9-2

Joint Commission Standards That Address Culture

2010 Leadership Standards

Overview

Leaders shape the hospital's culture, and the culture affects how the hospital accomplishes its work. A healthy, thriving culture is built around the hospital's mission and vision, which reflect the core values and principles that the hospital finds important. Leaders ask some basic questions to provide this focus: How does the hospital plan to meet the needs of its population(s)? By what ethical standards will the hospital operate? What does the hospital want to accomplish through its work? Once leaders answer these questions, the culture of the hospital will begin to take shape. Leaders also have an obligation to set an example of how to work together to fulfill the hospital's mission. By dedicating themselves to upholding the values and principles of the hospital's mission, leaders model to others how to collaborate, communicate, solve problems, manage conflict, and maintain ethical standards, essential practices that contribute to safe health care.

Specific Standards

LD.03.01.01 Leaders create and maintain a culture of safety and quality throughout the hospital

2010 Rights and Responsibilities of the Individual

Overview

When the hospital recognizes and respects patient rights, it is providing an important aspect of care that has been shown to encourage patients to become more informed and involved in their care. The hospital shows its support of patient rights through its interactions with patients and by involving them in decisions about their care, treatment, and services. Recognizing and respecting patient rights directly affects the provision of care. Care, treatment, and services should be provided in a way that respects and fosters the patient's dignity, autonomy, positive self-regard, civil rights, and involvement in his or her care. Care, treatment, and services should also be carefully planned and provided with regard to the patient's personal values, beliefs, and preferences.

Specific Standards

RI.01.01.01 The hospital respects, protects, and promotes patient rights.

RI.01.01.03 The hospital respects the patient's right to receive information in a manner he or she understands.

RI.01.02.01 The hospital respects the patient's right to participate in decisions about his or her care, treatment, and services.

RI.01.03.01 The hospital honors the patient's right to give or withhold informed consent.

RI.01.03.05 The hospital honors the patient's right to give or withhold informed consent to produce or use recordings, films, or other images of the patient for purposes other than his or her care.

RI.01.03.05 The hospital protects the patient and respects his or her rights during research, investigation, and clinical trials.

RI.01.05.01 The hospital addresses patient decisions about care, treatment, and services received at the end of life.

RI.01.06.05 The patient has the right to an environment that preserves dignity and contributes to a positive self-image.

RI.01.07.03 The patient has the right to access protective and advocacy services.

2010 Provision of Care, Treatment, and Services

Overview

The provision of care, treatment, and services is composed of four core elements: assessing patient needs; planning care, treatment, and services; providing the care, treatment, and services; and coordinating care, treatment and services. The complexity of providing care, treatment, and services often requires an interdisciplinary collaborative approach. The activities are performed by a wide variety of staff and licensed independent practitioners. Communication, collaboration, and coordination are essential so that care, treatment, and services are provided at the highest level.

Specific Standards

PC.01.01.01 The hospital accepts the patient for care, treatment, and services based on its ability to meet the patient's needs.

PC01.03.01 The hospital plans the patient's care.

PS.02.01.01 The hospital provides care, treatment, and services for each patient.

BOX 9-2 *(continued)*

PC.02.02.13 The patient's comfort and dignity receive priority during end-of-life care.

PS.02.03.01 The hospital provides patient education and training based on each patient's needs and abilities.

PC.04.01.05 Before the hospital discharges or transfers a patient, it informs and educates the patient about his or her follow-up care, treatment, and services.

- Identifying patient communication needs
- Addressing patient communication needs
- Collecting race and ethnicity data
- Collecting language data
- Patient access to chosen support individual
- Nondiscrimination in patient care
- Providing language services

New and Revised Elements of Performance Anticipated for 2011

- Addressing qualifications for language interpreters and translators

Joint Commission Resources. (2010). *Comprehensive accreditation manual for hospitals.* http://amp.jcrinc.com. Accessed February 22, 2010.
Joint Commission. (January 2010). *The Joint Commission Perspectives,* 5–6.

BOX 9-3

Standards and Sources of Evidence That Address Culture

Select Standards from the Code of Nurses (American Nurses Association, 2001)

Standard 1
The nurse, in all professional relationships, practices with compassion and respect for the inherent dignity, worth, and uniqueness of every individual, unrestricted by considerations of social or economic status, personal attributes, of the nature of health problems.

Standard 2
The nurse's primary commitment is to the patient, whether an individual, family, group, or community.

Standard 3
The nurse promotes, advocates for, and strives to protect the health, safety, and rights of the patients.

Standard 8
The nurse collaborates with other health professionals and the public in promoting community, national, and international efforts to meet health needs.

Magnet Sources of Evidence Related to Providing Culturally Congruent Care (American Nurses Credentialing Center, 2008)

Organizational Overview
- Provide an ethnic profile of the nursing staff, client population, and community served.
- Provide a list of continuing education programs and the number of nurses completing each during the past 24 months. Include programs covering the following topics: research, including protection of human subjects; application of ethical principles; and cultural competence.

Transformational Leadership
- TL-1—How nursing's mission, vision, values, and strategic plans reflect the organization's current and anticipated strategic priorities.
- TL3—The strategic planning structure(s) and process(es) used by nursing to improve the health care system's effectiveness and efficiency.

(box continues on page 216)

BOX 9-3

Standards and Sources of Evidence That Address Culture (*continued*)

Structural Empowerment

- SE9—How nurses support community educational activities.
- SE11—The structure(s) and process(es) used to identify and allocate resources for affiliations with schools of nursing, consortiums, or community outreach programs.
- SE12—How the organization supports and recognizes the participation of nurses at all levels in service to the community.
- SE13—How the organization or nursing addresses the health care needs of the community by establishing partnerships.

Exemplary Professional Practice

- EP4—That the structure(s) and process(es) of the Care Delivery System involve the patient and/or his or her support system in the planning and delivery of care.
- EP16—Interdisciplinary collaboration across multiple settings to ensure the continuum of care.
- EP18—Interdisciplinary collaboration to develop, implement, and evaluate a comprehensive set of patient education programs and resources within the organization.

- EP23—How nurses use available resources, such as the ANA Code of Ethics for Nurses to address complex, ethical issues.
- EP25—How the organization identifies and addresses disparities in the management of the health care needs of diverse patient populations. Include the role of the nurse.
- EP26—How nurses use resources to meet the unique and individual needs of patients and families.
- EP27—How the organization promotes a non-discriminatory climate for patients.
- EP29—The organization's workplace advocacy for diversity.
- EP32—The nursing structure(s) and process(es) that support a culture of patient safety.

Empirical Evidence

- TL3EO—The outcome that resulted from nursing's strategic planning.
- SE11EO—The result(s) of the affiliations with schools of nursing, consortiums, or community outreach programs.

BOX 9-4

National Standards for Culturally and Linguistically Appropriate Services (CLAS) in Health Care

Culturally Competent Care

Standard 1

Health care organizations should ensure that patients/consumers receive from all staff members, effective, understandable, and respectful care that is provided in a manner compatible with their cultural health beliefs and practices and preferred language.

Standard 2

Health care organizations should implement strategies to recruit, retain, and promote at all levels of the organization a diverse staff and leadership that are representative of the demographic characteristics of the service area.

Standard 3

Health care organizations should ensure that staff at all levels and across all disciplines receive ongoing education and training in culturally and linguistically appropriate service delivery.

Language Access Services

Standard 4 (Mandate*)

Health care organizations must offer and provide language assistance services, including bilingual staff and interpreter services, at no cost to each patient/consumer with LEP at all points of contact, in a timely manner during all hours of operation.

BOX 9-4 *(continued)*

Standard 5 (Mandate*)

Health care organizations must provide to patients/consumers in their preferred language both verbal offers and written notices informing them of their right to receive language assistance services.

Standard 6 (Mandate*)

Health care organizations must assure the competence of language assistance provided to limited English proficient patients/consumers by interpreters and bilingual staff. Family and friends should not be used to provide interpretation services (except on request by the patient/consumer).

Standard 7 (Mandate*)

Health care organizations must make available easily understood patient-related materials and post signage in the languages of the commonly encountered groups and/or groups represented in the service area.

Organizational Supports for Cultural Competence

Standard 8

Health care organizations should develop, implement, and promote a written strategic plan that outlines clear goals, policies, operational plans, and management accountability/oversight mechanisms to provide culturally and linguistically appropriate services.

Standard 9

Health care organizations should conduct initial and ongoing organizational self-assessment of CLAS-related activities and are encouraged to integrate cultural and linguistic competence-related measures into their internal audits, performance improvement programs, patient satisfaction assessments, and outcomes-based evaluations.

Standard 10

Health care organizations should ensure that data on the individual patient's/consumer's race, ethnicity, and spoken and written language are collected in health records, integrated into the organization's management information systems, and periodically updated.

Standard 11

Health care organizations should maintain a current demographic cultural, and epidemiological profile of the community as well as a needs assessment to accurately plan for and implement services that respond to the cultural and linguistic characteristics of the service area.

Standard 12

Health care organizations should develop participatory, collaborative partnerships with communities and utilize a variety of formal and informal mechanisms to facilitate community and patient/consumer involvement in designing and implementing CLAS-related activities.

Standard 13

Health care organizations should ensure that conflict and grievance resolution processes are culturally and linguistically sensitive and capable of identifying, preventing, and resolving cross-cultural conflicts or complaints by patients/consumers.

Standard 14

Health care organizations are encouraged to regularly make available to the public information about their progress and successful innovations in implementing the CLAS standards and to provide public notice in their communities about the availability of this information.

*Mandate—indicates the standard is a current Federal requirement for all recipients of Federal funds.

Source: Office of Minority Health, Department of Health and Human Services. (March 2001). *National standards for culturally and linguistically appropriate services in health care final report.* Washington DC.

In addition, National Standards for **Culturally and Linguistically Appropriate Services** in Health Care (CLAS Standards), outlined in Box 9-4, were developed by the U.S. Department of Health and Human Services' Office of Minority Health (2001) to correct health care inequities that currently exist and to make health care services more responsive to the individual needs of all patients. All people entering the health care system should receive equitable and effective care in a culturally and linguistically appropriate manner. The CLAS standards are inclusive of all cultures and are especially designed to address the needs of racial, ethnic, and linguistic populations that experience unequal access to health services. Ultimately, the aim of the standards is to contribute to the elimination of racial and ethnic **health disparities** and to improve the health of all Americans.

The Need for Culturally Competent Organizations

Disparities in health have long been acknowledged. The National Institutes of Health (2010) define disparities in health as "differences in the incidence, prevalence, mortality, and burden of diseases and other adverse health conditions that exist among specific population groups in the United States." At the most basic level, disparities are evident in life expectancies. For example, the Centers for Disease Control and Prevention National Vital Statistics System (2009) reports the U.S. life expectancy is 77.9 years. However, life expectancy varies by race, with White males (75.8 years) and White females (80.7 years) higher than African American males (70.2 years) and African American females (77.0 years).

Annually, the Agency for Healthcare Research and Quality (AHRQ) tracks disparities in health care delivery as it relates to racial and socioeconomic factors (AHRQ, 2008a). Three themes emerged from the National Healthcare Disparities Report, 2008 (AHRQ, 2008b):

1. Disparities persist in health care quality and access
2. Some disparities exist across multiple populations
3. The magnitude and patterns of disparities are different within subpopulations

Access (getting into the health care system) and quality care (receiving appropriate, safe and effective health care in a timely manner) are key factors in achieving good health outcomes. Access to primary care is a key aspect of health care in the United States; research suggests that having a usual source of care increases the chances that people will receive adequate preventive care and other important health services. Yet evidence suggests that access disparities persist for all minority populations. Between 2000–2001 and 2005–2006, 20% to 80% of the access measures stayed the same or worsened for Black, Asian, American Indian/Alaskan Native, Hispanic, and the poor. Barriers include lack of health insurance and trouble getting appointments. For example, both Blacks and Hispanics are more likely than Whites to be unable to receive care or to delay care. In addition, between 2000–2001 and 2005–2006, 70% of quality of care measures stayed the same or worsened for Black, Asian, American Indian/Alaskan Native, Hispanic, and the poor.

Some disparities exist across multiple populations. For example, core measures for cancer screening (colonoscopy, sigmoidoscopy, or fecal occult blood test) have worsened for Black, Asian, American Indian/Alaskan Native, and Hispanic populations. Blacks and Asians are more likely to report poor provider–patient communication and are less likely to have received a pneumococal vaccination if age 65 or older. Blacks and Hispanics are less likely to have received treatment for a major depressive episode.

In addition, the magnitude and patterns of disparities are different within subpopulations. The three largest disparities are summarized in Box 9-5.

BOX 9-5

Three Largest Disparities in Quality of Care for Select Groups

Group	Measures
Black compared to White	• New AIDS cases per 100,000 population age 13 and over • Hospital admissions for lower extremity amputations in patients with diabetes per 100,000 population • Pregnant women who did not receive prenatal care in the first trimester
Asian compared to White	• Adults who can sometimes or never get care for illness or injury as soon as they wanted • Children ages 2 to 17 who did not receive advice about physical activity • Adults age 65 and over who never received pneumococcal vaccination
American Indian/Alaskan Native compared to White	• Pregnant women who did not receive prenatal care in the first trimester • Adults age 50 and over who did not receive colorectal cancer screening • Home health care patients who were admitted to the hospital
Hispanic compared to non-Hispanic White	• New AIDS cases per 100,000 population age 13 and over • Children whose parents reported poor communication with health provider • Pregnant women who did not receive prenatal care in the first trimester
Poor compared with higher income*	• Children whose parents reported poor communication with health provider • Adults who can sometimes or never get care for illness or injury as soon as they wanted • Women age 40 and over who reported they did not have a mammogram in the past 2 year

* Poor is defined as people living in families whose household income falls below specific poverty thresholds, established annually by the U.S. Bureau of the Census based on family size and composition. The number of people living in poverty increased from 31.6 million in 2000 to 36.5 million in 2006. Poverty rates vary by race and ethnicity, with 24% of Blacks, 21% of Hispanics, 10% of Asians, and 8% of Whites classified as poor in 2006.

Source: AHRQ (Agency for Healthcare Research and Quality). (2008b). *Disparities in health care quality among racial and ethnic minority groups.* Findings from the National Healthcare Disparities Report, 2008.

In Canada, with its National Health Insurance Model, many individuals experience similar disparities in access to preventative services. This implies that other factors may account for health disparities. Although these factors have not yet been identified, potential barriers that contribute to the disparities may be related to demographics, culture, and the health care system itself. Potential barriers are summarized in Box 9-6.

Although identifying disparities in care is important, it is not sufficient. To reduce health disparities, individuals must deliver culturally competent health care that focuses on risk reduction, vulnerability reduction, and promotion and protection of human rights (Flaskerud, 2007). A variety of projects are underway to develop tools to help eliminate racial and ethnic disparities.

Organizational culture is one area that may influence both cultural competence and health disparities. A culturally competent organization is extremely complex. Within the health care setting, practitioners must be aware of the effects of culture on individual behaviors. A culturally competent organization, however, goes beyond this awareness and calls for an understanding of the interplay among organizational culture, professional culture, and community culture.

BOX 9-6
Potential Demographic, Cultural, and Health System Barriers

Demographic Barriers

Age
Gender
Ethnicity
Primary language
Religion
Educational level and literacy level
Occupation, income, and health insurance
Area of residence
Transportation
Time and/or generation in the United States

Cultural Barriers

Age
Gender, class, and family dynamics
Worldview/perceptions of life
Time orientation
Primary language spoken
Religious beliefs and practices
Social customs, values, and norms
Traditional health beliefs and practices

Dietary preferences and practices
Communication patterns and customs

Health System Barriers

Differential access to high-quality care
Insurance and other financial resources
Orientation to preventive health services
Perception of need for health care services
Lack of knowledge and/or distrust of Western medical
   practices and procedures
Cultural insensitivity and incompetence in providers,
   including bias, stereotyping, and prejudice
Lack of diversity in providers
Western versus folk health beliefs and practices
Poor provider–patient communication
Lack of bilingual and bicultural staff
Unfriendly and cold environment
Fragmentation of care
Physical barriers (such as excessive distances)
Information barriers

Organizational Culture

Organizational culture has emerged as an important variable for behavior, performance, and outcome in the workplace. Nurses, while familiar with the concept of culture, may be less familiar with the area of organizational culture. Organizational culture is not consistently described in the literature, and multiple definitions exist. Many definitions center on enduring attributes of culture such as values, assumptions, and beliefs (Scott-Findlay & Estabrooks, 2006). Leininger (1996) defines organizational culture as the goals, norms, values, and practices of an organization in which people have goals and try to achieve them in beneficial ways.

Organizations are complex, with multiple and competing subcultures. For example, nurse specialties result in subcultures within hospitals that impact nurse and patient outcomes

(Mallidou, 2004). Organizations are subcultural systems with inherent values and beliefs, folklore, and language; these systems are organized in a hierarchy of authority, responsibilities, obligations, and functional tasks that are understood by members of the organization.

Organizational culture has been studied as it relates to accountability (O'Hagan & Persaud, 2009); change (Seren & Baykul, 2007); emotional intelligence (Momeni, 2009); effectiveness (Casida, 2008); implementation of best practices and research (Marchionni & Ritchie, 2007; Scott-Findlay, 2006); leadership and management (Carney, 2006; Casida & Pinto-Zipp, 2008; Kane-Urrabazo, 2006); mentoring (Bally, 2007); and patient safety (Dekker, 2007; Khatri, Brown, & Hicks, 2009; Singer et al., 2009; Sorra, Famolaro, Dyer, Nelson, & Khanna, 2008). However, organizational culture affects not only people working in the institution, such as employees, physicians, and volunteers, but also those who access the institution's services, such as patients, families, and community members. The social organization of hospitals and other health care facilities has a profound effect on patients, both directly through the care provided and indirectly through organizational policies and philosophy. Organizational culture has not been directly linked to patient or provider outcomes, or to the provision of culturally competent care.

Theories of Organizational Culture

A variety of definitions, methods of measurement, and theories for organizational culture exist. However, there is reasonable consensus on the following (Strasser, Smits, Falconer, Herrin, & Bowen, 2002):

- an organization's culture consists of shared beliefs, assumptions, perceptions, and norms leading to specific patterns of behaviors;
- an organization's culture results from an interaction among many variables, including mission, strategy, structure, leadership, and human resource practices;
- culture is self-reinforcing; once in place, it provides stability and changes are resisted by organizational members.

Strasser et al. (2002) describe four types of hospital culture: personal, dynamic, formal, and production oriented. A **personal hospital** is like an extended family. People share information about themselves. A **dynamic hospital** is entrepreneurial. People are willing to take risks. A **formal hospital** is structured. Bureaucratic procedures govern actions. A **production-oriented hospital** is concerned primarily with getting the job done. People are not personally involved. Studies suggest that teams in cultures perceived as personal and dynamic have higher ratings of team functioning (Strasser et al., 2002).

Bolman and Deal (1997) describe four organizational culture perspectives or "frames" that affect the way in which an organization resolves conflicts. The **human resource frame** strives to facilitate the fit between person and organization. When conflict arises, the solution considers the needs of the individual or group as well as the needs of the organization. The **political frame** emphasizes power and politics. Problems are viewed as "turf" issues and are resolved by developing networks to increase the power base. The **structural frame** focuses on following an organization's rules or protocols. This culture relies on its policies and procedures to resolve conflict. The **symbolic frame** relies on rituals, ceremony, and myths in determining appropriate behaviors.

To understand how these four perspectives will result in different outcomes, consider typical responses to the following situation. Hospital A is located on the border of two communities. One community is primarily African American. The other community is primarily Hispanic. The hospital has traditionally provided care to African Americans and is well regarded by that community. The hospital has noted, however, that few members of the Hispanic community use its services. The hospital's board of directors realizes that, to survive, the hospital must expand its patient base. The approach to this challenge will vary based on the organization's culture.

Hospital leaders in a human resource perspective culture are likely to approach the situation by assessing the needs of both communities and the staff. For example, a hospital with a human resource perspective culture may convene focus groups with members of the Hispanic community to identify why the hospital's services are not used by that community. At the same time, the hospital will assess the African American community's perspective on the hospital's expanding its services and becoming a more inclusive organization. The hospital will also provide opportunities for staff members to provide input and to express their feelings about the goals of the organization. In the end, the hospital with a human resource perspective culture will reach a decision that balances the needs of all of these groups while enhancing the goal of expanding the patient base.

Hospital leaders in a political perspective culture will take a different approach. They will identify key "power" leaders in the Hispanic community.

Perhaps they will invite a Hispanic leader to join their board of directors or serve in another advisory capacity, or ask a priest from a Hispanic congregation to serve as a hospital chaplain. In addition, they will actively recruit Hispanic physicians and other clinician leaders. They will build a Hispanic power base within the hospital and use it to reach out to the larger Hispanic community and expand the patient base.

Hospital leaders in a structural perspective culture will develop policies and procedures to attract more Hispanic patients. For example, they may make certain that all signage appears in both English and Spanish, or develop a policy that requires all patient educational materials to be available in both Spanish and English. They may require all staff to attend a session on Hispanic culture, and may strongly encourage or mandate Spanish-language training for key personnel.

Finally, hospital leaders in a symbolic perspective culture will use ceremony to meet their goal. They will make physical changes to the environment to attract more Hispanics. For example, they may create or alter a chapel, inviting a priest from a Hispanic congregation to say mass. They may display other religious symbols, such as a crucifix or a statue of Our Lady of Guadalupe, or alter their artwork to be more culturally inclusive. They may also include Hispanic stories and rituals in their internal communications. These leaders will draw on symbols and rituals that will make persons of Hispanic culture more comfortable in the hospital environment and that will attract a larger Hispanic patient base.

None of these organizational cultures are inherently good or bad, just different. Each presents both strengths and weaknesses, and more than one culture may exist in an organization. For example, an organization may be guided primarily by both human resource and symbolic perspectives.

Schein (2004) describes organizational culture at three levels: (1) observable artifacts, (2) values, and (3) basic underlying assumptions. Artifacts are visible manifestations of values. Artifacts may include signage, statues and other decorations, pictures, décor, dress code, traffic flow, medical equipment, and visible interactions. Values are explicitly stated norms and social principles, and are manifestations of assumptions. Underlying assumptions are shared beliefs and expectations that influence perceptions, thoughts, and feelings about the organization; they are the core of the organization's culture. Assumptions define the culture of the organization, but because they are invisible, they may not be recognized. At times, the assumptions of an institution are ambiguous and self-contradictory, especially when an institutional merger or acquisition has occurred.

The basic premises of an organization, reflected in its mission statement, provide insight into the presence or absence of a commitment to providing culturally competent care. Organizations are well aware of the need to identify a consistent vision and a set of values to guide their organizational culture. As seen in Table 9-1, the mission, vision, and values may also include specific behaviors demonstrated toward both customers and colleagues.

Organizational Culture and Employees

There is a significant relationship between race/ethnicity and beliefs about the quality of workplace relationships and career opportunities. For example, research suggests that African American nurses experience stressors such as racism and lack of teamwork and supervisory support that causes them to contemplate leaving the workplace or the profession (Gibson-Jones, 2009). Health care organization leaders are called upon to implement strategies to make diversity work in health care organizations.

Many organizations are aware of the impact of organizational culture on its employees. When filling positions, recruiters consider the "fit" between the organization and the potential employee, because a good "fit" results in better retention and satisfied employees. Nurses and other health care professionals also learn how to determine whether an organization will match their personal values. For example, a nurse who wants to provide care in a culturally competent manner to lesbians and homosexuals will not be

TABLE 9-1
Vision and Values

WE WILL...	
Mission	To support health and strengthen communities by providing outstanding health care services.
Vision	• Locally preferred
	• Regionally referred
	• Nationally recognized
Values	• Patients first
	• Integrity
	• Compassion
	• Responsibility
	• Collaboration
	• Passion

Behaviors

We will...

Commitments to our customers

Welcome you
We will welcome you immediately, introduce ourselves, and call you by name.
We will tell you our role and what we'll do for you.
We will offer you a personal escort to your destination.

Care for you
We will be caring and treat you as an individual.
We will coordinate your services among our coworkers.
We will assure your privacy and confidentiality.

Promote safety
We will ask you to speak up with questions and concerns.
We will listen and work with you to find the answers.
We will explain your plan of care.
We will involve you in decisions about your care.
We will provide a clean, safe environment.

Provide great service
We will provide on-time service or inform you promptly about any delays.

Together, we will...

Commitments to each other

Work as a team
We will support each other's individuality and value differing experiences, skills, and ideas.
We will treat each other kindly.
We will warmly welcome new employees to Edward.
We will help each other succeed.

Communicate openly
We will compliment and recognize each other.
We will approach our work in an honest and professional manner.
We will keep our sense of humor.

Promote a safe environment
We will speak up about errors and potential safety concerns.
We will work together to resolve safety concerns and prevent future errors.
We will focus on solutions rather than blame.
We will use safe practices in our work.

Strive to be the best
We will ensure quality and timeliness of work.
We will base our decisions on what is best for the customer.
We take pride in our work and celebrate each other's success.

(table continues on page 224)

TABLE 9-1
Vision and Values (*continued*)

WE WILL...

We will do everything reasonably possible to make you comfortable and relieve your pain.	We will use Edward resources efficiently and protect them against loss, theft, or misuse.
We will answer your calls and requests promptly.	We will foster an environment of optimal health and well-being.

Courtesy of Edward Hospital & Health Services (2010), Naperville, IL.

happy in a critical care unit that restricts visitors to nuclear family members.

Culturally caring organizations are needed for nurses and other staff members, and humans need care to survive, thrive, and grow. Historically, however, organizations have made few attempts to nurture and nourish the human spirit. According to Leininger (1996), organizations need to incorporate universal care constructs, including respect and genuine concern for clients and staff.

An inclusive workplace is characteristic of a caring organization. Such a workplace, however, is not satisfied simply by a diverse workforce. Instead, such an organization focuses on capitalizing on the unique perspectives of a diverse workforce, in essence "managing for diversity" rather than "managing diversity" (Chavez & Weisinger, 2008). An inclusive workplace also reaches out beyond the organization by encouraging members of the workforce to become active in the community and participate in state and federal programs, working with the poor and with diverse cultural groups. Rather than espousing the golden rule (treat others as you wish to be treated), an inclusive workplace treats others as they wish to be treated, in what is sometimes called the platinum rule (Alessandra, 2010). Organizations with inclusive workplaces draw staff members who are committed to cultural competence and who value diversity and mutual respect for differences.

Although the impact of organizational culture on employees has been acknowledged, the impact of organizational culture on the community being served has received less attention. For years, hospitals and other health care organizations have espoused the view that "If we build it, they will come" (i.e., all that is needed is to offer the services). Now, there is a growing recognition that health care services should be structured in ways to appeal to and meet the needs of various members of the community. Health care leaders recognize that cultural competence in organizations is essential if organizations are to survive, grow, satisfy customers, and achieve their goals. Image is critically important for an organization's survival. A variety of factors are needed to move an organization toward cultural competence.

Assessing the Organizational Culture

Organizational culture may be assessed in numerous ways. Various instruments have been summarized by Scott-Findlay and Estabrooks (2006). In addition, Dansky, Weech-Maldonado, De Souza, and Dreachslin (2003) describe a 64-item tool that measures the breadth and degree of diversity management practices. The Magnet Hospital Recognition Program for Excellence in Nursing Services also evaluates organizational climate or culture (American Nurses Credentialing Center, 2008) and is used by many organizations as a blueprint for achieving excellence (Schaffner & Ludwig-Beymer, 2003). Evidence-Based Practice 9-1 outlines the original research that resulted in the creation of **Magnet designation**.

The Magnet Model may be helpful in assessing the culture of an organization. Questions related to each element of the model are listed in Box 9-7.

Leininger's (1991) Theory of Culture Care Diversity and Universality is also helpful in assessing the culture of an institution. **Leininger's**

EVIDENCE-BASED PRACTICE 9-1

Magnet Research and the Forces of Magnetism

The Magnet Recognition Program for Excellence in Nursing Services grew out of a 1982 descriptive study conducted by the American Academy of Nursing's Task Force on Nursing Practice (McClure, Poulin, Sovie, & Wandelt, 1983). The study began by asking Fellows from the American Academy of Nursing to identify hospitals that attracted and retained professional nurses who experienced professional and personal satisfaction in their practice. The Fellows nominated 165 institutions. These institutions were viewed as "magnets." The task force then began narrowing the list based on specific criteria and the hospitals' willingness and availability to participate in the study.

Data were then collected from staff nurses and nursing directors in 41 hospitals. Nurses identified and described variables that created an environment that attracted and retained well-qualified nurses and promoted quality patient care. Nurses were asked nine questions, which remain valuable for structuring nursing input even today:

1. What makes your hospital a good place to work?
2. Can you describe particular programs that you see leading to professional/personal satisfaction?
3. How is nursing viewed in your hospital, and why?
4. Can you describe nurse involvement in various ongoing programs/projects whose goals are quality of patient care?
5. Can you identify activities and programs calculated to enhance, both directly and indirectly, recruitment/retention of professional nurses in your hospital?
6. Could you tell us about nurse–physician relationships in your hospital?
7. Describe staff nurse–supervisor relationships in your hospital.
8. Are some areas in your hospital more successful than others in recruitment/retention? Why?
9. What single piece of advise would you give to a director of nursing who wishes to do something about high RN vacancy and turnover rates in his or her hospital?

Staff nurses identified a variety of conditions that made a hospital a good place for nurses to work, specifically related to administration, professional practice, and professional development. Clustered together, a very clear culture of nursing emerged from this descriptive study.

Based on findings from the original magnet study, the Magnet Recognition Program was developed in 1990. The program was created to advance three goals:

- Promote quality in a milieu that supports professional practice;
- Identify excellence in the delivery of nursing services to patients/residents;
- Provide a mechanism for the dissemination of "best practices" in nursing services.

The Magnet model (American Nurses Credentialing Center, 2008), derived from the 1982 study and the original 14 forces of magnetism, may be used to assess organizational culture. The Magnet model is presented in Box 9-5.

Clinical Application

As they rotate to different facilities for their clinical experiences, nursing students are in an ideal position to evaluate organizational climate. Nurses and nursing students are encouraged to use the Magnet framework, presented in Box 9-7, to assess nursing subcultures and determine organizational fit.

BOX 9-7

Using the Magnet Model to Assess Organizational Culture

Transformational Leadership

Strategic Planning

- What are the mission, vision, values, and philosophy for the organization? For nursing? What are the strategic priorities?
- How do the chief nursing officer (CNO) and nurses at all levels advocate for resources?
- How does nursing improve the health care system's effectiveness and efficiency?

Advocacy and Influence

- How does the CNO influence organizational change?
- How do nurse leaders guide change?
- How does the organization support leadership development, performance management, mentoring activities, and succession planning for nurse leaders?
- How do nurse leaders value, encourage, recognize, reward, and implement innovation?

Visibility, Accessibility, and Communication

- How is the CNO visible and accessible to direct-care nurses? How does two-way communication take place?
- How do nurse leaders use input from direct-care nurses to improve the work environment and patient care?

Structural Empowerment

Professional Engagement

- How do nurses from all settings and roles participate in organizational decision-making groups?
- How do nurses at all levels participate in professional organizations at the local, state, and national levels?

Commitment to Professional Development

- How does the organization set expectations and support nurses at all levels who seek additional formal nursing education?
- How does the organization set expectations and support professional development and professional certification?

- How does the organization develop and provide continuing education programs for nurses at all levels and settings?
- How does the organization provide career development opportunities for non-nurse employees and community members interested in a nursing career?

Teaching and Role Development

- How does the organization promote the teaching role of nurses.
- How does nursing facilitate the effective transition of new graduates into the work environment?
- How do nurses support community educational activities?
- How do nurses support academic practicum experiences and serve as preceptors, instructors, adjunct faculty, or faculty?

Commitment to Community Involvement

- How are resources allocated for affiliations with schools of nursing, consortiums, and community outreach programs?
- How does the organization support and recognize the participation of nurses at all levels in service to the community?
- How does the organization address the health care needs of the community by establishing partnerships?

Recognition of Nursing

- How does the organization make visible and recognize the contributions of nurses?
- How does the community at large recognize the value of nursing in the organization?

Exemplary Professional Practice

Professional Practice Model

- How do nurses develop, apply, evaluate, adapt and modify the Professional Practice Model?
- How do nurses investigate, develop, implement, and evaluate standards of practice and standards of care?
- How do nurses track and analyze nurse satisfaction or engagement data? How satisfied or engaged are the nurses?

BOX 9-7 *(continued)*

Care Delivery Systems

- How does the care delivery system involve the patient and his or her support system in the planning and delivery of care?
- How do the nurses make patient care assignments that ensure continuity, quality, and effectiveness of care?
- How are regulatory and professional standards incorporated into the care delivery systems?
- How are internal experts and external consultants engaged to improve care?

Staffing, Scheduling, and Budgeting

- How do nurses use trended data to formulate a staffing plan? How do direct-care nurses participate in staffing and scheduling? How are guidelines, standards, and requirements incorporated into staffing and scheduling?
- How do nurses develop, implement and evaluate action plans for unit-based staff recruitment and retention?
- How do nurses use data to make decisions about unit and department budget formulation, implementation, monitoring, and evaluation?

Interdisciplinary Care

- What is the role of nurses in interdisciplinary collaboration?
- How do nurses participate in interdisciplinary collaboration?
- How do nurses have access to and use current literature, and professional standards to support autonomous practice?
- How do nurses at all levels use self-appraisal, peer review, and goal setting?
- How do nurses participate in shared leadership or participative decision making to promote nursing autonomy?
- How do nurses resolve issues related to patient care or operations?

Ethics, Privacy, Security, and Confidentiality

- How do nurses address complex ethical issues?
- How do nurses resolve issues related to patient privacy, security, and confidentiality?

Diversity and Workplace Advocacy

- How does the organization identify and address disparities in the management of health care needs of diverse patient populations?
- How do nurses use resources to meet the unique and individual needs of patients and families?
- How does the organization promote a nondiscriminatory climate for patients?
- How does the organization identify and manage incompetent, unsafe, and unprofessional conduct?
- What initiatives are in place to address caregiver stress, diversity, rights, and confidentiality?

Culture of Safety

- How is the organization improving workplace safety for nurses?
- How does the organization address proactive risk assessment and error management?
- How does nursing support a culture of patient safety?

Quality Care Monitoring and Improvement

- How does the organization allocate and reallocate resources to monitor and improve quality of nursing and total patient care? How does the nurse assure coordination of care among other disciplines and support staff?
- Do direct-care nurses review and act on quality and patient satisfaction data?

New Knowledge, Innovations, and Improvements

Research

- How do nurses evaluate and use published research findings in their practice?
- How do nurses participate in the Institutional Review Board or other body responsible for the protection of human subjects in research? How do direct-care nurses support the human rights of research participants?
- How does the organization develop, expand, and advance nursing research?
- How does the organization disseminate knowledge generated through nursing research internally and externally?

(box continues on page 228)

BOX 9-7

Using the Magnet Model to Assess Organizational Culture (*continued*)

Evidence–Based Practice
- How is existing nursing practice evaluated based on evidence?
- How is new knowledge translated into nursing practice?

Innovation
- What types of innovations are being tested by nurses?
- How are nurses involved in evaluating and allocating technology, information systems, and space design to support practice?

Empirical Outcomes
- What are the quantitative and qualitative results for the patient? For nurses? For the organization? For the community?
- What are the changes in individuals and populations that can be attributed to health care provided by the organization?

Adapted from American Nurses Credentialing Center. (2008). *Magnet recognition program. Recognizing excellence in nursing service.* Application manual. Silver Spring, MD: American Nurses Credentialing Center.

Culture Care Model may be used to conduct a cultural assessment of the organization, with dominant segments of the sunrise model identified. An example of such an assessment is provided in Table 9-2. Other cultural care assessment tools are available to assess the culture of an institution. This assessment is then compared with the values and beliefs of the groups who use the health care organization.

Andrews (1998) provides an assessment tool for cultural change that examines demographic/descriptive data; strengths; community resources; continued growth; perspectives of patients, families, and visitors; institutional perspective; and readiness for change. This tool allows organizational leaders to assess the needs of the community they serve and to use their findings to guide strategic planning for the future.

Roizner (1996) identifies a checklist for culturally responsive health care services. Health care services are considered for their availability, accessibility, affordability, acceptability, and appropriateness. When the organizational culture is assessed by this model, it is important to consider these "five A's":

- Are the health services that are needed by the community readily available? In a community with rampant illicit drug use, for example, one should expect to find a variety of types of drug abuse prevention and treatment programs offered that are readily available to the local population.

- Are health care resources accessible? A pediatrician's office, for example, might need to expand its hours of operation to accommodate the schedules of working parents. Geographic location should be considered in terms of proximity to public transportation, traffic patterns, and available parking. Structural changes may also be needed to accommodate specific types of clients, such as those who use wheelchairs.

- Are the services affordable? Partnerships between public and private organizations may be needed to ensure that services are affordable. A sliding scale might be developed to accommodate the needs of people with diverse financial resources.

- Are the services acceptable? Providers need to carefully consider this question. Do community members who use the services perceive the services to be of high quality? Do community members value the services? Are the waiting rooms stark, dimly lit, or untidy? Is the furniture worn or the reading material frayed and outdated? Providers need to understand what makes services acceptable to the community they seek to serve. Community members may avoid a particular

TABLE 9-2

Example of Leininger (1991) Culture Care Model Used to Conduct an Organizational Assessment in a Hypothetical Hospital

FACTOR	TYPES OF QUESTIONS	SAMPLE FINDINGS
Environmental context	What is the general environment of the community that surrounds the organization? Socioeconomic status? Race/ethnicity? Emphasis on health? Living arrangements? Access to social services? Employment? Proximity to other health facilities?	Hospital A is in a low-income urban setting. The majority of residents in the area are African Americans, with a few Asians and Whites. A public housing complex is located within a few blocks of the hospital. The economy is depressed, and many are out of jobs. Drug abuse and alcoholism are rampant. Families are challenged to survive, and they tend to view disease prevention as unimportant. There is a short-term perspective on health, which is defined as being able to do normal activities. Several social agencies nearby provide assistance with food pantries. There are no other hospitals within a 5-mile radius.
Language and ethnohistory	What languages are spoken within the institution? By employees? By patients? How formal or informal are the lines of communication? How hierarchical? What communication strategies are used within the institution? Written? Poster? Electronic? Oral? "Grapevine"? How did the institution come to be? What was the original mission? How has it changed over the years?	Patients primarily speak English. Employees typically speak English, although Polish and Russian are heard, particularly among the housekeepers. The grapevine is alive and well at Hospital A. Although memos are circulated, verbal communication is prized throughout the institution. The president/chief executive officer, chief nursing officer, and chief medical officer all maintain an open-door policy in their offices. Posters are also used to communicate, especially in the elevators. Electronic communication via e-mail has not been successful because computer workstations are in short supply throughout the institution. Hospital A was founded by a Roman Catholic religious order of nuns in 1885. The original mission was to provide care to immigrants and the poor. Immigrants from many nations, including Ireland, Poland, Hungary, and Russia, originally inhabited the area. The mission is still to provide the highest quality of care to the poor and underserved, although that is becoming increasingly difficult financially.
Technology	How is technology used in the institution? Who uses it? Is patient documentation electronic? Is electronic order entry in place? Is cutting-edge technology in place in the emergency department (ED), critical care units, labor	There are a few computer workstations on each nursing unit, which are primarily used by the clinical secretaries. Nurses do not document electronically, and physicians do not use electronic order entry. Hospital A received external funding several years ago to renovate

(table continues on page 230)

TABLE 9-2
Example of Leininger (1991) Culture Care Model Used to Conduct an Organizational Assessment in a Hypothetical Hospital (*continued*)

FACTOR	TYPES OF QUESTIONS	SAMPLE FINDINGS
	and delivery, radiology, surgical suites, and similar units? Is electronic mail used? Is web-based technology embraced?	their old ED. The new ED has state-of-the art equipment, as do the critical care units. The labor and delivery area is cramped and overcrowded. Equipment is well worn. Similarly, the surgical suites are dated. The radiology department is scheduled for a major capital investment next year.
Religious/philosophical	Does the institution have a religious affiliation? Are religious symbols displayed within the facility? By patients? By staff? Is the institution private or public? For-profit or not-for-profit?	Founded by a religious order, Hospital A is very clearly viewed as Roman Catholic. Outside, the hospital is marked with a large cross on its roof. Inside, a crucifix hangs in each patient room. A large chapel is used for daily mass. A chaplain distributes communion to patients and staff every evening. Nurses demonstrate a variety of religious symbols. One nurse is seen wearing a cross; another wears a Star of David. Patients adhere to a variety of faith traditions, including Southern Baptist and Black Muslim. Chaplains come from a variety of faith traditions and attempt to meet the needs of diverse groups.
Kinship and social factors	What are the working relationships within nursing? Between nursing and ancillary services? Between nursing and medicine? How closely are staff members aligned? Is the environment emotionally "warm" and close or "cold" and distant? How do employees relate to one another? Do they celebrate together? Turn to one another for support? Do employees get together outside of work?	RNs at Hospital A tend to be White and are often the children of immigrants. They are most often educated in associate degree or diploma programs. Aides tend to be African American. There is tension between the two groups especially as the role of the aide has expanded. Nurses tend to be somewhat in awe of physicians. Physicians' attitudes toward nurses range from respect to disrespect. Many physicians are angry about the erosion of their autonomy and economic security. Most units tend to be tight knit, with celebrations of monthly birthdays and recognition provided when staff members "go the extra mile." Nurses rarely socialize with one another outside of work. Staff nurses are middle-aged (mean age 45). Most of them commute from the suburbs to the hospital and are anxious to return home after their shift. On the other hand, many of the aides are from the immediate community, know each other, and socialize outside of work.

FACTOR	TYPES OF QUESTIONS	SAMPLE FINDINGS
Cultural values	Are values explicitly stated? What is valued within the institution? What is viewed as good? What is viewed as right? What is seen as truth?	The institution clearly identifies its mission and strives to fulfill it in economically difficult times. Its stated values are collaboration and diversity. Although diversity training has been provided to managers, tensions still exist between work groups, particularly because the work force tends to be racially divided.
Political/legal	How politically charged is the institution? Where does the power rest within the institution? With medicine? With finance? With nursing? With information technology? Is power shared? What types of legal actions have been taken against the institution? On behalf of the institution?	Historically, Hospital A has been politically naive. It has gone about its mission without regard to the external environment. Recently, the hospital has begun to lobby for better reimbursement for care provided under Medicaid. Institutional power rests with the strong medical staff and department chairs. Because the hospital houses its own diploma school of nursing, staff nurses are less likely to be BSN- and MSN-prepared.
Economic	What is the financial viability of the institution? Who makes the financial decisions? How do the salaries and benefits compare with those of competitors in the immediate environment?	Hospital A has a very low margin: 0.5%, compared with an industry standard of more than 2%. This means that little money is available for capital improvements, which results in less technology and some units being cramped. Community needs are considered, along with all financial decisions. People are valued, and efforts are made to keep salaries competitive. With the growing nursing shortage, starting salaries are increasing for new graduates and experienced nurses are complaining of salary compression.
Educational	How is education valued within the institution? What type of assistance (financial, scheduling, flexibility) is provided for staff seeking advanced degrees? Does the institution provide education for medicine, nursing, and other professions? Are advanced-practice nurses utilized? What is the educational background of staff nurses? Nurse managers? Nursing leaders? How does this compare with education of other professional groups? With competing organizations?	Nurses are most often educated at the diploma level. Although flexible scheduling and limited tuition reimbursement are provided, many nurses do not take advantage of the benefits because of the need to work extra shifts to ensure staffing and competing personal and family priorities. All new nurse managers are required to have a BSN; however, most existing managers are educated at the diploma level. New directors are required to have a master's degree and most have earned MBAs. Nursing students from five different programs rotate through the institution, with first priority given to the hospital's diploma program. In addition,

(table continues on page 232)

TABLE 9-2
Example of Leininger (1991) Culture Care Model Used to Conduct an Organizational Assessment in a Hypothetical Hospital (*continued*)

FACTOR	TYPES OF QUESTIONS	SAMPLE FINDINGS
		Hospital A has developed a relationship with one school of nursing and provides a summer preceptor program to those students. Faculty members are also employed during summers and holidays. Medical education is also provided at Hospital A: 150 residents and many third-year and fourth-year medical students rotate through the facility. The residents, while learning, also provide important service to the community, particularly through their clinic rotations. Students in respiratory, social work, dietitian, physical therapy, occupational therapy, speech therapy, and pastoral care also have clinical rotations at Hospital A.

agency or institution because services are delivered in a noncaring and patronizing fashion.

• Are the services appropriate? Community members may not use services if they do not perceive that these services meet their needs. For example, community members who struggle with day-to-day survival with limited financial and social resources may not use fitness classes. Programs that are disconnected from the daily life of community members constitute a recipe for failure.

Barriers to Creating Culturally Competent Health Care Organizations

Standards for providing culturally and linguistically appropriate health care services have been clearly articulated. Regulatory bodies, such as The Joint Commission, and certification groups, such as Magnet designation, require adherence to several mandates related to culturally competent health care organizations. Regardless, a variety of barriers exist.

Prejudice, racism, stereotyping, and ethnocentrism are present in all health care settings. The dominant subgroup is often ignorant of its own privilege. For example, services may be organized for the convenience of providers, and providers may be completely oblivious to the fact that inconvenient hours or locations are affecting the community members who seek services.

The identity of a group or organization is based on phenotype, culture, or any other characteristic that a group shares that sets it apart from others. The professional values espoused by nurses, for example, set us apart from other health care providers. Numerous boundaries exist in the health care professions; they may be based on gender, ethnic differences, class and hierarchy, licensure and certification, history, and tradition (Dreachslin, 1999).

Institutional racism may also exist in health care. The *MacPherson Report* (2001) defines **institutional racism** as "the collective failure of an organization to provide an appropriate and professional service to people because of their colour, culture or ethnic origin." In contrast with individual behaviors, institutional racism occurs when systematic policies and practices disadvantage certain racial or ethnic groups. Institutions may be overtly racist, as when they specifically exclude certain groups from service. More often, institutions are unintentionally racist. For example, a dress code that requires everyone to wear the same hat would institutionally discriminate against Sikh men, who are expected to wear turbans, and Muslim women, who wear the hijab or veil. Institutions don't necessarily adopt such policies with the intention of discriminating, and often revise their practice once the discrimination is pointed out.

This is an international concern. In Australia, for example, a government report in the 1990s identified that the exclusionary culture of the health care system was a major impediment to equity and access for people of non–English-speaking background. Health care providers tend to use their own cultural frameworks as the normative reference point and may view people of culturally and linguistically diverse backgrounds as a problem. Blackford (2003) found that a Melbourne, Australia, hospital was designed to deliver care to an Anglo-Saxon population rather than meeting the needs of the surrounding multicultural population. Blackford suggests that the interactions that occur between health professionals and non–English-speaking patients may result in systems of exclusions and repressions. For example, Blackford found that families were defined from an Anglo-Saxon perspective. This resulted in a physical environment that could not accommodate large family groups, policies that limited visitors to two at any time, and parental expectations that were culturally incongruent with non–Anglo-Saxon cultures.

In some cases, organizations may fail to correctly collect race and ethnicity data. Research conducted in California (Gomez, Le, West, Santariano, & O'Connor, 2003) suggests that while 85% reported consistently collecting data on race, approximately half of the hospitals obtained data on race by observing a patient's physical appearance. In addition, only 12% of the hospitals reported having a procedure for recording the race and/or

ethnicity of a patient with mixed ancestry, and 55% reported never collecting ethnicity data. According to a report from the Commonwealth Fund and the American Hospital Association's Health and Research Educational Trust (Hasnain-Wynia et al., 2004), fewer than 80% of hospitals collect data on race and ethnicity. Most often, data are collected because of a law or regulatory requirement. However, the information that is collected may not always accurate or valid. Frequently, the admitting clerk collects the data by asking questions of the patient and/or by observing patients. The report recommends that hospitals standardize who provides the information, when it is collected, which racial and ethnic categories should be used, and how the data are stored. Regenstein and Sickler (2006) also found that 78.4% of hospitals collect race information, 50.4% collect data on patient ethnicity, and 50.2% collect data on language preference. However, only 20% have formal data collection policies and fewer than 20% use the data to assess and compare care quality, health services utilization, health outcomes, or patient satisfaction.

The Institute of Medicine (2002) reports that 51% of providers believe that patients do not adhere to treatment because of culture or language. At the same time, nurses and other health care report having received no language or cultural competency training (Baldonado et al., 1998; Park et al., 2005). Many medical residents feel unprepared to treat patients who have religious beliefs that may affect treatment (20%), have LEP (22%), are new immigrants (25%), use complementary medicine (26%), or distrust the U.S. health system (28%) (Weissman et al., 2005). Similarly, while both nurses and baccalaureate nursing students perceive an overwhelming need for transcultural nursing, they report only 61% confidence in their ability to provide care to culturally diverse patients (Baldonado et al., 1998). Providing care to non-English-speaking patients is especially problematic.

Large health care organizations may have resources to secure trained professional interpreters and bilingual providers. Regardless of setting, however, Youdelman and Perkins (2005) suggest the following eight-step process for developing appropriate language services:

1. Designate responsibility
2. Conduct an analysis of language needs
3. Identify resources in the community
4. Determine what language services will be provided
5. Determine how to respond to LEP (limited English proficient) patients
6. Train staff
7. Notify LEP patients of available language services
8. Update activities after periodic review

The Physical Environment of Care

Organizational leaders must assess the physical environment of care to determine barriers and potentially negative messages. A flow chart is a helpful tool for determining such barriers. For example, in an effort to provide comprehensive women's health programs in a caring fashion, organizational leaders may examine the steps for admission to a particular hospital for the delivery of a baby. To determine this, staff members may walk through this care process at their site, and then create a flow chart that outlines the steps. Staff members may be alert, in particular, for possible sources of confusion for parents at this highly stressful time. The flow chart can then be used to design changes in the environment that can be implemented to decrease barriers and improve services.

The physical environment should also be assessed. Approaching this assessment as a potential client is helpful, and a variety of factors should be considered. What message does the organization send through its physical surroundings? How is the facility organized physically? How does the entryway present the culture of the organization to the public? Is the entrance warm and inviting?

Is the signage prominent? What languages are presented on signs? Is the patient at a loss for where to go to give or receive information? Are amenities available to patients and their family members? Are the doors open or closed? Do people talk with one another, and what language(s) are spoken? What is the traffic pattern, and what is the general flow of traffic? Does the environment appear calm or turbulent? Are the staff members attentive and courteous?

A physical environment may send unintentional messages. Several years ago, I visited a birthing unit in a city hospital. The hospital's service area was undergoing tremendous changes, with a large influx from African American, Hispanic, Indian, and Polish American communities. The birthing unit was beautifully and tastefully decorated with oak furniture and pastel prints. Every picture on the walls, however, showed a Caucasian family. This clearly sent a message of exclusivity rather inclusiveness. When I brought this to the attention of the nurse manager, she was completely dumbfounded and quickly took steps to rectify the situation. Ethnocentrism and stereotyping were in play here, but it took an outsider to identify this and bring it to recognition and resolution.

Community Context

Understanding what culturally competent health care means from the standpoint of patients is an important first step in building culturally competent organizations. Researchers (Napoles-Springer, Santoyo, Houston, Perez-Stable, & Stewart, 2005) conducted 19 community focus groups to determine the meaning of culture and what cultural factors influenced the quality of their medical visits. Culture was defined in terms of value systems, customs, self-identified ethnicity, and nationality. African Americans, Latinos, and non-Latino Whites all agreed that the quality of health care encounter was influenced by clinicians' sensitivity to complementary/alternative medicine, health-insurance discrimination, social class discrimination, ethnic concordance between patient and provider, and age-based discrimination. Ethnicity-based discrimination was identified as a factor for Latinos and African Americans. Latinos also described language issues and immigration status factors. Overall, participants indicated greater satisfaction with clinicians who demonstrated cultural flexibility, defined as the ability to elicit, adapt, and respond to patients' cultural characteristics.

Health care institutions exist to provide care. A variety of factors, summarized in Box 9-8, contribute to mortality in the United States and Canada. Confronting these factors will require individual behavioral change, community change, social change, and economic change. Health care organizations cannot confront these complex factors in isolation but must partner with their communities to build trust in their institutions and meet the needs of their local communities.

Community partnerships may be configured in a variety of ways. Hospitals and health care systems usually articulate their desire to improve the health of the communities they serve. Historically, hospitals have fulfilled this mission through charity care, health care provider education, research in health care, community education programming, and community outreach

---

BOX 9-8

Major Contributors to Mortality in the United States and Canada

Tobacco use
Alcohol
Poor diet and physical inactivity
Microbial agents
Toxins
Firearms
Sexual behaviors
Motor vehicle accidents
Illicit drug use
Poverty
Lack of access to medical care

(Pelfrey & Theisen, 1993). Recognition is growing that true improvements in the health of a community require the focused efforts of the entire community. Such improvement may occur only in partnerships with community members and other community organizations.

An ethnographic study of community (Davis, 1997) revealed five themes related to the experience of community caring. Of particular significance to this chapter are three themes: (1) reciprocal relationships and teams working together are central to building **healthy communities**; (2) education with a focus on prevention is key to enhancing health; and (3) understanding community needs is a primary catalyst for health care reform and change. The healthy communities program, with partnerships between communities and hospitals, is one example of this trend in health care. In a healthy communities program, health care professionals collaborate with surrounding communities to conduct community health assessments. In community mapping, staff collect a variety of data, including demographics, health status, community resources, barriers, and enablers. Both strengths and needs are identified from the perspective of the community. All these data are then used collaboratively with communities to set priorities. An example of such a community assessment is provided in Box 9-9. Data from these assessments are used to set priorities and guide the planning and implementation of key initiatives. These initiatives are most well accepted when they are sponsored by a variety of community organizations rather than by a single health care organization such as a hospital.

Focus groups may assist an organization in assessing how well they are meeting the needs of the populations they serve. For example, the Boston Pain Education Program worked collaboratively with community representatives to develop a culturally sensitive, linguistically appropriate cancer pain education booklet in 11 languages and for 11 ethnic groups. Focus groups were used to develop materials that would empower

---

BOX 9-9

Community Assessment Example

By using the assessment of the communities served by Advocate Lutheran General Hospital and by analyzing data from clinical practice, staff members realized that Hispanics made up an increasing proportion of the population and were the most frequently underserved population. As a result, a family practice physician initiated the idea for a community center for health and empowerment. A coalition composed of individuals from social services, health care agencies, schools, police, churches, businesses, city government, and other community services also identified the Hispanic community as underserved. This group provided an etic, or outsider, view of the Hispanic community.

To provide a local, or emic (insider), view, community members worked with health care personnel to design and conduct a door-to-door community assessment. As described elsewhere (Ludwig-Beymer, Blankemeier, Casas-Byots, & Suarez-Balcazar, 1996), Leininger's Theory of Cultural Diversity and Universality served to guide the assessment. The assessment process involved 2 focus groups, 15 community interviewers, and 220 door-to-door interviews. In addition, 5 meetings, attended by 180 community members, were held to report the findings to community members and solicit their input on how to maintain strengths and address needs. As a result, numerous task forces were formed to preserve strengths or mediate needs.

Major strengths were identified as access to friends and families to socialize and get support, prenatal and postnatal care, and pediatric care. Major needs were identified as affordable housing, programs to help immigrants, Spanish-speaking dentists, and activities for youth.

The community was involved in key decision making from the beginning, including selecting the site for the center, choosing the name for the center, and establishing a sliding scale for fees. The bilingual center provides primary health care services, a Women–Infant–Children program run by the county health department, and a community empowerment program. A salaried community outreach worker coordinates the community empowerment program. In collaboration with businesses, churches, and city services, community members have undergone training in group work and priority setting. Monthly dental services through a dental van were added at the center.

Activities for youth were identified as concerns in the community assessment. As a result, community members and center personnel have actively partnered with the park district, schools, churches, and the police to provide recreational activities for youth. The community also uses this as an opportunity to celebrate their cultural heritage. Health promotion materials and activities are also provided through collaboration.

---

patients and families to more effectively partner with health care professionals and mange pain in culturally competent ways (Lasch et al., 2000). To ensure valid focus group results, the organization must understand racial identity development theory, models of communication style differences, cultural archetypes, and ethnic markers (Dreachslin, 1998).

Community-based participatory research or **participatory action research** is a research strategy for understanding a community and developing health improvement initiatives with community members. The method uses collaborative, participatory approaches to develop

sustainable services (Koch & Kralik, 2006). Increasingly, such research is being funded. For example, the National Canter on Minority Health and Health Disparities (NCMHD), located within the National Institutes of Health, has funded disease intervention research in reducing and eliminating health disparities using community-based participation research that is jointly conducted by health disparity communities and researchers (NIH, 2010).

Conducting community assessments requires cultural awareness and sensitivity. Interpreting the data requires knowledge of the cultural dimensions of health and illness. Using the data to develop and implement programs in conjunction with the community requires the ability to plan and implement culturally competent care. The skill of a transcultural nurse or other culturally competent health care professional is invaluable in these situations.

Developing Culturally Competent Initiatives

Once the elements, outlined above, are in place, it is possible to develop culturally competent initiatives. Many important factors must be considered in planning programs across cultural groups. Before a program is planned, a cultural assessment of the target population should be a routine component of the needs assessment process (Huff & Kline, 1999). In many cases, cultural competence must be demonstrated with multiple cultures simultaneously. For example, one hospital in the Chicago area provides care for individuals who speak 64 different languages. This calls for much effort and creativity on the part of patients, health care providers, and interpreters. Culturally competent initiatives must reach out to multiple cultural groups. Case Study 9-1 describes the development and implementation of a culturally competent initiative.

This case study focuses on one culturally competent program provided to a community. Additional programs, targeting the needs of other age groups, may also be envisioned. For example, adult immunizations are also an issue for many communities, so a program might be developed that focuses specifically on older adults and their immunization needs. Similarly, programs might be instituted to deal with other health issues of concern to community members. The case study demonstrates the importance of incorporating an understanding of culture in every aspect of an initiative. To design and implement an effective program, the cultural values of patients must be understood and addressed.

CASE STUDY 9-1

Caring Hospital is a not-for-profit hospital serves clients who differ in multiple ways, including socioeconomic status, education, race, ethnicity, religion, language, and culture. Organizational leaders embrace Leininger's Theory of Culture Care. In particular, nursing leaders believe that nursing care must be congruent with the client's culture if nursing intends to promote the client's health and satisfaction.

Through a healthy community program, the hospital remains grounded in the reality of their clients. The healthy community program, developed and staffed by two nurses with community health backgrounds, is responsible for broadly defining community-based health promotion initiatives that address individual, social, and community factors. Their goal is to establish partnerships with community members and governmental and community organizations to ensure that everyone has access to the basics needed for health; that the physical environment supports healthy living; and that communities control, define, and direct action for health.

The nurses in the healthy community program bring together resources from settings both within and outside their hospital. For example, they work closely with other community-focused staff members, such as home care and parish nurses. They also work with multiple external organizations, such as local health departments and other government agencies, religious institutions, community businesses, schools, and other health care entities. These nurses work specifically with the communities surrounding their facility. In this way, they acknowledge the specific needs of diverse groups.

The healthy community nurses use Leininger's Culture Care Diversity and Universality model in their practice. They use data gathered from cultural assessments to assist them in understanding the communities they serve. They consider environmental context, ethnohistory, language, kinship, culture values and lifeways, the political and legal system, and technologic, economic, religious, philosophic, and educational factors. They understand the interactions among the folk system, nursing care, and the professional systems. They also understand the importance of using the three culture care modalities: preservation/maintenance, accommodation/negotiation, and repatterning/restructuring.

Because of their community health backgrounds, the nurses are knowledgeable about disparities in health. The nurses use data from a variety of sources, including hospital-specific data, census tract data, and health department data, to help them understand health and access disparities in their area. They also talk to community members and to health care providers to identify competing priorities. Using these processes, they discover that their communities have not achieved the Healthy People 2010 goal of 90% full immunization for children by the age of two years.

To address the lack of immunizations, the nurses acknowledge that the issues that affect immunizations are multifaceted. The immunization schedule changes frequently and is quite complex. Even health care providers have difficulty interpreting it. Communication with parents has been sketchy and has been complicated by controversy. Immunizations may not be seen by parents as essential for young children until they enter elementary school. Immunizations may not be easily accessible, available, and affordable. Parents may make decisions based on misinformation, rumor, or hearsay. The nurses know, however, that community members want to keep their children healthy and that immunizations have contributed greatly to reduced illness in individuals and better overall health for the community. They also know that community members prefer to have their children immunized in a consistent place, as part of an overall medical home.

Because the childhood immunization levels are suboptimal in the communities served by the hospital, childhood immunization is selected as a quality initiative. A group of consumers and clinicians is convened to implement a program with the goal of increasing immunization to the Healthy People 2010 goal of 90%. There is much discussion on the best way for increasing immunization rates, using a broad-based program. Both telephoned and mailed reminders are known to be effective in increasing immunizations in adults and children (Szilagyi et al., 2000). Because telephoned reminders are substantially more expensive than mailed reminders, the group opts to use mailed reminders.

Various materials are developed in both English and Spanish, and incentives are put into place to assist parents. Babies are automatically enrolled in the program when they are born in the hospital. Mailings occur at regular intervals and include a personalized letter indicating what vaccines are due, a vaccine record, vaccine information statements, and a growth and development newsletter. Additionally, incentives are mailed to help keep the parents motivated to use preventive services. Materials are written at a sixth-grade level. All materials are reviewed for cultural congruity, and the illustrations include babies from various ethnic groups.

New materials are developed as needed, based on a continuous assessment of the needs of the parents. For example, reproducing all the materials in all the languages used by patients is too expensive, so a multiple-language brochure is developed in the 11 most common languages. The brochure explains the program and asks that non–English-speaking and non–Spanish-speaking families obtain help in translating the materials. In addition, after families express a major concern about the multiple injections required to keep their babies fully immunized and their babies' resultant distress and crying, a "calming strategies" flyer is developed.

Because financial barriers still exist among parents seeking immunizations for their children, the healthy community nurses implement several additional strategies. First, they work with physicians and help them enroll in the Vaccines for Children program, making vaccines available at no cost or low cost right in their offices. They also work with the staff in physicians' offices to enhance their role in fostering childhood immunizations. In addition, they work with the health department to provide monthly immunizations on site at the hospital.

The Role of Individual Health Care Providers in Creating Culturally Competent Organizations

All of us play a role in creating culturally competent organizations. Individual health care providers are at the core of helping an institution attain cultural competence. If they listen and attend carefully, health care providers have a valuable window directly into the world of their patients. They can take what they learn and escalate it as needed to improve the cultural responsiveness of their organization. Speaking the language can also be an advantage.

When health care providers fail to take the patient's culture seriously, they misinterpret the patient's value system and, by doing so, elevate their own value systems. This posture is culturally destructive because it minimizes the other person's culture. A better approach is to take time to ask questions about what the patient prefers and to listen attentively. In the end, this will increase understanding, trust, collaboration, adherence, and satisfaction.

Even when serving a diverse patient base, health care providers can make a difference. Individuals and groups of clinicians can develop special programs to meet the needs of the specific populations they serve. For example, in our interfaith chapel, prayer materials are available from many faith traditions.

SUMMARY

As with individuals, the quest for organizational cultural competence is a lifetime journey. There is always room for improvement. To be truly effective in improving patient care for all, health care services and social services that take cultural diversity into account must make an organizational commitment to cultural competence. Cultural competence cannot live in one or two nurses; it must be systemic. It must involve all layers of the organization: the policy making level, the administrative level, the management level, and the provider level. In addition, an organization must have a mutually beneficial relationship with the community it serves to achieve cultural competence. As such, organizations must reach out to community members.

REVIEW QUESTIONS

1. What types of access, health care and health outcome disparities exist in the United States?
2. How does the culture of an organization affect the quality of care provided?
3. What tools or models are helpful for assessing organizational culture?
4. How does an organization's culture influence or affect its employees?

CRITICAL THINKING ACTIVITIES

1. An excellent way to understand a culturally competent organization is to assess the organizational culture using the "five A's" described in this chapter. With some of your classmates, compare and contrast the availability, accessibility, affordability, acceptability, and appropriateness of the organization. Discuss what actions could be taken by the organization to increase its cultural competency.

2. Then, use a different approach to assess the cultural competency of the same organization. Use Leininger's (1991) Theory of Culture Care Diversity and Universality to assess the culture of the organization. Table 9-2 in this chapter provides an example of how Leininger's Culture Care Model can be used. Compare and contrast the values and beliefs of the organization with the values and beliefs of the groups using the

health care organization's services. What areas would be most problematic, and why?

3. Many members of ethnic or minority communities lack adequate access to care because they do not have adequate health insurance. Often, these individuals use the emergency departments (EDs) of city hospitals for episodic care. Visit a busy ED. What types of patients do you see? Assess the physical environment to determine potential barriers to culturally competent care. Develop a flow chart that outlines the steps a patient takes when he or she seeks care in an emergency room. Identify the changes that would decrease barriers and improve services if they were implemented.

REFERENCES

Agency for Healthcare Research and Quality. (2008a). *National healthcare disparities report, 2008*. Rockville, MD: U.S. Department of Health and Human Services, Agency for Healthcare Research and Quality. Retrieve from http://www.ahrq.gov

Agency for Healthcare Research and Quality. (2008b). *Disparities in health care quality among racial and ethnic minority groups*. Findings from the National Healthcare Disparities Report, 2008. Rockville, MD: U.S. Department of Health and Human Services, Agency for Healthcare Research and Quality. Accessed February 14, 2010 at http://www.ahrq.gov

Alessandra, T. (2010). *The platinum rule*. Accessed February 21, 2010 at http://www.alessandra.com

American Nurses Association. (2001). *Code of ethics for nurses with interpretive statements*. Washington DC: American Nurses Association.

American Nurses Association Council on Cultural Diversity in Nursing Practice. (1991). Cultural diversity in nursing practice [position statement]. Washington DC.

American Nurses Credentialing Center. (2008). *Magnet recognition program. Recognizing excellence in nursing service*. Application manual. Silver Spring, MD: American Nurses Credentialing Center.

American Organization of Nurse Executives. (February 2005). AONE Nurse Executive Competencies. *Nurse Leader, 3*(1), 50–56.

Andrews, M. M. (October 1998). A model for cultural change. *Nursing Management, 66*, 62–64.

Baldonado, A., Ludwig-Beymer, P., Barnes, K., Starsiak, D., Nemivant, E. B. & Anonas-Ternate, A. (1998). Transcultural nursing practice described by registered nurses and baccalaureate nursing students. *Journal of Transcultural Nursing, 9*(2), 15–25.

Bally, J. M. G. (2007). The role of nursing leadership in creating a mentoring culture in acute care environments. *Nursing Economics, 25*(3), 143–149.

Betancourt, J. R., Green, A. R., Carrillo, J. E., & Park, E. R. (2005). Cultural competence and health care disparities: Key perspectives and trends. *Health Affairs, 24*(2), 499–505.

Blackford, J. (2003). Cultural frameworks of nursing practice: Exposing an exclusionary healthcare culture. *Nursing Inquiry, 10*(4), 236–244.

Bolman, L. G., & Deal, T. E. (1997). *Reframing organizations: Artistry, choice, and leadership* (2nd ed.). San Francisco: Jossey-Bass.

Carney, M. (2006). Understanding organizational culture: The key to successful middle manager strategic involvement in health care delivery? *Journal of Nursing Management, 14*, 23–33.

Casida, J. (2008). Linking nursing unit's culture to organizational effectiveness: A Measurement tool. *Nursing Economics, 26*(2), 106–110.

Casida, J., & Pinto-Zipp, G. (2008). Leadership-organizational vulture relationship in nursing units of acute care hospitals. *Nursing Economics, 26*(1), 7–15.

Centers for Disease Control and Prevention National Vital Statistics System. (2009). Deaths: Preliminary data for 2007. *National Vital Statistics Reports, 58*(1), 1–52.

Chavez, C. I., & Weisinger, J. Y. (2008). Beyond diversity training: A social infusion for cultural inclusion. *Human Resource Management, 47*(2), 331–350.

Clancy, C. M., & Stryer, D. B. (2001). Racial and ethnic disparities and primary care experience. *Health Services Research, 36*(6), 979–986.

Cox, T. (1994). *Cultural diversity in organizations*. San Francisco, CA: Berrett-Koehler.

Dansky, K. H., Weech-Maldonado, R., De Souza, G., & Dreachslin, J. L. (2003). Organizational strategy and diversity management: Diversity-sensitive orientation as a moderating influence. *Health Care Management Review, 28*(3), 243–253.

Davis, R. N. (1997). Community caring: An ethnographic study within an organizational culture. *Public Health Nursing, 14*(2), 92–100.

Dekker, S. (2007). *Just culture, balancing safety and accountability*. Burlington, VT: Ashgate.

Dreachslin, J. L. (1996). *Diversity leadership*. Chicago, IL: Health Administration Press.

Dreachslin, J. L. (1998). Conducting effective focus groups in the context of diversity: Theoretical underpinnings and practical implications. *Qualitative Health Research, 8*(6), 813–820.

Dreachslin, J. L. (1999). Diversity leadership. *Journal of Nursing Administration, 29*(6), 3–4, 21.

Flaskerud, J. H. (2007). Cultural competence: What effect on reducing health disparities? *Issues in Mental Health Nursing, 28*, 431–434.

Gibson-Jones, T. (2009). Perceived work and family conflict among African-American nurses in college. *Journal of Transcultural Nursing, 20*(3), 304–312.

Gomez, S. L., Le, G. M., West, D. W., Santariano, W. A. & O'Connor, L. (2003). Hospital policy and practice regarding the collection of data on race, ethnicity, and birthplace. *Journal of Public Health, 93*(10), 1685–1688.

Greiner, A. C., & Knebel, E. (Eds.), Institute of Medicine. (2003). *Health professionals education: A bridge to quality.* Washington DC: The National Academies Press.

Hasnain-Wynia, R., Pierce, D., & Pittman, M. A. (May, 2004). *Who, when, and how: The current state of race, ethnicity, and primary language data collection in hospitals.* The Commonwealth Fund and the American Hospital Association's Health Research and Educational Trust. Accessed February 20, 2006 at http://www.cmwf.org

Huff, R. M., & Kline, M. V. (1999). The cultural assessment framework. In *Promoting health in multicultural populations: A handbook for practitioners.* Thousand Oaks, CA: Sage Publications.

Institute of Medicine. (2002). *Unequal treatment: Confronting racial and ethnic disparities in health care.* Washington DC: National Academies Press.

Joint Commission. (January 2010). *The Joint Commission Perspectives,* 5–6.

Joint Commission Resources. (2010). *Comprehensive accreditation manual for hospitals.* http://amp.jcrinc.com. Accessed February 22, 2010.

Kane-Urrabazo, C. (2006). Management's role in shaping organizational culture. *Journal of Nursing Management, 14,* 188–194.

Khatri, N., Brown, G. D., & Hicks, L. L. (2009). From a blame culture to a just culture in health care. *Health Management and Informatics, 34*(4), 312–322.

Koch, T., & Kralik, D. (2006). *Participatory action research in health care.* Wiley-Blackwell.

Lasch, K. E., Wilkes, G., Montuori, L. M., Chew, P., Leonard, C., & Hilton, S. (2000). Using focus group methods to develop multicultural cancer pain education materials. *Pain Management Nursing, 1*(4), 129–138.

Leininger, M. (1991). *Culture care diversity and universality: A theory of nursing care.* New York: National League for Nursing Press.

Leininger, M. (1996). Founder's focus: Transcultural nursing administration: An imperative worldwide. *Journal of Transcultural Nursing, 8*(1), 28–33.

Ludwig-Beymer, P., Blankemeier, J. R., Casas-Byots, C., & Suarez-Balcazar, Y. (1996). Community assessment in a suburban Hispanic community: A description of methods. *Journal of Transcultural Nursing, 8*(1), 19–27.

MacPherson Report. (2001). http://news:bbc.co/uk/vote2001. Accessed December 29, 2006.

Mallidou, A. A. (2004). *The impact of hospital nurse specialty subcultures on nurse and patient outcomes.* University of Alberta, Canada: Doctoral Dissertation.

Malone, B. L. (1997). Improving organizational cultural competence. In J. A. Dienemann (Ed.). *Cultural diversity in nursing: Issues, strategies, and outcomes.* Washington, DC: American Academy of Nursing.

Marchionni, C., & Ritchie, J. (2007). Organizational factors that support the implementation of a nursing best practice guidelines. *Journal of Nursing Management, 16,* 266–274.

McClure, M. L., Poulin, M. A., Sovie, M. D., & Wandelt, M. A. for the American Academy Task Force on Nursing Practice in Hospitals. (1983). *Magnet hospitals. Attraction and retention of professional nurses.* Kansas City, MO: American Nurses Association.

Momeni, N. (2009). The relationship between managers' emotional intelligence and the organizational climate they create. *Public Personnel Management, 38*(2), 35–48.

Napoles-Springer, A. M., Santoyo, J., Houston, K., Perez-Stable, E. J., & Stewart, A. L. (2005). Patients' perceptions of cultural factors affecting the quality of their medical encounters. *Health Expectations, 8,* 4–17.

National Institutes of Health (2010). Accessed February 21, 2010 at http://www.nih.gov.

Office of Minority Health, Department of Health and Human Services. (March 2001). *National standards for culturally and linguistically appropriate services in health care final report.* Washington DC.

O'Hagan, J., & Persaud, D. (2009). Creating a culture of accountability in health care. *Health Care Manager, 28*(2), 124–133.

Park, E. R., Betancourts, J. R., Kim, M. K., Maina, A. W., Blumenthal, D., & Weissman, J. S. (2005). Mixed messages: Residents' experiences learning cross-cultural care. *Academic Medicine, 80*(9), 874–880.

Pelfrey, S., & Theisen, B. A. (1993). Valuing the community benefits provided by nonprofit hospitals. *The Journal of Nursing Administration, 23*(6), 16–21.

Regenstein, M., & Sickler, D. (2006). *Race, ethnicity, and language of patients.* The National Public Health and Hospital Institute. Accessed February 21, 2010 at http://www.naph.org

Roizner, M. (1996). *A practical guide for the assessment of cultural competence in children's mental health organizations.* Boston: Judge Baker's Children's Center.

Schaffner, J. W., & Ludwig-Beymer, P. (2003). *Rx for the nursing shortage.* Chicago, IL: Health Administration Press.

Schein, E. H. (2004). *Organizational culture and leadership* (3rd ed.). San Francisco: Jossey-Bass.

Scott-Findlay, S. D. (2006). *The Roles of Culture and Context in Nurses' Research Utilization.* Unpublished dissertation, University of Alberta.

Scott-Findlay, S., & Estabrooks, C. A. (2006). *Mapping the organizational culture research in nursing: A literature review.* Journal of Advanced Nursing, 56(5), 498–513.

Seren, S., & Baykal, U. (Second Quarter 2007). Relationships between change and organizational culture in hospitals. *Journal of Nursing Scholarship, 39,* 191–197.

Singer, S. J., Falwell, A., Gaba, D. M., Meterko, M., Rosen, A., Hartmann, C. W., & Baker, L. (2009). Identifying organizational cultures the promote patient safety. *Health Care Management Review, 34*(3), 300–311.

Sorra, J., Famolaro, T., Dyer, N., Nelson, D., & Khanna, K. (2008). *Hospital survey of patient safety culture: 2008 comparative database report.* AHRQ Publication Number 08-0039, Rockville, MD.

Strasser, D. C., Smits, S. J., Falconer, J. A., Herrin, J. S., & Bowen, S. E. (2002). The influence of hospital culture on rehabilitation team functioning in VA hospitals. *Journal of Rehabilitation Research and Development, 39*(1), 115–125.

Szilagyi, P. G., Bordley, C., Vann, J. C., Chelminski, A., Kraus, R. M., Margolis, P. A., & Rodewald, L. E. (2000). Effect of patient reminder/recall interventions on immunization rates. *Journal of American Medical Association, 284*(14), 1820–1827.

U.S. Department of Health and Human Services. (2000). *Healthy People 2010.* Washington, DC: DHHS.

Weissman, J. S., Betancourt, J. R., Campbell, E. G., Park, E. R., Kim, M., Clarridge, B., ..., Maina, A. W. (2005). Resident physicians' preparedness to provide cross-cultural care. *Journal of the American Medical Association, 294*(9), 1058–1067.

Youdelman, M., & Perkins, J. (2005). *Providing language services in small health care provider settings: Examples from the field.* The Commonwealth Fund. Accessed October 17, 2005 at http://www.cmwf.org

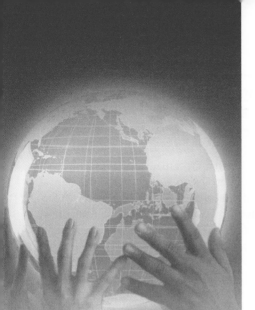

Transcultural Perspectives in Mental Health Nursing

Joanne T. Ehrmin

KEY TERMS

Acculturation
Cultural blindness
Cultural blind spot
Cultural competence
Culturally congruent care
Cultural norms
Cultural pain
Cultural values, beliefs, or practices
Culture-bound syndromes
    (folk illnesses, culture-specific
    illnesses, culture-specific
    syndromes)
Culture shock
Diversity
Ethnocentrism
Historical Unresolved Grief
    (Historical Trauma,
    American Indian Holocaust,
    Disenfranchised Grieving)
Illness/disease
Interpersonal communication
Mental health
Mental illness
Stereotyping

LEARNING OBJECTIVES

1. Evaluate the importance of cultural patterns of values, beliefs, and practices when planning and implementing nursing care.
2. Examine common facilitators and barriers encountered in caring for culturally diverse patients with mental health disorders.
3. Analyze the influence of culture on decisions about mental health care.
4. Assess strategies to provide competent transcultural mental health nursing care.
5. Understand the importance of evidence-based transcultural mental health nursing research to improve mental health care.

Mental health and mental illness have been described as two different positions on a continuum with "mental health problems," in between the two end positions. A mental health problem may be "feeling down" about a stressful job and many of us can relate to that situation. On the other hand, at the one extreme end of the continuum are debilitating mental illnesses such as schizophrenia and bipolar disorders. "Left untreated, these disorders erase any doubt as to their devastating potential" (p. 1). The prior statements were retrieved from *A Supplement to Mental Health: A Report of the Surgeon General: Cul-*

ture, Race, and Ethnicity (2001). This landmark document brought a focus to mental health and culture, race, and ethnicity for the first time in such an obvious and distinct manner (Manson, 2003).

This chapter will examine mental illnesses within a transcultural nursing perspective and will assist the reader in understanding how culture influences the way in which we interpret and behave with mental illnesses. The goal of this chapter is to help nurses gain the necessary knowledge and skills to improve the mental health and well-being of patients from all cultural backgrounds. As culture strongly influences how patients experience illness, and culture is the framework for the interpretation of that experience, transcultural mental health nursing knowledge is integral for culturally competent mental health care.

The concept of **cultural norms** is relevant to transcultural mental health nursing, as one's culture shapes what is considered normal and, by default, what is considered abnormal. Cultural norms are patterns, values, meanings, expressions, beliefs, practices, and experiences that are typical of specific cultural groups. Such norms are learned and passed down by family, friends, communities, and other members of the cultural group. Given the broad influence of culture, culture and mental health care are described as intricately related and dependent on one another. In fact, there is growing evidence that culture has a major influence on the expression of mental illness, particularly on depressive disorders for culturally diverse populations (Nicholas et al., 2007).

The distinction between **illness** and **disease** is relevant to mental health nursing care. Disease comes out of the medical model, is objective, physiologically based, and requires a "cure," whereas illness is subjective, comes from the perspective of the patient, is culturally based and requires "care." Interestingly, disease can occur without illness and illness can also occur without disease.

Defining Mental Health Within a Transcultural Nursing Perspective

The World Health Organization (WHO) (2007) proposed: "There is no health without mental health" and the influential organization incorporated mental well-being in their definition of health. According to WHO, "Health is a state of complete physical, mental and social well-being and not merely the absence of disease or infirmity" (p. 1). WHO further specified that **mental health** is "a state of well-being in which the individual realizes his or her own abilities, can cope with the normal stresses of life, can work productively and fruitfully, and is able to make a contribution to his or her community" (p. 1), and that this understanding of mental health can be interpreted "across cultures" (p. 1). For example, in the *Rural Healthy People 2010 Report*, survey results of state and local rural leaders indicated that mental health and mental disorders are the fourth most often identified rural health priority (Gamm & Hutchison, 2003). Taking into consideration the WHO definition of mental health, a definition of mental illness would then include one or more of the following: a lack of a sense of well-being in which the individual does not realize his or her own disabilities, is not able to cope with the normal stresses of life, is not able to work productively and fruitfully, and is not able to make a contribution to his or her community. It is important to remember there is a continuum of mental health on one end and mental illness on the extreme other end. An individual can fall on one end of the continuum or the other, or anywhere in between. Individuals' and communities' cultural beliefs and values about mental health and mental illness can influence one's placement on the continuum, as well.

It is a daunting task to know all there is to know about each cultural group that mental health nurses care for in their daily practice. Leininger (1991; Leininger & McFarland, 2002) in *Culture*

Care Diversity and Universality: A Theory of Nursing, theorized the importance of identifying what is common and universal among cultures, while at the same time understanding there is individual diversity within cultures. **Diversity** for transcultural mental health nurses would encompass not only culture and ethnicity, but also gender, sexual orientation, socioeconomic status, age, physical abilities or disabilities, religious beliefs, and political beliefs or other ideologies. Figure 10-1 shows a transcultural nurse working on promoting health and well-being with a patient from a culture different from her own.

In this chapter on Transcultural Perspectives in Mental Health Nursing, patterns of values, beliefs, and practices for mental health care are presented and can be used as one "tool" in caring for patients, families, and communities from diverse cultural groups. This is different from simplistic overgeneralizations that can lead to stereotyping

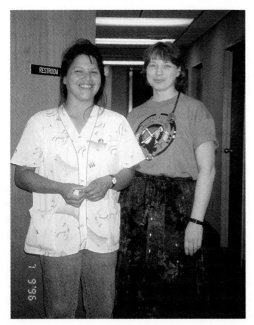

FIGURE 10-1 Transcultural nurses bring together sensitivity, knowledge and skill to promote health and care for the mentally ill in culturally competent ways.

a particular culture. Stereotyping can also lead to erroneous misrepresentations of mental health for multiculturally diverse patients. Stereotypes can be used as an underlying rationale to distort mental illness symptoms and misdiagnose multiculturally diverse individuals, families, and communities. Stereotypes can serve to exploit culturally diverse patients, particularly in the area of mental health care, where differences in group norms can sometimes be used to inappropriately label patients with a mental health diagnosis. It is not the intent of this chapter to reduce cultural groups to a limiting set of characteristics, but to identify cultural patterns and norms that can be used to assist the mental health nurse in caring for culturally diverse patients with mental health needs.

Transcultural nurses do not promote **stereotyping** of patients, families, and communities because of unique characteristics. Stereotyping labels people and is a form of prejudice that is damaging and harmful to any recipient, let alone a patient with a mental illness! Furthermore, stereotyping is generally inaccurate and is often based more on the individual expressing the stereotypical view than the cultural group being targeted. Stereotyping identifies a cultural group or members of that culture as identical and indistinguishable from each other. Some examples of common stereotyping are beliefs that African Americans are "better at sports" and "dancing" than other cultural groups. Other examples of stereotypes are that Irish Americans are "quick tempered," or Turkish women are "belly dancers." Identifying people as all looking the same or thinking the same is stereotyping. Transcultural mental health nursing does not promote applying a stereotypical "cookbook" approach to mental health care. One other concept that is important to consider in transcultural mental health nursing is ethnocentrism. In its mildest form, **ethnocentrism** presents as subconscious disregard for cultural differences; in its most severe form, it presents as authoritarian" (Sutherland, 2002, p. 280). Ethnocentrism can manifest as feelings of superiority or discrimination with respect to one's own group or culture over another group or culture. For example, ethnocentrism can manifest as a belief that one's own religious beliefs are superior to another group or culture's religious beliefs. One's own health care beliefs and practices are superior to another culture's health care beliefs and practices. U.S.-educated health care professionals are frequently guilty of the latter ethnocentric assumption.

Many cultural groups have distinct patterns of values, beliefs, and practices that can be used as a basis for providing mental health care in a culturally congruent and competent manner. However, many individuals and families belonging to specific cultural groups may have more diverse mental health care needs than those of the cultural group norm. The term "norm" is used to identify patterns of values, beliefs, and practices specific to mental health that have been identified through research and caring for culturally diverse patients, families, and communities.

Population Trends and Mental Health

The U.S. population is projected to increase in age and cultural diversity as we move toward the middle of the century. Given the increasing numbers of elderly in the United States, it is important to understand trends in utilization of mental health care services for older populations of all cultures. Day (1996) in a report developed for The U.S. Bureau of the Census predicts that by 2030, approximately 20% of the total population will be over 65 and those 85 and older will increase fivefold by 2050. By mid-century, African Americans will double in number. Those individuals of Hispanic origin, Asian, and Pacific Islander populations will have the highest rates of increase. By 2030, the non-Hispanic "White" population will be less than 50% of the population under age 18. However, in that same year, this group will comprise 75% of the population aged 65 and over. Native Americans (American Indians and Alaska Natives) will have the lowest number of those aged 65 and older. However,

there is evidence of underutilization of mental health services by many minority groups. Community education and outreach programs are needed to increase mental health service utilization in older ethnic minority populations (Jang, Kim, Hansen, & Chiriboga, 2007). Although mental health nurses care for clients of all age groups and all cultural groups, the current and future trends in population projections do have major implications for transcultural nursing and mental health services in the United States.

According to Kessler, Chiu, Demler and Walters (2005) approximately 26.2% of Americans 18 years old and older, or 1 in 4 adults, suffer each year from a mental disorder that is defined in the *Diagnostic and Statistical Manual*, 4th edition (DSM-IV) of the American Psychiatric Association (APA) mental disorders. Of those cases, more than one-third are mild. However, approximately 6%, or 1 in 17 individuals suffer from a "serious mental illness," including suicide, mental or substance abuse, nonaffective psychosis, bipolar I or II disorder, or acts of violence.

The institutionalized view of mental health care as portrayed in the movie "One Flew Over the Cuckoo's Nest" (1975) is no longer the norm for care today. Increasingly, mental health care is moving from state and general "mental" hospitals to community-based service centers. The U.S. Department of Health and Human Services' Center for Mental Health Services (CMHS) is the Federal agency within the U.S. Substance Abuse and Mental Health Services Administration (SAMHSA) charged with improving prevention and mental health treatment services in the United States. For 2008, CMHS statistics for utilization of community-based mental health treatment was 19.15%, as compared to treatment in state hospitals and other psychiatric inpatient settings just over 2%. So, not only is the cultural diversity of mental health patients increasing, but also the trends to community-based mental health treatment centers. These statistics can help to guide the direction nursing will take in meeting the needs of mental health patients.

Role of Consumers in Decision Making and Mental Health Care in Relation to Evidence-Based Practice

Consumers of mental health care (patients, families, and communities) are more knowledgeable now than they have ever been in the past. With the advent of the Internet, mental health care information is more widely available to those seeking knowledge. Continuous news broadcasts offer health care information to both consumers and professionals alike. National and international news and research breakthroughs are increasingly available to consumers, almost as soon as they are available to professionals. In addition, our society is more open to talking about depression and bipolar conditions in ways that would have been unthinkable just two decades ago.

Consumers want an active role in the decision making about their own mental health care and they use numerous resources to make those decisions. Mental health patients, particularly, can become agitated when their voice is not heard or taken into consideration with treatment decisions. For culturally diverse patients with mental health care needs, this can even be more frustrating and lead to misunderstandings on both sides. Patients may feel misunderstood and isolated in a health care system that can seem cold, frightening, rigid, and controlling. Offering support and clear communication can be key to bringing about favorable outcomes for all patients, but support and clear communication can be more challenging for those patients, families, and significant others from diverse cultural groups.

It has become important for mental health care professionals to attempt to include consumers and family members in care decisions. At times, this can be problematic for mental health care providers, particularly if the mental health status of the patient is considered to be questionable in making critical personal decisions regarding their own care. Consumer treatment input can also seem a daunting task for those care providers who have based practice decisions on a strictly authoritarian framework. Understanding and taking into account the patient's values, beliefs, and practices is crucial to ensuring favorable outcomes. Evidence-based or "best" practice options can be discussed with patients and family members who are able to participate in care decisions (Evidence-Based Practice 10-1). However, the ultimate decision lies with the patient and his or her family or relatives. It is important for nurses to assess the knowledge level of their patients, family members, and/or significant others regarding the patient's status and care the patient is receiving. Try to include the patient in decisions affecting his or her care whenever possible.

Disparities in Mental Health Care

Reducing and eliminating disparities in health care has been a focus of numerous initiatives in recent years. The Department of Health and Human Services (USDHHS, 2001a, 2001b, 2001c) began an initiative to eliminate disparities in health among minorities. Healthy People 2010 (USDHHS, 2001a, 2001b, 2001c) also specified strategies to reduce health disparities among minority groups. The National Institute of Nursing Research (NINR) identified strategies to reduce and eventually move toward elimination of health disparities among a number of underrepresented cultural groups. However, despite these important initiatives to reduce health disparities in diverse and underrepresented cultural populations, disparities in health continue (Phillips & Grady, 2002). When asking the question "What can nursing do about health disparities?" Smith (2007) suggested that nursing has lost its vision and capacity for caring, which qualifies the profession to address disparities. "It has also been seduced by the scientific model and does not always use its best judgment of truths about human suffering" (p. 285). It is imperative that all health

EVIDENCE-BASED PRACTICE 10-1

Role of Consumers in Decision Making and Mental Health Care in Relation to Evidence-Based Practice

Consumers of mental health care (patients, families, and communities) are more knowledgeable now than they have ever been in the past. With the advent of the Internet, mental health care information is more widely available to those seeking knowledge. Continuous news broadcasts offer health care information to both consumers and professionals alike. National and international news and research breakthroughs are increasingly available to consumers, almost as soon as they are available to professionals.

Consumers want an active role in the decision making about their own mental health care and use numerous resources to make those decisions. Mental health patients, particularly, can become agitated when their voice is not heard or taken into consideration with treatment decisions. For culturally diverse patients with mental health care needs, this can even be more frustrating and lead to misunderstandings on both sides.

Patients may feel misunderstood and isolated in a health care system that can seem cold, frightening, rigid, and controlling.

Clinical Application

Whenever possible, include the patient, family/significant other in care decisions. Consumer treatment input can seem a daunting task for those care providers who have based practice decisions strictly on an authoritarian framework. It is important for mental health care professionals to try to include consumers in care decisions when feasible. It is important to try to understand and take into account the patient's values, beliefs, and practices to try to ensure favorable outcomes. Evidence-based or "best" practice options can be discussed with patients and family members who are able to participate in care decisions. However, the ultimate decision lies with the patient and their family or kin.

---

care providers, including mental health nurses, care about and reach out to those individuals and families suffering from mental health care disparities.

The treatment of mental illness has been challenging and has been shaped by numerous difficulties. Disparities in mental health treatment have existed from the earliest historical recordings. Those with behavior that was considered to be "abnormal," were thought to be "deranged" or "mad" and in many cases they were sent to asylums, under the harshest of conditions, to live out the remainder of their lives. Psychiatric mental health nurses have been at the forefront in paving the way for the humane care and treatment of mental health patients today and, yet, mental health still remains wrought with disparities and

stigma that do not exist for many other health conditions (Evidence-Based Practice 10-2).

The first Surgeon General's Report on mental health identified disparities among diverse cultural groups in seeking and being treated for mental illness: "Even more than other areas of health and medicine, the mental health field is plagued by disparities in the availability of and access to its services. These disparities are viewed readily through the lens of racial and cultural diversity, age, and gender" (USDHHS, 1999, p. vi).

Historically, racism in America has led to difficulties in acknowledging and/or discussing differences in cultural values and lifeways for diverse cultural groups. Bell and Peterson (1992) indicated that slavery, segregation, and institutionalized racism have resulted in numerous problems

EVIDENCE-BASED PRACTICE 10-2

Emic & Etic "Patient" Perspectives

Consider Making It Crazy: An Ethnography of Psychiatric Clients in an American Community by Sue E. Estroff (1981), Los Angeles: University of California Press. Estroff's ethnography of psychiatric clients is a research study utilizing participant observation. Estroff showed both the emic (insider) perspective and etic (outsider) perspective of institutionalization and deinstitutionalization for individuals suffering with severe mental illness. Estroff gained access to the world of the mentally ill and was able to understand, from an emic perspective, how psychiatric clients attempted to survive in the community. She explored the daily lives of those involved in the struggle for mental health, from both the caregiver and patient perspectives. Her insights offer mental health care providers an emic view rarely presented or understood in this struggle.

Clinical Application

It is important for nurses and other health care providers, as outsiders (or etic perspective), to try to understand the "emic," or insider perspective of their patients, families and significant others, so that they can provide care to patients in a culturally competent manner.

Encourage consumers to ask questions about their care. This is especially important for patients and families who have difficulty speaking the dominant English language.

Use certified interpreters whenever possible and help patients understand treatment options.

Listen to patients describe treatment modalities that have helped them in the past, even if they have involved health care values, beliefs and practices that are not accepted practices in the dominant health care system.

Encourage shamans, medicine men and women, and other nontraditional healers to be active in the patient's care, if that is the choice of the patient and his or her family. Transcultural mental health nurses can facilitate the role of nontraditional healers' as cocare providers in the traditional Western health care system.

Encourage family input, if it is available, when mental health patients are not capable of making competent decisions about their care. Otherwise, nurses and other health care providers need to advocate for treatment options that are in the patient's best interest. Frequently nurses know the patient from past admissions (if in a hospital or community-based mental health care setting) and may know what has worked or has not worked for the patient in the past.

Explain scientific and new treatment options to consumers of mental health care and allow patients and their families to have an active role in new treatment decisions. Make sure the patient understands that if a new treatment option is started that the patient will have a voice in continuing that treatment option in the future. Finally, respect for all patients is crucial to mental health care with patients and families from all cultures.

Adams, J. R., & Drake, R. E. (2006). Shared decision-making and evidence-based practice. *Community Mental Health Journal, 42*(1), 87–105.

Tanenbaum, S. J., (2008). Consumer perspectives on information and other inputs to decision-making: Implications for evidence-based practice. *Community Mental Health Journal, 44,* 331–335.

faced by African Americans, resulting in what the authors labeled as "cultural pain." **Cultural pain** is defined as feeling "insecure, embarrassed, angry, confused, torn, apologetic, uncertain, or inadequate because of conflicting expectations of and pressures from being a minority" (Bell & Peterson, 1992, p. 8). Leininger (1995) identified cultural pain as "the suffering, discomfort, or unfavorable responses of an individual group towards an individual who has different beliefs or lifeways, usually reflecting the insensitivity of those inflicting the discomfort" (p. 67).

A number of diverse cultural groups have experienced what is called **historical unresolved grief**, sometimes referred to as **historical trauma, American Indian holocaust**, or **disenfranchised grieving**. Yellow Horse Brave Heart and DeBruyn (1998, p. 60) observed that "American Indians experienced massive losses of lives, land, and culture from European contact and colonization resulting in a long legacy of chronic trauma and unresolved grief across generations." Past emotional harm done to people of a diverse culture would include such examples as the Jewish holocaust, slavery of African American people in the United States, internment of Japanese Americans in America during World War II, and treatment of American Indians. In order to help individuals within the particular culture to heal from the historical unresolved grief or historical trauma, nurses need to understand how experiences of the past shape the present and future (Yellow Horse Brave Heart & DeBruyn, 1998; Struthers & Lowe, 2003). Helping patients to move through the process of unresolved grief is an important care measure nurses and other health care providers must consider when caring for individuals and families from cultures who have experienced horrific events or trauma in the past. Cultural groups honor life stages in diverse ways. A wreath made of tobacco ties and sage in a circular form that reflects unity marks a traditional Lakota grave (Figure 10-2). Often interventions are directed toward the community at large rather than focused on specific individuals. Working "with" patients, families, and communities and encouraging their voices to be heard are key to helping those who have experienced pain associated with racial, social, and economic disparities and oppression (Evidence-Based Practice 10-3).

Johnston (2008) in an ethnographic study with Northern British Columbian Aboriginal mothers with adolescents diagnosed with fetal alcohol spectrum disorder, observed that the mothers who

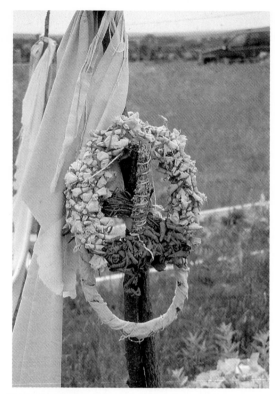

FIGURE 10-2   Cultural groups honor life stages in diverse ways. Here a wreath made of tobacco ties and sage, in a circular form that reflects unity, marks a traditional Lakota grave.

participated in the study lived within a marginalized and poverty-stricken context. Intergenerational alcohol abuse had played a major role in all of the women's lives. Johnston suggested that nurses need to take a leadership role to reduce health disparities with marginalized and poverty-stricken populations, particularly when there is evidence of prejudice, including stereotyping. Nurses can advocate on behalf of such individuals and communities thereby effecting change at the macro level.

Zayas, Torres, and Cabassa (2009) compared mental health diagnostic agreement in an outpatient unit with Hispanic and non-Hispanic health care providers. The non-Hispanic care providers rated patient's functional ability and the severity of symptoms significantly worse than the Hispanic care providers. The authors noted that because

EVIDENCE-BASED PRACTICE 10-3

Healthcare: Racial, Social, and Economic Disparities and Oppression

The fact that racial disparities do exist in the United States is deeply disturbing. Low socioeconomic status contributes to health care disparities, particularly in a society that values monetary success. Social disparities, based on race and economic status are an indication of a society that has failed to integrate its members into a caring and unified protective modality. The United States has a long history of racial discrimination and segregation and this includes health care. What is even more disturbing is that racial disparities in health care are sometimes perpetuated by the health care providers, themselves. If there are racial and economic disparities in health care, then health care providers and those academics and institutions educating the providers are perpetuating a societal disease.

(Freire, 1970/1990), over four decades ago, identified the pain of oppression, as a "Pedagogy of the Oppressed," and discussed the importance of working "with" the oppressed (individuals or peoples) in an "incessant struggle to regain their humanity" (p. 33). Racism and oppression,

including internalized oppression (Freire, 1970/1990), are continuous forces that exacerbate destructive behaviors such as suicide, and alcoholism in various oppressed cultural groups (Yellow Horse Brave Heart, & DeBruyn, 1998).

Clinical Application

Nurses can recognize that patients, families, and communities experience the effects of racial, social, and economic disparities and oppression.

Acknowledge that historical grief or cultural pain are very real to those persons who experience them. Transcultural mental health nurses are skilled at caring for and working "with" patients, families, and communities experiencing emotional pain associated with such oppression, disparity and discrimination.

Transcultural nurses work with many cultural groups who have experienced racial, social, and economic disparities and oppression. Encouraging patients, families, and communities to assume an active role in their own health care can be empowering.

Freire, P. (1970/1990). *Pedagogy of the oppressed.* New York: The Continuum Publishing Company.

Weisfeld, A., & Perflman, R. L. (2005). Disparities and discrimination in health care. *Perspectives in Biology and Medicine, 48,* S1–S9.

Yellow Horse Brave Heart, M., & DeBruyn, L. M. (1998). The American Indian holocaust: Healing historical unresolved grief. *American Indian & Alaska Native Mental Health Research, 8*(2), 56–78.

the mental health labor force is primarily "White" or non-Hispanic, Hispanic immigrants are likely to be assigned a non-Hispanic care provider. The authors questioned the possibility of the care provider's cultural and social biases, and wondered if those factors were responsible for the discrepancy in diagnoses. It is important for mental health professionals not only to identify but to understand racism and the role it plays in mental health at both a conscious and unconscious level, in order to eradicate racial inequalities in mental health care.

Immigrant Mental Health Care

There has been extensive debate about immigration policy during the past several years in the United States as well as internationally. In the United States, the debate has become heated politically with both Republicans and Democrats arguing the implications, from their standpoint, of immigration policies. Health care for those immigrants who are not in this country legally has also been extensively debated, again with both sides stating the merits of their views on whether such immigrants, or undocumented workers, have a right to health care in this country. At the same time, however, there has been minimal understanding of these issues from the perspective of the undocumented immigrants and the impact immigration has on their mental health.

Setting aside the political debate, transcultural mental health nurses have cared for both documented and undocumented immigrants for many years and are increasingly caring for those immigrants who are feeling the emotional pressures of such a political climate. The term **culture shock** was coined by the anthropologist Kalervo Oberg (1960) to describe individuals, such as immigrants, who enter a new culture (either legally or illegally). Culture shock is "precipitated by the anxiety that results from losing all our familiar signs and symbols of social intercourse" (p. 177). Oberg suggests that the "signs" or "cues" that people use within a culture--such as the words people speak, customs people follow, and even nonverbal communication such as gestures and facial expressions are not recognized by those who are new to the culture. This leads to feelings of frustration and anxiety even in those persons who would be considered "mentally healthy." Imagine how these negative feelings would be confounded for an individual who has entered the country illegally and fears arrest, detention, and deportation.

The concept of **acculturation** was initially defined by Redfield, Linton, and Herskovits (1936) as "those phenomena which result when groups of individuals having different cultures come into continuous first-hand contact, with subsequent changes in the original cultural patterns of either or both groups" (p. 149). Acculturation can be a stressful and complex process, particularly for immigrants who experience difficulty adjusting to the new culture. Frequently, children become acculturated sooner than their parents (Boyle, 2008). Some individuals may find themselves unable to work through the stress of acculturation and have great difficulty in modifying their **cultural values, beliefs, or practices** and feel isolated from their new

culture or even from their culture of origin. Depression is the most common mental health problem among immigrants in the United States and has been associated with the process of acculturation (Al-Omari & Pallikkathayil, 2008; Choi, Miller, & Wilbur 2009). Immigrants and refugees may be fleeing war and other traumatic political environments and may exhibit symptoms of posttraumatic stress disorder as well as depression (Boyle, 2008).

Immigration stress can be a result of economic adversity in the new country, language difficulties, loss of support networks, even loss of family members as well as prejudice and discrimination. These difficulties may place immigrants at higher risk for mental health problems. Walsh, Shulman and Maurer (2008) studied immigration distress in young adults immigrating to Israel from Eastern Europe and found young immigrants experienced immigration distress, including feelings of guilt and shame, failure, and incompetence and not feeling wanted, understood, or a sense of belonging. Because of the difficulties faced by immigrant families, their children are at higher risk for depression, anxiety disorders, substance abuse, and other mental health problems. Mental health nurses working with immigrants and their families need to be aware of the risk for mental health problems. Many immigrants may express their anxiety as somatic complaints, so nurses working with immigrant populations need to be aware of the linkages between somatic complaints such as headaches, backaches, and the like, and mental health problems (Lamberg, 2009).

Culture-Bound Syndromes

Various mental health symptoms are experienced by people all over the world. Cultural meanings, beliefs, and practices regarding specific symptoms may vary depending on one's culture and socioeconomic status within the culture. Although specific identifying terms, manifestations and meanings within different cultures may vary, a diagnosis such as depression is similar around the world. Cultural values, beliefs, and practices also shape how various groups interpret symptoms and identify causality and determine appropriate treatment.

In contrast, "**Culture-Bound Syndromes**," (also called **folk illnesses, culture-specific illnesses**, or **culture-specific syndromes**) often are localized to a particular cultural group. As population trends have indicated, the United States is becoming an increasingly multicultural country and it is necessary, then, for mental health nurses to become familiar with culture-bound syndromes. Mental health nurses will most likely, during their professional practice, encounter patients with symptoms and patterns of behavior that are not commonly observed in the United States and other Western countries, and these symptoms and behaviors have been referred to as culture-bound syndromes. Many mental health nurses must practice within a health care system based on the medical model and use the DSM-IV (2000) of the APA to obtain health insurance reimbursement. In fact, the APA included culture-bound syndromes for the first time in the 2000 DSM-IV edition. This step indicates the extent to which mental health care providers are caring for patients

from diverse cultures with unique symptoms that do not fit into the traditional Western diagnostic medical categories. According to APA (2000), culture-bound syndromes are described as recurrent, locality specific patterns of aberrant behavior and troubling experience that may or may not be linked to a particular DSM-IV diagnostic category. Many of these patterns are indigenously considered to be "illnesses," or at least afflictions, and most have local names. Culture-bound syndromes are generally limited to specific societies or culture areas and are localized, diagnostic categories that frame coherent meanings for certain repetitive, patterned, and troubling sets of experience and observations (p. 898).

As mental health care is changing to meet the increasing multicultural diversity of the patient population, it is important for mental health nurses to recognize the culture-bound syndromes. As you review the table listing culture-bound syndromes (Table 10-1), keep in mind the cultural context in which the syndromes have evolved. Since values, beliefs, and practices of people are culturally constructed, the syndromes can only

TABLE 10-1
Culture–Bound Syndromes

SYNDROME	CULTURE	SYMPTOMS
Amok Cafard, Cathard Mal de Pelea lich'aa	Malaysia Polynesia Puerto Rico Navajo	Period of brooding with subsequent aggressive behavior followed by amnesia or exhaustion Typically occurs in young to middle-aged males who have experienced recent loss.
Ataque de nervios	Latino cultures Puerto Rico	Uncontrollable shouting, crying, trembling, and aggressive behavior Sensation of heat in the chest Possible fainting or seizure-like activity Triggered by stressful familial event and buildup of anger Typically occurs in women 45 years and older
Bilis, Colera, Muina	Latino cultures	Acute nervous tension, trembling, screaming, gastrointestinal disturbances Cause is thought to be unexpressed anger or rage

(table continues on page 254)

TABLE 10-1
Culture–Bound Syndromes (*continued*)

SYNDROME	CULTURE	SYMPTOMS
Boufee Delirante	West Africa, Haiti	Abrupt outburst of agitation, aggression, and confusion May be associated with hallucinations (visual and auditory) and paranoia
Brain fag, Brain fog	West Africa	Brain "fatigue," difficulty concentrating or sleeping, weakness Crawling sensation under skin Feelings of depression Most often afflicts high school or college students
Dhat, Jiryan *Sukra Prameha* *Shen k'uei*	India Sri Lanka China, Taiwan	Somatic complaints of dizziness, fatigue, weakness, loss of appetite, guilt, and sexual dysfunction associated with semen-loss anxiety
Falling out, Blacking out	Southern United States, Caribbean	Spinning sensation and dizziness prior to collapse Visually impaired Difficulty interacting with environment
Ghost sickness	Navajo	Weakness, pending sense of "doom," loss of appetite, feeling of suffocation, fainting, dizziness, and hallucinations Preoccupation with death
Hwa-byung	Korea	Insomnia, chest discomfort, dizziness, headaches, fearful, sadness, suicidal ideation, and guilt Typically occurs in middle-aged or elderly women
Koro *Shuk yang, Shook yong, Suo yang* *Jinjinia bemar* *Rok joo*	Malaysia China Assam Thailand	Fear that the penis in men and vulva and nipples in women are retracting into the body and will possibly cause death
Latah *Amurakh, Irkunii, Olan, Myriachit, Menkeiti* *Bah tschi, Bah tsi, Baah ji* *Imu* *Mali-mali, Silok* *Locura*	Malaysia Siberia Thailand Ainu, Sakhalin, Japan Phillipines Latin America and Latinos in the United States	Exaggerated startle response, screaming, cursing, laughing echopraxia, echolalia Typically occurs in women
Mal de ojo, Evil eye	Mediterranean	Typically occurs with children and can also affect women Sleep disturbances, crying, diarrhea, vomiting, and fever

SYNDROME	CULTURE	SYMPTOMS
Nervios	Latino cultures	Feeling of vulnerability and emotional distress to stressful life experiences Irritability, sleep disturbances, nervous, difficulty concentrating, tearfulness, and dizziness
Pibloktoq, Arctic hysteria	Inuit	Fatigue, depressive silences, confusion Typically follows a major loss
Qi-gong psychotic reaction	Chinese	Dissociation and paranoia Headache, dizziness, disorientation Can occur following Qi-gong meditation
Rootwork	Southern U.S. Caribbean	Witchcraft, voodoo, hexing, or evil influence are responsible for illnesses
Mal puesto, Brujeria	Latino cultures	GI disturbances, anxiety, afraid of being poisoned or killed ("voodoo death")
Sangue dormido	Portuguese Cape Verde Islanders	Pain, numbness, paralysis, convulsions, stroke, heart attack, infection and miscarriage
Shenjing	Chinese	Depression, anxiety, dizziness, headaches, GI and sleep disturbances, and sexual dysfunction
Shin-byung	Korean	Anxiety, weakness, dizziness, fear, sleep, and GI disturbances Somatic complaints are followed by dissociation and feeling possessed by ancestral spirits
Spell	Southern United States	Trance-like state, communication with deceased spirits May be misdiagnosed as psychosis
Susto, Fright, Soul loss *(Espantro, Pasmo, Tripa Ida, Perdida del alma chibih)*	Latinos in the United States Mexico Central America South America	Actual "fright" Sleep and appetite disturbances, sadness, lack of motivation, low self-esteem, muscle aches, headache and GI disturbances Typically follows a frightening event resulting in the soul leaving the body Symptoms can occur immediately following event or years later
Taijin kyofusho	Japan	Intense fear that one's body (appearance, odor, nonverbal communication) embarrasses or offends others
Zar	North Africa Middle East	Feeling possessed by a spirit Dissociation (laughing, hurting self, singing, crying), withdrawal, difficulty caring for self May develop relationship with spirit

Data from American Psychological Association. (2000). *Diagnostic and statistical manual of mental disorders* (4th ed.); and Hales, Yudofsky, & Gabbard (Eds.). (2008). *The American Psychiatric Publishing Textbook of Psychiatry* (5th ed.).

be interpreted within the context of the specific culture in which they exist.

Cultural Values, Beliefs, and Practices of Specific Cultural Groups as They Relate to Mental Health

Immigration trends have been important factors in the cultural diversity and history of the United States. Nurses have always cared for diverse populations of patients and in particular, community-based nurses have focused on newly arrived immigrant populations. A century ago, nurses and other health professionals were concerned about contagious diseases and malnutrition. Currently, there is a great deal of research being conducted to better understand nursing care for culturally diverse patients and their family members who are seeking care. Many of these studies focus specifically on mental health care, particularly helping patients, families, and communities adjust to life in the United States. In addition, health care services for immigrant communities also place an emphasis on mental health as many current immigrants have experienced war, displacement, and other associated traumas.

Nurse researchers and other health-related disciplines have continued to explore the health beliefs and practices of culturally diverse patients specific to mental health. An overview of mental health beliefs and practices of selected cultural groups will be presented in this chapter. The overviews are not intended to stereotype or generalize the specific cultures. They are only intended as a resource for transcultural nurses and others to increase the awareness of patterns of values, beliefs, and practices related to mental health of the selected cultural groups. However, the transcultural nurse is also encouraged to understand the diversity within cultural groups with respect to mental health beliefs and practices. Many patients and families of specific cultural groups may not exhibit traditional patterns of values, beliefs, and practices of any specific

cultural group. Transcultural nurses should conduct a thorough history and cultural assessment to ensure competent cultural care for each patient.

Transcultural mental health nurses and other mental health care providers want to help patients of all cultures to achieve their optimal level of human functioning. However, it is important to note that an individual's optimal level of human functioning can have different meanings and expressions based on that individual's culture (Lopez et al., 2006, p. 224). Current trends on psychologic functioning of individuals from diverse cultures are focused on positive constructs and models (Constantine & Sue, 2006a, 2006b). The majority of research on psychologic functioning with immigrants, persons from diverse cultures, and people of color has relied on the deficit model. According to the deficit model, hostile environmental factors such as prejudice and inequality in social conditions lead to increased rates of stress among minority populations, which ultimately lead to inferior or self-destructive methods of coping (Kaplan & Sue, 1997). Although the deficit model drew attention to the effects of prejudice and inequality in social conditions, there was a tendency to equate one's psychologic functioning with negative rather than positive forces. This focus of research—upon the deficit model—has changed in the last few years as researchers now seek more positive frameworks to describe diverse experiences, beliefs, and transitions. This latter approach has emphasized the strengths of immigrants and minority populations.

According to Constantine and Sue (2006a, 2006b) an individual's optimal level of human functioning is dependent upon the cultural context in which it is being defined. In fact, Western goals associated with optimal human functioning, and grounded in a Eurocentric cultural value system such as happiness and self-determination may differ greatly with individuals from diverse cultures. Optimal human functioning of culturally diverse persons may be better understood by studying the values, beliefs, and practices of the cultural group. For example in the United States, optimal level of human functioning for African Americans and Native Americans may include such concepts as collectivism, racial and ethnic pride, spirituality, religion, holistic health, and family/kin and community or tribal importance. In addition, overcoming such adversity as racism may serve as a strength and helps mental health care providers better understand optimal human functioning for diverse cultural groups (Constantine & Sue, 2006a, 2006b).

It is important to be flexible, open, and adapt to culturally congruent ways of knowing and doing when working with patients from diverse cultural groups in providing mental health care. Ahnallen, Suyemoto, and Carter (2006) emphasized the importance of health care providers recognizing patterns of self-identification for patients from diverse cultural groups. In addition, health care providers should acknowledge that patients may have varied expressions of either a sense of belonging or feeling excluded in certain situations and contexts and with different social and cultural groups.

Modern medical care may not be viewed the same as traditional health care in reservation or immigrant communities. Native Americans, as well as newly arrived immigrants, may experience some difficulty in trusting modern-day (allopathic) health care providers. For example, some Native Americans may be reluctant to consult professionally educated mental health care workers as they perceive that the mental health professionals are attempting to "brainwash" them into accepting the cultural values, beliefs, and practices of the Western health care system (Gone & Alcantara, 2007, p. 356). It is important for health care providers to be open to the values, beliefs, and practices of patients from diverse cultural groups. That is not to say one must adopt all the cultural values, beliefs, and practices of multiculturally diverse patients, but one should be open to and incorporate when possible, the values, beliefs, and practices of our patients.

African Americans: An Overview of Some Mental Health Concerns

Individuals of African descent comprise 12.8% of the total U.S. population (U.S. Census Bureau,

2008). The concept of African Americans as a distinct group in the United States is grounded historically in their shared social and environmental contexts, historical events, as well as family and kin memories of those experiences. Bell and Peterson (1992) noted that slavery, segregation, and institutionalized racism created a climate that resulted in health disparities, structural inequalities, marginalization, and cultural pain for African Americans. Acknowledging and understanding this cultural context is an important first step prior to providing transcultural mental health care to African American individuals, families, and communities.

Although numerous health disparities are of great concern in the African American population, mental health issues have often gone unnoticed, taking a back seat to other health concerns. While there is an equal percentage of Black and White males who suffer from depression, Black men experience a higher rate of suicide (NPR: Recognizing Depression and Suicide Risk in Black Men, 2005). Black men, in particular, often are uninsured and have little or no access to mental health care. They may receive a poorer quality of care even if they are able to access the mental health system. Furthermore, minorities are underrepresented in mental health research (USDHHS, 2001a, 2001b, 2001c). Over time, all of these factors lead to more untreated depression and eventually to higher rates of suicide. In addition, there has been little outreach to the Black community about the availability of mental health care and education about what mental health is and what depression is all about, as well as targeted education about other kinds of mental disorders. Many in the Black community, especially young Black males, may believe that depression is not really an illness or that it is a sign of weakness, so they tend not to seek help. There is a notion that is prevalent among young Black men (as well as others) that because of machismo, being macho or tough . . . then Black men cannot be suicidal. It is one of the most pervasive and damaging falsehoods within and outside of the

African American community. Some studies have shown that that some African Americans believe that depression is a personal weakness and the result of improper lifestyles (e.g., too much worry, working too hard, not being religious enough) (Shellman & Mokel, 2010).

Black men, as in other diverse cultural groups, often express their depression through bodily symptoms, that is, headaches, stomach aches, pains, and so on. Within the Black community, there can be considerable stigma about mental illnesses. Prevention of depression and suicide is extremely important and education is the key to early prevention. Although the Black church has traditionally viewed suicide as a sin, many religious organizations are now starting to create mental health programs. The Black church is a major institution in the community and pastors can be educated to recognize signs of depression among parishioners and refer troubled individuals to the proper professionals (Taliaferro, 2006). In addition, mental health providers need to be attuned and realize that depression occurs in Blacks, particularly young men. It can often be overlooked, but sometimes cultural insensitivity to what Black people are trying to say or how they might say it leads health care providers to overlook symptoms of depression.

There are other mental health issues within the African American community that lead to premature mortality or morbidity. The societal costs of substance abuse can be calculated in terms of violence, disease, and death. There is a close relationship between substance abuse and HIV/AIDS as well as other sexually transmitted diseases. In a grounded theory study focused on understanding the use of street drugs among older African Americans, Pope, Wallhagen, and Davis (2010) found that a close relationship with family members was often the precipitating factor for entrance into rehabilitation. Close relationships and the context of those relationships are sometimes a precipitating factor for beginning substance abuse. Respondents in this study also identified several media images that negatively portrayed African American culture and influenced the use of illegal substances. The negative images portrayed by "harmful one-dimensional characterizations surrounding criminal culture/drug culture, negative characterizations and comedic renderings" were profoundly described by the sample (p. 251). These images have two major effects: for African Americans, they glamorize a drug lifestyle and for White Americans, they portray crime, violence, and deviant behavior. Evidence-Based Practice 10-4 describes some of the

EVIDENCE-BASED PRACTICE 10-4

The Challenge of Recovery for African American Women

Alcohol and substance abuse is a national and transcultural phenomenon in epidemic proportions in many cultures. Substance abuse within the African American culture and communities has been a significant challenge for health care providers who care for the patients, families and communities wrought with this debilitating epidemic. Battle (1990) identified that "alcohol has been consumed by Blacks since the period of slavery to ease the effects and pressures of racism and oppression; to tune out physical and emotional pain" (p. 251).

Refer to *No Hiding Place, Empowerment and Recovery for Our Troubled Communities* (Williams, 1992). Reverend Williams at Glide Memorial Church in San Francisco's Tenderloin neighborhood, identified the epidemic of drug abuse in inner cities today as a new form of slavery, "a slavery of addiction" (p. 3). Reverend Williams began a recovery program based on what he called a "smell of death" (p. 2). The "smell of death" came from many people, especially young mothers, strung out on crack cocaine, and the Reverend declared a "war on addiction" (p. 3).

EVIDENCE-BASED PRACTICE 10-4 *(continued)*

Since most of the individuals attending services at Glide memorial were African Americans, Williams developed a recovery program in conjunction with the church and community members. The recovery program was "culturally based" (p. 7) and included acts of recognition, self-definition, rebirth, and community, and eventually formed the basis of the recovery program. Williams stressed that recovery was a process in which everyone needed to participate. He was able to help a community begin to deal with their cultural pain and move through the process of recovery from their drug and alcohol abuse.

In a transcultural ethnonursing research study conducted using Leininger's Culture Care Diversity & Universality Theory of Nursing, Ehrmin (2000, 2001, 2002, 2005) entered the African American women's emic world to study the women living in an inner-city transitional home for substance abuse. Transcultural nursing concepts and principles were valuable to gain insight about the women and their cultural experiences, with respect to their values, beliefs, meanings, and practices that influenced their use and abuse of substances and their cultural care needs in recovery. In order for substance-dependent African American women to successfully move through treatment and recovery for their substance abuse, they needed to feel respected, cared for, listened to and treated in a nonjudgmental manner. The women wanted to be guided and directed in their treatment to learn to be productive members of society. The women also needed to resolve past cultural pain experiences. The predominant reason that women sought treatment and recovery for their addiction was their children. For many of the women, their children had either been taken away from them by Children's Services Board (CSB) or were currently living with family or other relatives. The women expressed unresolved maternal feelings of guilt and shame for their use of alcohol and drugs. Dealing with those feelings was key to women moving successfully through the process of recovery for substance abuse.

Clinical Application

African American families are generally matriarchal families and women have strong gender roles within the family. To facilitate the success of women in recovery, transcultural mental health nurses can help women learn to trust and develop positive supportive relationships with female care providers, other recovering women and with female members of their families.

Substance-dependent women need to be supported in a nonjudgmental manner as they resolve past painful life experiences, particularly those having to do with perceived maternal failures during their active addiction.

Assess substance-dependent women for comorbid depression, which can increase a woman's risk for relapse.

Battle, S. (1990). Moving targets: Alcohol, crack and Black women. In E. C. White (Ed.). *The Black women's health book: Speaking for ourselves.* Seattle: The Seal Press.

Ehrmin, J. T. (2000). Cultural implications of the 12-approach in addictions treatment and recovery. *Journal of Addictions Nursing, 12,* 37–41.

Ehrmin, J. T. (2001). Unresolved feelings of guilt and shame in the maternal role with substance-dependent African-American women. *Journal of Nursing Scholarship, 33,* 53–58.

Ehrmin, J. T. (2002). Family violence and culture care with African and Euro-American cultures in the United States. In M. Leininger & M. R. McFarland (Eds.). *Transcultural nursing: Concepts, theories, research & practice* (3rd ed., pp. 333–346). New York, NY: McGraw-Hill.

Ehrmin, J. T. (2005) Dimensions of culture care for substance-dependent African American women. *The Journal of Transcultural Nursing, 16,* 117–125.

Williams, C. (1992). *No hiding place, empowerment and recovery for our troubled communities.* San Francisco: Harper San Francisco.

challenges that African Americans face in recovering from alcohol and substance abuse.

Although major health disparities affect the African American community, mental health issues need immediate attention as these issues are complex and require creative and substantive interventions. There is clearly a need for concerted action as the core issues of substance abuse and suicide cannot be addressed by just one discipline alone; the environmental and larger societal forces must be attended to by multidisciplinary actions on numerous fronts. There are several important factors to keep in mind when providing transcultural mental health care to African Americans. First, family and kin networks, while perhaps not as strong as in the past, are still extremely important in assisting the recovery process. Outreach and education to family members about depression, suicide, and substance abuse are extremely important. For many African Americans who have experienced difficulty with mental health issues of substance and drug abuse and serious and persistent mental illnesses, such as depression, *family* and *community* are very important components in the recovery process. Maintaining a connection with family members and others in the community assists patients to feel accepted and demonstrates to themselves and others that they can move forward in the recovery process (Ehrmin, 2005; Armour, Bradshaw, & Roseborough, 2009). Secondly, the African American church is a key player in changing community perceptions about depression and suicide as well as a leading player in substance abuse programs. The Black church is a major institution where many African Americans choose to go for help. Spirituality has been a traditional cultural norm in African cultures and the modern African American church has incorporated the spiritual component into healing and care.

Native Americans: An Overview of Some Mental Health Concerns

Native Americans (American Indians and Alaska Natives) comprise 1.0% of the total population in the United States (U.S. Census Bureau, 2008). There are 562 Federally Recognized Native American Tribes and Nations in the United States (Federally Recognized Indian Tribes. Federal Register: July 12, 2002).

The need to improve care for Native Americans has been known for some time. The U.S. DHHS received a 9% increase from Congress in 2001 to boost the budget of the Indian Health Services (IHS) to $2.6 billion. Funds for diabetes and improved living quarters were included in the increase. There was also an increase in mental health services to increase the overall health of Native Americans (USDHHS, 2001a, 2001b, 2001c). Still, much work remains to be accomplished in the overall health care for Native Americans.

The Native American culture believes in holistic health care and generally has a holistic outlook in all aspects of their lives. Holism is a belief that the physical, mental, emotional, and spiritual dimensions of an individual are perceived as one. Native Americans, as a cultural group, are also perceived as one, although bear in mind that each tribe may have unique characteristics. The mind–body separation of Western health care is not present in the Native American culture (Yurkovich & Lattergrass, 2008). Traditional peoples bring cultures together in contemporary life in many ways. Ideally, individuals with more than one cultural affiliation can bring parts of each culture together without conflict. Figure 10-3 shows tipis at a Lakota Nation Powwow, Pine Ridge, South Dakota.

For Native Americans, acknowledging positive cultural strengths such as spirituality in all aspects of their lives, resiliency and positive identity are necessary for healing within a cultural care perspective (Yurkovich & Lattergrass, 2008). It is important for nurses working with Native American patients to focus on such strengths as spirituality, resiliency and positive identity to help patients in the healing process. Gone (2009) conducted a study on the legacy of Native American historical trauma with staff and patients in a Native American Healing Lodge. Findings suggested connecting evidence-based and culturally

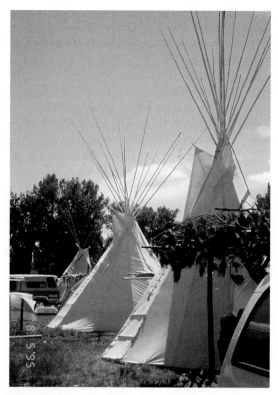

FIGURE 10-3 Traditional peoples bring cultures together in contemporary life in many ways. Ideally, individuals with more than one cultural affiliation can bring parts of each culture together without conflict. Tipis at a Lakota Nation Powwow, Pine Ridge, South Dakota.

Trauma." Nurses can help specific cultural groups grieve the past traumatic event(s) and resolve some of the past pain associated with such grief and trauma (Evidence-Based Practice 10-5).

Alcohol has had an overwhelming impact on the mental health of Native Americans. Forced into a harsh reservation system, Native Americans were forced to give up their native lands and ways of life. Yellow Horse Brave Heart and DeBruyn (1998) suggest that, for many individuals, the resulting anger and oppression are acted out upon oneself and others like the self, such as members of one's group. Native Americans have repeatedly suffered losses of family and community members to alcohol-related accidents, homicides, and suicide. Abuse, such as domestic violence and child abuse are leading mental health concerns among Native American communities throughout the country. "These layers of present losses in addition to the major traumas of the past fuel the anguish, psychologic numbing, and destructive coping mechanisms related to disenfranchised grief and historical trauma" suffered by Native Americans (Yellow Horse Brave Heart, & DeBruyn, 1998, pp. 68–69).

Kasl (1992) observed an anniversary celebration of a Native American healing center. She suggested that the Native Americans in attendance drew from several belief systems and referred to this phenomena as an "integrated faith." Other examples of integrated faith may be an informal Catholic mass integrating Native American wisdom and then followed by an Alcoholics Anonymous (AA) meeting. Many Native American tribes have developed their own mental health centers, including those that specifically treat chemical dependencies (alcohol and drugs). These treatment centers (both inpatient and outpatient) are fully accredited by appropriate accreditation agencies and employ certified and licensed counselors, who are often Native Americans themselves. The services combine traditional beliefs with professional treatment. The services focus on wellness and healing; they may include spiritual retreats, talking circles, sweats, burning sage, smudge, and other practices that are specific to the patients' tribes.

sensitive treatment options with indigenous programs, to create culturally sensitive interventions congruent with community values and norms. Program staff identified the importance of embracing the Native American indigenous heritage, identity, and spirituality in order to begin healing the detrimental effects of historical trauma and colonization. In order to provide culturally competent care, health care professionals should work closely with native healers to integrate spirituality and other indigenous beliefs into treatment processes (Yurkovich & Lattergrass, 2008). Many minority and underrepresented cultural groups have experienced what is called "Historical Unresolved Grief" or "Historical

EVIDENCE-BASED PRACTICE 10-5

"Historical Unresolved Grief" or "Historical Trauma"

Certain cultural groups, such as American Indians, have experienced what is called "**Historical Unresolved Grief**" or "**Historical Trauma**". They have experienced loss of people, land and their culture as a result of European colonization. This phenomenon "contributes to the current social pathology of high rates of suicide, homicide, domestic violence, child abuse, alcoholism and other social problems among American Indians" (p. 60). Other cultural groups experiencing the phenomenon of historical unresolved grief or historical trauma include such examples as the Jewish holocaust, slavery of African Americans, and the internment of Japanese Americans during World War II. Nurses can help specific cultural groups grieve the past traumatic event(s) and allow them to acknowledge the events that occurred. It is important to help individuals, groups and communities identify methods and solutions to move forward in the healing process.

Clinical Application

As individuals, families, and communities continue to grieve the emotional pain associated with cultural pain, historical trauma/ historical unresolved grief/disenfranchised grieving, it is important for transcultural mental health nurses to acknowledge the emotional feelings (insecurity, embarrassed, angry, confused, torn, apologetic, uncertain, or inadequate) associated with such grief and the conflicting expectations of and pressures from being a minority.

It is important for transcultural mental health nurses to facilitate a safe and healing environment for individuals, families, and communities to work through the feelings associated with cultural pain, historical trauma/historical unresolved grief/disenfranchised grieving.

Bell, P., & Peterson, D. (1992). *Cultural pain and African Americans: Unspoken issues in early recovery.* Hazeldon Pub.

Yellow Horse Brave Heart, M., & DeBruyn, L. M. (1998). *The American Indian holocaust: Healing historical unresolved grief by,* 8(2), 60–82.

Native Americans frequently communicate through storytelling. So, allowing Native American patients to tell their story is an important and useful way to get information. Use of broad, open-ended questions facilitates obtaining a health history and other information in a culturally competent manner. As there is a focus on tribal and family viewpoints, how one views himself or herself is frequently based on how others in their tribe or family view them. So, rather than discourage tribal and family inclusion in treatment approaches, it may be important to help the patient form an "interdependent" view of themselves, acknowledging the impact of treatment on the tribe and family is important to the patient (DeCoteau, Anderson, & Hope, 2006).

Asian/Pacific Islander Cultural Groups: An Overview of Some Mental Health Concerns

Asian Americans and Pacific Islanders are one of the fastest growing minority groups in the United States, second only to the Hispanic or Latino cultural groups. Individuals of Asian ancestry are 4.5% of the total U.S. population (U.S. Census Bureau, 2008). Asian Americans and Pacific Islanders of Asian ancestry represent 43 diverse cultural groups from Korea, Japan, China, India, Cambodia, Vietnam, Indonesia, Philippines, and Papua New Guinea to name only a few (U.S. Census Bureau, 2008).

In some Asian Americans and newly arrived immigrants from China and Japan, stigma related to mental health problems can be a stumbling block in seeking appropriate care. For example, a study by Gilbert et al. (2007) focused on Asian and non-Asian young women's shame related to mental health care and identified three components of shame. They were external shame or a belief that an individual will be viewed negatively for mental health problems; internal shame that is evaluating oneself negatively; and reflected shame, a belief that having mental health problems could bring shame to an individual's family or community. Results of this study suggest that Asian women had higher external and reflected shame beliefs than non-Asian women. Asians also expressed concerns about confidentiality when talking about personal feelings/anxieties. This study suggests that stigma may play a role in seeking mental health care and may encourage individuals to seek care among friends and family. These same individuals may not seek professional mental health services at all, as they would risk feelings of shame for themselves and others if mental health services were utilized.

Asian Americans' core cultural values of honor and pride and patriarchal obligations, particularly with elders, are important to understanding the Asian American culture. Collective group harmony, including family and kin, rather than individual concerns are significant cultural values (Leininger, 1995). Understanding core cultural values of the Asian American culture, particularly the importance of maintaining harmony, will help transcultural nurses plan care for patients with mental health problems in a culturally competent manner.

In a study of older Korean Americans exploring cultural attitudes toward mental health services, Jang et al. (2007) found that individuals who had been in the United States for a shorter time frame and had more severe levels of depression were more likely to have negative attitudes about mental health services. Cultural values and beliefs of older Korean Americans seemed to have a major influence on whether or not they viewed mental health services in a negative manner. Those individuals who identified mental illness with personal weakness or shame held more

negative attitudes about utilizing mental health services. However, if the individual associated depression as a health condition, then he or she had a more positive attitude about mental health services. Cultural values and beliefs about mental illness, including stigma associated with mental illness were also found to be influential in individual's attitudes toward mental health services.

Community agencies have often provided mental health services specifically to Asian Americans. With recent cuts in funding for health care, many of these community agencies have suffered a severe cut-back in services and are unable to provide the level and kinds of care that they have provided in the past. Recognition of cultural barriers such as language that has a direct effect on communication between nurses and other health care providers and patients and their family/ significant other(s) can be preemptive and lead to more positive patient outcomes (Evidence-Based Practice 10-6).

Hispanic/Latino Cultural Groups: An Overview of Some Mental Health Concerns

Individuals of Hispanic or Latino descent are the fastest growing cultural group in the United States and make up 15.4% of the total population of the United States (U.S. Census Bureau, 2008). By 2050 approximately 97 million people, or one-fourth of the U.S. population, will self-identify as Hispanic Americans (U.S. Department of Health and Human Services, 2009). Hispanic countries include such diverse places as Mexico, Puerto Rico, Cuba, South and Central America, Spain, and various states in the United States. It is important to keep in mind that Hispanic/Latino groups may contain tremendous cultural diversity.

In general, Mexican Americans (those who have traditionally lived within the U.S. borders or who have immigrated to the United States from Mexico) tend to rely on their family and extended family networks. Family and the extended family members are viewed as a whole and are highly valued. Family members rely on each other for

EVIDENCE-BASED PRACTICE 10-6

Lessons Learned: Or Have They Been?

The spirit catches you and you fall down: A Hmong child, her American doctors, and the collision of two cultures (Fadiman, 1999) is required reading in many universities nationally. This book has helped students learn the importance of recognizing cultural diversity in an increasingly multicultural nation as well as the devastating results that can ensue when one's cultural values and beliefs are misunderstood and are compounded by difficult language barriers. The book is an actual narrative account about two cultures with very different values, beliefs, and practices and about health care for 3-month-old Lia Lee, who was diagnosed with epilepsy. Everyone wanted the best for Lia Lee; however, Lia Lee's parents and the pediatricians who treated her had very different ideas about what was best for Lia Lee.

In keeping with the strongly held traditions and rituals of the Hmong people, Lia Lee's parents believed that their daughter's illness was linked to spiritual matters. In the Hmong culture her illness is called "quag dab peg," which means "the spirit catches you and you fall down." Translated into English, this means "epilepsy." Her parents believed that one of Lia Lee's three souls had wandered and it was replaced by the spirit "Dab." Within the Hmong culture, those afflicted with "quag dab peg" frequently become shamans, a highly valued and respected position. Her parents believed that animal sacrifice was the "treatment" of choice. On the other hand, her physicians, in keeping with the Western medical belief system, did not take the family's beliefs about the soul into account when treating Lia Lee's epilepsy. They prescribed anticonvulsants, the accepted "best practice" of Western medicine for epilepsy.

Lia Lee's parents sought help at the local emergency department for their daughter as her epilepsy progressed to more frequent and severe seizure activity. Given the difficulty in communication and the inability of Western health care providers to understand the Hmong beliefs about quag dab peg, the results were devastating to all concerned. Her parents did not understand the treatment or the instructions provided by the health professionals. The health care providers didn't understand the choices being made by Lia Lee's parents and complained that her parents were not caring for her as instructed. Cultural misunderstandings and difficulty with comprehending the importance of cultural values and beliefs that influence health care decisions and actions led to a painful and disastrous outcome for all those involved, but especially for Lia Lee and her parents. Unfortunately, this is not an isolated incident and similar experiences happen here in this country and internationally as immigrants and others move to countries with totally different cultures and health care systems.

Clinical Application

Transcultural mental health nurses can increase skills to recognize cultural barriers, including language and difficulty with communication. They can understand the significance of diverse cultural perspectives, such as those that occurred in the clinical experiences with Lia Lee, her parents and the health-care providers.

Transcultural nursing involves trying to understand the patient's perspective, in other words, trying to understand the patient's cultural values, beliefs, experiences, expressions, practices, and cultural norms.

socialization, support (emotional and monetary), childcare and often, they expect loyalty from other members. Mexican Americans have a lower incidence of mental illness, possibly due to strong extended family connections and the role family networks play in dealing with anxiety and stresses as well as the role of religion (Leininger, 1995).

For Hispanic immigrants (who may be Mexican American) use of mental health services in the United States is low when compared to use of health care services for general health concerns. According to a report by The U.S. Department of Health and Human Services (2009) less than 1 in 11 Hispanic Americans with a mental health illness contact a mental health care provider, while less than 1 in 5 contact a health care provider for a general health concern. For Hispanic immigrants with a mental health illness, less than 1 in 20 contact a mental health care provider, while 1 in 10 contact a health care provider for general health concerns. Hispanic Americans may use a greater variety of folk treatments than seeking specific services from folk healers, known as *curanderos* or *herbalistas*.

The bonds in the traditional Mexican American family are often very strong and the father is the authority figure. Male *machismo* may encourage men to consume too much alcohol in order to express their masculinity and power (Leininger, 1995), although obviously life stressors related to poverty and living conditions often play a part. Stereotypically, machismo is viewed as "exaggerated male pride," however, in the Latino culture it is a respected position of honor vital to one's self-esteem and manhood. The father or oldest male relative is the power figure in most families and may make health decisions for other family members. In public, women show respect for their husbands, while in private, some women may hold more power. Although, family violence associated with male dominance in the Mexican American culture may be prevalent, as in other cultural groups it may be frequently underreported (Kemp, 2005).

Many Hispanic Americans use cultural folk medicine, remedies and healers, neighborhood women, naturalist shops or naturalist doctors,

called *doctora naturalista*, and naturopaths, who have gained the people's trust, are frequently used for illness, in addition to prayer and healing. Western health care is accessed for more specific purposes. Some Hispanic Americans may perceive a lack of holistic care and unnatural medicines in the U.S. health care system and this prevents a wider use of health care in the United States (Zapata & Shippee-Rice, 1999).

Religion is very influential in Hispanic communities and may play a major role in the health and illness of Hispanic Americans. Many Hispanic Americans are Roman Catholics and faith and church activities are an influential part of their daily life activities (Kemp, 2005). Some studies have identified religious and cultural barriers to professional health care as some Hispanic Americans report that they trust in God, and "if I am sick, it is his will" (Carter-Pokras et al., 2008). These attitudes often delay appropriate preventive care as well as treatment of disease and illness.

The hot and cold system is one of the most prevalent folk systems found in Mexican American cultural groups. The hot and cold system is based on balancing substances in the body and the outside environment. Various substances including food, water, and different herbs and medications are considered hot or cold. Lack of balance is thought to be the cause for illness: the mind and body are viewed as intertwined and balance is sought in all aspects of life (Berry, 2002).

Arab Muslim Cultural Groups: An Overview of Mental Health Concerns

There are over 48 countries, where at least 50% of the population is Muslim including Pakistan, Turkey, Egypt, Iran, Afghanistan, Iraq, Saudi Arabia, Syria, Libya, and Jordan to name only a few. The Arabic language is spoken in Arab Muslim countries and Islam is the main religion of the people. Islam is growing more rapidly than any other religion in the world. Those who practice the Islamic faith are considered Muslim. There are two major religious orthodoxies of Muslims, the Sunni and the Shi'a (Luna, 2002). Ramadan is the ninth month of the Islamic calendar and was the month in which the Koran was revealed to the Prophet Muhammad. During the month of Ramadan, Muslims are required to abstain from food and drink from dawn until dusk. Devout Muslims pray five times each day. Prior to prayer, each person must perform a cleansing of the body, which signifies a pure soul. In some Muslim countries, there is a preference for male children and it has been documented that female children may receive inferior care from birth (Douki, Ben Xineb, Nacef, & Halbreich, 2007).

There are a number of Islam religious requirements specific to men and women such as an un-related male should not touch females, including shaking hands, make direct eye contact with each other, or be alone in a room with one another (Simpson, 2008). In the Arab Muslim culture, women are required to avoid raising their voices so they will not be overheard by strangers (Abushaikha & Oweis, 2005). Talking in a manner in which other patients and observers can overhear what is being communicated would then seem to be incongruent with the women's needs of privacy. In a study conducted by Simpson and Carter (2008), on Muslim women's experiences with health care in the rural United States, one participant described writing a letter to her physician prior to her health care appointment to identify her religious needs. She stated: "I don't shake hands and I would prefer not to be examined by a male. I don't speak with a male unnecessarily either, and conversations with males will be succinct and to the point" (p. 19). When Arab Muslim women believed their religious beliefs were violated, they experienced feelings of guilt and viewed the health care experience as negative and when no religious beliefs were violated, they viewed their experience as more positive. However, the women also expressed an understanding that it is difficult for health care providers outside of their culture to understand all of their cultural beliefs and practices. Several women identified being treated differently by health care providers because they wore the Islamic head covering (*hijab*) (Simpson & Carter, 2008).

Seventy to 80% of mental health patients in Arab countries tend to present with somatic symptoms for psychologic issues. There is a stigma about mental health problems and the patient who presents with somatic complaints is protected from the stigma of being diagnosed with a mental health illness. However, this creates difficulties for the patient as they are treated for physical rather than psychologic problems (Okasha, 2003). Nurses and other health care providers in emergency departments need to be aware of this phenomenon and assess the patient for any mental health concerns. The subordinate position of Arab women places them at risk for developing mental health disorders such as depression, anxiety, and suicidal behaviors (Douki et al., 2007).

Prior to seeing health care professionals, Arab Muslims may seek traditional healers for mental health problems. Traditional healers hold special importance to Arab Muslim people because of their affiliation and connection to the community. Traditional healers also deal with the "'mystical,' the 'superstitious,' and the 'unknown,' all of which are still powerful cognitive constructions" in Arab Muslim countries (Okasha, 2003).

Following the terrorist attacks on 9/11, there is evidence to suggest that the experience of prejudice, intolerance, and hostility toward Arab Americans has increased in the United States. Arab Americans have been victims of racism, aggression, insulting speech, and discrimination on the basis of their cultural religious beliefs and practices and national origin (Kulwicki, Khalifa, & Moore, 2008). Arab American nurses in Detroit participated in a study to explore the influence of the terrorist attacks on 9/11 on their profession as nurses. Overall, the Arab American nurses had not experienced hate crimes or major work-related retaliation, such as termination. The discrimination the nurses did experience was in the form of verbal insults about their cultural and religious practices such as wearing a hijab, the traditional head covering worn by Muslim women. One in seven of the nurse participants had experienced a situation wherein patients and their families refused their care (Kulwicki et al., 2008).

Culturally Competent Mental Health Care

The interpretation of behavior generally transpires within the context of the specific culture in which it occurs. However, when patients and families from diverse cultural groups come to institutions of the dominant culture, the behavior is identified and interpreted by the dominant culture. Frequently, that interpretation can be misinterpreted and/or distorted if health care providers are not competent in caring for patients from diverse cultural groups. Particularly with mental health, diagnoses can be applied to patients that may be inaccurate and if the cultural behavior were understood and interpreted within the context of the specific culture, a different diagnosis might be made with different treatment or no diagnosis at all. Inaccurate mental health labels can be applied that will have a negative impact on an individual and family for years and may not be congruent with the values, beliefs, practices, and norms of the patient's culture.

Process of Cultural Competence (Cultural Awareness, Cultural Sensitivity, and Cultural Knowledge)

Most nurses understand that developing a mutually trusting relationship with patients improves plans of care and increases the likelihood of more optimal health outcomes. Developing a trusting relationship with patients is particularly important in mental health nursing care. Because of difficult experiences with past family and other relationships, it may be difficult for some patients with mental health needs to trust others, including health care providers. An understanding of the patient's culture increases the likelihood of improved health outcomes. As one's culture shapes an individual's health care values, meanings, expressions, beliefs, practices and experiences, or cultural norms, it becomes difficult to separate health care from culture. The shared values, beliefs, and practices, including how one perceives mental health, are determined to a great extent by one's culture.

Nurses are increasingly caring for patients from diverse cultures and are expected to have a broad understanding of culture in order to provide culturally competent mental health care. Culturally competent nursing care for patients from diverse cultures becomes crucial in caring for patients with mental health needs. Some questions that nurses may be asking are what exactly does **culturally congruent care** mean? How can a transcultural mental health nurse understand the cultural values, beliefs, and practices of all the culturally diverse patients a nurse will care for over the lifetime of his or her career? Well, one answer may be that, of course, you cannot understand the values, beliefs, and practices of all of the patients you will care for in your career. However, nurses can become familiar with the values, beliefs, and practices of the culturally diverse groups to whom they do provide care. This will enable them to acknowledge and recognize common cultural needs of all patients with mental health care needs.

Because of the need to understand the values, beliefs, and practices of patients with mental health care needs, a number of theories and models of culturally competent care have been developed. One of the most prominent culture-specific nursing theory is Leininger's (1991) Culture Care Diversity and Universality Theory of Nursing. Leininger theorized that understanding the patient's social structure factors (technological, religious and philosophical, kinship and social, cultural values and lifeways, political and legal, economic and educational) in addition to generic or folk systems could lead to nursing care decisions and actions that would facilitate culturally congruent nursing care and improved health and well-being of patients. Leininger (1967, 1991) identified cultural congruent care was "care that was congruent with people's lifeways" (p. 41).

Nurses have identified the importance of culturally sensitive care. Although learning to be sensitive to patient's cultural values, beliefs, and practices is important, it has became obvious that transcultural nurses needed to move beyond being "sensitive" to competency-based cultural care. **Cultural competence** is defined as a process in which nurses strive to work successfully within the cultural context of individuals, families, and communities (Andrews & Boyle, 1997; Campinha-Bacote, 2002). Campinha-Bacote (2009) identified that cultural competency "requires nurses to see themselves as becoming culturally competent rather than being culturally competent" (p. 49).

Buchwald et al. (1994) used the term "**cultural blind spot,**" sometimes referred to as **cultural blindness** to describe the assumption that if a person is similar in appearance and behaviors as the care provider, then there are no perceived cultural differences or potential barriers to giving appropriate care. The cultural blind spot supports people's beliefs that they understand the culture and have had similar cultural encounters. Thus, a person could conclude he or she has culturally competent skills. However, it is this lack of awareness of differences that creates the cultural blind spot. Transcultural mental health nurses need to be aware of the phenomenon of cultural blind spot/cultural blindness because of the unintended influence it can have on care of diverse populations of mental health patients.

Important Factors to Consider in Transcultural Mental Health Nursing Communication and Language

As most mental health nurses know, both verbal and nonverbal communications are some of the most important skills used with patients. Communication is even more important with multiculturally diverse mental health patients, where language may serve as a barrier and make the process of communication more difficult. **Interpersonal communication** helps mental health nurses assess each patient's values, beliefs, and practices about their mental health care. Communicating with each patient is important in caring for clients in a culturally congruent and competent manner.

Communication between the mental health nurse and the patient and family generally brings together the exchange of two diverse cultures, that of the nurse and that of the patient. Therefore, it is also important for nurses to have an understanding of their own cultural values, beliefs, and practices, so they can better understand the diversity between their own cultural values, beliefs, and practices and those of the patient and family, particularly as these phenomena relate to mental health care.

Culture influences each interaction we, as nurses, have with our patients. If we are not knowledgeable about the cultural context in which our communication is being interpreted, there is a possibility that our message can be misunderstood. Rosenberg (2003) described how cultural conditioning, a socialization process that influences how we think and behave, has a major impact on each of us. Becoming consciously aware of our individual cultural conditioning is a key to lessening the effect it has on us. Communication is crucial when nurses are caring for culturally diverse patients with such mental health problems as schizophrenia, bipolar disorder, or major depression, where patients and their family or kin may be confused or even fear a health care system in which they have no previous experience. Effective transcultural communication skills are particularly important when caring for mental health patients (Figure 10-4). Developing lasting meaningful relationships across potential social barriers such as ethnicity and culture contributes to improved communication.

Mental health nurses understand the importance of developing trust with patients and their family/kin networks. Taking time to develop trust with patients who do not speak English or minimal English can be very challenging, particularly given the increasingly culturally diverse population seeking mental health care. Sometimes health care providers can become irritated that patients and family members do not speak the dominant English language. When there is a possibility to have a certified translator/interpreter serve as an interpreter, that is the ideal

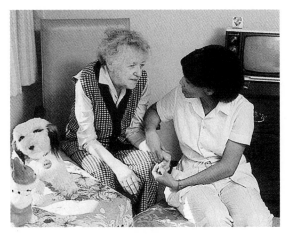

FIGURE 10-4   Effective transcultural communication skills are particularly important when caring for mental health patients. Developing lasting meaningful relationships across potential social barriers such as race contributes to improved communication.

choice rather than use family members or other staff who may not understand complex health situations. Family members should be encouraged to offer family support rather than serve as an interpreter.

People who do not speak English identify care as less supportive and more rushed than those individuals who do speak English (Simpson & Carter, 2008). However, Bowes and Domokos (1995) found that speaking the same language, while important, is not the most important element in communicating with patients from diverse cultural backgrounds. The attitude of the care provider is instrumental in helping the patient be open to treatment options. Communicating an understanding of cultural diversity helps facilitate the patient–nurse relationship. On the other hand, authoritarian care providers have a negative impact on treatment services.

Bowes and Domokos (1995) make a distinction between language and communication suggesting that language has more to do with the technical aspect of speech, while communication consists of both verbal and nonverbal elements, including the provider's attitude. For a number of cultur-

ally diverse patients and their families/kin, there are cultural values that influence what subjects are appropriate to discuss with health care providers. Some topics (sexual activities, for example) may be considered inappropriate to discuss with health care providers. Other topics that most of us consider appropriate to discuss with a health care provider in the United States are not necessarily viewed that way by persons from different cultures. For example, in Asian and Latino cultures, individuals would not communicate dissatisfaction with services. In a study on Latino health disparities, one nurse participant in the study stated "If someone does not like the doctor or does not agree, they will not speak up or say anything because they are taught that it is rude to do this" (Carter-Pokras et al., 2008, p. 163). Even in conducting a health history and assessment, what are culturally acceptable questions to ask in the United States may not be acceptable in other countries and cultures. There are other factors that may have a profound influence on the communication between patients and health care providers. Undocumented migrants may fear that health care providers would turn them in to the authorities if providers learned that their patients were in the United States illegally (Carter-Pokras et al., 2008).

Empathy is one of the most important communication skills that transcultural mental health nurses and other health care providers can use with patients from diverse cultural backgrounds. In using empathy in communicating with patients, health care providers are attempting to understand what a patient is experiencing or has experienced. You are trying to put yourself in the patient's place and feel and experience what they are feeling and experiencing. You are then communicating that understanding back to the individual patient (Egan, 2009). Empathic communication helps the health care provider to better understand the situation or context of the patient as well as the cultural norms and values that structure that context and influence the patient. For example, if a patient was sitting in his or her hospital room crying, the nurse would know to further explore that patient's feelings.

According to Rasoal, Jungert, Hau, Stwine, and Andersson (2009) the ability to use "ethnocultural empathy" (p. 300) has become crucial for health care providers in their interactions with patients. It is important to communicate back to the patient and family your understanding of their experience so they may clarify whether you have accurately identified the patient's perception of a particular experience (Egan, 2009).

Empathy becomes very important in trying to understand the experience and feelings of mental health patients and their families. Attempting to understand the experience of abuse, schizophrenia, depression, bipolar disorders, and other mental health issues is crucial to understand the perspectives of the patient and family. In communicating with patients from diverse cultures, perceptions of both the nurse and patient specific to "time, space, distance, touch, modesty, and other factors" are necessary (Andrews, 2008, p. 21). When communicating with patients from other cultures, particularly for those who do not speak English or English is a second language, there is an increased risk of miscommunication (Andrews, 2008).

Transcultural Mental Health Nursing and Spirituality

Sometimes people tend to have some difficulty differentiating spirituality and religion. In fact, frequently the terms spirituality and religion are used interchangeably. Spirituality tends to refer to a broad sense of the inner experience of the self and a search for meaning. Religion generally involves an institution with a given set of rules and observances involving devotion and ritual (see Chapter 13, Religion, Culture, and Nursing, pages 351–402). There are many spiritual and religious themes to mental health disorders such as schizophrenia, bipolar disorder, psychosis, hallucinations, and delusions. Transcultural mental health nurses care for patients who have diverse cultural values, beliefs, meanings, and practices many of which are grounded in spiritual and religious beliefs. At times, an individual's religious and spiritual beliefs may be difficult to separate from their cultural values, beliefs, meanings, expressions, and practices. This applies to patients and families from all of the world's major religious systems, Jewish, Christian, Islam, and others.

A phenomenological research study attempted to answer the question with Australian mental health patients from a community mental health center: "What does spirituality mean for people with a mental illness?" (Wilding, Muir-Cochrane, & May, 2006, p. 144). Patients were not recruited to the study if they were experiencing psychosis or exacerbation of symptoms. Findings indicated that spirituality became increasingly important in patient's lives after being diagnosed with a mental illness. Spiritual experiences of the patients could be interpreted as signs and symptoms of mental illness, depending on who was interpreting the experiences. Patients expressed a fear that mental health nurses would label them as mentally ill when their spiritual beliefs and experiences were similar to symptoms of mental illness. As we have previously discussed, the interpretation of one's cultural values, beliefs, and practices takes place within the dominant culture or power structure in which the situation or event occurs. Therefore, it is quite likely that within a mental health setting, values, beliefs and practices would be interpreted according to the mental health professional's views rather than those of the patient.

Spirituality and religious practices can play a very influential role in enhancing mental health and emotional stability. For example, many African Americans view their church as the focal point of their lives. Within the African American church emotions can be released that cannot be expressed in many other social situations and friendships established that last throughout a lifetime. The African American church functions in promoting a high level of self-esteem, particularly for those individuals and communities in poverty-stricken environments. The role of the African American church "as a cornerstone for optimal health care cannot be emphasized enough" (Geiger, Appel, Davidhizar, & Davis, 2008, p. 382). The church can often connect the African American and health care communities and play an integral role in increasing positive health outcomes for African Americans even those who do not attend church on a regular basis. In fact, the important role the African American church plays in the lives of parishioners is a clue for health care providers to partner with churches and develop culturally congruent interventions to improve care for a particular church population. Blank, Mahmood, Fox, and Guterbock (2002) found that African American churches offered more mental health services than did more mainline or European American churches. Findings also indicated that African American churches played a key role in mental health service referrals.

Bonifield (2009) in a report for CNN about African American churches fighting mental health "demons" described how African American church leaders were taking a lead in reaching out to those who need mental health services. In an effort to change attitudes about mental illness, concerned Black clergy of Atlanta established a connection with the National Alliance on Mental Illness to educate their church members about the signs and symptoms of mental illness. The church leaders suggested that it may be helpful for an individual to go to a church pastor if he or she was experiencing minor depression. Pastors were trained to recognize early signs and symptoms of depression and how to refer parishioners with major depression to mental health facilities. In another example, the Tennessee Department of Mental Health and Magellan Health Services, in collaboration with African American churches in various Tennessee communities, initiated "Emotional Fitness Centers" to screen for signs and symptoms of mental illness with parishioners seeking emotional support. Listening was stressed as the most important skill a pastor can use with someone seeking emotional support.

Mental health nurses need to practice culturally competent communication skills to improve care for an ever-increasing population of culturally diverse mental health patients. Becoming aware of the importance of communication is key to caring for this patient population. Taking into account the cultural values, beliefs, meanings, practices, expressions, and cultural norms of specific cultures takes knowledge, experience, and patience in acquiring these skills. In addition, basic verbal and nonverbal communication skills such as tone of voice, use of probes and clarification, listening, empathy, facial expressions and body gestures, for both the nurses themselves and for the patients and family members will help to improve overall communication and patient care.

Intrapersonal Reflection

Several transcultural nursing leaders identified the importance of conducting a personal inventory of one's own cultural values, beliefs, and practices to begin to identify, understand, and remove personal cultural bias, ethnocentrism, and prejudice (Andrews & Boyle, 1997; Leininger, 2000). It is important for nurses to explore and reflect on their own cultural values, beliefs, practices, expressions, meanings, and own cultural norms in order to identify and begin to understand personal biases, prejudices, and other barriers to caring for patients in a culturally congruent and competent manner. Although tolerance may be the opposite of prejudice, it is clearly an inadequate benchmark in caring for patients in a culturally competent manner. Nurses and other health care providers need to celebrate diversity and recognize the challenge to continually explore areas within themselves or others that may block or serve as barriers to caring for patients in a culturally competent manner. Each nurse needs to explore his or her own personal values, beliefs, and practices in order to recognize areas of prejudice, bias, stereotyping, and ethnocentrism of culturally diverse individuals, families, and communities.

Gordijn, Koomen, and Stapel (2001) studied whether an individual's level of knowledge of cultural stereotypes about minority groups was universal or whether that knowledge was influenced by that individual's level of prejudice. Findings indicated that an individual's level of prejudice was related to that individual's level of knowledge about cultural stereotypes with minorities. Findings such as these should encourage transcultural mental health nurses to explore their personal prejudices and biases toward people from diverse cultures and peel away and expose stereotypes that impede caring for culturally diverse patients.

Transcultural Mental Health Experiences of Pain

In mental health nursing, the patient's experience of pain can be manifested in many different ways. Unlike other somatic symptoms frequently associated with mental health issues, pain has a component that includes emotional elements. Psychosocial factors have been found to influence pain. In a study by Palmer et al. (2008) on somatic complaints, mood and self-rated health as predictors of arm pain, mental health was found to be a strong predictor of complaints of arm pain in adults from a British community. Beliefs about causation and prognosis of arm pain were also associated with persistence of symptoms.

There is increasing evidence to suggest that pain can be a physical symptom of depression and that pain and depression are common comorbidities (Williams, Jacka, Pasco, Dodd, & Berk, 2006). It seems to be extremely difficult to separate the somatic, physical component of pain from the psychologic component of pain. In a study conducted by Bonnewyn et al. (2009) researchers found that chronic pain and mood disorders were common in elderly populations. Elderly individuals with a 12-month major depressive episode were more likely to have painful physical symptoms than those persons without major depression.

There is the concept of psychosomatic pain or pain with psychologic components and this pain is expressed differently by cultural groups. One of the distinct types of depression with Haitian women is *"Douluer de Corps* (pain in the body)" (Nicholas et al., 2007, p. 87). Barkwell (2005) studied Native Americans (Ojibwa) with cancer pain; they described their pain as "all that was

most painful in life" and included the following properties in their description of cancer pain: "physical sensation, threatening cognitions, emotional, social and spiritual anguish, and intuitive sensing" (p. 454). In a study to differentiate somatic versus psychologic symptoms as a cultural expression of depression, Chinese outpatients reported more somatic symptoms compared to Euro-Canadians, who reported more psychologic symptoms specific to the diagnosis of depression (Ryder et al., 2008).

Lee, Kleinman, and Kleinman (2007) have suggested that current knowledge about depression and other mental illnesses is based on research conducted with Western populations. In a study with Chinese patients in Guangzhou (Canton), China, in an outpatient mental health service, patients experiencing symptoms of depression identified numerous affective symptoms, including sadness, preverbal pain, social disharmony, and sleeplessness. The authors emphasized how important it is to study depression transculturally, in order to be more sensitive and appropriate with culturally diverse populations.

SUMMARY

This chapter has explored perspectives on transcultural mental health nursing care. The goal is to help nurses provide culturally competent care that improves the health and well-being of culturally diverse mental health patients. Nurses can increase their competency by understanding cultural values, beliefs, practices, meanings, expressions, and cultural norms of diverse cultures specific to the mental health and well-being of individuals, families/kin, and communities. Competency-based transcultural knowledge is essential in today's complex mental health environment.

REVIEW QUESTIONS

1. Describe the influence of culture on mental health care values, beliefs, and practices.
2. Identify specific cultural values, beliefs, and practices of three diverse cultural groups

and how transcultural mental health nurses might facilitate culturally congruent care in a mental health care system.

3. Compare and contrast your cultural values, beliefs, and practices about mental health care with that of another cultural group.

4. Critically explore and reflect on any personal or familial biases, prejudices, and other culturally specific barriers that would impact your ability to provide culturally congruent care.

5. Identify five communication skills that facilitate culturally competent mental health care.

CRITICAL THINKING ACTIVITIES

1. Describe a personal clinical experience you have had or observed where a cultural misunderstanding occurred. How did you feel either as a participant or as an observer? How do you believe the other individual(s) involved in the situation felt? How might the situation have been resolved in a culturally congruent manner?

2. Role play several clinical situations in which cultural misunderstandings occurred. Then role play how you would resolve the cultural misunderstandings in a culturally congruent manner?

3. Describe several cultural spiritual/religious beliefs and practices that may be incorrectly interpreted as signs and symptoms of a mental health diagnosis. Describe the impact an incorrect mental health diagnosis and label might have on individuals' lives.

4. An activity to collect data on knowledge and skills for culturally congruent transcultural mental health nursing involves interviewing someone from a culture that is very different from your own. Practice some basic interpersonal communication skills to get to know the person and establish some basic trust, ask the individual about their values, beliefs, and practices related to mental health and mental illness. Then search the literature for information to read about that individuals cultural group. Regardless of whether your interviewee is from Haiti, Japan, or another cultural group, is gay, young, or elderly, consider if what you have read either represents

or does not represent the individual you have interviewed.

5. Talk about various times in your life that you have been involved with a group of people with whom you have felt comfortable, connected to, and shared similar values, beliefs, and practices. Talk about the times in your life that you have been involved with a group of people with whom you did not feel comfortable with, connected to, and did not share similar values, beliefs, and practices. Compare and contrast those different experiences in your life. Talk about how it might feel for an individual from a different culture to come into the group you felt comfortable with, connected to, and shared similar values, beliefs, and practices.

6. You are working with several nurses who imitate patients and their families who have difficulty speaking English and make fun of some of the cultural values, beliefs, and practices of culturally diverse individuals and families who are different from their own. How might you deal with this situation? Try role playing the situation from different perspectives and different communication skills not only to challenge the actions of your coworkers, but to help them begin to understand the impact of their behavior on others.

7. You are working with a patient and his or her extended family who do not speak English. Talk about some ways you might communicate with your patient and the family. Role play some options you might try to communicate with your patient and family.

8. You are caring for a patient from an Arab Muslim culture in a clinical setting and the patient is exhibiting behaviors that you believe may be signs and symptoms of mental illness. Describe some of the signs and symptoms you might be observing. Describe some of the techniques you might use to differentiate whether the behavior is a manifestation of cultural values, beliefs, and practices you are not familiar with or are a result of a mental illness?

REFERENCES

Abushaikha, L., & Oweis, A. (2005). Labor pain experience and intensity: A Jordanian perspective. *International Journal of Nursing Practice, 11*(1), 33–38.

Adams, J. R., & Drake, R. E. (2006). Shared decision-making and evidence-based practice. *Community Mental Health Journal, 42*(1), 87–105.

Ahnallen, J. M., Suyemoto, K. L., & Carter, A. S. (2006). Relationship between physical appearance, sense of belonging and exclusion, and racial/ethnic self-identification among multiracial Japanese European Americans. *Cultural Diversity and Ethnic Minority Psychology, 12*, 673–686.

Al-Omari, H., & Pallikkathayil, L. (2008). Psychological acculturation: A concept analysis with implications for nursing practice. *The Journal of Transcultural Nursing, 19*, 126–133.

American Psychiatric Association. (2000). *Diagnostic and statistical manual of mental disorders* (4th ed.-text revision). Washington, DC: American Psychiatric Association.

Andrews, M. M. (2008). *Culturally competent nursing care*. In M. M. Andrews & J. S. Boyle (Eds.). Transcultural concepts in nursing care (5th ed.). New York, NY: Wolters Kluwer/Lippincott Williams & Wilkins.

Andrews, M. M., & Boyle, J. S. (1997). Competence in transcultural nursing care. *American Journal of Nursing, 98*(8), 16AAA–16DDD.

Armour, M. P., Bradshaw, W., & Roseborough, D. (2009). African Americans and recovery from severe mental illness. *Social Work in Mental Health, 7*(6), 602–622.

Barkwell, D. (2005). Cancer pain: Voices of the Ojibway people. *Journal of Pain and Symptom Management, 30*(5), 454–464.

Battle, S. (1990). *Moving targets: Alcohol, crack, and Black women*. In E. C. White (Ed.). *The Black women's health book: Speaking for ourselves*. Seattle: The Seal Press.

Bell, P., & Peterson, D. (1992). *Cultural pain and African Americans: Unspoken issues in early recovery*. Hazeldon Pub.

Berry, A. (2002). Culture care of the Mexican American family, In Leininger, M. & McFarland, M. R. (Eds.), *Transcultural nursing: Concepts, theories, research & practice* (3rd ed., pp. 363–373). New York, NY: McGraw-Hill.

Blank, M. B., Mahmood, M., Fox, J. C., & Guterbock, T. (2002). Alternative mental health services: The role of the Black Church in the South. *American Journal of Public Health, 92*(10), 1668–1672.

Bonifield, J. (2009). African-American churches fighting mental health 'demons.' *CNN: Paging Dr. Gupta*, July 17, 1–6. URL: http://pagingdrgupta.blogs.cnn.com/2009/07/17/african-american-churches-fighting-mental-health-demons

Bonnewyn, A., Katona, C., Bruffaerts, R., Haro, J. M., de Graaf, R., Alonso, J., & Demyttenaere, K., (2009). Pain and depression in older people: Comorbidity and patterns of help seeking. *Journal of Affective Disorders, 117*(3), 193–196.

Bowes, A., & Domokos, T. (1995). South Asian women and their GPs: Some issues of communication. *Social Sciences in Health: International Journal of Research & Practice, 1*(1), 22–33.

Boyle, J. S. (2008). Transcultural perspectives in the nursing care of adults. In M. M. Andrews & J. S. Boyle (Eds.). *Transcultural concepts in nursing care* (5th ed.). New York, NY: Wolters Kluwer/Lippincott Williams & Wilkins.

Buchwald, D., Caralis, P. V., Gany, F., Hardt, E. J., Johnson, T. M., Muecke, M. A., & Putsch, R. W. (1994). Caring for patients in a multicultural society. *Patient Care, 28*, 105–123.

Campinha-Bacote, J. (2002). The process of cultural competence in the delivery of healthcare services: A model of care. *Journal of Transcultural Nursing, 13*(3), 181–184.

Campinha-Bacote, J. (2009). A culturally competent model of care for African Americans. *Urologic Nursing, 29*(1), 49–54.

Carter-Pokras, O., Brown, P., Martinez, I., Solano, H., Rivera, M., & Pierpont, Y. (April 2008). Latin American–trained nurse perspective on Latino health disparities. *Journal of Transcultural Nursing, 19*(2), 161–166.

Choi, J., Miller, A., & Wilbur, J. (2009). Acculturation and depressive symptoms in Korean immigrant women. *Journal of Immigrant Minority Health, 11*, 13–19.

Constantine, M. G., & Sue, D. W. (2006a). Factors contributing to optimal human functioning in people of color in the United States. *Counseling Psychologist, 34*, 228–244.

Constantine, M. G., & Sue, D. W. (Eds.). (2006b). *Addressing racism: Facilitating cultural competence in mental health and educational settings*. Hoboken, NJ: John Wiley & Sons.

Day, J. C. (1996). *Population projections of the United States by age, sex, race, and Hispanic origin: 1995 to 2050*, U.S. Bureau of the Census, Current Population Reports, P25–1130, Washington, DC: U.S. Government Printing Office. Available online at http://www.census.gov/prod/1/pop/p25-1130/p251130a.pdf

DeCoteau, T., Anderson, J., & Hope, D. (2006). Adapting manualized treatments: Treating anxiety disorders among Native Americans. *Cognitive and Behavioral Practice, 13*, 304–309.

Douki, S., Ben Xineb, S., Nacef, F., & Halbreich, U. (2007). Women's mental health in the Muslim world: Cultural, religious, and social issues. *Journal of Affective Disorders, 102*(1–3), 177–189.

Egan, G. (2009). *The skilled helper: A problem management and opportunity development approach to helping*, Belmont, CA: Thomson Brooks/Cole.

Ehrmin, J. T. (2000). Cultural implications of the 12-approach in addictions treatment and recovery. *Journal of Addictions Nursing, 12*, 37–41.

Ehrmin, J. T. (2001). Unresolved feelings of guilt and shame in the maternal role with substance-dependent African-American women. *Journal of Nursing Scholarship, 33,* 53–58.

Ehrmin, J. T. (2002). Family violence and culture care with African and Euro-American cultures in the United States. In M. Leininger& M. R. McFarland (Eds.). *Transcultural nursing: Concepts, theories, research & practice* (3rd ed., pp. 333–346). New York, NY: McGraw-Hill.

Ehrmin, J. T. (2005). Dimensions of culture care for substance-dependent African American women. *The Journal of Transcultural Nursing, 16,* 117–125.

Estroff, S. E. (1981). *Making it crazy: An ethnography of psychiatric clients in an American Community.* Los Angeles: University of California Press.

Fadiman, A. (1999). *The spirit catches you and you fall down: A Hmong child, her American doctors, and the collision of two cultures.* New York: The Noonday Press, Farrar, Straus and Giroux.

Federally Recognized Indian Tribes. Federal Register: July 12, 2002 (volume 67, no. 134) Notices (pp. 46327–46333).

Freire, P. (1970/1990). *Pedagogy of the oppressed.* New York: The Continuum Publishing Company.

Gamm, L. D., & Hutchison, L. L. (2003) *Rural Healthy People 2010: A companion document to healthy people 2010* (Vol. 1). College Station, TX: The Texas A&M University System Health Science Center, School of Rural Public Health, Southwest Rural Health Research Center. Available online at http://www.srph.tamhsc.edu/centers/rhp2010/Volume_3/Vol3rhp2010.pdf.

Geiger, J. N., Appel, S. J., Davidhizar, R., & Davis, C. (2008). Church and spirituality in the lives of the African American community. *Journal of Transcultural Nursing, 19*(4), 375–383.

Gilbert, P., Bhundia, R., Mitra, R., Mcewan, K., Irons, C., & Sanghera, J. (March, 2007). Cultural differences in shame-focused attitudes towards mental health problems in Asian and Non-Asian student women. *Mental Health, Religion & Culture, 10*(2), 127–141.

Gone, J. P. (2009). A community-based treatment for Native American historical trauma: Prospects for evidence-based practice. *Journal of Consulting and Clinical Psychology, 77*(4), 751–762.

Gone, J. P., & Alcantara, C. (2007). Identifying effective mental health interventions for American Indians and Alaska Natives: A review of the literature. *Cultural Diversity an Ethnic Minority Psychology, 13*(4), 356–363.

Gordijn, E. H., Koomen, W., & Stapel, D. A. (2001). Level of prejudice in relation to knowledge of cultural stereotypes. *Journal of Experimental Social Psychology, 37,* 150–157.

Hales, R., Yudofsky, S., & Gabbard, G. (Eds.). (2008). *The American Psychiatric Publishing Textbook of Psychiatry* (5th ed.). Arlington, Virginia: American Psychiatric Publishing, Inc.

Jang, Y., Kim, G., Hansen, L., & Chiriboga, D. A. (2007). Attitudes of older Korean Americans toward mental health services. *Journal of the American Geriatric Society, 55,* 616–620.

Johnston, M. S. (2008). *Northern British Columbian Aboriginal mothers: Raising adolescents with fetal alcohol spectrum disorder.* Doctoral Dissertation. The University of Arizona, Tucson, AZ.

Kaplan, J. S., & Sue, S. (1997) Ethnic psychology in the United States. In D. F. Halpern & A. E. Voiskounsky (Eds.). *States of mind: American and post-Soviet perspectives on contemporary issues in psychotherapy* (pp. 349–369). New York: Oxford University Press.

Kasl, C. D. (1992). *Many roads one journey: Moving beyond the 12 steps.* New York, NY: Harper Collins.

Kemp, C. (2005). Mexican and Mexican-Americans: Health beliefs & practices, URL, http://bearspace.baylor.edu/Charles_Kemp/www/hispanic_health.htm

Kessler, R. C., Chiu, W. T., Demler, O., & Walters, E. E. (2005). Prevalence, severity, and comorbidity of twelve-month DSM IV disorders in the National Comorbidity Survey Replication (NCS-R). *Archives of General Psychiatry, 62,* 617–627.

Kulwicki, A., Khalifa, R., & Moore, G. (2008). The effects of September 11 on Arab American nurses in metropolitan Detroit. *Journal of Transcultural Nursing, 19*(2), 134–139.

Lamberg, L. (2009). Children of Immigrants may face stresses, challenges that affect mental health. *Journal of the American Medical Association, 300*(7), 780–781.

Lee, D. T. S., Kleinman, J., & Kleinman, A. (2007). Rethinking depression: An ethnographic study of the experiences of depression among Chinese. *Harvard Review of Psychiatry, 15,* 1–8.

Leininger, M. M. (1967). The culture concept and its relevance to nursing. *Journal of Nursing Education, 6*(2), 27–39.

Leininger, M. M. (1991). The theory of culture care diversity and universality. In M. M. Leininger (Ed.). *Culture care diversity and universality: A theory of nursing* (pp. 5–68). New York, NY: National League for Nursing Press.

Leininger, M. M. (1995). *Transcultural nursing: Concepts, theories, research and practices.* New York: McGraw-Hill.

Leininger, M. M. (2000). Founders focus: Transcultural nursing is discovery of self and the world of others. *The Journal of Transcultural Nursing, 11,* 312–313.

Leininger, M. M., & McFarland, M. R. (2002). *Transcultural nursing: Concepts, theories, research and practice* (3rd ed.). New York: McGraw Hill.

Lopez, S. J., Magyar-Moe, J. L., Petersen, S. E., Ryder, J. A., Krieshok, T. S., O'Byrne, K. K., & Fry, N. A. (2006). Counseling psychology's focus on positive aspects of human functioning. *The Counseling Psychologist, 34,* 205–227.

Luna, L. J. (2002). Arab Muslims and culture care. In M. Leininger & M. R. McFarland (Eds.). *Transcultural nursing: Concepts, theories, research & practice* (3rd ed., pp. 301–332). New York, NY: McGraw-Hill.

Manson, S. M. (2003). Extending the boundaries, bridging the gaps: Crafting mental health: culture, race, and ethnicity, a supplement to the Surgeon General's Report on Mental Health. *Culture, Medicine and Psychiatry, 27,* 395–408.

NPR: Recognizing Depression and Suicide Risk in Black Men. (December 27, 2005). Retrieved October 2, 2010, from http://www.npr.org/templates.story///story.php?storyId=5070636

Nicholas, G., Desilva, A. M., Subrebost, K., Breland-Noble, A., Gonzalez-Eastep, D., Manning, N., . . ., Prater, K. (2007). Expression and treatment of depression among Haitian immigrant women in the United States: Clinical observations. *American Journal of Psychotherapy, 61*(1), 83–98.

Oberg, K. (1960). Cultural shock: Adjustment to new cultural environments. *Practical Anthropology, 7,* 177–182.

Okasha, A. (Fall 2003). *Arab studies quarterly.* URL: http://findarticles.com/p/articles/mi_m2501/is_4_25/ai_n6129825

Palmer, K. T., Reading, I., Linaker, C., Calnan, M., & Coggon, D. (2008). Population-based cohort study of incident and persistent arm pain: Role of mental health, self-rated health and health beliefs. *Pain, 136,* 30–37.

Phillips, J., & Grady, P., (2002). Reducing health disparities in the twenty-first century: Opportunities for nursing research, *Nursing Outlook, 50,* 117–120.

Pope, R. C., Wallhagen, M., & Davis, H. (2010). The social determinants of substance abuse in African American baby boomers: Effects of family, media images, and environment. *Journal of Transcultural Nursing, 21,* 246–256.

Rasoal, C., Jungert, T., Hau, S., Stwine, E. E., & Andersson, G. (2009). Ethnocultural empathy among students in health care education. *Evaluation & the Health Professions, 32*(3), 300–313.

Redfield, R., Linton, R., & Herskovits, M. (1936). Memorandum on the study of acculturation. *American Anthropologist, 38,* 149–152.

Rosenberg, M. B. (2003). *Nonviolent communication: A language of life.* Encinitas, CA: PuddleDance Press.

Ryder, G., Yang, J., Zhu, X., Yao, S., Yi, J., Heine, S. J., & Bagby, M. R. (2008). The Cultural shaping of depression: Somatic symptoms in china, psychological symptoms in North America? *Journal of Abnormal Psychology, 117* (2), 300–313.

Shellman, J., & Mokel, M. (2010). Overcoming barriers to conducting an intervention study of depression in an older African American population. *Journal of Transcultural Nursing, 21*(4), 361–369.

Simpson, J. L., & Carter, K. (2008). Muslim women's experiences with health care providers in a rural area of the United States. *Journal of Transcultural Nursing, 19*(1), 16–23.

Smith, G. R. (2007). Health disparities: what can nursing do? *Policy, Politics & Nursing Practice, 8,* 285–291.

Struthers, R., & Lowe, J. (2003). Nursing in the Native American culture and historical trauma. *Issues in Mental Health Nursing, 24*(3), 257–272.

Sutherland, L. L. (2002). Ethnocentrism in a pluralistic society: A concept analysis. *Journal of Transcultural Nursing, 13*(4), 274–281.

Taliaferro, P. (2006). The myth about black men and suicide. Retrieved October 2, 2010, from http://www.blackvoices.com/blacklifestyle/health_headlines_features advice/canvas/feat

Tanenbaum, S. J., (2008). Consumer perspectives on information and other inputs to decision-making: Implications for evidence-based practice. *Community Mental Health Journal, 44,* 331–335.

United States Census Bureau. (2008). quickfacts.census.gov/qfd/states/00000.html

U.S. Department of Health and Human Services. (1999). *Mental health: A report of the surgeon general.* Rockville, MD: U.S. Department of Health and Human Services, Substance Abuse and Mental Health Services Administration, Center for Mental Health Services, National Institutes of Health, National Institute of Mental Health. Available online at http://www.surgeongeneral.gov/library/mentalhealth/home.html

U.S. Department of Health and Human Services. (January, 2001a). HHS Reshaping the Health of Minority Communities and Underserved Populations, Available online at http://www.hhs.gov/news/press/2001pres/01fsminhlth.html

U.S. Department of Health and Human Services. (2001b). *Mental health: Culture, race, and ethnicity—A supplement to mental health: A report of the surgeon general.* Rockville, MD: U.S. Department of Health and Human Services, Substance Abuse and Mental Health Services Administration, Center for Mental Health Services. August, Inventory Number: SMA-01-3613. Available online from: http://www.surgeongeneral.gov/library/mentalhealth/cre/

U.S. Department of Health and Human Services. (October, 2001c). *Healthy people 2010: Understanding and improving health* (2nd ed.). Washington: Government Printing Office, Document Stock No.: 017-001-00550-9. Available online from http://www.healthypeople.gov/Document/pdf/uih/uih.pdf

U.S. Department of Health and Human Services. (2009). Office of the Surgeon General, SAMHSA, Fact sheet: Latino / Hispanic Americans. Retrieved October 25, 2009, from http://mentalhealth.samhsa.gov/cre/fact3.asp

Walsh, S., Shulman, S., & Maurer, O. (2008). Immigration distress, mental health status and coping among young immigrants: A 1-year follow up study. *International Journal of Intercultural Relations, 32,* 371–384.

Weisfeld, A., & Perflman, R. L. (2005). Disparities and discrimination in health care. *Perspectives in Biology and Medicine, 48,* S1–S9.

Wilding, C., Muir-Cochrane, E., & May, E. (2006). Treading lightly: Spirituality issues in mental health nursing. *International Journal of Mental Health Nursing, 15,* 144–152.

Williams, C. (1992). *No Hiding Place, Empowerment and Recovery for Our Troubled Communities,* San Francisco: Harper San Francisco.

Williams, L. J., Jacka, F. N., Pasco, J. A., Dodd, S., & Berk, M. (2006). Depression and pain: An overview. *Acta Neuropsychiatrica, 18,* 79–87.

World Health Organization. (September 2007). *Fact sheet no 220.* Retrieved from http://www.who.int/mediacentre/factsheets/fs220/en/

Yellow Horse Brave Heart, M., & DeBruyn, L. M. (1998). The American Indian holocaust: Healing historical unresolved grief. *American Indian & Alaska Native Mental Health Research, 8*(2), 56–78.

Yurkovich, E. E., & Lattergrass, I. (2008). Defining health and unhealthiness: Perceptions held by Native American Indians with persistent mental illness. *Mental Health, Religion & Culture, 11*(5), 437–459.

Zapata, J., & Shippee-Rice, R. (1999). The use of folk healing and healers by six Latinos living in New England: A preliminary study. *Journal of Transcultural Nursing, 10*(2), 136–142.

Zayas, L. H., Torres, L. R., and Cabassa, L. J. (2009). Diagnostic, symptom, and functional assessments of Hispanic outpatients in community mental health practice. *Community Mental Health Journal, 45,* 97–105.

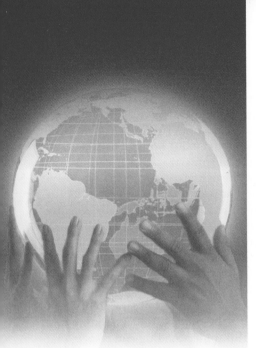

Culture, Family, and Community

Joyceen S. Boyle and
Martha B. Baird

KEY TERMS

Acculturation
Aggregates
Alternative therapies
Assimilation
Asylee
Community-based nursing
Community-based settings
Community health nursing
Community nursing
Community settings
Cultural assessment
Cultural health care systems
Cultural knowledge
Culturally competent care
Dinka culture
Epidemiologic model
Immigrants
Kinship
Levels of prevention
Primary prevention
Refugee
Secondary prevention
Specialized community interventions
Subcultures
Sudanese culture
Tertiary prevention
Traditional health beliefs
   and practices
Worldview

LEARNING OBJECTIVES

1. Use cultural concepts to provide care to families, communities, and aggregates.
2. Understand the necessary components of a cultural assessment of an aggregate group.
3. Explore interactions of community and culture as they relate to concepts of community-based practice and specialized community interventions.
4. Analyze how cultural factors influence health and illness of groups.
5. Critically evaluate potential health problems and solutions in refugee and immigrant populations.
6. Assess factors that influence the health of diverse groups within the community.

An understanding of culture and cultural concepts enhances the nurse's knowledge and facilitates culturally competent nursing care in **community-based settings**. Currently, many nurses practice in community settings with clients from a wide variety of cultural backgrounds, and this trend is expected to increase with more nurses moving from acute care institutions to community settings. The care of clients in the community can be extremely complex, calling for a high level of nursing skill. In addition, it is predicted that cultural diversity will increase in the

United States. Trends in the health care delivery system as well as an increased emphasis on health promotion and disease prevention have influenced nurses to make changes in their practice as well as the setting in which care is delivered. Concepts such as partnership, collaboration, empowerment, and facilitation now form the basis for community-based nursing practice with individuals, families, and **aggregates** in the community. For some time, national nursing associations, including the National Institute of Nursing Research (NINR), have urged a community focus in both nursing research and practice. For example, NINR defines community-based services as those services requiring "active involvement of clients and communities in assessing the needs for care, designing service programs, implementing interventions, and evaluating outcomes" (NINR, 1995, p. 2). Although it is possible to provide community-based nursing services to individuals and families in communities as well as to provide community-oriented nursing care to either the community or groups within the community, for **culturally competent care** to be provided, clients and populations must be involved in all aspects of the care or services. Indeed, it is this focus—involving clients in planning for and providing nursing services that is the foundation of culturally competent care.

Specialized community interventions that are culturally relevant to the people served are built on collaboration and partnerships between community leaders, health consumers, and health care providers. When community residents or health consumers are involved as partners, community-based services are more likely to be responsive to locally defined needs, are better used, and are sustained through local action. The NINR has stated that "until recently...research tended primarily to address the needs of the majority population, with little examination of cultural or gender-based influences on disease incidence or health outcomes often seen among diverse communities" (NINR, Specialized Community Interventions, p. 1, September 2007). Specialized community interventions are complex and often fragile. They require a high level of nursing

knowledge and skill in working with and relating to different individuals and groups. In many instances, the complexity is increased when clients and their families come from diverse cultures. Nurses must understand how to help persons from various cultures work with community leaders and health care providers to form partnerships that are responsive and can structure nursing care in ways that are culturally sensitive and appropriate. It is often the cultural factors that determine whether a particular population or group will choose to participate in community-based health services. There is always a need for continuing communication among health care providers and community residents that is characterized by mutual understanding and respect. It is this understanding and respect that forms the basis for culturally relevant and competent nursing care.

In this chapter, the terms **community nursing**, **community-based nursing**, and **community health nursing** are used interchangeably, even though they have different meanings in some settings and in different contexts (Clark, 2008). Whether the nurse is employed as a community health nurse in a health department or practices in a community-based setting, he or she needs the knowledge and skills to provide culturally competent care. The practice of nursing in a community setting requires that nurses be comfortable with clients from diverse cultures and the broader socioeconomic context in which they live. As the U.S. population continues to grow in diversity, health disparities have become more apparent in diverse populations and are now a vital area of focus for researchers and practitioners alike.

Care that is not congruent with the client's value system is likely to increase the cost of care because it compromises quality and inhibits access to services. Furthermore, members of diverse cultural groups, such as the officially designated minority groups in the United States, tend to experience greater health disparities than do members of the general population. This was the impetus for targeting the four ethnic minority groups in *Healthy People 2000*

(U.S. Department of Health and Human Services, 1990) and *Healthy People 2010* (U.S. Department of Health and Human Services, 2000) because cultural diversity must be respected and taken into account by health care professionals. Equally important, we must address the stark disparities that exist in health status between minority groups and the wider American society.

Overview of Culturally Competent Nursing Care in Community Settings

Nurses practice in many settings within the community, including work sites, schools, physicians' offices, health care program sites, churches, and the community itself (Figure 11-1). The use of **cultural knowledge** in community-based nursing practice begins with a careful assessment of

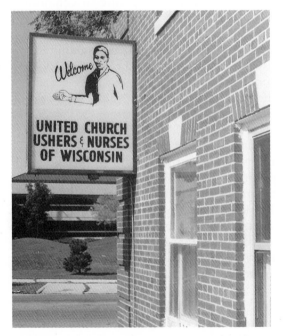

FIGURE 11-1 Some African American churches are organized to meet health, social, and emotional needs of church members.

clients and families in their own environments. Cultural data that have implications for nursing care are selected from clients, families, and the environment during the assessment phase and are discussed with the client and family to develop mutually shared goals.

Community nurses are particularly challenged when they frequently encounter clients and families who must change behaviors and living patterns to maintain health or promote wellness. Nursing interventions based on cultural knowledge help clients and families to adjust more easily and assist nurses to work effectively and comfortably with all clients, especially those from different cultural backgrounds.

Cultural data are important in the care of all clients; however, in community nursing, they are a prerequisite to successful nursing interventions. Community nursing is practiced in a community setting, often in the home of the client, and frequently requires more active participation by the client and family. Usually, the client and family must make basic changes in lifestyle, such as changes in diet and exercise patterns. Cultural competence requires that the nurse understand the family lifestyle and value system, as well as those cultural forces that are powerful determinants of health-related behaviors. Nurses often work closely with clients with chronic diseases or those who have other health problems and nursing interventions must include aspects of counseling and education as well as anticipatory guidance directed toward helping clients and families adjust to what may be lifelong conditions. Nursing care must take account of the diverse cultural factors that will motivate clients to make successful changes in behavior because improvement in health status requires lifestyle and behavioral modifications.

Transcultural nursing practice has the potential to improve the health of the community as well as the health of individual clients and families. An additional consideration of the nurse who is involved in community-focused planning is the health needs of populations at risk. Special at-risk groups can be found in all communities: the homeless, the poor, persons with HIV/AIDS and/ or tuberculosis, refugees, prison populations, and even the elderly are groups at risk for decreased health status. From a community standpoint, an understanding of culture and cultural concepts will increase the skill and abilities of the nurse to work with diverse groups within the community. Identification of high-risk groups and appropriate community-based strategies to reduce health risks requires considerable knowledge about cultural and ethnic groups and their place in the community.

Consider if you will, what problems might arise if one were to design a health program for a community composed primarily of Somali refugees who recently arrived in the United States. They may have spent years in refugee camps in other countries and lost many family members, or their family members may be still in Somalia and they are now making a life for themselves in a strange country. Certainly language would be a major problem, but so could many other cultural differences, from nuances in communication to differences in beliefs of what constitutes health and illness, as well as treatment and cure. A failure to understand and deal with these differences would have serious implications for the success of any health or nursing intervention. Nurses, who have knowledge of, and an ability to work with, diverse cultures are able to devise effective community interventions to reduce risks that are consistent with the community and group, as well as individual values and beliefs of community members.

A Transcultural Framework

A distinguishing and important aspect of community-based nursing practice is the nursing focus on the community as the client (Nies & McEwen, 2007; Stanhope & Lancaster, 2006). Effective community nursing practice must reflect accurate knowledge of the causes and distribution of health problems and of effective interventions that are congruent with the values and goals of the community. An **epidemiologic model** can be used by the community nurse to collect, organize, and analyze information about high-risk groups that are encountered in community practice.

An epidemiologic model emphasizes human biology, environment, lifestyle, and the health care system; however, with modifications, the nurse can use this model to collect cultural data that influence the health of the community (Clark, 2008). The epidemiologic model focuses on the community or on aggregate groups rather than on individuals or families. Using a cultural overlay with the epidemiologic model enhances nurse-community interactions in numerous ways.

Identifying Subcultures and Devising Specialized Community-Based Interventions

A transcultural framework for nursing care helps the nurse to identify subcultures within the larger community and to devise community-based interventions that are specific to community health and nursing goals. For example, in the multicultural societies of the United States, it is common to speak of "the Black community," "the Hispanic community," or "the Francophone community." We might also speak more broadly of "the immigrant community" or the "refugee community" or of other unique groups within or near a local community. A cultural focus allows this variety and facilitates data collection about specific groups based on their health risks. A cultural/epidemiologic framework facilitates a view of the community as a complex collective yet allows for diversity within the whole. Interventions that are successful in one subgroup may fail with another subgroup of the same community, and often the failure can be attributed to cultural differences or barriers that arise because of these differences.

Identifying and Analyzing Various Components of the Community

Transcultural concepts often are useful in identifying and analyzing various components of the community, such as social structure and religious and political systems. A cultural approach allows the nurse to identify **cultural health care systems**, which are made up of individuals who experience illness as well as those who provide care for them. Anderson and McFarlane (2008) suggest that each cultural health care system can have as many as three recognized sectors, most commonly referred to as popular, folk, and professional. We often forget that alternative health systems as well as **alternative therapies** exist side by side with the professional system. How individuals organize themselves to meet group and individual needs within cultural health care systems is important information for community and transcultural nurses. An assessment of whether social institutions such as churches and schools meet the health, social, and emotional needs of their members, and whether the health and political systems are responsive to the needs of all residents, can sometimes pinpoint critical needs and identify gaps in care. Cultural traditions within a community often determine the structure of community support systems as well as how resources are organized and distributed.

Identifying the Values and Cultural Norms of a Community

A transcultural framework is essential to the community nurse's identification of the values and cultural norms of a community. Although values are universal features of all cultures, their types and expressions vary widely, even within the same community. Values often serve as the foundation for a community's acceptance and use of health resources or a group's participation in community-based intervention programs to promote health and wellness. Just as nurses share data and collaborate with clients and families to establish mutually acceptable goals for nursing care, the community-based nurse works with the community or aggregates within the community to plan community-focused health programs. In addition to forming partnerships with communities, the community nurse considers the influences of social, economic, ecologic, and political issues.

Larger policy issues directly and profoundly affect many, if not all, community health issues. These larger policy issues are, in turn, influenced by the wider national and/or international culture. An example of this can be seen in the recent emphasis on bioterrorism, now a focus and concern of local and state health departments as well as at the national level.

Cultural Issues in Community Nursing Practice

The need for nurses to be sensitive to clients who are culturally different is increasing as we become more aware of the complex interactions between health care providers and clients and how these interactions might affect the client's health. Diverse client groups who have limited access to health services, along with barriers resulting from language and cultural differences often suffer a variety of health disparities (NINR, Specialized Community Interventions, September, 2007). The material in this chapter will assist nurses to be aware of cultural factors that affect health, illness, and the practice of nursing in community settings. Several cultural assessment tools or guides are available that provide comprehensive frameworks to guide the nurse in the assessment of cultural factors in the care of individuals, families, and groups. The Andrews/Boyle Transcultural Nursing Assessment Guides (see Appendices A and B) provide outlines for the nurse to collect and assess cultural data relevant to individuals, families, and communities. The majority of cultural assessment guides are oriented to individuals and occasionally to families. Only a few have the comprehensive view necessary for assessing cultural factors for intervention at the community level. Because individual clients and their families constitute larger communities, nurses who work in community settings must understand cultural issues as they relate to individuals and families as well as communities. We shall begin with a discussion of cultural influences on individuals and families before moving to a discussion of cultural factors within communities.

Cultural Influences on Individuals and Families

Cultural influences—those values, norms, beliefs, and behaviors—have a profound effect on health. When assessing individuals and families, the community health nurse should carefully examine the following:

1. Family roles, typical family households and structure, and dynamics in the family, particularly communication patterns and decision making
2. Health beliefs and practices related to disease causation, treatment of illness, and the use of indigenous healers or folk practitioners and other alternative/complementary therapies
3. Patterns of daily living, including work, school, and leisure activities
4. Social networks, including friends, neighbors, kin, and significant others, and how they influence health and illness
5. Ethnic, cultural, or national identity of client and family, for example, identification with a particular group, including language
6. Nutritional practices and how they relate to cultural factors and health
7. Religious preferences and influences on well-being, health maintenance, and illness, as well as the impact religion might have on daily living and taboos or restrictions arising from religious beliefs that might influence health status or care
8. Culturally appropriate behavior styles, including what is manifested during anger, competition, and cooperation, as well as relationships with health care professionals, relationships between genders, and relations with other groups in the community.

A cultural assessment of individuals and families includes all the preceding factors. This list is by no means exhaustive; rather, it is presented as a guide for community nurses as they assess cultural aspects of individuals and families. Cultural values shape human health behaviors and determine what individuals and families will do to maintain their health status, how they will care for themselves and others who become ill, and where and from whom they will seek health care. Most importantly family members are often the ones who decide on the course of treatment. Families have an important role in the transmission of cultural values and learned behaviors that relate to both health and illness. It is in the family context that individuals learn basic ways to stay healthy and to ensure the well-being of themselves and their family members.

One commonality shared by members of functioning families is a concern for the health and wellness of each individual within the family because the family has the primary responsibility for meeting the health needs of its members. The nurse not only must assess the health of each family member, but also define how well the family can meet family health needs. Just how well families function in relation to this will determine how, when, and where interventions will take place; by whom; and what the specific approach to the family will be. A cultural orientation assists the nurse in understanding cultural values and interactions, the roles that family members assume, as well as the support system available to the family to help them when health problems are identified.

The family is usually an individual's most important social unit and provides the social context within which illness occurs and is resolved and within which health promotion and maintenance occur. Most **traditional health beliefs and practices** promote the health of the family because they are generally family and socially oriented. Frequently, traditional beliefs and practices reinforce family cohesion. Some values are more central and influential than others; given a competing set of demands, these central values will typically determine a family's priorities. In families that adhere to traditional cultural values, the families' (or tribe's and/or community's) needs and goals often will take precedence over an individual's needs and goals. The culturally competent nurse can recognize and use the family's role in promoting and maintaining health. This requires an appreciation of the family context in health and illness and how this varies among diverse cultures. Box 11-1 provides some ideas on how to develop the cultural competence and sensitivity that are necessary for successful health promotion programs for diverse cultural groups.

Cultural Factors Within Communities

In addition to identifying and meeting the cultural needs of clients and families, the community health nurse must consider social and cultural factors on a community level to respect cultural values, mobilize local resources, and develop culturally appropriate health programs and services. Important cultural factors include demographics in the United States, with detailed data on specific states and cities; cultural diversity in communities; subpopulations in the United States; refugee and immigrant populations, with special consideration given to newly arrived refugee communities; maintenance of traditional cultural values and practices; and access to health and nursing care for diverse cultural groups.

Demographics and Health Care

During the 21st century, the United States and many other countries will face enormous demographic, social, and culture change. North America is becoming more diverse, not less so, and thus it is incumbent on

---

BOX 11-1

Developing Cultural Competence to Promote Health in Diverse Cultural Groups

- Learn about the history of the cultural group or diverse population with which you are working. For example, an understanding of African American culture would not be complete without considering the effect of slavery on this group of Americans.
- Make an effort to understand the African American cultural values beliefs and ways of life of the community. Read some of the works of noted African American authors such as James Baldwin, Malcolm X, Langston Hughes, Maya Angelou, and so on.
- Incorporate as many of the traditional values, beliefs, and ways of life into the design and use of any educational materials. Whereas Chinese American teenagers might prefer a comic book or video in English, their grandparents might prefer a health magazine or a news article in the Chinese language.
- Become familiar with the appropriate verbal and nonverbal communication patterns within the group as well as many of the communication nuances that are contextual in nature. An example might be that a traditional Afghan woman would never speak to a strange man outside of her own kinship circle.

- Become familiar with beliefs and practices related to religion, gender, food preferences, and other related cultural differences that might lead to the quick success or failure of a health program. Be aware that the most effective health programs are those that foster community ownership and involvement. This implies that they must be planned and implemented with community input.
- Spend as much time as possible within the community, attending local events. Examples might be churches, school programs, fairs, and meetings with leaders. Taking an intervention into the community rather than having the community come to the intervention might be more effective over time.
- Seek the community's input and feedback for any health program that is planned for the community. Be aware that the use of peer educators, such as *promotoras* or the Native American community health workers (CHRs) from within the community, have been found to be effective in delivering health promotion programs and other health services to diverse communities.

Adapted from Huff, R. M., & Kline, M. V. (1999). *Promoting health in multicultural populations.* Thousand Oaks, CA: Sage.

nurses to be prepared to respond appropriately. Since the 1990s and 2000s, there has been a steady growth in cultural diversity in the United States. The health status of individuals in the United States differs dramatically across cultural groups and social classes. Certain population groups in the United States face greater challenges than the general population in accessing timely and needed health care services, and national goals have been adopted in Healthy People 2010 to address these health disparities (U.S. Department of Health and Human Services, 2000). Major indicators such as morbidity and mortality rates for adults and infants show that the health status of minority Americans in the United States is substantially worse than that of White Americans. Health status is worse among those who are medically underserved. Medically underserved populations are defined as those who have inadequate access to quality health care. These include low-literacy, low-income, rural, tribal, isolated and non-English-speaking groups (NINR, Specialized Community Interventions, September 2007). Thus, community nurses must assess groups within the community in a very sensitive manner; often those characteristics that we assume are related to the group's culture may be caused by other factors instead.

Cultural Diversity Within Communities

The United States has many diverse cultures as a result of the history of immigration to this country by a variety of cultural and ethnic groups and because of the indigenous populations of Native Americans, Native Alaskans, and Native Hawaiians. If current trends continue, the United States will consist of an even greater variety of cultural groups. In 2007, minority groups accounted for 33% of the population (U.S. Census Bureau, May 17, 2007). Although most people in this country share broad cultural values, a rich diversity of cultural orientations does exist, including those with considerable variations in health and illness practices.

Subcultures in the United States

Subcultures are aggregates of people that establish certain rules of behavior, values, and living patterns that are different from mainstream culture. Leininger described subcultures as having "distinctive patterns of living with sets of rules, special values and practices that are different from the dominant culture" (1995, p. 60). Obviously, there can also be diversity within each subculture. Hispanic culture as a group is very broad and includes Mexican Americans, Puerto Ricans, Cubans, and Central and South Americans, as well as undocumented individuals. There is diversity within each of these groups as well.

Certain geographic areas of the country, such as Appalachia, can be singled out as containing subcultures. Persons born and reared in the southern states or in New York City can often be identified by their language and mannerisms as members of a distinct subculture. We used to believe that the United States had a "melting pot" culture in which new arrivals gave up their former languages, customs, and values to become Americans. It is now agreed that the "melting pot" or "blending" concept may not be appropriate, at least not for everyone. A more accurate metaphor would be to view the U.S. population as a rich and complex tapestry of colors, backgrounds, and interests (Figure 11-2).

Refugee and Immigrant Populations

Immigrants are persons who voluntarily and legally immigrate to the United States to live. Immigrants come of their own choice, and most plan to eventually become citizens of their new host country. Of course, many persons also come to the United States, Canada, and Western Europe illegally or without the proper documentation. Although terms differ for these persons, in the United States they usually are referred to as "undocumented" or, perhaps in a more pejorative sense, "illegal immigrants."

Under international law, *refugee* is a special term that describes a person who is outside of his or her country of nationality or habitual residence and who has a well-founded fear of persecution if he or she returns to his or her own country. By definition then, refugees are persons escaping persecution based on race, religion, nationality, or

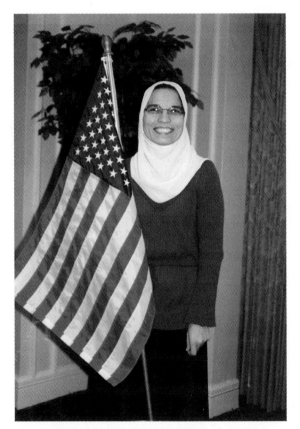

FIGURE 11-2 Communication between people from different cultures can help to break down misunderstandings, stereotypes, and other cultural barriers. Immigrants from other cultures have contributed much to enrich American culture.

political stance (United Nations High Commissioner for Refugees [UNHCR], 1966. Evidence-Based Practice 11-1 presents a study about the barriers to human rights that women encountered in southern Sudan. Violence against women is considered the most pervasive human rights violation in the world. Violence against women is exacerbated in war-torn countries with a high incidence of rape and other physical/sexual abuse during armed conflicts. Women and girls, often unaccompanied by family members, are particularly at high risk. Many refugee women who come to the United States have experienced these human rights violations.

Barnes, Harrison, and Heneghan (2004) suggested that there is a need for research about refugees that is distinct from other categories of immigrants. The circumstances that lead to forced migration of refugees are very different from those that influence an immigrant to relocate and these differences can have distinct health implications. Currently, immigration of undocumented individuals, or those who do not have the appropriate documentation to immigrate, can be a contentious issue in the industrialized nations of the world. Many of the key issues in the debate on immigration policy are economic (U.S. Chamber of Commerce, n.d.).

One well-known group of refugees was made up of persons who came to the United States from Southeast Asia after the Vietnam War. Primarily, these refugees came from Vietnam, Laos, and Cambodia. In more recent times, refugees have come to the United States from countries in Africa, including Sudan and Somalia, Eastern Europe, Afghanistan, the Middle East, and other countries undergoing violent transitions; refugees are fleeing war, famine, and other social upheavals. They are fleeing for their lives and safety rather than personally choosing to leave their homeland. The term refugee and the status of an individual who is a refugee have legal meanings and designations that differ from those of ordinary immigrants. Another classification of newcomers is that of **asylees**—persons who come to a particular country seeking political asylum from some sort of persecution in their home country. These various types of classification—immigrant, refugee, asylee, or undocumented or illegal immigrant—often determine the rights of individuals (e.g., the granting of work permits or residency status, or the types of social and health services that newcomers may obtain). In addition, those who are undocumented, or without appropriate residency status may face arrest and deportation to their country of origin.

The United States has grown and achieved its success as a nation of immigrants and foreigners. Immigration is a continuing phenomenon in this country. Many recent immigrants

EVIDENCE-BASED PRACTICE 11-1

Human Rights Barriers for Displaced Persons in Southern Sudan

This is a community-based research study that explores community perspectives on barriers to human rights that women encounter in a postconflict setting of southern Sudan. Violence against women is considered the most pervasive human rights violation in the world. Violence against women is exacerbated in war-torn countries with high incidence of rape and other physical/sexual abuse during armed conflicts; women and girls are particularly at high risk. Violence against women is often rooted in social values and mores and potential success of change depends on learning more about local priorities regarding gender relationships, practices, and rights.

The region of southern Sudan is the site of a 40-year civil war that has had a horrific effect on the population as well as the social, economic, and physical infrastructures and health care services. Focus groups and key informant interviews provided the data for this ethnographic study. Themes found in human rights structures and barriers are described in this article. Most human rights situations are dealt with by the traditional clan system and then go on to the more formal court and police system. Customary behavior often prevails and often women are disadvantaged because of their social positions and power differentials. Although some police officials receive procedural training in law enforcement and occasionally informal training in human rights, key informants reported that the police might actually perpetuate human rights abuses. The formal court system is still "developing" and do not always offer protection to women. Numerous barriers exist to extending human rights and protection to women. These barriers include (1) shifting legal frameworks that create a lack of knowledge about what constitutes a human rights violation; (2) mistrust and doubt about human rights; (3) weak government infrastructure; and, (4) poverty.

Clinical Application

1. Nurses should be aware of the everyday struggle for justice and human dignity that refugees from the Sudan have experienced. Similarly, nurses must consider the broader historical and cultural factors that contribute to human rights abuses when working with displaced or refugee communities.

2. Given their advocacy role and direct contact with communities, nurses can help educate community members regarding the health effects of human rights violations. Furthermore, by questioning social practices (domestic violence, for example) that violate women's rights, nurses can create opportunities for social change.

3. Research results also indicated that enacting human rights was frequently associated with a sense of connectedness and community responsibility, suggesting that nurses can work with local residents and service providers in addressing violence against women and promoting human rights.

4. Nurses are in a key position to help refugee communities analyze and address human rights barriers thus advancing women's health and well-being.

Clinical Resources

- Ending violence against women: http://www.unfa.org
- Prevent gender-based violence (GBV) in Africa: http://www.preventgbvafrica.org
- Gender-based violence in conflict situations: http://www.rhrc.org

Reference: Pavlish, C. & Ho, A. (2009). Human rights as barriers for displaced persons in southern Sudan. *Journal of Nursing Scholarship, 41*, 284–292.

and refugees are not acculturated to prevailing Western norms of health beliefs or behaviors. Many arrive with scant economic resources and must learn English and become economically self-sufficient as quickly as possible. Certain factors such as settlement patterns or living near friends or family, communication networks, social class, and education have helped many immigrants maintain their cultural traditions. Immigrant or refugee communities provide support for newcomers and opportunities for cultural continuity because these ethnic communities reflect the identities of the home countries. At the same time, belonging to such a community tends to set immigrants and refugees apart and isolate them from the larger community. For example, newcomers from Mexico realize that they need to learn English to get better jobs, but they often join expanding Latino communities where most residents speak Spanish. Learning English well enough to obtain employment in the English-speaking world is difficult, and it is to their credit that most immigrants and refugees do learn English and make significant contributions to their new country. Nevertheless, where immigrants live and how they participate should remain individual choices and privileges rather than prescribed options.

In addition to the legal entrance of immigrants and refugees, many other persons seeking political asylum have entered the United States from all over the world. Often those seeking asylum or those who enter the country both legally and illegally are at considerable risk for health and social problems. Health care along the U.S.–Mexico border where many individuals are undocumented, poses special problems and challenges for residents who live there (McEwen & Boyle, 2007). Table 11-1 shows terms used for individuals residing in a country who are not citizens. In addition to language and employment barriers, immigrants and refugees may have scant economic resources, some have experienced rapid change and traumatic life events, their coping abilities have been overwhelmed, and few resources are available to assist them. Immigrants in general, whether they are here legally or illegally, have special health risks.

TABLE 11-1
Terms Used for Individuals Residing in a Country Who Are Not Citizens

TERMS	DESCRIPTION OF TERMS
Illegal immigrant or illegal alien	A person who is in a country without the appropriate documentation and permission
Immigrant	A person who comes to a country to take up permanent residence
Refugee	A person who is escaping persecution based on race, religion, nationality, or political persuasion
Emigrant	A person departing from a country to settle elsewhere
Émigré	A person forced to emigrate for political reasons
Asylee	A person seeking political asylum from persecution in his or her home country
Temporary stay migrant	A person who moves to another country with the intention of staying there for only a limited time, usually for occupational reasons
Undocumented	A person without the required documents that provide evidence of status or qualification, such as nationality or specified length of time a person may legally reside within a country

Aroian (2001) conducted an extensive literature review about immigrant and refugee women's health and found that most research focused on reproductive and childbearing issues. Although these issues are certainly important, they provide only a limited glance at the lives of women and they do not capture the experience of resettlement to another country. More recently, the trend is the psychologic study of refugee women's response to trauma that is often focused on posttraumatic stress disorders (PTSD), but once again this focus tells us very little about refugee women's health or the strategies they use to cope and manage health-related issues.

Special Considerations: A New Refugee Community—The Dinka of Southern Sudan*

Sudan is one of the largest refugee-producing countries in Africa and the world today (UNHCR, 2006). Forced migration and displacement have been occurring in Sudan for decades, as Sudan's civil war began in 1955 and is now the longest lasting civil war in the world. This civil war is the result of religious and ethnic conflict between the predominantly Muslim north and the minority indigenous, and Christian south. It is estimated that some 2 million people have died and 4 million others have been displaced as a result of the civil war (Adar, 2000). For some time now, Sudan has gained worldwide attention for documentation of human rights violations, including genocide and slave trade (UNHCR, 2006). Both sides of the conflict are thought to be involved in these violations, although it is evident for some time that the government-backed northern militia has targeted the minority south. It is estimated that over 80% of the southern Sudanese population are either internally displaced or refugees in other countries and one of every five southern Sudanese has died as a result of the civil war (Adar, 2000, p. 18). Most Sudanese are displaced in neighboring African countries such as Ethiopia, Kenya, Uganda, and Egypt.

*With special assistance and contributions to this section from Martha B. Baird, PhD, ARNP, CTN

In particular, Sudanese refugees have undergone stressful, traumatic, and even catastrophic experiences such as war, torture, refugee camps, death of family members, and loss of homeland. Many of the health problems experienced by the Sudanese refugees are the result of prolonged civil war, and the lack of nutrition and basic medical care. Refugees arriving from Sudan may suffer a variety of problems including severe malnutrition and diseases endemic to Sudan, including gastrointestinal diseases, tuberculosis, schistosomiasis, sleeping sickness, and HIV/AIDS (Brown, 2004; Pinto et al., 2005). Given the horrendous scale of human rights abuses that Sudanese refugees have experienced, many of them suffer PTSD. Studies have indicated that many refugees experience PTSD, which follows a psychologically traumatic event outside of the range of usual human experiences. The symptoms may include nightmares, depression, withdrawal, hopelessness, sleep disorders, and other somatic complaints (American Psychiatric Association, 1987).

The Sudanese refugees were forced out of their communities and often traveled many miles, some on foot, adapting to temporary environments, and often harsh conditions. Many have lost close family members in the conflicts as well as all that is familiar to them, thus losing a sense of identify and community. Many others have witnessed and/or experienced the worst kind of human atrocities, including forced slavery, torture, rape, and genocide. Refugee Sudanese women were especially vulnerable during migration when they did not have the protection and support of their families and communities. However, trying to make a new life in a new host country has also been very stressful for Sudanese refugees. Factors such as unemployment, decreased family income, changes in lifestyle, lack of ability to speak English, cultural conflict, and separation from family and loved ones continue to add to stress and decrease the quality of life for many Sudanese refugees.

The Dinka tribe is one of the largest tribes in southern Sudan and its members are some of the most persecuted. Their Christian faith and practices have made them a target of ethnic persecution by the Islamic northern militia. Many Dinka have come to the United States as refugees and large communities can be found in Georgia, Florida, and Kansas. The Dinka refer to themselves as *Monyjang,* which means "The lord of all people" (Deng, 1984, p. 2). In general, the Dinka have a tall, thin, and graceful appearance. This following section will discuss the traditional Dinka culture, health care for Dinka communities, as well as presenting a Dinka family health case study. Although the focus is on Dinka refugees, many of the issues, challenges, and topics identified here have relevance to other refugee groups as well.

Traditional Dinka Culture

Traditional **Dinka culture** is very community-oriented, and kinship and family ties extend beyond blood relatives. A husband may have more than one wife, and the wives and their children exist as one extended family. Although Dinka women are traditionally subservient to men, it is not uncommon for jealousy and competition to arise between a Dinka man's wives. Cattle hold special significance in Dinka culture and traditions as well as providing a livelihood for the tribe. In addition, cattle are also considered an important aspect of Dinka marriage rituals. Bridewealth (or a bride's value) depends on the amount of cattle her union will bring to her family (Deng, 1984).

The Dinka are considered very religious and spirituality is an integral part of Dinka life. They have a belief in an inseparable connection between the natural and supernatural world. Even as refugees in the United States, the Dinka have established a strong Christian church presence within their communities. Health and illness are closely linked to spirituality and supernatural forces. Illness is considered a community affair and family and friends often gather at the bedside of a sick member to pray or to sit in watchful silence. Dinka women have been the center of family life and responsible for the transmission of the cultural values and beliefs to the children. There is still tremendous social pressure from family members and the Dinka community to continue these cultural traditions after resettlement

to the United States. This sometimes causes problems as Dinka women are also coping with tremendous role changes as we shall see in the case study.

Although marriage and childbearing have traditionally been the only acceptable roles for women, now there are considerable variations, given that Dinka family life here in the United States is in transition. Many Dinka women now work to help support their children; they have learned to drive cars, speak English and to provide for their families. Dinka traditions such as patriarchy, bridewealth, and polygamy, which have perpetuated the family clan system in Sudan for centuries, have created conflict for some Dinka women who resettle in the United States. When Dinka women come to the United States, they are encouraged to find employment and learn English; they begin to experience the freedoms and autonomy that benefit American women and this sometimes causes difficulties within the extended family as roles and expectations change very rapidly. Polygamy, a long-standing Dinka tradition, which has served to extend family lineage and promote large families, creates problems for both Dinka women and men when they come to the United States as refugees. The practice of polygamy conflicts with the cultural values and laws in the United States and when polygamous Dinka families are resettled to the United States, the husband must choose only one wife and their children. This obviously leads to dissolution and separation of families.

Dinka refugees living in the United States remain very close to their family members back in Sudan, particularly now with the availability of cell phones. Frequent phone calls enable the resettled Dinka to keep in touch with their extended families back in Sudan and this contact sometimes reinforces traditional practices and values. As an example, Dinka women learn very quickly that domestic abuse is against the law in the United States. When a Dinka woman experiences domestic violence, she can call the police and threaten divorce. Divorce is simply not an acceptable option for traditional Dinka and the husband's family back in Sudan might arrange for him to take another wife to replace the one who they believe is causing all of the marital problems. If the wife actually pursues a divorce, the husband's family back in Sudan may ask for the bridewealth to be returned. This could place a considerable financial hardship on the woman's family. Thus, although some traditional practices can be deterrents to the well-being of women and disrupt the family system, it is very important to remember that traditional customs also serve as a form of protection and they buffer the stress of being a refugee in a new country.

Characteristics of a Dinka Refugee Community

A community assessment of a Dinka community within the United States requires that the nurse assess cultural factors such as **kinship**, religious practices, family roles and patterns, language use, and cultural health beliefs and practices. Obviously, other parameters of a community assessment such as population trends, environment, industry, education, employment opportunities, recreation, and health care services are important to assess also. However, the composition of refugee and other immigrant communities requires that nurses study and interpret cultural data and understand how these data influence health and wellness. Several years ago, DeSantis observed "that interventions that are not built on an understanding of the concept of culture will always limit the effectiveness of nursing" (1997, p. 184). This is certainly true now more than ever in our multiethnic/ multicultural and pluralistic society.

There is no "one" Dinka refugee community in the United States; however, several cities have significant communities of Dinka refugees who have settled there. Traditionally, the Dinka are basically a tribal society and are very community-oriented. A tribal society simply refers to a social group, often with a territorial affiliation, which has a strong cultural and ethnic identity. Traditional Dinka society was further divided along gender and generational lines. The experiences of men, women, and children who have grown up outside of Sudan may be strikingly different from their elders. Many Dinka adults, as well as their children, have spent years in refugee campus or countries of

transit before arriving in the United States. It is also quite possible that they have experienced traumatic events prior to relocation and such factors may have a profound experience on transition to life in the United States. In essence, any attempt to bring health care services to the community or to address the community's health problems must take into account the tremendous diversity within the whole community. This obviously requires flexibility and ingenuity on the part of health care professionals. Further complicating this situation is language. Some Dinka may have learned English in their homeland due to postcolonial British occupation. Most Dinka speak the tribal language, named after their ethnic clan, the Dinka, and many speak Arabic, although few are literate in either. It goes without saying that as Dinka are resettled in the United States, they are learning English as they seek employment, interact with Americans, and send their children to school during the resettlement process. Many of the Dinka families live in apartment complexes with large concentrations of Dinka and other African refugees. Although this practice may isolate newly arrived refugees from other Americans, close association with persons from their own culture and tribe can form a supportive network for new arrivals.

Refugee communities that facilitate healthy transitions include support from family, friends, and health care professionals. Social support has been identified in the resettlement process as one of the most critical factors that promotes health and well-being. The cultural values and traditions that refugees maintain after resettlement such as a sense of communality, hope, and religious practices are resources that enable them to develop healthy strategies to cope with resettlement experiences.

The Dinka Family

The Dinka are very proud of their traditional tribal culture and their identification of being "Dinka." The traditions of communality, the bonds of family kinship, respect for elders, and a strong Christian lifestyle are some of the important traditions that the Dinka women strive to maintain and pass on to their children. Both men and women take a "Christian" or "Biblical" name in keeping with a common practice among the Dinka who are given this name at birth as well as a traditional Dinka name. Common Christian names might be John, James, Rachel, Sarah, and so forth. The Christian name reflects their strong affiliation with their Christian faith.

Family life is at the core of Dinka culture. Although many health care professionals are familiar with strong family systems among the family groups that they care for, they still may have difficulty comprehending the differences inherent in Dinka culture. The Dinka family life has a profound influence on well-being. The Dinka tend to socialize almost exclusively with other Dinka and with extended family members. This can cause conflict when they live in the United States because there may be geographic distances between the family members, thus making frequent visits very difficult. The Dinka also go to considerable efforts to maintain ties with family members back in the Sudan. Modern technology, for example, the use of cell phones as we mentioned earlier, has greatly enhanced communication with family members back home.

This group communality provides an important buffer for the refugees, especially new arrivals. Dinka communities usually have a Sudanese community church, which serves as the religious and social center for the members. During weekly services, traditional cultural practices including chanting Christian hymns in the Dinka dialect, accompanied by tribal drums, is a common practice. Social events held at the church might include birthday celebrations, baby showers, as well as memorial services for those family members who have died in Sudan. In addition, the church provides updates on the current political and social situation in Sudan. Newly arrived refugees came to the church services and stand before the congregation to announce which village in Sudan they were from and how long they had been in the United States. Women are able to continue the Dinka traditions of language, dress, food, and music through their association with the church. The weekly events at the church allow the Dinka to stay connected with each other and give them a sense of belonging and familiarity.

Many social concerns that are relevant to the Dinka community are addressed through the Sudanese church. Sermons might include lessons about issues that face Dinka families such as the importance of continuing education or methods to resolve domestic disputes. Often there is a women's group at the church that provides help to Dinka families when there is illness or financial problems; they collect money or cook food for a family in need. It is through attendance at the Sudanese Church that the Dinka values of respect for the elderly is reinforced in the socialization of Dinka children.

Dinka Women's Roles

The Dinka are strong Christians and the Sudanese churches provide an important buffer against the changes that refugee women face when they are resettled in the United States. Dinka traditions such as patriarchy, bridewealth, and polygamy, which have been a part of the family clan system in Sudan for centuries, have created conflict for Dinka women (and Dinka men, too) who resettle in the United States. Women experience conflict over their freedom, conflict between maintaining traditional values and becoming Americanized, role overload from adding new American roles to Dinka roles, a lack of suitable spouses for single women, and parenting difficulties.

In the traditional patriarchal culture of the Dinka, women are dependent and subservient to men. The family clan system in the Dinka culture continues to subjugate women, even after they are resettled in the United States. At the same time that women are learning English, learning to drive, and taking jobs outside of the home, the families back in Sudan as well as Dinka men (usually the husbands) are trying to control and manage those very women. If difficulties arise between a husband and wife, the husband is likely to communicate with his family back in Sudan by telephone and soon, the family members will call the recalcitrant wife and apply pressure on her to maintain traditional ways. For example, the Dinka culture values large families and encourages women to have many children as children are a sign of prosperity. However, refugee women soon learn that large families are not affordable or practical in the United States. Baird (2009) described an interaction that occurred between a husband and wife at a hospital after the birth of their fourth child. The physician broached the subject of a tubal ligation. The woman was interested, but it was the husband who said "No". When the physician persisted, saying that the woman should have input into the decision, the husband replied again "No. We will talk with her at home."

If a woman is reluctant to have another child or refuses outright, the family back in the Sudan might arrange for a second wife for the husband. Often resettlement to the United States leads to dissolution and separation of families as husbands must choose only one wife and their children. This, of course, poses difficulties for the wives as well as the husband. Children are affected by these situations as well. Women who pursue a divorce because of domestic violence or polygamy are discouraged by their families back in Sudan as well as the Dinka community in the United States. When a woman seeks a divorce, her family may be expected to return the bridewealth that was paid to her husband's family as part of the marital contract. The loss of the bridewealth can lead to serious financial problems for the woman's family back in Sudan. If a Dinka woman should seek a divorce in the United States, she will face considerable stigma and she will be censored by friends and her community. Baird (2009) described a situation wherein a divorced woman was shunned at her Sudanese church because of her divorce. This left her very isolated and without friends at a very difficult time in her life.

Resettlement to the United States provides the Dinka refugee women with opportunities that were not possible back in Sudan. Like many American families, it is necessary to have two breadwinners to adequately support a family, so women seek work outside of the home. They learn new skills that are necessary to parent children in the foreign U.S. culture. They struggle to learn a new set of rules and social norms for themselves as well as for their children. Taking a job usually means a woman has to learn to speak English to her coworkers, and she must find transportation to work—either by taking public transportation by herself or by learning to drive an automobile. For the first time ever, she must learn how to earn and manage money, including the use of credit and debit cards as well as their monthly payments. When Dinka mothers work outside of the home, they find that arranging for adequate child care can be very difficult. They have been accustomed to extended family members who were able to help with child-care arrangements. Many Dinka women reported that placing their children with strangers made them very uncomfortable (Baird, 2009).

The freedoms and opportunities that Dinka women gain when they come to the United States may create conflict and power imbalances in their marriages. Husbands are sometimes threatened by their wives' newfound sense of equality and independence, and this often leads to marital discord and sometimes to domestic violence. Women learn very quickly that they do not have to tolerate beatings from their husbands and that they can call 911 and the police will intervene. Dissolution of marriage and the breakup of families has been a grave concern to Dinka communities and in many instances, community elders have met with local police departments to discuss alternatives to arresting Dinka husbands and removing them from their homes. Sudanese churches have also become involved, encouraging men to support women as they learn to be American wives and mothers. Couples are encouraged to discuss their problems openly with each other and work out their differences among themselves. This means learning new skills and coping strategies for both men and women.

Raising children in the American culture has proved challenging for Dinka mothers. They struggle to help their children with their homework, and it is a struggle as often the mothers' English reading skills are limited and they do not have the background or education to help their children. Mothers can experience pressure from their children to cook "American food," such as apple pie. Children want to participate in Halloween activities and they want toys from Santa Claus at Christmas time; all celebrations and activities that are unknown and strange to Dinka parents. Disciplining children by using corporal punishment is not acceptable in America, and mothers are afraid that they might be reported to authorities who would then take their children away from them. Dinka mothers and father soon learn that in the United States, children are expected to express their feelings and opinions openly and to question rules and authority. This is rather shocking to Dinka parents. Many mothers are concerned that their children will identify with the antisocial behaviors they see in their neighborhood or on television—smoking cigarettes, drinking alcohol, and sexual promiscuity.

In summary, Dinka women, like other women refugees, have experienced profound role changes. In traditional **Sudanese culture**, a woman's proper place is in the home. However, in the United States, it has been necessary for many Dinka women to work outside the home. As women's roles have changed, their husbands have often reacted with frustration. Of course, their roles have been changing too. Some men have begun to drink heavily or abuse family members, increasing the stress and pressure on women and families. Dinka parents worry about raising their children in the United States. As children are exposed to American culture at school and on television, sex, violence, and other controversial aspects of American life are pervasive and difficult to avoid. Children tend to acculturate more rapidly than their parents, learning English more quickly and, in general, adapting to new social roles and gender identities as well as establishing roots in American culture. This does not imply

that Dinka childhood is free from conflict. On the contrary, the cultural clash between generations can be profound, given that Dinka parents are often opposed to many of the American cultural values and behaviors their children have acquired. This can be a source of great conflict and dissension.

Health Care for Dinka Refugee Communities
Case Study 11-1 describes a Dinka refugee family struggling with the difficulties of adjusting to a new and different life. The case study serves as the basis for a discussion on health care for Dinka refugee communities.

CASE STUDY 11-1

Health Care for Dinka Families and Communities

The Deng family came to the United States in 2001 after an extended stay in Egypt. Rachel and Paul had fled their Dinka village during an attack by an Arab militia, known as the *Janjaweed*. Like other Dinka refugees who experienced similar circumstances, they fled the village with their two young children, a 4-year-old boy and an 8-month-old baby girl. They hid in "the bush" until after dark when the attackers had left the area. When they made their way back to their village, they found it destroyed and their neighbors and family members dead. They originally fled to Kenya where Paul had relatives who were living there. They applied to the UNHCR for refugee status in Kenya and were denied. The family then migrated to Egypt where Rachel helped to support the family by working as a domestic housekeeper. They again applied for refugee status and this time were successful. In 2003, Rachel and Paul were resettled with their two children in California. Three years after living in the United States, Paul decided to return to the Sudan because he was unable to find suitable employment. This left Rachel alone in a new country to support herself and the two children. Even though the family has lived in the United States for more than 6 years, they still struggle with the difficulties of adjusting to a new and different life. Resettlement and adjustment in the United States have not been easy for them.

Rachel was immediately confronted with the markedly different roles of women in the United States. American gender roles are much more egalitarian and American women fill roles that only men were traditionally allowed in Sudan. Rachel became the head of household after Paul returned to the Sudan. She struggled to learn English in classes offered at the local refugee center. With the social worker's help, she found a job working as a maid in a large hotel. Constant contact with coworkers enabled her to improve her English. She took a city bus to work but after several months, she was able to save up sufficient money for a down payment on a used car. The pastor at the Sudanese community church and his wife were helpful new friends and Rachel relied on them for advice and support. Rachel developed confidence in her ability to depend on herself and to take care of her children. She explained how depending on herself has changed the way that she perceives herself since coming to the United States. "I don't depend on anything. I don't relay on anybody now. I depend on me to do something."

Still, without the social support and interaction of her family, she feels lonely and has experienced some depression, which is not uncommon for refugee women. She has learned through family members that Paul has taken another wife back in Sudan. This has been upsetting to her. The Sudanese Community church has been a source of support and comfort for Rachel and she attends services and the many social activities that the church sponsors. She has been able to maintain close and consistent ties with other Dinka refugees who have been resettled in the United States.

Although many Dinka men and women had horrific experiences in Sudan and the subsequent escape from their village and county, they are adjusting to life in the United States and are coping as well as possible with their past experiences. Their lives are not stress free by any means, but Rachel, her friends, and other refugees have demonstrated considerable strength in adjusting to traumatizing experiences and the stress of adapting to life in the United States.

Rachel does worry a great deal about her children: her son, James, is now 12 years and her daughter, Ester, is 8 years old. Rachel is worried about raising the children in American society. She is distressed by what she sees on television, and she is shocked by the explicit sex and violence portrayed in the media. She is told by other Dinka refugees that drugs are easily available and that she should warn James about them. Rachel and her children live in a poor urban neighborhood and James is exposed to boys his age who smoke, swear, and occasionally are in trouble with the law. Rachel often calls the boy's father, Paul, in Sudan and he talks to his son, encouraging him to mind his mother and to do well in school. Rachel believes that she must work very hard to instill traditional Dinka values and norms in her children. Sometimes her son says: "Mom! You don't understand. I am not Dinka. I am an American from San Diego!" Rachel worries that her children are exposed to negative aspects of American culture at school and on television as controversial aspects of American life are difficult to avoid. James learned English at school and from his classmates, and he has acculturated much more rapidly than his mother. Ester is also in school and has learned English very quickly too. Ester was recently invited by a classmate to a "sleep over". Rachel could not understand what such an event might be and she refused to allow Ester to accept the invitation. This precipitated a minor crisis in family relations.

Planning Nursing Care for Refugee Families

Careful assessment of cultural backgrounds and individual factors can help nurses anticipate and work with difficulties that are experienced by refugees and immigrants who seeking health care. The Andrews/Boyle Transcultural Nursing Assessment Guide for Individuals and Families used in this text (see Appendix A) is recommended for use with clients and their families. We have listed topics discussed by Lipson and Meleis (1983) below to provide minimum information for the nurse to plan culturally competent care.

- Length of time the client and family have been here, and where the client was raised. Not only is the country important, but rural and urban

differentiation may also be important, as well as social, political, and economic levels
- Language spoken in the home and language skill in English
- Nonverbal communication style
- Religious practices
- Ethnic affiliation or identity
- Family roles and how they are influenced by the resettlement experience
- Social support or networks, especially relatives or family members in the new country

Assessment of these factors will assist the nurse in planning health care for Rachel and her children as well as other refugee and/or immigrant families. Health services, preventive care, and health education have been identified as important needs in health surveys that have been conducted in refugee communities (Lipson, Omidian, & Paul, 1995).

The stress of resettlement is often a significant problem for members of refugee communities. Stress is related to the refugee experience and also to inadequate income, work-related problems, and loss of culture and tradition. The lack of mental health services is a grave concern in refugee and immigrant communities and should be addressed by creative and innovative solutions. In refugee communities, a church, synagogue, or mosque can play a positive and important role as religion is often identified as a protective factor by refugees in facilitating wellness and increasing quality of life. Refugee men may be reluctant to seek mental health services because of the stigma of mental illness as well as their traditional male roles. Postmigration stress may be exacerbated by unemployment or underemployment and may contribute to depression, PTSD, alcohol abuse, and poor general health status.

Preventive care in the areas of dental health, breast self-examination, mammography, and Papanicolaou (Pap) smears are important for refugee women. Refugee men have dental problems too, and need regular prostrate and testicular exams. Many of these procedures may be new to refugees who are not familiar with them. However,

many barriers to good preventive care are environmental and social rather than cultural. Constraints are based on the refugees' individual situations as well as language, economic, occupational, and transportation problems. Cultural groups differ in regards to the priority given to individual goals versus those of the larger group. For example, many refugee communities, such as those of the Dinka, are a collectivist society that values the good of the group, traditional values and group loyalty. This often conflicts with the individualistic American society. Many African refugees may suffer from racism and discrimination when they resettle in the United States and this too, impacts mental health and successful resettlement.

As many refugee women may have experienced gender-based violence including torture, rape and human rights abuses, nurses and other health professionals must learn sensitive ways of broaching these subjects and helping refugee women access culturally appropriate care. Health care professionals, especially women physicians and nurses, can design programs that consider problems in access and appropriate language as well as culturally sensitive health care for women who have experienced gender-based violence.

Health education, including information about access to care, is always important in planning services for refugee and immigrant communities. Many refugees and immigrants do not use health education services, not necessarily because of cultural barriers but because of difficulties with language and access, the need for translation and transportation, and the desire for women health care providers, as well as other barriers such as child care.

Health care institutions and agencies, from the beginning, should include bicultural health care providers on their staff. Community health workers could be trained to serve as interpreters and translators. It is always problematic for health care providers to use various family members as interpreters because of divisions along age and gender lines. Children do learn English more quickly than their parents, but it would be very insensitive to expect a young boy to interpret a conversation about results of his mother's pap smear. The health care provider's gender is important as many refugee women are not comfortable with male doctors or nurses and might avoid health care altogether if female care providers are not available. Obviously, health care providers must be knowledgeable about the refugees' or immigrants' experiences and background, cultural and social factors, and other unique aspects of the population they serve. Refugees and new immigrants need access to language-appropriate and culturally sensitive health care. Many refugees from community-oriented societies prefer to receive such information in a group or social setting rather than a one-to-one basis that is common in the U.S. health care setting. For many refugee or immigrant communities, churches, mosques, and/or synagogues are appropriate settings for health education.

The traditional or classic definition of community uses a geographic boundary, such as a village, town, or an urban settlement such as a city. This sense may be conveyed somewhat in terms such as Little Havana, Little Kabul, and Little Saigon, but such designations do not really convey the nature or quality of the refugee or immigrant experience, which tends to cross geographic boundaries. Although refugees from certain geographical areas such as Sudan tend to be sent to common locations, they may later move to be closer to relatives or families who came from the same village back home. The sense of shared displacement or "uprootedness" that serves to unite and distinguish immigrant or refugee communities from other groups or communities is quite profound and cannot be ignored when planning for community-based health services.

Immigrants are often seen by health professionals as dominated by psychoemotional experiences and consequences of relocation. In other words, we focus on the effects of stress, relocation, and human rights violations. Indeed, much of the literature on immigrants and refugees focuses on PTSD. Although many immigrants and refugees have endured horrific experiences, this focus alone is not holistic. This view, according to DeSantis (1997), focuses on the primacy of the individual (an American value) rather than the community and thus prescribes psychiatric treatment instead of addressing the sociocultural and economic barriers at the macro level. It is at the macro level that transcultural health care providers must be engaged if they are to be effective participants in building healthy refugee and immigrant communities. This does not mean that individual health care should be ignored; it simply acknowledges that it can be more effective when incorporated within a community focus, especially when dealing with immigrant or refugee communities.

Maintenance of Traditional Cultural Values and Practices

An important aspect of transcultural nursing is the collection of cultural data and the assessment of traditional values and practices and how they are maintained over time. The processes of **assimilation** and **acculturation** can be briefly defined as those ways in which individuals and cultural groups adapt and change over time. Yet, at the same time, both individuals and groups may be resistant to some changes and retain many traditional cultural traits. Hispanics are the largest cultural/ethnic group in the United States, and in several large American cities, they constitute large percentages of the population. Obviously, in these ethnic communities, it is easier to speak Spanish and to maintain other traditional cultural practices. Because traditional health beliefs and practices influence health and wellness, it is important for the nurse to understand the degree to which clients, families, and communities adhere to traditional health values and how nursing practice should reflect those values. Spector (2008) suggests that a person's health care and behavior during illness may well have roots in that person's traditional belief system. Unless community health nurses understand the traditional health beliefs and practices of their clients and communities, they may intervene at the wrong time or in an inappropriate way.

Many factors influence the likelihood that clients, families, and communities will maintain traditional health beliefs and practices. For example, the length of time a person lives in the new host country will influence factors such as language and the use of media such as radio and television. Teenagers may quickly adjust to American culture and prefer headphones with a CD player or an iPod. The ability to speak English and to communicate with members of the majority culture is crucial to acculturation. The size of the ethnic or cultural group is also important; obviously, if the group is small, individuals from that group are more likely to be exposed to outsiders and will not spend all their time within their own group or community. Although this may hasten their acculturation, it deprives members of an immigrant or refugee community the social support and presence of a large ethnic community.

Generally, children acculturate quicker because they are exposed to their peer group through schooling and they learn cultural characteristics through that association. The need to work outside

the household often exposes women from traditional cultures to others of the majority culture; thus, they learn English more quickly than if they remain isolated at home. When individuals from other cultures seek health care in their Western host country, they become familiar with its health care system. This does not necessarily mean that they comply with all health advice, but contact with the system decreases anxiety and confusion, and individuals are more likely to seek care again. In addition, if individuals or groups have distinguishing ethnic characteristics such as skin color, they may be more isolated because of discrimination and thus retain traditional values, beliefs, and practices over a longer time. Some factors that influence the likelihood that clients, families, and communities will maintain traditional health beliefs and practices are shown in Box 11-2.

Access to Health and Nursing Care for Diverse Cultural Groups

Members of diverse cultural groups, especially those who are poor and without health insurance

---

BOX 11-2

Factors Influencing Traditional Beliefs and Practices

1. Length of time in the new host country.

2. Size of the ethnic or cultural group with which an individual identifies and interacts.

3. Age of the individual. As a general rule, children acculturate more rapidly than adults or seniors.

4. Ability to speak English and communicate with members of the majority culture.

5. Economic status. For example, if the family economic situation necessitates that a Salvdoran woman work outside the home, she may learn English more quickly than if she remains within the household and speaks only Spanish with her family members.

6. Educational status. In general, higher levels of education lead to faster acculturation.

7. Health status of family members. If individuals and their families seek health care in their host

country, they begin to "learn the system," so to speak. This does not mean that they comply with all of the health advice by any means, but contacts with the system should decrease anxiety and confusion.

8. Individuals and groups who have distinguishing ethnic characteristics, such as skin color. These individuals may be more isolated because of discrimination and thus may retain traditional values related to health beliefs and behavior.

9. Intermarriage. Ethnic intermarriage is associated with a greater loss of traditional ethnic identity.

10. Rigidity or flexibility of the host society. This refers to the extent to which the host society is willing to allow members of different ethnic groups, along with their traditions, beliefs, and practices, into their structure, culture, and identity.

face special problems in accessing health and nursing care. Access to care is often determined by economic and geographic factors. Community nurses who focus on the care of aggregates face the challenge of promoting the health of populations even when there are new and different causes of morbidity and mortality (such as HIV/AIDS or the "new" influenza, H_1N_1) as well as underserved populations who are more likely to experience health problems. Certain cultural groups have faced discrimination and poverty, and their ability to access care has been compromised. Sensitivity to cultural factors has often been lacking in the health care of traditional communities and identified minority groups. In addition to economic status and discriminatory factors that limit access to care, geographic location plays an important role. Many rural areas lack medical personnel and the variety of health facilities and services that are available to urban populations. For example, Native Americans, living in sparsely settled and isolated reservations in the western part of the United States, must travel long distances over primitive roads to obtain health care services. Individuals who have type 1 diabetes and live on the Navajo or Hopi reservations may be picked up very early in the morning by a shuttle van that takes them into Tuba City for renal dialysis. The van takes them home later in the afternoon; this arduous routine may take place as often as three days each week. Other factors may also limit access to care. Many clients from culturally diverse backgrounds seek the services of health care professionals who speak their language. When this is not possible, they are reluctant to seek care or may not understand the importance of following medical advice.

Another common and significant factor that limits access to health services is a lack of understanding by clients of how to use health resources. This lack of understanding may be due in part to cultural factors. Often this lack of understanding means that members of diverse cultural groups are less able to adequately cope with health problems than are other members of the community. Nurses can develop sensitivity to diverse groups within communities and reach out

---

BOX 11-3

Factors to Consider in the Nursing Care of Culturally Diverse Groups

1. Lack of employment opportunities and finances for health care services

2. Different traditional belief systems as well as different norms and values

3. Lack of cultural sensitivity on the part of social service and health care workers

4. Lack of bilingual personnel or staff members or the lack of interpreters to assist clients and care providers

5. Rapid changes in the U.S. health care system, where clients are "lost" in the gaps between agencies and services

6. Inconvenient locations or hours that preclude clients from accessing care

7. Lack of understanding, trust, and commitment on the part of health care providers

---

to them with culturally specific health programs. Box 11-3 lists some important factors that nurses must take into account for culturally appropriate community-based care.

Assessment of Culturally Diverse Communities

A **cultural assessment** is the processes used by nurses to assess cultural needs of individual clients (Leininger, 1991, 1995; see also Appendix A). In general, all successful cultural assessments have at their foundation the extensive data base to help health professionals better understand and address the specific health needs and interests of their target populations. Individual cultural assessments are accomplished through the use of a systematic process. In community health nursing, the community is considered the client, and several models have been proposed to help nurses assess the community (Clark, 2008;

Stanhope & Lancaster, 2006), including the Andrews/Boyle Transcultural Nursing Assessment Guide for Individuals and Families in Appendix A. A community nursing assessment requires gathering relevant data, interpreting the database (including problem analysis and prioritization), and identifying and implementing intervention activities for community health (Stanhope & Lancaster, 2006). Although the community nursing assessment focuses on a broader goal, such as improvement in the health status of a group of people, it is important to remember that it is often the characteristics of people that give every community its uniqueness. These common characteristics, which influence norms, values, religious practices, educational aspirations, and health and illness behaviors, are frequently determined by shared cultural experiences. Thus, adding the cultural component to a community nursing assessment strengthens the assessment base. Box 11-4 provides basic principles underlying all cultural assessments.

Nurses find cultural data extremely helpful in planning care for individual clients as well as diverse groups within communities. Leininger (1978, 1995) presented assessment domains within which to seek data to understand culture, and she developed a tool to assess clients' cultural patterns by broadly looking at lifeways (Leininger, 1991). Inherent in most definitions of culture is the concept of shared cultural backgrounds, a way of life or a **worldview**. The concept of culture may be more easily applied to a community or a group of persons rather than just an individual as it is easier to identify patterns of behavior and beliefs within a group rather than just an individual. An overview of selected cultural components is presented in Table 11-2. These components can be used to assess diverse cultural groups within a community. For example, using these components, a cultural assessment of a Native American would provide much of the general data detailed in Appendix B shown at the end of this text.

BOX 11-4

Basic Principles of Cultural Assessment

1. **All cultures must be viewed in the context in which they have developed.** Cultural practices develop as a "logical" or understandable response to a particular human problem, and the setting as well as the problem must be considered. This is one reason why environmental and/or contextual data are so important.

2. **The underlying premises of the behavior must be examined.** For example, the Hispanic client's refusal to take a "hot" medication with a cold liquid is understandable if the nurse is aware that many Hispanic patients adhere to hot/cold theories of illness causation. There is often a range or spectrum of illness beliefs, with one end encompassing illnesses defined within the Western biomedical model and the other end firmly anchored within the individual culture (Huff & Kline, 1999). Obviously, the more widely disparate the differences between the biomedical model and the beliefs within the cultural group, the greater

the potential for encountering resistance to biomedical interventions.

3. **The meaning and purpose of the behavior must be interpreted within the context of the specific culture.** An example would be the close relationship that is often seen in Hispanic cultures between mother and son; such an intense relationship might be viewed as abnormal in European American families.

4. **There is such a phenomenon as intracultural variation.** Not every member of a cultural group displays all the behaviors that we might associate with that group. For instance, not every Hispanic client will adhere to hot/cold theories of illness, and not every Hispanic mother will have a close personal relationship with her son. It is only by careful appraisal of the assessment data, and validation of the nurse's assessment with the client and family, that culturally competent care can be provided.

TABLE 11-2
Components of the Cultural Assessment

CULTURAL COMPONENT	DESCRIPTION
Family and kinship systems	Is the family nuclear, extended, or "blended"? Do family members live nearby? What are the communication patterns among family members? What is the role and status of individual family members? By age and gender?
Social life	What is the daily routine of the group? What are the important life cycle events such as birth, marriage, and death? How are the educational systems organized? What are the social problems experienced by the group? How does the social environment contribute to a sense of belonging? What are the group's social interaction patterns? What are its commonly prescribed nutritional practices?
Political systems	Which factors in the political system influence the way the group perceives its status vis-à-vis the dominant culture, for example, laws, justice, and cultural heroes? How does the economic system influence control of resources such as land, water, housing, jobs, and opportunities?
Language and traditions	Are there differences in dialects or language spoken between health care professionals and the cultural group? How do major cultural traditions of history, art, drama, and so on, influence the cultural identity of the group? What are the common language patterns in regard to verbal and nonverbal communication? How is the use of personal space related to communication?
Worldview, value orientations, and cultural norms	What are the major cultural values about the relationships of humans to nature and to one another? How can the groups' ethical beliefs be described? What are the norms and standards of behavior (authority, responsibility, dependability, and competition)? What are the cultural attitudes about time, work, and leisure?
Religion	What are the religious beliefs and practices of the group? How do they relate to health practices? What are the rituals and taboos surrounding major life events such as birth and death?
Health beliefs and practices	What are the group's attitudes and beliefs regarding health and illness? Does the cultural group seek care from indigenous health (or folk) practitioners? Who makes decisions about health care? Are there biologic variations that are important to the health of this group?

Community Nursing Interventions

Cultural Competence in Health Maintenance and Health Promotion

Leininger (1978, 1995) suggested that cultural groups have their own culturally defined ways of maintaining and promoting health. Nursing interventions to improve the health of individu-als, groups, and communities can best be planned and implemented by considering persons within their social, cultural, and environmental contexts Community nurses who have direct access to clients in the context of their daily lives should be especially aware of the importance of cultural knowledge in promoting and maintaining health because the promotion and maintenance of health occurs in the context of everyday lives rather than in the doctor's office or in a hospital. The range of cultural influences on health maintenance and promotion is considerable. Major cultural issues and considerations must be addressed before health maintenance and promotion programs are implemented for culturally diverse groups.

First, it is important to involve local community leaders or "elders" who are members of the cultural group being targeted to promote the acceptance of health promotion programs. Such a leader, for example, might be the pastor of an African American church in the rural south or a member of the tribal council for a Native American tribe. The nurse must also be sensitive to cultural differences in leadership styles. For example, the African American pastor may not speak in favor of the health education program from his or her pulpit but might choose instead to work through more informal networks. Numerous nurse researchers (Abrums, 2004; Shambley-Ebron & Boyle, 2006) have found that many African Americans rely on spirituality and/or religious practices when they are ill and in general, a health program that has the support of the church pastor would be favorably viewed by the church community. In addition to local community and religious leaders, it is important in the planning process to involve those who are most affected by the health-related problem. Those involved in planning and participating in the program's activities should likewise participate in its evaluation. Collaboration between the planner and the participants is often the key to success in community-based health programs (Clark, 2008).

Second, family members, churches, employers, and community work sites need to be involved in supporting health promotion/education programs through the use of networks that already exist. For example, a health education program about the importance of having a routine screening such as a mammography can be established at a work site that employs mostly women. A display could be set up in the cafeteria, dining room, or other accessible site. Women could view the educational material during breaks or after lunch. Providing information about sites where women could obtain a mammography would be an important component of such a program.

Third, health messages are more readily accepted if they do not conflict with existing cultural beliefs. If the nurse plans to talk about prevention of teenage pregnancy to mothers and daughters at a local conservative church, he or she could discuss these plans in advance with some of the mothers and the pastor and ask for ways to strengthen the church's support of abstinence programs. This is not the appropriate time to focus on contraception methods but to be sensitive to the group's religious values.

Fourth, language barriers and cultural differences are very real problems in many large U.S. cities as well as rural areas. For example, in the U.S.–Mexico border areas, *promotoras* (community health workers) are used to disseminate messages in their own language (Spanish) and to help organize and present information that is culturally appropriate and understood by community members. Many Native American tribes make use of community health representatives (CHRs) to assist native individuals to improve their health and/or access care. The health care professional should not be afraid to ask for help and suggestions, and should make it a point to find educational material such as brochures or videotapes in the appropriate language as well as with the "culturally acceptable" message.

Last of all, sensitivity is essential to meeting health needs that exist within diverse cultural groups. For example, HIV/AIDS is spreading rapidly in some Hispanic and African American populations and is associated with intravenous drug use, violence, and the use of crack cocaine. In addition, the root causes of poverty and unemployment should be examined, and programs that improve overall economic status of culturally diverse communities should be developed. Culturally relevant treatment programs should be implemented. Many minority women who seek treatment programs for cocaine addiction encounter barriers that seem

EVIDENCE-BASED PRACTICE 11-2

Cultural Care for Substance-Dependent African American Women

Substance abuse is in epidemic proportions in the United States and is currently defined as the nation's number one public health problem. Caring for members of diverse cultural groups who abuse drugs and alcohol can be challenging. High rates of recidivism, relapse, and inadequate psychologic support as well as lack of treatment facilities are among some of the issues in addressing substance dependence. In addition, health care providers have failed to address issues of culturally sensitive treatment strategies or gender issues. Clients from diverse cultural backgrounds have tended to be "treated" from a unicultural perspective, with limited approaches to fit the client's cultural background or needs.

This ethnonursing qualitative research study explored the meanings and expressions of care from 14 key and 18 general participants, all of whom were African American women. Four universal culture care themes were identified in the data.

1. Culture care for substance-dependent African American women meant taking time to listen and to understand them in a nonjudgmental manner, showing respect for and understanding of their traditional family, religious, spiritual, and cultural lifeways.

2. Culture care for African American women meant learning reciprocal support with other recovering women while forming alliances with adult females in developing recovery care networks.

3. Culture care was viewed as guidance and direction through suggestions by care providers.

4. Cultural care for African American women reflected concern for or about resolving past cultural pain experiences and ameliorating anger, guilt, fear, and shame.

Clinical Application

1. Understand and value that to be effective in providing culture care to African American women, health care providers must be knowledgeable about African Americans' religious, spiritual, philosophical, and cultural values and lifeways.

2. Recognize the influence of spirituality on health and incorporate spirituality in the provision of health care.

3. Assist African American women who are in treatment facilities to maintain family and kinship networks.

4. Spent time with African American women who are undergoing treatment for drug and alcohol abuse, to listen to and understand them and to show respect and concern for them.

5. Become knowledgeable about addictions and understand that recovery from substance abuse is a process.

Reference: Ehrmin, J. T. (2005). Dimensions of culture care for substance-dependent African American women. *Journal of Transcultural Nursing 16*(2), 117–125.

insurmountable. Treatment programs are not available in many areas, and child-care facilities are not provided—even in day-treatment programs. Thus, a young mother living in a rural area with children would not be able to find a treatment center that meets her needs. If she seeks admittance to a residential treatment program, she might have to agree to place her children in foster care.

Evidence-Based Practice 11-2 discusses culturally appropriate care for substance-dependent African American women.

Family Systems

Because the family is the basic social unit, it provides the context in which health promotion and maintenance are defined and carried out by family members within culturally diverse communities. The nurse can recognize and use the family's role in altering the health status of a family member and in supporting lifestyle changes. This requires an appreciation of the role of the family in diverse culture groups. African American families, for example, may demonstrate interchangeable roles for their male and female members, extended ties across generations, and strong social support systems, including the African American church, all of which can be tapped by a community health nurse to activate health and wellness in families (Abrums, 2004). Immigrant and refugee families also tend to have strong extended ties with their kin and changes in lifestyle, diet, and other established patterns of daily life that influence health status will need the understanding and support of all family members.

Coping Behaviors

Culturally diverse clients often have distinct behaviors to cope with illness as well as to maintain and promote health. These behaviors may be traced to the health–illness paradigms that were discussed earlier in Chapter 4. Beliefs about hot and cold, yin and yang, harmony and balance may underlie actions to prevent disease and maintain health. Community nurses who understand their clients' cultural values and beliefs can assess their understanding of health and illness. These assessment data serve as the basis for planning health guidance and teaching strategies that focus on incorporating cultural beliefs and practices in the nursing care plan. It seems likely that clients in the process of coping with illness and seeking help may involve a network of persons, ranging from family members and select laypersons to health care professionals.

Seeking social support is often seen as a means of coping. It is now evident that social support varies widely across people, cultural groups, and circumstances. An individual's coping behaviors during an illness of a family member may differ remarkably at any one time during the illness, depending on intrapersonal, interpersonal, and environmental factors. Certainly, nurses working with diverse cultural populations will want to learn and understand how coping styles are used by individuals and family members as well as how these coping styles change over time as these factors are often influenced by culture.

Lifestyle Practices

Cultural influences have a significant impact on such health-promoting practices as diet, exercise, and stress management. Community health nurses should assess the implications of diet planning and teaching to clients and family members who adhere to culturally prescribed practices concerning foods. Some cultural groups believe that certain foods maintain or promote health. Some foods often are restricted during illness, just as there are "sick foods"—special dishes served to an ill person, such as the proverbial chicken soup. Cultural preferences determine the style of food preparation and consumption, the frequency of eating, the time of eating, and eating utensils. Milk is not always considered a suitable source of protein for Native Americans, Hispanics, Blacks, and some Asians because of their relatively high incidence of lactose intolerance.

Nurses who work with culturally different clients must evaluate patterns of daily living as well as culturally prescribed activities before they suggest forms of physical activity or exercise to clients. Exercise is often defined in terms of White middle-class values. Not everyone has access to the tennis court at a local country club or a gym and many individuals would not feel comfortable in such surroundings or in aerobics classes regardless of the setting. Some men might feel more comfortable playing basketball or hiking. Traditional tribal dancing has become popular on some reservations for Native Americans. In the past, members of the Hopi tribe were superb distance runners and the tribe still sponsors running events for its members. Helping clients plan physical activities that are culturally acceptable is only the first step in implementing a program of physical activity.

Another aspect of lifestyle that must be understood for the successful promotion of health and wellness is the manner in which culturally

EVIDENCE-BASED PRACTICE 11-3

Youth Suicide Prevention in a Pacific Northwest, American Indian Tribe

Suicide rates among American Indian youth in the United States are two to three times higher than the national average. Risk factors include abuse of alcohol, depression and hopelessness, family conflict and violence, and divorce and poverty. Community risks include discrimination, prejudice, and rapid change and instability. Researchers interviewed American Indian parents and elders to obtain their perspectives on community needs and to identify strengths within the community that might reduce suicide risk.

Parents and elders voiced concern about the vicious cycle of fractured families that contributes to difficulties in school and in obtaining employment, both of which perpetuate the further fracturing of families. Parents and elders worried about the loss of traditions and the effect of modern-day life on traditional family values and cultural practices. Cultural revitalization efforts were valued. Parents and elders believed that certain action would strengthen the community and reduce suicide risk. For example, youth mentoring programs, more cultural activities, support for economic development, and greater opportunities for youth recognition were identified.

Clinical Application

1. Accept and be sensitive to historical and contextual conditions under which stress, depression, and suicide ideation occur.
2. Use culturally relevant interventions as appropriate, such as story telling, demonstration, and role modeling.
3. Strengthen cultural values that enable youth to be strong and have hope for the future.
4. Recognize that the concept of family is remarkably different for American Indian people.
5. Direct community interventions to families, communities, and the larger systems in which social injustice and racial discrimination occur.

Reference: Strickland, C. J., Walsh, E., & Cooper, M. (2006). Healing fractured families: Parents' and elders' perspectives on the impact of colonization and youth suicide prevention in a Pacific Northwest American Indian Tribe. *Journal of Transcultural Nursing, 17,* 5–12.

different clients manage stress. Stress management is learned from childhood through our parents, our social group, and our cultural group. Smoking and/or chewing tobacco, although not healthy habits, are often used to manage stress. Persons who choose to use tobacco products greatly increase the risk of the development of heart disease and cancer. Debates currently rage about smoking in public places and the use of tobacco, although the trend is toward banning the use of tobacco in public places.

The use and abuse of alcoholic beverages are also related to lifestyle practices. Families coping with multiple stressors often feel overwhelmed by the challenges of everyday living, and individuals within families may develop dysfunctional ways of coping, such as alcohol abuse and domestic violence. Although many of these lifestyle practices are not associated with a group's culture per se, they are often found in groups whose members do not have appropriate options and/or alternatives and who are poor and unable to access other options. Evidence-Based Practice 11-3 describes the problems and concerns aroused by youth suicide in a Native community. Studies such as this one by Strickland, Walsh, and Cooper (2006) help us to understand the views and experiences of parents and elders in tribal communities about youth suicide, a particular concern for American Indian people.

Many cultural groups tend to express psychologic distress through somatic symptoms, and some studies have found that women are at high risk for depression and somatic complaints. Indeed, for many immigrants and refugees, stress-related disorders such as PTSD are relatively common. The presence of large numbers of families with altered family processes and unhealthy lifestyles within the community may create problems for all members of the larger community or society. The nurse who works in **community settings** will frequently encounter these families and is in an ideal position to act as their advocate, to refer them to appropriate care, and, in effect, to improve the health of the community at large.

The nurse may find that in some cultural groups, such as Mexican Americans, traditional healers, such as *curanderos*, can be helpful for persons with some emotional or psychologic disorders. In addition, health professionals such as physicians, dentists, and nurse practitioners may be more acceptable if they share the same ethnic heritage or at least speak the language of the client. In some aggregate ethnic settings, such as the Chinatown area in San Francisco, there are practitioners of traditional Chinese medicine as well as Western medicine, acupuncturists, neighborhood pharmacies, and herbalists, all of which are available to meet the diverse needs of that particular neighborhood.

Cultural Competence in Primary, Secondary, and Tertiary Preventive Programs

Nurses working in community settings use health-related concepts that are identified with the practice of community health nursing. Concepts such as "community as client" and "population-focused practice" were discussed briefly in the first sections of this chapter. Another important concept to community nurses is that of **levels of prevention**. Preventive care, consisting of primary, secondary, and tertiary activities, is directed toward high-risk groups or aggregates within a community setting. **Primary prevention** is composed of activities that prevent the occurrence of an illness, disease, or health risk. The preventive actions take place before the disease or illness occurs. **Secondary prevention** involves the early diagnosis and appropriate treatment of a condition or disease. **Tertiary prevention** focuses on rehabilitation and the prevention of recurrences or complications. The major aim of community-based preventive programs is to reduce the risk for the population at large rather than to prevent illnesses in specific individuals. As long as preventive actions are directed toward a given population rather than toward individuals, there is a chance of altering the general balance of forces so that even though not all will benefit, many will have a chance to avoid illness. This last section of this chapter discusses the use of cultural knowledge to plan community-nursing interventions for diverse cultural groups at the primary, secondary, and tertiary levels of prevention.

Primary Prevention: Prenatal Services in Mexican American Communities

Overview of the Health Concern
When viewed as a group, racial and ethnic minorities suffer from worse health compared to their U.S. counterparts. Differences in the incidence, prevalence, mortality, and burden of diseases and other adverse health conditions exist among ethnic population groups in the United States (Minority Health: Health Quick Facts, 2009). This is certainly the case for maternal and infant health. For many years, public health agencies have tried to improve maternal and infant services to high-risk populations. As long ago as 1985, a special government report on minority health reported that many minority women do not begin prenatal care during the first trimester (Heckler, 1985a, 1985b) and that this has serious consequences for mothers and infants. The risk factors of pregnancy include age (both extremes), parity, low socioeconomic status, as well as other factors such as diabetes, and alcohol and tobacco use. In addition, numbers of children within the family (need for child care), transportation problems, and less assistance from a support system influence use of prenatal care and other health services. Many women of Mexican American origin fall in these categories. Furthermore, an infant with health concerns is at risk for further

problems as there may be negative and long-term consequences for the child and the mother as well as other family members. Obtaining early and regular prenatal care greatly enhances a young woman's chance of delivering a healthy, full-term baby. A program of primary prevention would focus on preventing infant morbidity and mortality and other health problems in Mexican American mothers and their infants. Early prenatal care may enhance pregnancy outcome and maternal health by assessing risk, providing health advice, and managing chronic and pregnancy-related health conditions (Martin et al., 2009). Nursing care must be broadly focused, providing some specific services but also helping clients access other resources in the community.

Access to Care

There are various reasons why Mexican American women might not seek care during pregnancy. Cost is often a factor, and in many areas of the country, Mexican Americans have tended to belong to poorer socioeconomic groups. Mexican Americans are concentrated in blue-collar jobs, farm work, and service occupations; lower status jobs translate into lower income and higher poverty rates (ERIC Digest, 1990). In 2005, the Pew Hispanic Center estimated that nearly 11 million undocumented immigrants live in the United States, 6 million of who are from Mexico (Passel, 2009). Undocumented immigrants face special problems with access to care: They lack health insurance, language, and knowledge regarding health services, and they fear that they may be arrested and deported because of their legal status.

The value of routine prenatal visits to a health care provider should be repeatedly emphasized by nurses, otherwise some Mexican American women may stop their regular visits because they are feeling well and are not accustomed to seeing a health care provider unless they are ill. The community health nurse can provide information about community resources and help clients access care early in pregnancy by referral to appropriate agencies. Nearly all states now provide programs that provide funds and services for low-income pregnant women, al-

though in the financial crises of the late 2000s, these services are being reduced or eliminated in some states. Although not a health program specifically, the Women, Infants, and Children (WIC) Program provides nutritious food and nutrition education to low-income pregnant and breast-feeding mothers, their infants, and their children under age 5 (U.S. Department of Agriculture, Food and Nutrition Service, 1999). The rate of low birth weight babies among infants born to women on WIC is 25% lower than for infants born to similarly situated women not on WIC. WIC is an example of one of the most popular, successful, and cost-effective public health programs (U.S. Department of Agriculture, Food and Nutrition Service, 1999; U.S. Department of Agriculture, Food and Nutrition Service, n.d.). Referring pregnant women to WIC services is a strong primary prevention intervention by community nurses.

Many Mexican Americans are more comfortable accessing health educational services in a setting that is known to them and where they feel comfortable. Neighborhood churches are excellent settings for health education as women know where they are located and are familiar with them in contrast to a hospital or clinic setting away from their neighborhood. Often churches can provide child care so that mothers can leave their children in a safe place while they are attending prenatal classes.

Cultural Views About Modesty

Any prenatal program that serves Mexican American women may be underused unless consideration is given to some Mexican American women's modesty and reluctance to be examined by male health care providers. The use of female nurse practitioners and midwives is ideal for this population. In addition, some consideration should be given to incorporation of the traditional *parteras* (lay midwives) or *promotoras* (health workers) into the preventive educational services. *Promotoras*, those community health workers who speak Spanish, are especially effective in delivering primary health care services to expectant mothers either in community settings or in the client's home.

Language Barriers

It is absolutely essential in a prenatal program for a Mexican American population that the majority of health care professionals in the program be bilingual. If that is impossible, interpreters must be employed to facilitate the professional services. All prenatal classes should be offered in Spanish and English. This sometimes means that two classes must be offered concurrently; many Mexican American women speak predominantly either Spanish or English and would choose the class where they understand the language. The availability of health education material in Spanish is critical to reinforce teaching and anticipatory guidance. Videos may be more effective than brochures or other written material. In Berry's study (1999) of Mexican American women and prenatal care, the key informants who were bilingual spoke only Spanish within their homes because they did not want their children to forget their heritage. In some border communities such as Nogales, Arizona, the Hispanic population is high (93.6%), and most residents speak Spanish in their homes (Arizona Department of Health Services, Office of Health Systems Development, 2005).

Cultural Views of Motherhood and Pregnancy

Some evidence indicates that women of Mexican American culture may adhere to slightly different value orientations and cultural views of motherhood and pregnancy than those found in mainstream American culture (Burk, Wieser, & Keegan, 1995). The Mexican American culture traditionally values motherhood, and young women are encouraged to prepare themselves for this role. Community health nurses, nurse practitioners, and professional midwives are in important positions to help pregnant women prepare for motherhood and its associated responsibilities. Understanding and reinforcing the approved cultural views of pregnancy will be helpful for clients because trust and mutual goal setting can develop more rapidly. All nursing interventions should incorporate family members, especially mothers and sisters, for support of the pregnant woman. Emphasizing the responsibility for the mother to be healthy for her baby's health and welfare is appropriate for this cultural group.

Traditional Pregnancy-Related Folk Beliefs of Mexican Americans

Many Mexican Americans may adhere to some traditional beliefs and practices related to pregnancy and childbirth. Additionally, children are greatly valued and are desired soon after marriage. Census data indicate that Mexican Americans tend to marry and have children at earlier ages (ERIC Digest, 1990). As in many other cultures, Mexican Americans consider pregnancy, birth, and the immediate postpartum period as a time of great vulnerability for women and their newborns. Box 11-5 shows selected beliefs and practices of pregnancy and childbirth in traditional Mexican

---

BOX 11-5

Selected Beliefs and Practices of Pregnancy and Childbirth in Traditional Mexican American Culture

- Avoid strong emotions such as anger and fear during pregnancy.
- Cool air is dangerous during pregnancy and should be avoided.
- Bathe often during pregnancy; be active so that the baby will not grow too big and hinder delivery.
- Eat a nutritious diet; "give in" to food cravings.
- Massage is helpful to place the baby in the right position for birth.
- Don't raise your arms above your head or sit with your legs crossed during pregnancy because these actions will cause knots in the umbilical cord.
- Moonlight should be avoided during pregnancy, especially during an eclipse, because it will cause a birth defect.
- After delivery, a 40-day period known as *la diet* or *la cuarentena* is observed. Certain activities and foods are restricted.
- Chamomile tea will relieve nausea and vomiting in pregnancy.
- Heartburn can be treated with baking soda.
- Laxatives and purges may be used to "clean" the intestinal tract.

American culture. It is important for the culturally sensitive nurse to assess each client because each generation of childbearing women perceives pregnancy and birth differently (Nichols & Zwelling, 1997). In the Mexican American culture, it is important for the nurse to assess the views of members of the pregnant mother's support system, especially her mother, who belongs to an earlier generation and may adhere to more traditional values. It is always necessary to assess intracultural variation as not every member of any given culture adheres to the same beliefs and behaviors typical of that culture.

Mexican American Cultural Networks

Traditionally, the family is very important in Mexican American culture, and nursing care should be family focused. The most important social structural factor in the Mexican American culture is family and kinship ties. These ties often go beyond the family to a wide network of kin. If nursing care is to be effective, nurses must tap these kinds of cultural networks to ensure the support of family members, neighbors, or friends. Nurses face challenges such as language barriers, literacy levels, socioeconomic and educational levels, cultural backgrounds, and other subtle differences when they work with the varied Hispanic groups in the United States. It is also critically important to remember that there is tremendous diversity within Hispanic groups living in the United States. Mexican Americans are but one example, other major Hispanic groups include Puerto Ricans, Cubans, and Central and South Americans.

Using Cultural Competence at the Primary Level of Prevention

The community health nurse should target certain high-risk behaviors for change during pregnancy, such as smoking, using drugs, consuming alcohol, and maintaining poor nutritional habits. Although there is no set rule of thumb, a Mexican American mother-to-be may respond to suggestions for change if she is convinced that her behavior will cause harm to her baby. Family and social support groups in Mexican American culture can also be helpful and supportive to expectant mothers wishing to make lifestyle changes. Some researchers have found that pregnant Latin women will attempt to stop smoking and will be successful with the help, support, and assistance of their families (Pletsch & Johnson, 1996). Family members can play important supportive roles in terms of primary prevention that requires behavioral and lifestyle changes.

Prenatal services should go beyond the birth of the baby to include information about breast-feeding and family-planning services. Traditionally, some health care professionals have assumed that family-planning services will not be accepted in a Mexican American population because of religious opposition and machismo—the need of the man to prove his manhood by having children or to believe in the biologic superiority of men. However, it may be that Mexican American men as well as women are interested in family planning and are concerned about the number of children they can support. This issue should be validated with individual clients and their spouses. During la cuarentena, the 40 days after the birth of the baby, women kin of the new mother often help with infant care, household tasks, and preparation of special foods for the mother (Berry, 1999). Many Hispanic families believe that chili and other spicy foods should be avoided during and immediately after pregnancy.

Strategies for promoting breast-feeding should be identified and encouraged. For example, educational levels, family experiences with breast-feeding, the husband's attitude, the need to return to work, and feelings of embarrassment are associated with infant-feeding choices among Mexican American women as well as other groups. These factors need to be explored with individual women to help them make the best choices for themselves and their babies. Fortunately, breast-feeding is becoming commonplace in the United States and mothers realize the advantages that breast-feeding can provide for a new baby. Traditionally, Hispanic mothers may bind their abdomen as well as their baby's abdomen during the postpartum period. These customs should be supported by nurses who work with postpartum Mexican American women and their babies.

Secondary Levels of Prevention: Type 2 Diabetes and Native Americans

Overview of the Health Concern

Non–insulin-dependent diabetes (NIDD), or type 2 diabetes, is seen commonly among many Native Americans, and certain tribes have extremely high rates of the disease. At nearly 17%, Native Americans and Alaska Natives have the highest adjusted prevalence of diabetes among all U.S. racial and ethnic groups (American Diabetes Association, Native American Programs, 2009). By all accounts, the high rate of diabetes in Native North American groups is a leading health concern because diabetes is a leading cause of outpatient visits at Indian Health Service facilities. Equally of concern, Indian deaths resulting from renal failure alone were reported to be 290% higher than the national average in the United States (U.S. Department of Health and Human Services, 1993). Type 2 diabetes has become an epidemic and a national tragedy among many Native peoples.

The reasons for the epidemic of type 2 diabetes among some Native North Americans are not clear. It has long been believed that some Native North American tribes have an underlying genetic propensity for the disease that is triggered by major changes in dietary practices, a sedentary lifestyle, and increasing obesity (Neel, 1962; Young, 1994). These factors have been complicated by social conditions such as poverty, inadequate access to health care, as well as by problems of compliance or lack of adherence to medical regimens.

Because of the high rate of diabetes on some reservations, numerous secondary preventive services that focus on early diagnosis and treatment have been initiated. Many of them are modeled after programs that have been successful with White middle-class North Americans. Box 11-6 shows culturally related factors that could influence the success of secondary preventive programs for diabetes. Readers are cautioned that validation of beliefs and practices should always take place

with individual clients and families, and stereotyping (thinking that all Native Americans are the same) should be avoided.

Using Cultural Competence at the Secondary Level of Prevention

Nursing interventions at the secondary level of prevention should focus on the implementation of healthful lifestyle changes that will ultimately decrease the complications of diabetes. Most of these are related to what health professionals call diet and exercise, but what is appropriate for Native North American culture is an emphasis on health and a healthy lifestyle.

Nurses should emphasize health and a healthy lifestyle rather than negative factors such as control of diabetes, prevention of complications, weight reduction, and exercise. The choice of words, as well as the emphasis, is important. For example, when teaching the client and family about diabetic diets, the nurse can substitute the word "nutrition" for "diet," thus removing the negative perceptions and leading to a nursing plan that emphasizes substitution of healthy foods rather than deprivation. Substituting fruits for candy bars and packaged pastries, whole grains for French fries, potato chips or doughnuts, and vegetables for sugared snacks will improve the client's nutritional status and lead to a healthier lifestyle. Special traditional foods, even fried bread, can be eaten on special occasions, and other types of bread can be substituted during regular meals.

Health education can be oriented toward individual clients and directed toward the family rather than provided in an impersonal clinic situation. Physical activities that are culturally congruent can be encouraged; again, the value of health and a healthy lifestyle should be stressed over exercise and weight reduction. Physical activities that are congruent with overall lifestyle and cultural context will be easier to incorporate into daily living situations.

Usually, the Native American family system is an extended family that includes several households of closely related kin. Family members become exceedingly important during times of crisis

---

BOX 11-6

Beliefs and Practices Related to Diabetes in Some Native Americans

---

Nutritional Practices

- Diets are high in calories, carbohydrates, and fats.
- Sharing communal meals is a common and valued cultural practice.
- Some groups have a high incidence of obesity.
- Food preparation often adds fats and calories.
- Snack foods (potato chips, carbonated beverages, prepackaged pastries) are common.
- High intake of alcohol seriously compromises the treatment of diabetes.

Activity Levels/Fitness Practices

- Sedentary lifestyles have become common.
- Many reservations lack recreational facilities.
- Formal exercise activities are associated with the White man's culture and are not thought to be appropriate for Native Americans.

Beliefs and Values Related to Diabetes

- Ideal body image favors a heavier physique, and weight gain is considered normal; thinness is a cause for worry and concern.
- Concept of "control of one's body," that is, weight, glucose levels, blood pressure, may conflict with values and norms of Native American culture. For example, Native American clients may be uncomfortable with comparison of individual performance against others or against the norms and standards of biomedical care.
- Many Native Americans are uncomfortable with discussing or exposing private body functions, such as providing urine samples or participating in blood testing in a public situation.
- Illness is a personal and unpleasant topic, and Native American clients may be uncomfortable when asked to talk about it.
- Diabetes is a "White man's disease"; Native Americans did not have diabetes until Whites came to this continent.
- The term "diabetic" may be offensive to some, and the label "diabetic clinic" may discourage clients from seeking health care services.
- White health professionals may be viewed with some suspicion and distrust, given the history of cultural contact between Whites and Native Americans.
- Because diabetes is so common in some tribal groups, there is a fatalism about the disease, especially if a family member already has diabetes.
- Beliefs and health practices surrounding diabetes may vary according to the Native American tribe.

---

because they are a source of support, comfort, assistance, and strength. The importance of cultural ties with kin and other members of the reservation community always must be considered in planning for early diagnosis and treatment programs. It is in this context (family and community) that clients are encouraged and supported not only to seek care but also to institute lifestyle changes that are congruent with cultural practices and that will enhance the health status of all members of the family and, ultimately, the tribal community.

The increasing rates of type 2 diabetes are of great concern to Native American communities. Introducing preventive health programs requires great sensitivity to cultural traditions and to the past experiences that native communities have had with health care and health research. Understanding the needs of community members is essential for the development of culturally appropriate programs, and each Native American community has its own cultural traditions and beliefs that make up the details of daily life. Understanding the needs of Native communities begins by asking them what they want and need from preventive programs rather than imposing ideas upon them. The best way to find out what matters to people is to get out into the community and talk to them. In Native American communities, it is wise to begin with respected and esteemed members of the tribal council.

Serious behavioral and social problems contribute to the high-risk factors in American

Indian groups. Suicide rates are rising, and deaths resulting from homicide, accidents, and injuries have resulted in increased American Indian mortality (Strickland et al., 2006). In fact, suicide is the third leading cause of death among American Indian youth, ages 15 to 24 years (CDC, 2004). Evidence-Based Practice 11-3 shown earlier in this chapter offers both community- and family-based recommendations to reduce suicide risk. Newer threats to Indian health such as cancer, diabetes, nutritional diseases, and other illnesses caused by changing behaviors and environmental contaminants are on the rise. These problems contribute significantly to death and disease in Native communities. A Cultural Assessment for Traditional Indian Healing is shown in Appendix B at the end of this text. The Assessment guide provides a framework that can be used to assess traditional healing beliefs and practices in Native communities.

Tertiary Levels of Prevention: Hypertension and African Americans

Overview of the Health Concern

African Americans are a highly heterogeneous group and display considerable variation in health beliefs and behaviors. For the most part, this section will discuss a more traditional, rural African American culture, and the reader is advised to validate beliefs and behaviors with individual clients and communities.

Hypertension is a major risk factor for heart disease and stroke. Mean blood pressure levels are higher in Blacks than in White Americans, with a marked excess in Blacks. A decade ago, in a government study on minority health, the chairperson pointed out improvements in the treatment of hypertension in Blacks. In reviewing the data, she stated, "Hypertensive Blacks were at least as likely as Whites of the same sex to be treated with antihypertensive medication and nearly as likely to have their blood pressure controlled" (Heckler, 1985a, p. 110). Heckler also noted that from 1968 to 1982, stroke mortality in Blacks declined 5%, and coronary heart disease also had decreased dramatically. Control of hypertension has certainly been one factor responsible for this

improvement. It is critical that efforts to treat hypertension in African American populations be continued. Unfortunately, appropriate care often has been complicated by discrimination, poverty, and limited access to care.

The goal of tertiary prevention is to reduce disability and prevent complications from developing further. A major aim of nursing care in the implementation of tertiary activities is to help clients adjust to limitations in daily living, to increase their coping skills, to control symptoms, and in general to minimize the complications of disease by reducing the rate of residual damage in a given population. Cultural factors that should be considered in tertiary prevention programs for African Americans are shown in Box 11-7.

Using Cultural Competence at the Tertiary Level of Prevention

Community nurses have demonstrated competence in the management of community hypertension programs. Although these programs are vital to the early diagnosis and management of hypertension, they also include a component that focuses on helping clients manage a chronic disease—an aspect of tertiary prevention. Numerous studies have shown that African American churches are excellent sites for community-based health programs such as hypertension clinics. The African American community should be involved in every aspect of community-based programs. The goals, objectives, and interventions of the services should reflect the expressed needs of the community target group as well as their values, beliefs, and interests.

Poverty is often a problem in rural African American communities and, combined with the lasting effects of racism and discrimination, African Americans often experience severe economic deprivation. In 2007, 24.5% of all African Americans were living below the national poverty level (Poverty in the United States, 2007). Forty percent of African American households are headed by females, often another contributing factor to families having insufficient socioeconomic resources (U.S. Census Bureau, 1998). Community health nurses are in the

BOX 11-7

Cultural Factors to Consider in Planning Tertiary Prevention for a Traditional African American Population

Language

African American communication concepts and patterns can be identified and used in community education programs.

Cultural Health Beliefs

Good health comes from good luck.
Health is related to harmony in nature.
Illnesses are classified as "natural" or "unnatural."
Illness may be God's punishment.
Maintenance of health is associated with "reading the signs," for example, phase of the moon, seasons of the year, position of the planets.

Cultural Health Practices

The use of herbs, oils, powders, roots, and other home remedies may be common.

Cultural Healers

Older woman ("old lady") in the community who has knowledge of herbs and healing.
 Spiritualist who is called by God to heal disease or solve emotional or personal problems.
 Voodoo priest/priestess who is a powerful cultural healer who uses voodoo, bone reading, and so on, to heal or to bring about desired events.
 Root doctor who uses roots, herbs, oils, candles, and ointments in healing rituals.

Time Orientation

May be present-time oriented, which makes preventive care more difficult to implement and maintain.

Nutritional Practices

Soul food takes its name from a feeling of kinship among Blacks and may be served at home, provided at church dinners, or served at home-style restaurants.
 Diets may reflect traditional rural Southern foods such as fried chicken, greens, grits, corn bread, and chickpeas. Dessert may be peach cobbler.

Economic Status

African Americans account for many persons in the lower socioeconomic strata in American society.

Educational Status

High aspirations for education, but socioeconomic status and other complex factors limit educational opportunities.

Family and Social Networks

Often strong extended family networks with a sense of obligation to relatives.

Self-concept

The importance of race has been a continual issue for the self-identity of African Americans.

Impact of Racism

Unfortunately, racism is still present, and a negative perception of the African American's skin color by health professionals will seriously interfere with efficacious health care.

Religion

African American churches have tremendous influence on the daily lives of their members because they serve as a source of spiritual and social support.
 The African American church acts as a caretaker for the cultural characteristics of Black culture.

Biologic Variations

There is a high incidence of lactose intolerance and lactase deficiency; this has implications for diet planning if Black clients cannot tolerate milk or milk products.
 There is a higher prevalence of hypertension among African Americans than among Americans of European heritage. Sickle cell anemia is more common among African Americans.

Adapted from Andrew, M. M., & Bolin, L. (1993). The African American community. In J. M. Swanson & M. Albrecht (Eds.). *Community health nursing: Promoting the health of aggregates* (pp. 443–458). Philadelphia: W.B. Saunders.

advantageous position of assessing clients and families in their own homes and neighborhoods. This provides an understanding of the daily life situation faced by clients that other health care professionals often lack. Community health nurses can bring this understanding to bear on helping clients with tertiary preventive activities.

SUMMARY

Cultural concepts related to community health nursing practice were discussed. A framework for providing culturally competent nursing care was introduced to help nurses and other health professionals provide care to individuals and groups with diverse cultural backgrounds. Such frameworks help nurses use cultural knowledge in assessing, planning, and implementing nursing care. This chapter explored the role of the family in transmitting beliefs and practices concerning health and illness. Cultural diversity within communities was addressed, and various subcultures, including refugees and immigrants, were discussed. A community case study of Dinka Sudanese refugees was provided. Special concerns related to refugee populations were described. Cultural data about traditional Dinka culture were related, and examples of culturally competent care were provided.

Cultural concepts were explored as they relate to the community at large. A cultural assessment was described as an integral component of a community nursing assessment. Culturally competent nursing interventions for community health maintenance and health promotion were presented. Preventive care in the community is of particular importance to community health nursing. The use of cultural knowledge in primary, secondary, and tertiary levels of prevention was introduced. Examples of cultural diversity and levels of prevention were described to illustrate how cultural knowledge can be used in community health nursing practice.

REVIEW QUESTIONS

1. Describe four cultural concepts and discuss how they can be used to provide transcultural nursing care to families and community aggregates.
2. Describe an example of how cultural factors influence the health of an aggregate group within the community. How do cultural factors influence illness levels in an aggregate group?
3. List the major cultural considerations in implementing preventive programs for culturally diverse groups. How can cultural considerations be used to identify barriers and facilitators for preventive programs?
4. Identify special health considerations in immigrant groups within the community.
5. Describe an approach to primary preventive health care for several cultural groups, for example, Hispanics, African American, Amish, and Bosnian populations.
6. Describe secondary and tertiary programs targeting hypertension for elderly Chinese Americans living in San Francisco's Chinatown.
7. Describe similarities and differences between folk and scientific health care systems. Give an example of each.

CRITICAL THINKING ACTIVITIES

1. Describe sociocultural factors and their impact on health care for a cultural group within your community. Evaluate the access to, availability of, and acceptability of various health care services. Is this cultural group at risk? Why?

2. Conduct a community cultural assessment of a group within your community. Critically analyze the cultural knowledge and/or information that should be considered when planning care for the group. Use the outline provided in Table 11-2 to identify and collect cultural assessment

data, that is, family and kinship, social life, political systems, language, worldview, religious behaviors, health beliefs and practices, and health concerns. Compare and contrast the assessment of other groups in your community.

3. For a cultural group in your community, develop a program plan or intervention that has components of primary, secondary, and tertiary prevention.

4. Attend religious services at a church, temple, mosque, synagogue, or place of worship to learn about a religion different from your own. Assess how each church meets the unique needs of its congregation.

5. Identify alternative health care practitioners within your community. Which subcultures do they serve? Describe the kinds of care that they offer to residents.

REFERENCES

Abrums, M. (2004). Faith and feminism: How African American women from a storefront church resist oppression in healthcare. *Advances in Nursing Science, 27*(3), 187–201.

Adar, K. G. (2000). *SUDAN: The internal and external contexts of conflict and conflict resolution*. Retrieved January 13, 2006, from http://unher.ch/cgi-bin/texis/vtx/country?iso=sdn

American Diabetes Association, Native American Programs. (2009). Retrieved December 1, 2009, from http://www.diabetes.org/community-events/programs/native-american-programs/

American Psychiatric Association. (1987). *Diagnostic and statistical manual of mental disorders* (3rd ed., rev.). Washington, DC: Author.

Anderson, E. T., & McFarlane, J. M. (2008). *Community as partner: Theory and practice in nursing* (5th ed.). Philadelphia: Walters Kluwer/Lippincott Williams & Wilkins.

Andrew, M. M., & Bolin, L. (1993). The African American community. In J. M. Swanson & M. Albrecht (Eds.). *Community health nursing: Promoting the health of aggregates* (pp. 443–458). Philadelphia: W.B. Saunders.

Arizona Department of Health Services, Office of Health Systems Development. (2005). *Nogales primary care area statistical profile. Arizona Primary Care Area Program*. Retrieved January 12, 2006, from http://www.azdhs.gov/index.htm

Aroian, K. J. (2001). Immigrant women and their health. In N. Woods & D. Taylor (Eds.), *Annual review of nursing research* (Vol. 19, pp. 179–226). New York: Springer.

Baird, M. B., (2009). *Resettlement transition experiences among Sudanese refugee women*. Ph.D. dissertation, The University of Arizona, United States, Tucson, Arizona. Retrieved September 11, 2009, from Dissertations & Theses. University of Arizona (Publication No. AAT 3352364).

Barnes, D. M., Harrison, C., & Heneghan, R. (2004). Health risks and promotion behaviors in refugee populations. *Journal of Health Care for the Poor and Underserved, 15*, 347–356.

Berry, A. B. (1999). Mexican American women's expressions of the meaning of culturally congruent prenatal care. *Journal of Transcultural Nursing, 10*, 203–212.

Brown, H. (2004, August 21–27). Disease and hunger in Sudan. *Lancet, 364*, 654.

Burk, M. E., Wieser, P. C., & Keegan, L. (1995). Cultural beliefs and health behaviors of pregnant Mexican American women: Implications for primary health care. *Advances in Nursing Science, 17*(4), 37–52.

CDC. (2004). *Suicide fact sheet*. Retrieved January 29, 2006, from http://www.cdc.gov/ncipe/factsheets/suifacts.htm

Clark, M. J. (2008). Community health nursing as advocacy. In M. J. Clark (Ed.). *Community health nursing* (5th ed., pp. 3–24). Upper Saddle River, NJ: Pearson Prentice Hall.

Deng, F. M. (1984). *The Dinka of Sudan*. Prospect Heights, IL: Waveland Press.

DeSantis, L. (1997). Building healthy communities with immigrants and refugees. *Journal of Transcultural Nursing, 9*, 20–31.

Ehrmin, J. T. (2005). Dimensions of culture care for substance-dependent African American women. *Journal of Transcultural Nursing, 16*(2), 117–125.

ERIC Digest. (1990). *Demographic trends of the Mexican-American population: Implications for schools*. Retrieved December 1, 2009, from http//www.ericdigests.org/pre-9217/trends.htm

Heckler, M. M. (1985a). *Report of the Secretary's Task Force on black and minority health, Vol. I: Executive summary*. Washington, DC: U.S. Department of Health and Human Services.

Heckler, M. M. (1985b). *Report to the Secretary's Task Force on black and minority health, Vol. 2: Crosscutting issues in minority health*. Washington, DC: U.S. Department of Health and Human Services.

Huff, R. M., & Kline, M. V. (1999). *Promoting health in multicultural populations*. Thousand Oaks, CA: Sage.

Leininger, M. (1978). *Transcultural nursing: Concepts, theories and practices*. New York: John Wiley & Sons.

Leininger, M. (1991). Leininger's acculturation health care assessment tool for cultural patterns in traditional and nontraditional lifeways. *Journal of Transcultural Nursing, 2*(2), 40–42.

Leininger, M. (1995). *Transcultural nursing: Concepts, theories, research and practice*. New York: McGraw-Hill.

Lipson, J., & Meleis, A. (1983). Issues in health care of Middle Eastern patients. *Western Journal of Medicine, 139*(6), 854–861.

Lipson, J., Omidian, P., & Paul, S. (1995). Afghan health education project: A community survey. *Public Health Nursing, 12*, 143–150.

Martin, J. A., Hamilton, B. E., Sutton, P. D., Ventura, S. J., Menacker, F., Kirmeyer, S., & Mathews, T. J. (2009). *Births: Final data for 2006.* National Vital Statistics Report; Vol. 57, No 7, Hyattsville, MD; National Center for Health Statistics.

McEwen, M., & Boyle, J. S. (2007). Resistance, health and latent tuberculosis infection: Mexican immigrants at the U.S.-Mexico border. *Research and Theory for Nursing Practice: An International Journal, 21*(3), 185–197.

Minority Health: Quick Facts About Health Disparities. (December 1, 2009). Retrieved December 1, 2009, from http://www.familiesusa.org/issues/minority-health/facts/minority-health-health-quick-facts

Neel, J. V. (1962). Diabetes mellitus: A "thrifty" genotype rendered detrimental by progress. *American Journal of Human Genetics, 14,* 353–362.

Nichols, F. H., & Zwelling, E. (1997). *Maternal-newborn nursing: Theory and practice.* Philadelphia: W.B. Saunders.

Nies, M. A., & McEwen, M. (2007). *Community health nursing: Promoting the health of populations* (4th ed.). Philadelphia: W.B. Saunders.

National Institute of Nursing Research. (1995). *Community-based health care: Nursing strategies.* Bethesda, MD: U.S. Department of Health and Human Services.

National Institute of Nursing Research. (September 2007). *Specialized community Interventions.* Retrieved January 1, 2010, from http://www.docstoc.com/docs/7131604/Specialized-Community-Interventions

Passel, J. S. (2009). *A portrait of unauthorized immigrants in the U.S.* Pew Research Center Publications. Retrieved December 3, 2009, from http://pewresearch.org/pubs/1190/portrait-unauthorized-immigrants-states

Pavlish, C., & Ho, A. (2009). Human rights as barriers for displaced persons in Southern Sudan. *Journal of Nursing Scholarship, 41,* 284–292.

Pinto, A., Saeed, M., El Sakka, H., Rashford, A., Colombo, A., Valenciano, M., Sabatinelli, G. (2005). Setting up an early warning system for epidemic-prone diseases in Darfur: A participative approach. *Disasters, 29*(4), 310–322.

Pletsch, P. K., & Johnson, M. A. (1996). The cigarette smoking experiences of pregnant Latinas in the United States. *Health Care for Women International, 17,* 549–562.

Poverty in the United States. (2007). Retrieved December 1, 2009, from http://www.infoplease.com/ipa/AO104520.html

Shambley-Ebron, D., & Boyle, J. S. (2006). Self-care and the cultural meaning of mothering in African American women with HIV/AIDS. *Western Journal of Nursing Research, 28*(1), 42–60.

Spector, R. E. (2008). *Cultural diversity in health and illness* (7th ed.). New York: Appleton-Century-Crofts.

Stanhope, M., & Lancaster, J. (2006). *Community health nursing: Promoting health of aggregates, families and individuals* (6th ed.). St. Louis, MO: C.V. Mosby.

Strickland, C. J., Walsh, E., & Cooper, M. (2006). Healing fractured families: Parents' and elders' perspectives on the impact of colonization and youth suicide prevention in a Pacific Northwest American Indian tribe. *Journal of Transcultural Nursing, 17,* 5–12.

United Nations High Commissioner for Refugees. (1966). Convention and protocol relating to the status of refugees. Retrieved January 1, 2010, from http://www.unhcr.org

United Nations High Commissioner for Refugees. (2006). Populations of Concern to UNHCR: Statistical Snapshot Sudan Retrieved November 25, 2009, from http://unhcr.org

U.S. Census Bureau. (1998). *Country of origin and year of entry into the U.S. of the foreign born, by citizenship status.* Available at http://www.bis.census.gov/cps/pub/1998/foreign born.htm

U.S. Census Bureau News. (2007, May 17). *Minority populations tops 100 million.* Retrieved September 2007, from http://www.census.gov/Press-Release/www/releases/archives/population/010048.html

U.S. Chamber of Commerce, Labor, Immigration & Employee Benefits Division. (n.d.). *Immigration: Myths and the Facts behind the fallacies.* Retrieved November 24, 2009, from http://www.uschamber.com/NR/rdonlyres.e33skwh6f

U.S. Department of Agriculture, Food and Nutrition Service. (n.d.). *About WIC: How WIC helps.* Retrieved December 8, 2006, from http://www.fns.usda.gov/wic/aboutwic.howwichelps.htm

U.S. Department of Agriculture, Food and Nutrition Service. (1999). Washington, DC: U.S. Government Printing Office.

U.S. Department of Health and Human Services. (1990). *Healthy people 2000 review.* Washington, DC: U.S. Government Printing Office.

U.S. Department of Health and Human Services. (1993). *Healthy people 2000 review.* Washington, DC: U.S. Government Printing Office.

U.S. Department of Health and Human Services. (2000). *Healthy people 2010. National health promotion and disease prevention objectives.* Retrieved July, 2002, from http://www.health.gov.healthypeople/document

Young, K. (1994). *The health of Native Americans.* New York: Oxford University Press.

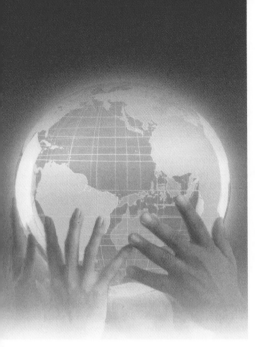

Cultural Diversity in the **Health Care Workforce**

Margaret M. Andrews and
Patti Ludwig-Beymer

KEY TERMS

Attitude change
Barriers
Bigotry
Collectivism
Conflict
Corporate culture
Cross-cultural communication
Cultural diversity
Cultural self-assessment
Cultural values
Discrimination
Dress code
Emic
Ethnoviolence
Etic
Etiquette
Facilitators
Family obligations
Formal attitude change approach
Group dynamics approach
Hatred
Human relations
Hygiene
Individual cultural self-assessment
Individualism
Moral and religious beliefs
Multicultural workforce

(key terms continue on page 317)

LEARNING OBJECTIVES

1. Analyze past, present, and future trends in the racial and ethnic composition of the health care workforce.
2. Identify the cultural meaning of work and its influence on the corporate culture and organizational climate of health care organizations.
3. Critically examine the manner in which hatred, prejudice, racism, discrimination, and ethnoviolence manifest themselves in the health care workplace.
4. Critically analyze the cultural origins of conflict in the health care workforce.
5. Evaluate strategies for promoting effective cross-cultural communication and preventing conflict in the multicultural workplace.
6. Examine the process and content of cultural self-assessment for nurses and for health care organizations, institutions, and agencies.

According to the World Health Organization, the United States is home to 16.6% of the nurses and midwifery personnel in the world (World Health Organization, 2009). Every 4 years, the U.S. Department of Health and Human Services conducts a national survey of registered nurses (RNs). Based on the 2008 survey, 3,063,163 RNs are licensed in the United States, a 5.3% increase from 2004. An estimated 14.5% (44,668 RNs) received their first RN license between 2004 and 2008.

K E Y   T E R M S (continued)

Multicultural workplace
Organizational climate
Organizational cultural
    self-assessment
Prejudice
Race relations
Racism
Resistance to change
Role
Social amnesia
Time orientation
Transcultural nursing administration

As seen in Figure 12-1, White, non-Hispanics comprise 83.2% of licensed RNs, a decrease from 2004 when 87.5% of RNs were White. According to the 2008 survey, 5.8% of RNs are Asian, Native Hawaiian other Pacific Islander, non-Hispanic; 5.4% are African American, non-Hispanic; and 3.6% are Hispanic or Latino of any race; 0.3% of RNs are American Indian or Alaska Native; and 1.7% are from two or more racial backgrounds. Nursing is becoming more diverse. The percentage of non-White or Hispanic nursing graduates has increased steadily, from 12.0% of the 1981–1985 graduates to 22.5% of the 2005–2008 graduates (U.S. Department of Health and Human Services, Bureau of Health Professionals, March 2010). Because of a change in definitions, comparisons of the racial/ethnic composition of the RN population to surveys prior to 2000 should be used with caution. In accordance with the Office of Management and Budget (OMB), the question regarding racial and ethnic background in the March 2000 survey was changed from the previous surveys. Nurses were asked to identify their ethnic background and then asked to identify all races that could best describe them. The information was aggregated to categories similar to those reported in previous years, with one additional grouping of non-Hispanics that reported being of mixed race (two or more races). In surveys prior to 2000, nurses had to choose from one of the racial/ethnic categories presented.

The number of internationally educated RNs licensed in the United States increased between 2004 and 2008, from 3.7% to 5.6% (an estimated 170,235 RNs). Internationally educated RNs licensed in the United States were most frequently from the Philippines (48.7%), Canada (11.5%), India (9.3%), United Kingdom (5.8%), U.S. Territories (2.8%), Korea (2.6%), and Nigeria (2.0%). Women comprise 93.4% of RNs. However, the percentage of male RNs is much higher for more recent nursing graduates. Only 4.1% of nurses who graduated in 1990 or earlier were male, while 9.6% of those who completed their initial nursing education after 1990 were male (U.S. Department of Health and Human Services, Bureau of Health Professionals, March 2010).

In the 2008 survey, 2,596,599 RNs (84.8%) were employed in nursing. This is the highest rate of employment in nursing since the survey began in 1977. There has also been an increase in full-time employment, rising from 58.4% in 2004 to 63.2% in 2008. The most common employment settings for RNs in the United States are hospitals (62.2%), ambulatory care (10.5%), public or community health (7.8%), home health (6.4%), and nursing home/extended care (5.3%). Reported satisfaction with their job increased between 2004 and 2008, with 78% extremely or

Distribution of Registered Nurses by Racial/Ethnic Background

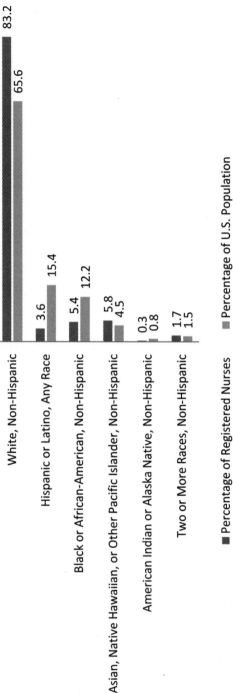

FIGURE 12-1 Distribution of registered nurses by racial/ethnic background compared to United States population, 2008 National Sample Survey.

Sources: U.S. Department of Health and Human Services (March 2010). *The registered nurse population. Initial findings from the 2008 national sample survey of registered nurses.* http://bhpr.hrsa.gov/healthworkforce/rnsurvey. Accessed March 22, 2010 and U.S. Census Bureau. (February 2007). Race and Ethnicity http://www.census.gov/population/www/pop-profile/ files/dynamic/RACEHO.pdf.

moderately satisfied in 2004 and 81.1% extremely or moderately satisfied in 2008 (U.S. Department of Health and Human Services, Bureau of Health Professionals, March 2010).

The average age of the RN population has been rising over the past two decades. Between 2004 and 2008, the average age of all licensed RNs rose from 46.8 to 47 years, and that of employed RNs rose from 45.4 to 45.5 years. Between 2004 and 2008, the share of nurses under the age of 40 grew for the first time since 1980. At that time, 54% of RNs were under 40 years of age but by 2004, only 26.6% of the RN population was under 40 years of age. According to the 2008 RN Survey, 29.5% of RNs are under the age of 40. The percentage of RNs employed in nursing drops for each age group after age 50 and the percentage working full-time drops rapidly after age 60 (U.S. Department of Health and Human Services, Bureau of Health Professionals, March 2010).

The most commonly reported initial nursing education for RNs remains associate degree (45.4%) followed by baccalaureate or higher (34.2%) and diploma (20.4%). Highest educational attainment is also collected, with 36.8% reporting a bachelor's degree and 13.2% reporting a master's or doctorate degree. Advanced practice nurses (APNs) have met additional educational and clinical practice requirements beyond initial nursing education and include clinical nurse specialists, nurse anesthetists, nurse midwives, and nurse practitioners. In 2008, 250,527 RNs were licensed as APNs; this represents 8.2% of RNs (U.S. Department of Health and Human Services, Bureau of Health Professionals, March 2010).

Additional results from the 2008 survey are expected in 2010 (U.S. Department of Health and Human Services, 2010). In 2004, considering both initial and postlicensure RN education, Asian, Pacific Islander, and Black nurses were more likely than White and Hispanic nurses to have at least baccalaureate nursing preparation and Black RNs were most likely to hold master's or doctoral degrees. Non-White, Hispanic or Latino nurses constituted 8% of APNs. The distribution by APN specialty is summarized in Figure 12-2 (U.S. Department of Health and Human Services, 2006).

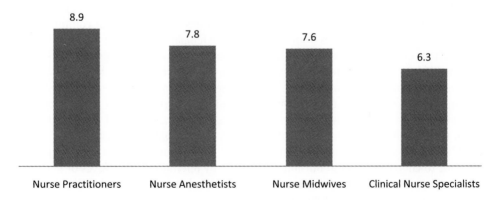

Distribution of Registered Nurses by Racial/Ethnic Background

■ Percentage Non-White and Non-Hispanic or Latino Nurses

FIGURE 12-2   Non-White and non-Hispanic or Latino nurses by Advanced Practice Nurse specialty.

Source: U.S. Department of Health and Human Services, Health Resources and Services Administration. (June 2006). *The registered nurse population: Findings from the March 2004 national sample survey of registered nurses.* ftp://ftp.hrsa.gov/bhpr/ workforce/0306rnss.pdf. Accessed March 6, 2010.

In contrast to the United States, the total supply of RNs in Canada was 279,399 in 2008, with 93.7% of the RN workforce employed in nursing, and 58.1% employed full time. Hospitals employed 62.7% of the RN workforce, followed by the community health sector at 14.2% and nursing home or long-term care at 10.1%. Like the United States, almost all RNs in Canada are female (94%); the average age is 45.1 years. RNs are quite mobile, both within Canada and across the world. Of the Canadian RNs practicing outside of their jurisdiction of registration, 52.6% are practicing in the United States.

At 8.4%, the proportion of foreign-educated nurses working in Canada is higher than that in the United States (Canadian Institute for Health Information, 2010). Like the United States, Canada's nursing workforce is not representative of current national demographics. For example, data from the 1996 Canadian Census indicate that only 10.7% of RNs employed in Canada identify themselves as members of a visible minority (Human Resources and Social Development Canada, 2001).

However, in both Canada and the United States, there continues to be an increasingly diverse workforce. In many health care settings there is diversity in race, ethnicity, religion, age, sexual orientation, and national origin. Recent strides in the women's movement have called attention to important gender differences and the manner in which changing societal roles of both men and women influence relationships in the **multicultural workplace**, as seen in Evidence-Based Practice 12-1. The interrelationship between culture and the physical, mental, and emotional handicaps and disabilities of some health care workers must also be considered in the complex web called the **multicultural workforce**.

Women have historically constituted the majority of personnel in nursing and in many allied health disciplines. For the past two decades, women

EVIDENCE-BASED PRACTICE 12-1

Motivations and Experiences of Males in the Nursing Profession

This pilot study of the motivations and experiences of males in the nursing profession examines and critiques the available literature on males in nursing from both a historical and contemporary, present-day perspective and provides the foundation for a pilot study of 30 male nurses prior to professional registration and 30 male nurses after they have earned their professional registration. Preliminary data based on 42 male nurses who completed a mailed survey revealed the following themes: (1) initial motivation for choosing nursing, including the influence of parents (particularly mothers); (2) lack of career advice for young men who might want to choose a career in nursing; (3) importance of altruism and caring in choosing a nursing career, with informants frequently reporting that they had experienced some form of a caring family situation prior to entering the profession; (4) age and cultural variations, for example, attitude of Black males toward senior female colleagues, with some expressing concern at being "given orders by a woman"; (5) exclusion of males from certain specialties such as maternal–child nursing, and from certain gender-specific procedures; (6) high level of comfort caring for "older female patients," but discomfort caring for female patients who are about their same age; (7) preference of some male patients for the presence of male nurses, especially when shaving, bathing, or performing intimate procedures (e.g., catheterization); and (8) a need to convey their own sexuality and sexual orientation in subtle ways, for example, confirming heterosexuality by referring to their wives or making negative remarks about homosexual male nurses.

Clinical Implications

Despite their historical significance to the nursing profession, the numbers of male nursing students and nurses have seldom exceeded 10% in the

EVIDENCE-BASED PRACTICE 12-1 (continued)

United States, Canada, or the United Kingdom. Findings from this preliminary pilot study confirm that some of the historic stereotypes about male nurses continue to exert a negative influence on young men as they make career choices. The major themes identified by the investigators need to be examined because they have implications for recruitment and retention strategies employed by schools of nursing and by employers of nurses. Limiting the clinical practice settings that are considered appropriate for males and excluding them from participating in specialties such as obstetric nursing or from performing certain procedures on female patients contributes to the perception by males that they are unwelcome in schools of nursing and in the nursing profession. Given the current shortage of nurses, the nursing profession collectively needs to explore how and where it markets itself to young men and the image of male nurses portrayed by the media.

Reference: Whittock, M., & Leonard, L. (2003). Stepping outside the stereotype. A pilot study of the motivations and experiences of males in the nursing profession. *Journal of Nursing Management, 11,* 242–249.

and members of racially and ethnically diverse groups have made significant inroads into health professions that were once overwhelmingly the province of White men. The largest gains for most culturally diverse groups, however, occurred during the mid- to late 1970s. Since that time, with the exception of Asians and Hispanics, **cultural diversity** in the health care fields has been relatively stable.

The Challenges and Opportunities of a Growing Multicultural Population and Health Care Workforce

A significant number of the U.S. and Canadian national health goals for the current decade and beyond involve specific objectives for improving the health status of members of minority groups identified by both countries' federal governments, particularly those with low incomes. Meanwhile, culturally diverse cohorts of children, women of childbearing age, and the elderly are expected to grow, exacerbating the need for culturally competent providers of health care.

Since 1972 there has been an explosion in the numbers of people migrating to the United States and Canada, both with and without legal documentation. In 2007, the total population of the United States was 301.6 million, which included 38.1 million foreign born, representing 12.6% of the total population. The top 10 countries of origin for the foreign-born population are Mexico (30.3%), China (5.1%), Philippines (4.5%), India (3.9%), El Salvador (2.9%), Vietnam (2.9%), Korea (2.7%), Cuba (2.6%), Canada (2.2%), and the Dominican Republic (2.0%) (U.S. Census Bureau, January 2010).

Foreign-born individuals constitute 19% of the overall population in Canada. The nearly 6.2 million foreign-born people in Canada reported over 200 countries of origin on the 2006 Census. Immigration was responsible for two-thirds of the population growth in Canada between 2001 and 2006. The source of immigrants has changed considerably over the past 20 years, as seen on Table 12-1 (Statistics Canada, November 2009).

Because the health care workplace is a microcosm of the changing demographic patterns in society at large, the growing diversity among nurses and other members of the health care team frequently poses challenges and opportunities in the multicultural work setting. These challenges and opportunities are summarized in Case Studies 12-1 through 12-5.

TABLE 12-1
Top 10 Countries of Birth for Recent Immigrants, Canada

RANK ORDER	2006 CENSUS	2001 CENSUS	1996 CENSUS	1991 CENSUS	1981 CENSUS
1	People's Republic of China	People's Republic of China	Hong Kong	Hong Kong	United Kingdom
2	India	India	People's Republic of China	Poland	Vietnam
3	Philippines	Philippines	India	People's Republic of China	United States of America
4	Pakistan	Pakistan	Philippines	India	India
5	United States of America	Hong Kong	Sri Lanka	Philippines	Philippines
6	South Korea	Iran	Poland	United Kingdom	Jamaica
7	Romania	Taiwan	Taiwan	Vietnam	Hong Kong
8	Iran	United States of America	Vietnam	United States of America	Portugal
9	United Kingdom	South Korea	United States of America	Lebanon	Taiwan
10	Columbia	Sri Lanka	United Kingdom	Portugal	People's Republic of China

Source: Statistics Canada (November 2009).

CASE STUDY 12-1

When a Black patient was admitted to a small rural hospital with predominantly White staff and patients, nurses from one shift would include "Black male" in their report to the oncoming shift. When one of the few Black nurses began using "White male" or "White female" in her report, she was accused of "having an attitude" and "trying to instigate racial trouble."

CASE STUDY 12-2

When informed that a patient was requesting medication for pain, a Lutheran nurse of German heritage responded to a fellow nurse, "She's just a Jewish princess who complains about pain all the time." A Jewish laboratory technician overheard the remark and demanded to know what the nurse manager was going to do about the "blatant anti-Semitism" on the unit.

CASE STUDY 12-3

A slightly built Black male nurse asked to meet with the operating room nurse manager about a surgeon who had recently immigrated from Russia. The nurse complained, "Dr. Ivanovich keeps asking me why I became a nurse. He asks very personal questions about my sexual orientation and wants to know if I'm 'queer.' I consider this a hostile work environment and refuse to scrub for his surgical cases any more."

CASE STUDY 12-4

After receiving a report on a critically ill victim of a motor vehicle accident, Dr. Juan Valdez-Rodriguez, the physician on call, asked for the patient's name. The reporting nurse said, "I don't know. Martinez, Hernandez, something like that. You'll recognize him when you see him—just another drunk Mexican who ran his pickup truck into a tree."

Upon entering the examination room, the physician immediately recognized the victim as his cousin.

CASE STUDY 12-5

A nurse entered into a conversation with a Chinese American food service worker. Ms. Chin remarked that for the past 4 days she had been asked to be the interpreter for an elderly Chinese man on one of the units where she delivers food. "I don't want to offend the nurse manager who asked me to translate, but it is not right for a younger woman to speak for an older man. It is not our custom. Besides, my supervisor scolded me for being so slow to do my work. She thinks I have become lazy. Would you talk to the nurse manager for me?"

Cultural Perspectives on the Meaning of Work

The earliest recorded ideas about work refer to it as a curse, a punishment, or a necessary evil needed to sustain life. People of high status did not work, whereas slaves, indentured servants, and peasants worked. In contemporary society, the concept of work must be considered in its historical and cultural context. Cultural views about caring for the sick also must be considered because such care may be perceived as a divine calling for those with supernatural powers (some African tribes), a religious vocation (some ethnic Catholic groups), or an undignified occupation for lower-class workers (some Arab groups such as Kuwaitis and Saudi Arabians).

Cultural norms influence a staff member's consideration of group interest as opposed to individual interests in the multicultural workplace. Scholars have identified two major orientations embraced by people: individualism and collectivism. With **individualism**, importance is placed on individual inputs, rights, and rewards. Individualists emphasize values such as autonomy, competitiveness, achievement, and self-sufficiency. Most English-speaking and European countries have individualist cultures.

Collectivism entails the need to maintain group harmony above the partisan interests of subgroups and individuals. In collectivist cultures, values such as interpersonal harmony and group solidarity prevail. A staff member whose ethnic heritage is Asian or South American is likely to be influenced by collectivism. Amish and Mennonite groups also are considered collectivist cultures.

One of the most notable distinctions between people from individualist and collectivist cultures is the meaning of work. Individualists work to earn a living. People are expected to work; they need not enjoy it. Leisure or recreational activities frequently are pursued to alleviate the monotony of work. People from individualist cultures tend to dichotomize work and leisure. Individualist concepts of work reflect an orientation toward the future.

It also is useful to understand cultural differences about appropriate and desired behavior in the workplace. People from most individualist cultures are typically achievement oriented. Stereotypically, they want to do better, accomplish more, and take responsibility for their actions. They tend to develop personality traits such as assertiveness and competitiveness that facilitate these goals. In many collectivist cultures, however, qualities such as commitment to relationships, gentleness, cooperativeness, and indirectness are valued.

Some researchers have suggested that the motivational strategies of Japanese managers must appeal to the Japanese worker's sense of loyalty, commitment, and group orientation, whereas the motivation strategies of North American managers must appeal to the worker's sense of contract, rules, and individuality. Although some individuals have a combination of the two qualities, most staff members will display either an individualistic or a collectivistic orientation in the workplace. Nurses in leadership positions need to recognize the fundamental value system embraced by their staff members to understand why they behave as they do at work.

Corporate Cultures and Subcultures

As described in Chapter 9, health care organizations are mini societies that have their own distinctive patterns of culture and subculture. One organization may have a high degree of cohesiveness, with staff working together like members of a single family toward the achievement of common goals. Another may be highly fragmented, divided into groups that think about the world in very different ways or that have different aspirations about what their organization should be. Just as individuals in a culture can have different personalities while sharing much in common, so can groups and organizations. This phenomenon is referred to as **corporate culture**. Corporate culture is a process of reality construction that allows staff to see and understand particular events, actions, objects, communications, or situations in distinctive ways. These patterns of understanding help people cope with the situations they encounter and provide a basis for making behavior sensible and meaningful.

Shared values, beliefs, meaning, and understanding are components of the corporate culture. The corporate culture is established and maintained through an ongoing, proactive process of reality construction. It is an active, living phenomenon through which staff members jointly create and re-create their workplace and world. One of the easiest ways to appreciate the nature of corporate culture and subculture is to observe the day-to-day functioning of the organization. Observe the patterns of interaction among individuals, the language that is used, the images and themes explored in conversation,

and the various rituals of daily routine. Historical explanations for the ways things are done will emerge in discussions of the rationale for certain aspects of the culture.

The corporate culture metaphor is useful because it directs attention to the symbolic significance of almost every aspect of organizational life. Structures, hierarchies, rules, and organizational routines reveal underlying meanings that are crucial for understanding how organizations function. For example, meetings carry important aspects of organizational culture, which may convey a sense of conformity and order or of causal informality. The environment in which the meetings are held reflects the formality or informality of the organization.

Box 12-1 poses several questions that might be considered in the determination of the corporate culture of a health care organization, institution, or agency. The answers to the questions will provide a beginning understanding of the corporate culture of the organization.

Health care work environments are social settings that encompass many elements of a social system. It is useful to distinguish between the **organizational climate** of the work environment and the corporate culture. The organizational climate usually measures perceptions or feelings about the organization or work environment. The corporate or organizational culture, on the other hand, is what its members share—their

---

BOX 12-1

Determining Corporate Culture

It is useful to pose the following questions when determining the corporate culture of an organization.

- Does the person presiding over the group stand or sit?
- Does the presider encourage discussion among group members or engage in a monologue?
- Are group members encouraged to express opinions freely, or is there pressure to silence those who express opposing points of view?
- How do group leaders and members dress?
- What message does the institutional dress code convey about the acceptance of cultural diversity?
- Do policies allow for cultural expressions in clothing, accessories, hair style, and related areas?
- Although most institutions require employees to wear identification badges or name tags, what flexibility does the individual have for self-expression and expression of cultural identity and affiliation?

beliefs, values, assumptions, rituals—often unconsciously. Culture provides the community, the sameness, and the consensus that makes those people unique and special.

Managing the delivery of care within complex corporate and organizational cultures requires astute **transcultural nursing administration**. As discussed on Chapter 9, transcultural nursing administrative perspectives are essential for survival, growth, satisfaction, and achievement of goals in the multicultural workplace.

In the contemporary health care industry, nurse administrators sometimes focus their time and energy on issues such as cost–benefit outcomes, downsizing, territorial struggles with members of other disciplines, appropriate use of technology, and other important topics. With increasing frequency, nurse administrators are realizing the critical importance of transculturally based administrative practices that positively influence cost and quality outcomes. With the increasing diversity among members of the health care workforce, nurses are challenged to develop and practice this new type of administration.

Negative Attitudes and Behaviors in the Multicultural Workplace

A variety of negative attitudes and behaviors may emerge in a multicultural workplace, including hatred, prejudice, bigotry, discrimination, racism, and violence. The formation of strategies for changing these attitudes and behaviors must be considered.

Hatred

In some organizations, the use of racial, ethnic, sexual, and other derogatory remarks signals a disturbing underlying problem in the workplace. Why does hatred exist in the workplace? Although the reasons are complex and interconnected, some contributing factors include the early socialization of children to cultural and gender stereotypes, personal experiences (or lack of them) with people from diverse backgrounds, and exposure to negative societal attitudes.

According to Henderson (1994), **hatred** in the workplace is exacerbated during times of rapid immigration, periods of economic recession or depression, and high unemployment. Competition for sexual partners also is cited as a cause for hatred. Hatred can be the cause of tremendous hostility in the workplace. In some organizations, technology is used to transmit derogatory remarks electronically to individuals or targeted groups by e-mail or fax. Sites on the Internet that allow free expressions of hatred have proliferated. Those responsible justify their actions by citing either the Canadian Charter of Rights and Freedoms or the U.S. Constitution's First Amendment rights to freedom of expression.

Prejudice, Bigotry, and Discrimination

The term **prejudice** refers to inaccurate perceptions of others. Prejudice results in conclusions that are drawn without adequate knowledge or evidence. All people are prejudiced for or against other people. Prejudices in the community at large are acted out in the workplace. **Bigotry** connotes narrow-mindedness and an obstinate or blind attachment to a particular opinion or viewpoint. The bigot blames members of outgroups for various misfortunes. In their efforts to make expedient decisions, bigots react to concepts rather than to people.

Whereas prejudice and bigotry refer to attitudes, **discrimination** refers to behaviors and is defined as the act of setting one individual or group apart from another, thereby showing a difference or favoritism. Discriminatory behaviors, not attitudes, constitute the majority of intergroup problems. Although there are many laws against discriminatory behaviors, especially in the workplace, there are none against prejudice or bigotry (Henderson, 1994).

The nurse in Case Study 12-1 who points out in the report that the patient is Black may not have any conscious discriminatory intent. By departing from the usual practice of not mentioning race, however, she makes a statement that race is a variable that needs to be mentioned. In turn, this gives an opportunity for prejudices in the minds of the other nurses to surface. Keeping people of color exploitable is a foundation of racial inequality.

Contrary to popular writings, prejudices in the workplace are not limited to Black–White conflicts and confrontations. There is prejudice against various members of the workforce, including women, older workers, individuals with disabilities, foreign-born workers, and White workers.

In Case Study 12-2, the nurse's characterization of the patient experiencing pain as a "Jewish princess" is a transparently anti-Semitic remark. The ability to control the lives of people is a psychological aspect of nursing that is often unconsciously manifested. The nurse in the case study may be exercising a certain degree of power over the patient, knowing that she is at the nurse's mercy for the relief of her pain. It also may reflect an underlying "scientific racism," that is, that there are biologic differences between certain groups. The nurse may believe that there are different pain thresholds among persons of diverse backgrounds and that Jewish patients tend to have a relatively low tolerance for pain.

The nurse's own ethnic background, religious affiliation, and personal experience with pain may contribute to her perceptions of the patient's need for pain relief. Although the nurse may be using "scientific racism" to rationalize her beliefs that a patient is requesting more pain relief than the average person, there is no excuse for the racist reference to her patient as a "Jewish princess." The nurse's racism adversely affects not only the patient, but also a fellow nurse and a laboratory technician. The racial slur is an example of an implicit cue passed on to others, in which the nurse perpetuates both prejudice against and stereotypes about Jewish people. The laboratory technician is likely to view the nurse, and perhaps by extension the entire multicultural workplace, as being hostile to Jews.

Prejudice is also based on sexual orientation, as illustrated in Case Study 12-3. The Black nurse expresses his concern with the hostile work environment created by the imposing Russian surgeon, who asks inappropriate questions about his sexual orientation. Because the offender is a recent immigrant, he may be unaware of cultural differences concerning appropriate topics for discussion in the workplace—though it is doubtful that his behavior would be widely accepted in a Russian operating room setting, either. Furthermore, the surgeon may have a limited English vocabulary and/or may be unaware of the negative connotation of the slang term "queer." These explanations for the surgeon's inappropriate behavior in the workplace do not excuse him; rather, they are offered as factors worthy of the nurse manager's consideration in an attempt to address the problem.

Racism

Racism implies that superior or inferior traits and behavior are determined by race. Racism connotes prejudice and discrimination. To understand racism in the workplace, distinctions need to be made among (1) institutional structures and personal behavior, and the relationship between the two; (2) the variation in both degree and form of expression of individual prejudice; and (3) the fact that racism is merely one form of a larger and more inclusive pattern of ethnocentrism that may be based on various factors, both racial and nonracial (Henderson, 1994; Williams & Rucker, 2000).

Racism is caused by a complex web of factors, including ignorance, apathy, poverty, historic patterns of discrimination against particular groups, and social stratification. In a classic work on racism, Brown (1973) posits that society "is racially divided and its whole organization...promotes racial distinctions" (p. 8). With this frame of reference, racial bias and discrimination have been built into most U.S. and Canadian institutions, and every citizen is a product of institutional racism. According to Henderson, "What is commonly called racism is part of the larger problem of ethnic identification, of power and powerlessness, and of the exploitation of the weak by the strong. . . . What most writers commonly call **race relations** should be properly understood in the larger context of **human relations**" (1994, p. 21) (emphasis added).

In the multicultural workplace, the expression of negative attitudes and behaviors by people toward others according to their identification as members of a particular group is of particular concern. The expression of these attitudes and behavioral patterns is learned as part of the cultural process. Negative group attitudes and destructive group conflicts are less likely to arise when employees treat each other as individuals and respond to each other on the basis of individual characteristics and behaviors (Williams & Rucker, 2000).

In Case Study 12-4, the nurse's remark "just another drunk Mexican" is an example of a stereotype that may have an element of truth in it but is nevertheless inaccurate. Although it is true that the majority of motor vehicle accidents are alcohol related, and that in this hospital a large proportion of those involved are Mexican Americans, it is untrue that all Mexican American men are alcoholics. By overgeneralizing in this way, the nurse fails to assess important information about the individual person and depersonalizes him through the stereotype. The nurse's apparent insensitivity to Dr. Valdez-Rodriguez's ethnic heritage is appalling. The pathos of the situation is further realized when the physician learns that the "just another drunk Mexican" accident victim is his cousin.

The career potential of staff from diverse backgrounds is frequently undermined by the relative lack of access to informal networks and mentors and by the expectation that these persons will assimilate into organizational cultures that are often intolerant of the cultures with which these staff members identify. These manifestations of discrimination can be expected to undermine the functioning of the health care organization. Paradoxically, the victims of mistreatment are often the perpetrators as well. The victim of mistreatment may, in turn, mistreat others. One explanation for this phenomenon is that people are likely to experience a form of internalized oppression as a result of low self-esteem.

Violence in the Workplace

Although not all hatred leads to violence, the number of reported attacks on gays and anti-Muslim and anti-Semitic incidents has increased significantly. **Ethnoviolence** is also increasing, not only in the United States and Canada, but worldwide. Blacks, Hispanics, homosexual men, Muslims, and Jews are the primary targets of hate crimes, many of which occur in the workplace. Although it is impossible to protect all employees and patients from violence in health care settings, reasonable steps must be taken to protect those believed to be at risk. Verbal threats and/or assaults by or against staff members should not be tolerated.

Health care administrators have a moral imperative to take reasonable steps in ensuring the physical safety of staff, patients/clients, and visitors. The institution's security officers and/or local police should be notified whenever violence is threatened. Some institutions require staff and visitors to pass through a metal detector when entering the premises, whereas others have posted security officers at entrances to ensure that only authorized persons are admitted. In extreme cases, it may be necessary to obtain a court order to prohibit an individual or group from the premises or to establish a safe perimeter so patients and staff may have safe access to the facility.

In recent years, attorneys representing health care institutions have sometimes found it necessary to obtain a court order to ensure a safe work environment during times of racial, ethnic, religious, and social discord. Unfortunately, some demonstrators with strong convictions have violated others' civil liberties and engaged in violent acts against those who disagreed with their point of view. The shooting of staff at clinics where abortions are performed is an extreme example of hatred that has resulted in violence. This violence is caused by a complex web of interconnected factors, including religious, moral, ethical, social, political, and cultural differences.

Formation of Attitudes

Attitudes are learned, not innate. Researchers have found that as children grow older they tend to forget that they were instructed in attitudes by their parents and significant other people. Around the age of 10, most children regard their attitudes toward people from different cultural backgrounds as being innate. Seldom do they recall being coached, resulting in **social amnesia**. When social amnesia develops, the individual tends to create elaborate rationalizations in an effort to account for learned attitudes toward certain groups of people in a society.

The superiority or inferiority of a group (versus an individual) is usually less obvious than an individual's behavior. Most staff members bring their cultural baggage to work with them, and their actions are molded and shaped by peer pressure. The values, behaviors, and customs of those in the outgroup are labeled as "strange" or "unusual." As children, many staff learned to reject people who were culturally different and to view differences as being synonymous with inferiority. In the insightful words of Carl Jung:

> We still attribute to the other fellow all the evil and inferior qualities that we do not like to recognize in ourselves, and therefore have to criticize and attack him, when all that has happened is that an inferior soul has emigrated from one person to another. The world is still full of betes noirs and scapegoats, just as it formerly teemed with witches and werewolves (1968, p. 65).

Changing Attitudes

Although some argue that the focus should be on behavior change rather than **attitude change**, others maintain that hatred, prejudice, bigotry, racism, discrimination, and ethnoviolence begin with an individual's attitudes toward certain groups. Staff members' attitudes can be changed in several ways, but they require commitment by all levels of management within an organization. They also require a certain degree of openness and receptivity by the individual.

Efforts to change staff members' attitudes about people from culturally diverse groups should

center on communication. Several approaches have been used by organizations. The first, called the **formal attitude change approach**, is based on learning theories: on the assumption that people are rational, information-processing beings who can be motivated to listen to a message, hear its content, and incorporate what they have learned when it is advantageous to do so. There is an actual or expected reward for embracing diversity.

The second, known as the **group dynamics approach**, assumes that staff members are social beings who need culturally diverse coworkers as they adjust to environmental changes. The amount of change depends on people's attitudes toward diversity, their attention to the message and to the communicator, their understanding of the message, and their acceptance of the message. Acceptance of diversity is likely to be enhanced by activities that provide tangible rewards for staff. It is seldom enough for top management to urge staff members to embrace diversity as a moral imperative.

Cultural Values in the Multicultural Workplace

Cultural values frequently lie at the root of cross-cultural differences in the multicultural workplace. Values form the core of a culture. Time orientation, family obligations, communication patterns (including etiquette, space/distance, touch), interpersonal relationships (including long-standing historic rivalries), gender/sexual orientation, education, socioeconomic status, moral/religious beliefs, hygiene, clothing, meaning of work, and personal traits exert influences on individuals within the multicultural health care setting.

What is the importance of learning about the values of people from diverse cultural groups? Values exert a powerful influence on how each person behaves, reacts, and feels. In the multicultural workplace, values affect people's lives in four major ways. Values underlie *perceived needs, what is defined as a problem, how conflict is resolved,* and *expectations of behavior*. When cultural values of individual staff members conflict with the organizational values or those held by coworkers, challenges, misunderstandings, and difficulties in the workplace become inevitable. You must use these inevitable conflicts as opportunities to foster cross-cultural understanding among staff members from diverse backgrounds and to enhance cross-cultural communication.

Cultural Perspectives on Conflict

The term **conflict** is derived from Latin roots (*confligere*, "to strike against") and refers to ac-tions that range from intellectual disagreement to physical violence. Frequently, the action that precipitates the conflict is based on different cultural perceptions of the situation. According to some social scientists, when participants in a conflict are from the same culture, they are more likely to perceive the situation in the same way and to organize their perceptions in similar ways.

By examining proverbs used by members of various cultural groups, it is possible to better understand differences in the way conflict is viewed. Table 12-2 summarizes selected proverbs that relate to conflict and its resolution. The dominant

TABLE 12-2
Cross-Cultural Perspectives on Proverbs and Conflict

PROVERB	VALUE
Dominant Culture	
The squeaky wheel gets the grease.	Aggressiveness Direct confrontation
Tell it like it is.	Direct confrontation Honesty even if it hurts the other
Take the bull by the horns.	Direct confrontation
Shoot first, ask questions later.	Aggressiveness Direct confrontation Protection of individual rights (versus good of the group)
Might makes right.	Aggressiveness Dominance
Japanese	
The nail that sticks out gets hammered.	Not calling attention to oneself Going along with the group Harmony and balance
Senegalese	
Misunderstandings do not exist; only the failure to communicate does.	Strive to understand the other's point of view Harmony and balance is normal state, not conflict and confrontation
Zen	
He who knows does not speak, and he who speaks does not know.	Listen to the other's side during conflict Silence
Arab	
The hand of Allah is with the group. Haste comes from the devil.	Primacy of group good (versus individual) Patience Conflict resolution takes time

culture's proverbs emphasize that people should behave assertively and deal with conflict through direct confrontation. Other cultures—particularly collectivist groups—may promote avoidance of confrontation and emphasize harmony (e.g., Native North Americans, Alaskan Natives, Amish, and Asians). The culture-based choices that lead people in these opposite directions are a major source of conflict in the workplace.

Many people from individualist cultures view conflict as a healthy, natural, and inevitable component of all relationships. People from many collectivist cultures, on the other hand, have learned to internalize conflict and to value harmonious relationships above winning arguments and "being right." To many people of Native North American and Asian descent, conflict is not healthy, desirable, or constructive. In the Arab world, mediation is critical in resolving disputes, and confrontation seldom works. Mediation allows for saving face and is rooted in the realization that all conflicts do not have simple solutions.

The assertive, confrontational, direct style of communicating is characteristic of people from individualistic cultures, whereas the cooperative, conciliatory style is a more collectivist or Eastern mode of managing conflict. When attempting to influence others during a disagreement, for example, nurses from China, Japan, and other collectivist cultures may use covert conflict prevention strategies to minimize interpersonal conflicts. Nurses from individualistic cultures are more likely to rely on the overt confrontation of ideas and argumentation by reason.

In Case Study 12-5, the Chinese food service worker demonstrates the cultural value for harmonious relationships, indirect communication, and nonconfrontational resolution of conflict. The nurse manager has inadvertently placed Mrs. Chin in an awkward position by violating Chinese norms concerning gender and age. In traditional Chinese culture, it is inappropriate for a younger person to speak for an older one and for a female to speak for a male. Serving as an interpreter for the elderly Chinese man has been uncomfortable for both Mrs. Chin and the patient. Mrs. Chin's value for harmonious relationships in the workplace prevents her from speaking directly to the nurse manager and food service supervisor about the problem. By involving the staff nurse as an intermediary with the nurse manager, she is attempting to convey her dissatisfaction with the situation in a nonconfrontational, indirect, and polite manner. She also attempts to avoid appearing like a complaining, disgruntled employee who is unwilling to cooperate with other workers. For these reasons, she is reluctant to bring the problem to her food service supervisor's attention. She believes that she must please those in authority, foster harmonious relationships, and avoid direct confrontation if she is to be a valuable employee of the hospital.

Cultural Origins of Conflict

Let's examine some cultural values and the manner in which they may result in conflict in the multicultural workplace. The origins of cultural conflict result from influences on the organization and on individuals. As indicated in Figure 12-3, political, economic, technologic, and legal factors influence the corporate culture and the organizational climate of both organizations and their employees. For organizations owned and operated by religious groups, religious influences must be considered. For example, in a hospital owned and operated by a Roman Catholic religious order, therapeutic abortions, tubal ligations, and other gynecologic procedures may be prohibited. Factors such as educational background, socioeconomic status, culture, moral and religious beliefs, and personal traits of employees must also be considered when determining the cultural origins of conflict. Staff members contribute to the perception that values are in conflict. Although there are many conflicting values that underlie problems, the following areas will be explored in the remainder of this chapter: cultural perspectives on family obligations, personal hygiene, cross-cultural communication (including etiquette and touch), clothing and accessories, time orientation, interpersonal relationships (including historic rivalries between groups),

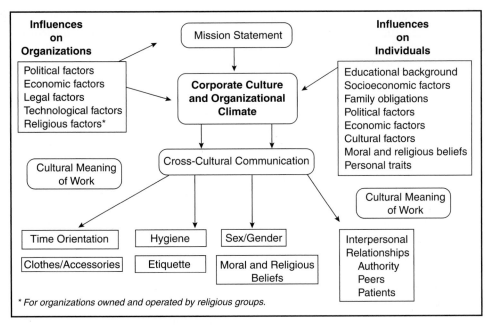

FIGURE 12-3   Origins of conflict in the multicultural health care setting.

gender/sexual orientation, and moral and religious beliefs (including dietary practices).

Cultural Perspectives on Family Obligations

Although family is important in all cultures, the constellation (e.g., nuclear, single-parent, extended, same-sex), emotional closeness among members, social and economic commitments among members, and other factors vary cross-culturally. Both staff nurses and those in administrative positions frequently report difficulty with requests from nurses of diverse cultural backgrounds that pertain to **family obligations**.

Some nurses from different cultures have been labeled as uncommitted to their work and/or disinterested in their nursing careers because family is a higher priority than job or career. The so-called appliance nurse has long been recognized among members of the dominant culture as well. Given that it is highly unlikely (and undesirable) that the nurse manager will be successful at changing fundamental family-related values, the most useful approach is to focus on the problematic behavior. For example, if excessive

absenteeism is the undesirable behavior, the nurse manager should arrange for a face-to-face meeting in which the problematic behavior is discussed. In addition, the use of peer pressure by coworkers also can be helpful in changing the undesirable behavior as fellow workers communicate to the individual why his or her behavior is troublesome. It is generally useful to identify the reason(s) for the excessive absenteeism and to explore culturally appropriate strategies for resolving the problem, such as use of the natural social support that is culturally expected of extended family members. The solution is seldom simple, as the following case analysis illustrates.

Independence from the family, for example, is highly valued by many from the dominant cultural groups in the United States and Canada, but it ranks very low in the hierarchy of people from most Middle Eastern and Asian cultures. In the latter groups, the family is highly valued, and the individual's lifelong duties toward the family are explicit. Thus, absence from work for family-related reasons may be considered legitimate and important by workers from some cultures but may be perceived as an unnecessary inconvenience to the supervisor. For example, a Mexican American staff member may submit a last-minute request for vacation time to visit with a distant cousin who has unexpectedly arrived in town after traveling a great distance. The Mexican American staff member thinks, "What a great opportunity to develop a stronger relationship with a distant member of my mother's family. How nice that cousin Juan has traveled so far to see me. I've been thinking about making a trip to Mexico next year, so perhaps I can stay with Juan during my visit. Surely my nurse manager understands how important it is for me to spend time with my family and will be able to rearrange the unit schedule to accommodate my request." The nurse manager may think, "What's wrong with these Mexican Americans? Don't they want to work? This vacation request means that I'll have to redo the schedule for the entire unit. If I permitted everyone to submit last-minute vacation requests, I'd go crazy. What's the big deal about a distant cousin coming to visit, anyway?"

Ideas about the importance of anticipating and controlling the future vary significantly from culture to culture. Whereas some staff members place a high priority on planning for retirement, accumulating sick days, and purchasing insurance, others, particularly recent immigrants with family obligations in their homelands, may be more concerned with current obligations and living in the present. Similarly, some workers in high-risk jobs will participate actively in preventive immunization programs aimed at hepatitis and influenza, whereas others bewilder managers by saying, "What will be, will be. I can't spend time worrying about something that may or may not happen in the future."

Cultural Perspectives on Personal Hygiene

Another value that influences behavior is found in the proverb "cleanliness is next to godliness." This proverb highlights the value for cleanliness, including an obsession with eliminating or minimizing natural bodily odors—as evidenced by the plethora of deodorants, douches, body lotions, mouthwashes, and the like with hundreds of different fragrances. Members of the dominant culture sometimes have difficulty with staff members from other cultures who are not unduly bothered by body odors and see no reason to mask nature's original smells. In some cases, the staff member may come from a country in which water is scarce and bathing is restricted. Other staff members may be following religious or cultural practices that prohibit bathing during certain phases of the menstrual cycle, after the delivery of a baby, and at other times. Nurse managers and other supervisors frequently find the sensitive topic of **hygiene** difficult to discuss with staff from diverse cultural backgrounds.

Cross-Cultural Communication

Underlying the majority of conflicts in the multicultural health care setting are issues related to effective **cross-cultural communication**, both verbal and nonverbal. Even when one is dealing with staff members from the same cultural background, it requires administrative skill to decide whether to speak with someone face to face, send an electronic or paper memorandum, contact the person by telephone, or opt not to communicate about a particular matter at all. The nurse must exercise considerable judgment when making decisions about effective methods for communicating with staff members and patients from diverse cultural backgrounds; as summarized in Figure 12-4, a variety of factors including a sense of timing, tone and pitch of voice, choice of location for face-to-face interactions, and related matters must be considered. Communication difficulties caused by differences in language and accent become compounded on the telephone. It is sometimes necessary to counsel recent immigrants from non–English-speaking countries to refrain from giving or receiving medical orders by telephone until their English language skills have developed (Nixon & Bull, 2006; Samovar, Porter, & McDaniel, 2006).

In the United States, approximately 18% of the total U.S. population has a primary language other than English. In rank order, the most frequently spoken languages are English (82%), Spanish or Spanish Creole (10%), Chinese (0.77%); French (0.63%), German (0.53%), Tagalog (0.47%),

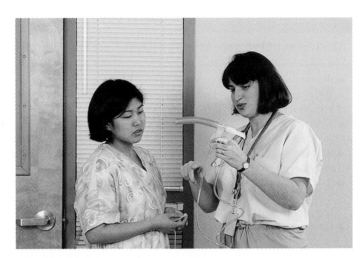

FIGURE 12-4 Effective cross-cultural communication among staff is necessary to ensure optimal patient care. (Copyright B. Proud)

Vietnamese (0.38%), Italian (0.38%), Korean (0.34%), and Russian (0.27%). Although the percentage seems small, the absolute numbers are large. For example, while only 0.27% of the U.S. population speaks Russian as their primary language, this represents 706,242 individuals (Modern Language Association, March 2006).

In Canada, 65.8% of the total population speaks English most often, and 21.2% speaks French most often. The remainder speak Chinese, Punjabi, Italian, Spanish, Portuguese, Aboriginal languages (such as Cree and Inukitut), Arabic, and German (Statistics Canada, 2010a, 2010b).

It is estimated that the United States will continue to attract about two-thirds of the world's immigration and that 85% of the immigrants will come from Central and South America. Immigration rates to Canada are also predicted to remain proportionally high, with approximately 250,000 immigrants being admitted each year. Box 12-2 suggests strategies for promoting effective cross-cultural communication in the multicultural workplace.

Cultural Perspectives on Touch

Differences in behavioral norms in the multicultural workforce are often inaccurately perceived. Typically, people from Asian cultures are not as overtly demonstrative of affection as are Whites or Blacks. Generally they refrain from public embraces, kissing, and loud talking or laughter. Affection is expressed in a more reserved manner.

Whites and Blacks may be perceived as boisterous, loud, ill mannered, or rude by comparison. In some cases, staff members from different cultures may send messages through their use of touch that are not intended. Special attention to male–female relationships is warranted in the multicultural workplace. In general, it is best to refrain from touching staff members of either sex unless necessary for the accomplishment of a job-related task, such as the provision of safe patient care. For nurses who tend to be more tactile, it is important to consciously refrain from placing one's hand on another's arm or shoulder, as frequently happens during ordinary conversation. For a further discussion of this topic, please see Chapter 2.

Cultural Perspectives on Etiquette

Values frequently underlie cultural expectations of behavior, including matters of **etiquette**, the conventional code of good manners that governs behavior. For example, some people from Hispanic, Middle Eastern, and African cultures expect the nurse manger to engage in social conversation and to establish personal and social rapport before giving assignments or orders for the day's work. In developing interpersonal relationships, a high value is placed on getting to know about a person's family, personal concerns, and interests before discussing job-related business. The nurse manager's reluctance to engage in self-disclosure about personal matters may leave the impression that he or she is uncaring and is

BOX 12-2

Strategies to Promote Effective Cross-Cultural Communication in the Multicultural Workplace

- Pronounce names correctly. When in doubt, ask the person for the correct pronunciation.
- Use proper titles of respect: "Doctor," "Reverend," "Mister." Ask permission to use first names, or wait until you are given permission to do so.
- Be aware of gender sensitivities. If uncertain about the marital status of a woman or her preferred title, it is best to refer to her as Ms. initially, then ask how she prefers to be addressed at the first opportunity.
- Be aware of subtle linguistic messages that may convey bias or inequality, for example, referring to a White man as Mister while addressing a Black female by her first name.
- Refrain from Anglicizing or shortening a person's given name without his or her permission. For example, calling a Russian American "Mike" instead of Mikhael, or shortening the Italian American Maria Rosaria to Maria. The same principle applies to the last name, or surname.
- Call people by their proper names. Avoid slang such as "girl," "boy," "honey," "dear," "guy," "fella," "babe," "chief," "mama," "sweetheart," or similar terms. When in doubt, ask people if they are offended by the use of a particular term.
- Refrain from using slang, pejorative, or derogatory terms when referring to persons from ethnic, racial, or religious groups, and convey to all staff that this is a work environment in which there is zero tolerance for the use of such language. Violators should be counseled immediately.
- Identify people by race, color, gender, and ethnic origin only when appropriate.
- Avoid using words and phrases that may be offensive to others. For example, "culturally deprived" or "culturally disadvantaged" imply inferiority, and "non-White" implies that White is the normative standard.
- Avoid cliches and platitudes such as "Some of my best friends are Mexicans" or "I went to school with Blacks."
- Use language in communications that includes *all* staff rather than excludes some of them.
- Do not expect a staff member to know all the other employees of his or her background or to speak for them. They share ethnicity, not necessarily the same experiences, friendships, or beliefs.
- Communications describing staff should pertain to their job skills, not their color, age, race, sex, or national origin.
- Refrain from telling stories or jokes demeaning to certain ethnic, racial, age, or religious groups. Also avoid those pertaining to gender-related issues or persons with physical or mental disabilities. Convey to all staff that there will be zero tolerance for this inappropriate behavior. Violators should be counseled immediately.
- Avoid remarks that suggest to staff from diverse backgrounds that they should consider themselves fortunate to be in the organization. Do not compare their employment opportunities and conditions with those people in their country of origin.
- Remember that communication problems multiply in telephone communications because important nonverbal cues are lost and accents may be difficult to interpret. Be patient.
- Provide staff with opportunities to explore diversity issues in their workplace; celebrate the strength that differences bring and constructively resolve conflicts.

not interested in the staff member. These behaviors by the manager are not conducive to building productive, harmonious relationships and may be misunderstood by staff members from diverse backgrounds. Similarly, some cultures value formal greetings at the start of the day or whenever the first encounter of the day occurs—a practice found even among close family members. For example, it is important to say, "Good morning, Mr. Okoro. There has been a change in your patient's insulin orders," rather than immediately "getting to the point" without recognizing by name the person to whom you are speaking.

Cultural Perspectives on Clothing and Accessories

Most health care institutions have a **dress code** or policy statement about clothing and accessories worn by staff in various parts of the facility (e.g., delivery room, operating room, specialty units). It is important to review these documents periodically from a cultural perspective. For example, modification of the dress code may be necessary to accommodate Hindu women dressed in saris, Sikh men who wear turbans, Amish and Mennonite women who wear bonnets and men who wear straw or black felt hats, Muslim women and Roman Catholic nuns who cover their heads with veils, and Arab men who wear kaffiyehs. Special consideration may need to be given to some Blacks and others who wear jewelry and other accessories in their hair, particularly when the hair is braided.

Cultural Perspectives on Time Orientation

In some cases, cultural differences in **time orientation** create difficulty in the workplace. This may manifest itself when staff members from diverse cultures are tardy, take excessive time for breaks, and fail to complete assignments within the expected time frame. These differences may be interrelated with the cultural meaning of work, religious practices, and cross-cultural communication issues. It is important to be explicit in the job-related expectations about punctuality, the schedule for breaks, and time allotted for assignments.

If a staff member develops a pattern of tardiness, the reason(s) should be explored. Although a uniform standard of punctuality needs to be applied to all staff members, it may be useful to listen to the staff member's explanation and ask what he or she thinks will rectify the problem. The reasons for problems with punctuality may range from child care to car repair needs. Solutions may include the mobilization of cultural resources, such as using extended family members to look after dependents, or networking with coworkers who might be able to recommend a reliable auto mechanic. It is important to listen attentively without rendering judgment or dictating solutions with which the person has not agreed.

It is sometimes useful to divide an assignment into subtasks with specific time lines for each activity. If the staff member has difficulty completing the assignment within the allotted time, it is important to follow up with a discussion of the reasons why there were problems. This follow-up discussion should be conducted in a positive, proactive manner and viewed as an opportunity to promote cross-cultural communication, not as a punitive or disciplinary measure.

Cultural Perspectives on Interpersonal Relationships

Authority Figures, Peers, Subordinates, and Patients

As indicated in Figure 12-5, there are cultural differences in interpersonal relationships involving authority figures, peers, subordinates, and patients. To examine these cultural differences, consider the following example. Dr. Kelly, an Irish American physician, gave an order for vital signs to Kim Li, a Chinese American nurse. The nurse perceived the order as unnecessary (but not harmful) to the patient; that is, she thought the physician was requesting vital signs more frequently than was warranted by the patient's condition. Nurse Li refrained from questioning the physician or negotiating with him out of respect for his position of authority and the value she placed on maintaining harmony in the relationship. Nurse Li said nothing and carried out the physician's order.

At the change of shift, the charge nurse became angry because she concurred with the assessment that Dr. Kelly had ordered vital signs too frequently and thought that Nurse Li should

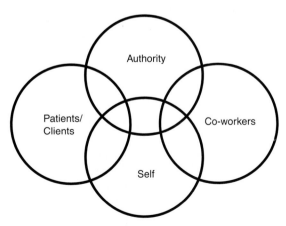

FIGURE 12-5 Cultural perspectives on interpersonal relationships.

have confronted the physician about the order. Nurse Li intentionally chose to avoid questioning Dr. Kelly's order because she perceived him as an authority figure and wanted to foster harmony and balance. In her cultural value system, causing conflict through direct confrontation would be perceived negatively. She would have experienced lowered self-esteem and "loss of face" if she had been responsible for causing disharmony in the nurse–physician relationship. The charge nurse, on the other hand, perceived the physician as a colleague whose respect would be earned by assertive, direct communication with him.

Long-Standing Historic Rivalries

The U.S. and Canadian media are replete with news, documentaries, human-interest stories, and related programs pertaining to nations with long-standing historic rivalries. Within nations there might be intergroup conflict such as the rivalries and civil war involving the Sunni and Shia Islamic groups in Iraq. At any given moment, there are numerous armed conflicts between two or more nations or between factions within nations. On occasion, the multicultural workplace becomes a battleground, where long-standing historic rivalries and more recent geopolitical differences are reenacted in the form of interpersonal conflict between two or more staff members. After ruling out other potential sources of conflict, it may be worth examining the ethnic heritage and national origins of staff members for possible reasons. For example, the nurse manager may observe a pattern of strained relationships between an Israeli physician and Palestinian physicians, nurses, laboratory technicians, physical therapists, and other health care providers. Similar observations may be made concerning staff members from countries known to be rivals, such as North and South Korea, Russia and Afghanistan, Iran and Iraq, India and Pakistan, and so forth.

Cues that may signal underlying historic rivalries include (1) the expression of high levels of emotional energy when a staff member is interacting with a person from a rival group and the topic does not seem to warrant it; (2) sudden, uncharacteristic behavior changes when the staff member is in the presence of a person from the rival group, for example, an ordinarily cordial staff member unexpectedly becomes acrimonious for no apparent reason; (3) the repeated expression of strong opinions about historical, political, and current events involving rival nations or factions; and (4) inappropriate attempts to persuade others to adopt the staff member's partisan views about the rivalry.

Cultural Perspectives on Gender and Sexual Orientation

Women have historically constituted the majority of personnel in nursing and in many allied health disciplines. Currently, women constitute 93.4% of the nursing profession in the United States (U.S. Department of Health and Human Services, Bureau of Health Professions, 2010) and 94% of the nursing profession in Canada (Canadian Institute for Health Information, 2010). Although Chapter 2 provides information about gender and sexual orientation, a few remarks about issues in the multicultural workplace will be made here. The complex interrelationship between gender and culture has been studied extensively. In the health care setting, nurses of both genders may face the biases and preconceptions of physicians, fellow nurses, and other health care providers. The issue is further complicated by cultural beliefs about relationships with authority figures and cross-national perspectives on the status of various health care disciplines. For example, in many less developed nations, nursing is a low-status occupation. In some oil-rich Arab countries (e.g., Saudi Arabia, Kuwait), care for the sick is carried out by health care providers who are hired from abroad for the purpose of caring for the bodily needs of the sick—an activity that is considered unacceptable in its cultural context.

Men in nursing and other health care disciplines dominated by women continue to struggle as minority members of their professions. In the multicultural health care workplace, both men and women face the gender biases that exist in society. These issues frequently emerge in verbal and nonverbal communication and in interpersonal relationships. Our language also betrays covert gender biases and preconceptions. For example, the expression "male nurse" is sometimes used, but seldom does one hear about the "female nurse" because that term is considered redundant and unnecessary. An extensive analysis of workplace issues concerning gay, lesbian, bisexual, and transgendered staff members is beyond the scope of this text, but these types of diversity must be considered in the multicultural workplace.

Cultural Perspectives on Moral and Religious Beliefs

In some circumstances, **moral and religious beliefs** may underlie conflicts in the multicultural workplace. Consider the following dilemmas:

- A nurse who believes that it is morally wrong to drink alcohol refuses to carry out a physician's order for the therapeutic administration of alcohol as a sedative–hypnotic or to administer medicines with an alcohol base (e.g., cough syrup).
- A nurse who believes that humankind should not unleash the power of nuclear energy refuses to care for cancer patients undergoing irradiation.
- A Roman Catholic nurse working in the operating room refuses to scrub for abortions, tubal ligations, vasectomies, and similar procedures because of religious prohibitions.
- A Jehovah's Witness nurse refuses to hang blood or counsel patients concerning blood or blood products.
- A Seventh-Day Adventist nurse who cites biblical reasons for following a vegetarian diet is unwilling to conduct patient education involving diets that contain meat.
- Muslim and Jewish staff members express concern that the hospital cafeteria fails to serve foods that meet their religious requirements.

These moral and religious issues reflect the diversity that characterizes staff members in the health care workplace. The challenge is to balance the health care needs and rights of patients with the moral and religious beliefs of health care providers. In some instances, it may be impossible to provide the services demanded by the organization's mission statement if all nurses refuse to engage in a particular activity. There may be legal implications for refusing to provide patients with certain services, for example, those related to reproductive health. In the clinical world, the options available to accommodate the diverse moral and religious beliefs of staff members frequently depend on the size of the organization, the moral and religious proclivities of workers, the attitudes and beliefs of managers, the organizational climate, fiscal constraints, and other factors. The challenge faced by nurse managers is to balance the conflicting moral and religious beliefs of diverse groups with the achievement of organizational goals. This must be accomplished in a manner that is respectful of the moral and religious beliefs of staff members.

Conflicting Role Expectations: Staff Educated Abroad

Many graduates of foreign nursing programs are currently practicing as RNs in the United States and Canada. Foreign-educated RNs practicing in the Unites States most commonly come from the Philippines (48.7%), Canada (11.5%), India (9.3%), and the United Kingdom (5.8%) (U.S. Department of Health and Human Services, 2010). Smaller numbers have come from Ireland, Australia, New Zealand, Nigeria, India, Jamaica, Israel, and South Korea. In Canada, internationally educated nurses most often graduated from schools in the Philippines (30.2%), United Kingdom (17.9%), United States (7.3%), India (5.7%), and Hong Kong (4.6%) (Human Resources and Social Development Canada, 2001). Similar trends prevail for foreign-educated physicians, laboratory technicians, and other health care providers in the United States and Canada.

Role is defined as the set of expectations and behaviors associated with a specific position. Considerable research has been conducted on the patient sick role and on the roles of nurses, physicians, and other health care providers. Furthermore, it is suggested that persons entering the United States or Canada from a similar culture (e.g., Australia,

England, Ireland) with English as the primary language may experience a lesser degree of culture shock than someone from a more diverse culture. For example, it is suggested that staff members from Australia or the United Kingdom will experience less difficulty with cultural adjustment to the United States or Canada than will persons from the Near and Middle East, Asia, or Africa, where language, religion, dress, and many other components of culture may be markedly different. Although social scientists speculate that people from similar cultures are more readily able to relate to one another, health care providers must be able to transcend cultural differences and to recognize that there are differences in role expectations.

Discrepancies in role expectations tend to create intrapersonal and interpersonal conflict. For example, nurses in Taiwan, the Philippines, and many African nations expect the families of patients to participate significantly in caregiving during the patient's hospitalization. Family members, who may be encouraged to remain with the patient around the clock, provide all aspects of personal hygiene often sleeping on the floor or in uncomfortable lounge chairs. This may result in conflict, as families are less involved in the care of hospitalized patients in the United States.

In many countries, nurses have considerably expanded roles, and their scope of practice is correspondingly broader. For example, in Nigeria it is clearly stated by the Board of Nursing and Midwifery that nurses diagnose and treat common illnesses such as malaria, typhoid, cholera, tetanus, and similar maladies. To graduate from a nursing program in the Philippines, nursing students must deliver a minimum of 25 babies unassisted and also assist at major and minor surgical procedures. In Haiti, nurses routinely perform episiotomies, and repair lacerations. In the mastery of technical skills, recent graduates of many foreign nursing programs have logged a considerable number of hours of clinical experience, often as apprentices mentored by experienced nurses who serve as their clinical faculty.

Some British and Irish nurses perceive U.S. and Canadian nurses as "junior physicians," second-guessing and anticipating therapy. Many perceive that in Great Britain and Ireland, nurses have greater freedom in ordering nursing modalities without a physician's orders. For example, decubitus ulcer care, ambulation, dressings, and nutritional therapy are all nurse-initiated activities based on nursing assessment. British and Irish nurses also expect that the nursing role includes activities that are defined by U.S. and Canadian nurses as nonnursing activities. For example, in many British hospitals, nurses are expected to clean patient rooms after discharge and prepare them for the next admission.

In many nations, nurse midwives are primarily responsible for obstetric care. In some ways, the United States and Canada are anomalous with so much emphasis on the medically dominated specialty of obstetric medicine. Viewing childbirth as a medical problem, rather than a normal physiologic process, reveals an underlying philosophic difference between the U.S. and Canadian health care delivery systems and those in other nations. Some nurses who have been educated abroad are both nurses and midwives; thus, the transition to the medically dominated U.S. and Canadian models may leave them feeling underutilized and confused about the roles of the obstetrician and the maternal–child nurse or nurse midwife.

Because of the shortage of qualified health care providers in many less developed countries, there usually are fewer interdisciplinary differences about the nature and scope of practice for various health care disciplines. There are also various categories of licensed and unlicensed health care providers who contribute to the overall health and well-being of people in countries around the world. For example, there are feldshers in the former Soviet Union, barefoot doctors in China, and herbalists in nearly every nation.

Cultural Assessment in the Multicultural Workplace

Cultural self-assessment in the multicultural workplace may focus on the individual or the organizational culture. **Individual cultural self-assessment** focuses on staff members and their beliefs about multiculturalism in the workplace. **Organizational cultural self-assessment** focuses on the entire health care organization, institution, or agency, or a particular unit or division of the organization.

Individual Cultural Self-Assessment

As indicated in Chapter 1, it is important for nurses to be aware of their own ethnocentric tendencies. This is best accomplished when individuals review their cultural attitudes, values, beliefs, and practices. Figure 12-6 shows the importance of cultural values in the workplace, and Table 12-3 contains the individual cultural assessment instrument, which is one instrument used for gathering cultural data about staff members and their beliefs about multiculturalism in the workplace. By gathering responses to the individual cultural assessment instrument, nurse managers can identify staff perceptions about diversity issues and determine what management strategies might be useful. A culturally diverse workforce should strengthen the organization's ability to meet the needs of culturally diverse patients and should be viewed as an asset. Nurse managers, however, need to recognize and encourage the cultural talents of this workforce.

Cultural Self-Assessment of Health Care Organizations, Institutions, and Agencies

Before engaging in a cultural self-assessment of a health care organization, institution, or agency, it is necessary to consider both content and process. A variety of tools may be used to assess organizational culture; several are provided in Chapter 9. Box 12-3 provides another instrument, which may be used to assess an entire organization or a particular unit or division. For example, staff in the operating room, specialty units, home health care division, ambulatory care area, and so forth may perceive a need to engage in an organizational self-assessment because of changing demographics in populations served or concerns with quality of care for diverse patients. Figure 12-7 provides a schematic representation of the cultural self-assessment of a health care organization, institution, or agency.

The Process of Cultural Self-Assessment by Organizations, Institutions, and Agencies

Although the manner in which the cultural self-assessment is carried out will vary for each institution, organization, or agency and for different units or divisions within it, the process remains fundamentally the same. After identifying key staff members to lead the institutional

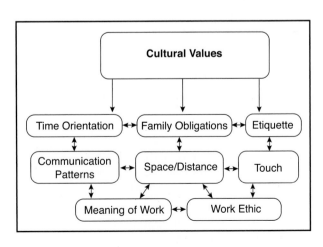

FIGURE 12-6 Influence of cultural values in the multicultural workplace.

TABLE 12-3
Individual Cultural Assessment Instrument

	STRONGLY AGREE	AGREE	NO OPINION	DISAGREE	STRONGLY DISAGREE
1. Open acknowledgment and/or general discussion of cultural diversity occurs in my work environment.	1	2	3	4	5
2. It is important that openness and general discussion of cultural diversity take place in my work setting.	1	2	3	4	5
3. Multicultural education or awareness programs are emphasized in my work environment.	1	2	3	4	5
4. Multicultural education and awareness program emphasis is important in my work environment.	1	2	3	4	5
5. I have personally experienced communication or interaction difficulties with a manager because of my ethnic, cultural, gender, or racial values.	1	2	3	4	5
6. It is important that various cultural values are understood and respected by all managers working in a multicultural environment.	1	2	3	4	5
7. Coworkers in my work environment tend to "hang out" during lunch or breaks with workers from the same cultural background.	1	2	3	4	5
8. It is important for management to facilitate work and to plan culturally mixed social activity for the workers and my work environment.	1	2	3	4	5
9. Members of my own culture are participants on existing work committees or task forces that help set direction for the work environment.	1	2	3	4	5
10. It is important for management to ensure that the cultures of all workers in my work environment are represented on work committees.	1	2	3	4	5
11. In my work environment, I have access to work-related growth and development opportunities like my coworkers.	1	2	3	4	5
12. It is important for managers to recognize and encourage growth opportunities equally for all workers.	1	2	3	4	5

	STRONGLY AGREE	AGREE	NO OPINION	DISAGREE	STRONGLY DISAGREE
13. In my work environment, coworkers communicate verbally and/or through body language in ways that demean my culture or race.	1	2	3	4	5
14. It is important for managers to work with staff to increase sensitivity to cultural values and perceptions that will help to reduce or eliminate racial and cultural barriers.	1	2	3	4	5
15. All workers in my work environment are held to the same standards of job performance regardless of gender, race, or cultural background.	1	2	3	4	5
16. It is important for managers to have systems to identify and analyze which employees receive promotions and growth experiences, and to consider biases that influence performance standards so that they are achievable for all groups of staff.	1	2	3	4	5
17. Staff in my work environment are more successful if they share the same cultural values and ancestry as the manager.	1	2	3	4	5
18. It is important for the administration to recognize, reward, and value the managers who successfully promote, manage, and retain a harmonious multicultural work force.	1	2	3	4	5
19. When bicultural or multicultural conflict occurs in my work area, cultural, gender, and racial influences are openly discussed as part of the conflict resolution steps.	1	2	3	4	5
20. It is important for managers to facilitate, promote, and participate in open dialogue about cultural influences and diverse perceptions that occur because of differences in ethnicity or gender.	1	2	3	4	5

Modified and used with permission. From Davis, P. D. (1995). Enhancing multicultural harmony. *Nursing Management, 26*(7), 32D–32E, © Springhouse Corporation.

BOX 12-3

Cultural Assessment of an Organization, Institution, or Agency

Demographics/Descriptive Data

- What types of cultural diversity are represented by clients, families, visitors, and others significant to the clients? Indicate approximate numbers and percentages according to the conventional system used for reporting census data.
- What types of cultural diversity are represented? What types of diversity are present among patients, physicians, nurses, X-ray technicians, and other staff? Indicate approximate numbers and percentages by department and discipline.
- How is the organization, institution, or agency structured? Who is in charge? How do the administrators support cultural diversity and interventions to foster multiculturalism?
- How many key leaders/decision makers within the organization, institution, or agency come from culturally diverse backgrounds?
- What languages are spoken by patients, family members or significant others, and staff?

Assessment of Strengths

- What are the cultural strengths or positive characteristics and qualities?
- What institutional resources (fiscal, human) are available to support multiculturalism?
- What goals and needs related to cultural diversity already have been expressed?
- What successes in making services accessible and culturally appropriate have occurred to date? Highlight goals, programs, and activities that have been successful.
- What positive comments have been given by clients and significant others from culturally diverse backgrounds about their experiences with the organization, institution, or agency?

Assessment of Community Resources

- What efforts are made to use multicultural community-based resources (e.g., community organizations for ethnic or religious groups, anthropology and foreign languages faculty and students from area colleges and universities, and similar resources)?
- To what extent are leaders from racial, ethnic, and religious communities involved with the institution (e.g., invited to serve on boards and advisory committees)?
- To what extent is there political and economic support for multicultural programs and projects?

Assessment of Weakness/Areas for Continued Growth

- What are the organization's weaknesses, limitations, and areas for continued growth?
- What could be done to better promote multiculturalism?

Assessment from the Perspective of Clients and Families

- How do clients (and families/significant others) evaluate the multicultural aspects of the organization, institution, or agency? Do patient satisfaction data indicate that clients from various cultural backgrounds are satisfied or dissatisfied with care? How are the quality outcomes the same and different for individuals of various races and ethnicities?
- How adequate is the system for translation and interpretation? What materials are available in the client's primary language (in written and other forms such as audiocassettes, videotapes, computer programs)? How is the literacy level of clients assessed?
- Are educational programs available in the languages spoken by clients?
- Are cultural and religious calendars used in determining scheduling for preadmission testing, procedures, educational programs, follow-up visits, or other appointments?
- Are cultural considerations given to the acceptability of certain medical and surgical procedures (e.g., amputations, blood transfusions, disposal of body parts, and handling various types of human tissue)?

BOX 12-3 *(continued)*

- Are cultural considerations a factor in administering medicines? How familiar are nurses, physicians, and pharmacists with current research in ethnopharmacology?
- If a client dies, what cultural considerations are given during postmortem care? How are cultural needs associated with dying addressed with the family and others significant to the deceased? Does the roster of religious representatives available to nursing staff include traditional spiritual healers such as shamans and medicine men/women as well as rabbis, priests, elders, and others?

Assessment from an Institutional Perspective

- To what extent do the philosophy and mission statement support, foster, and promote multiculturalism and respect for cultural diversity? Is there congruence between philosophy/mission statement and reality? How is this evident?
- To what extent is there administrative support for multiculturalism? In what ways is support present or absent? Provide evidence to support this.
- Are data being gathered to provide documentation concerning multicultural issues? Are there missing data? Are data disseminated to appropriate decision makers and leaders within the institution? How are these data used?
- Are opportunities for continuing professional education and development in topics pertaining to multiculturalism provided for nurses and other staff?
- Are there racial, ethnic, religious, or other tensions evident within the institution? If so, objectively and nonjudgmentally assess their origins and nature in as much detail as possible.
- Are adequate resources being allocated for the purpose of promoting a harmonious multicultural health care environment? If not, indicate areas in which additional resources are needed.
- What multicultural library resources and audiovisual and computer software are available for use by nurses and other staff?
- What efforts are made to recruit and retain nurses and other staff from racially, ethnically, and religiously diverse backgrounds? What other types of diversity (e.g., sexual orientation) are fostered or discouraged?
- How would you describe the cultural climate of the institution? Are ethnic/racial/religious jokes prevalent? Are negative remarks or comments about certain cultural groups permitted? Who is doing the talking and who is listening to negative comments/jokes?
- Are human resources initiatives pertaining to advertising, hiring, promotion, and performance evaluations free from discrimination?
- Are cultural and religious considerations reflected in staff scheduling policies for nursing and other departments?
- Are policies and procedures appropriate from a multicultural perspective? What process is used for reviewing them for cultural appropriateness and relevance?

Assessment of Need and Readiness for Change

- Is there a need for change? If so, indicate who, what, when, where, why, and how.
- Who is in favor of change? Who is against it?
- What are the anticipated obstacles to change?
- What financial and human resources would be necessary to bring about the recommended changes?

cultural self-assessment process, the leaders should communicate the purpose of the cultural self-assessment to those who will be participating in it. It is important to involve grassroots members of the staff and to solicit input from the patient population served through interviews, focus groups, written surveys, or other methods.

The process of cultural self-assessment by organizations, institutions, and agencies involves collecting demographic and descriptive data, identifying strengths and limitations, assessing the need and readiness for change, identifying community resources, evaluating the effectiveness of changes, and implementing any necessary revisions.

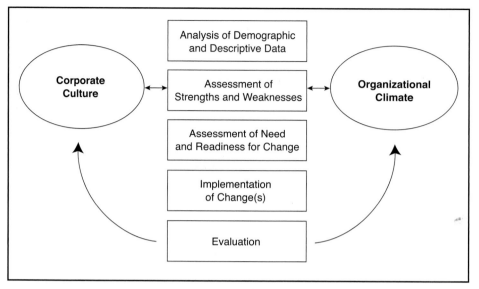

FIGURE 12-7   Cultural self-assessment of health care organization, institution, or agency.

Demographic and Descriptive Data

As with any assessment, begin by gathering demographic and descriptive data. It is highly likely that some of these data have already been collected and stored centrally. If reports containing the necessary data are available, the group should review and discuss them as part of the cultural assessment process. Data such as types and numbers of diverse patients and staff members should be determined. There should be an assessment of the predominant languages spoken and of the effectiveness of the system being used for translation and interpretation.

Strengths and Limitations

After the data have been gathered, a team of key leaders should convene to critically review and analyze them. Because this will be an active working group, membership should be limited to approximately 12 people. If the group is larger, consideration should be given to division into smaller subgroups. The purpose of the review is to assess the strengths, limitations, and areas for continued growth in terms of promoting a harmonious multicultural

environment for patients and staff members of diverse backgrounds. It is important to identify strengths and limitations from both an **emic** (insider) and an **etic** (outsider) perspective. This incorporates the viewpoints of health care providers (insiders) and patients, those significant to them, and visitors (outsiders). For example, although the staff may believe the system is structured adequately to meet the needs of linguistically diverse persons, it would be important to compare that perception with the patients' point of view. From their perspective, examine the ways in which cultural aspects are part of the care provided. From the institutional perspective, critically examine the infrastructure for philosophic, fiscal, and human resources that reflect a commitment—or lack of one—to promoting harmony in the multicultural workplace. Throughout the process, comparative analyses are made between input from staff members and that from patients to identify strengths and limitations.

Need and Readiness for Change

Once the strengths and limitations have been identified, there should be an assessment of the need and readiness for change. If changes are needed, it is important to identify why, who, what, when, where, and how. Identify the fiscal and human resources that will be needed to bring about the recommended change(s).

Be sure to anticipate staff **resistance to change**. Determine who is likely to favor and oppose the proposed change, anticipate obstacles to it, and develop contingency plans. Different people will see different meanings in activities by organizations to become more culturally diverse. Members of the federal minority groups may see job opportunities, whereas White men may complain of reverse discrimination. Depending on the nature of the recommendation and the corporate culture of the organization, an action plan should accompany the recommendation, that is, specifically what does the group believe ought to be done? Although most staff members will support the change, it is insufficient for nurse managers and supervisors to say, "A new law has been passed mandating diversity" or "Hospital policy requires diversity." Resistance can be expected to increase to the degree that staff members influenced by the changes have pressure on them to change, and it will decrease to the degree they are actively involved in planning diversity activities. Resistance can be expected if the changes are made on personal grounds rather than as requirements, sanctions, or policies. Finally, resistance can be expected if the organizational culture is ignored. There are informal as well as formal norms within every organization. An effective change will neither ignore old customs nor abruptly create new ones. As with most change, timing is important.

Community Resources

In developing an action plan for change, be sure to assess the community resources available to assist with goal achievement. For example, it may be possible to invite leaders from ethnic communities to provide staff in-service programs aimed at increasing understanding of the health care needs of persons from diverse backgrounds. A second example might be to involve foreign-language faculty and students from area colleges and universities to assist with translation for linguistically diverse patients and clients. A final example might be to invite clergy to discuss health-related religious beliefs and practices (Parsons & Reiss, 1999). If organizational resources are limited, it may be possible to identify community-based resources that are available at low cost.

Evaluation of the Effectiveness of Changes and Implementation of Revisions

After implementation of the recommended changes, an evaluation of their effectiveness should be conducted, and revisions should be made as needed. In recognition of the rapid pace of change in contemporary health care, the process of institutional cultural self-assessment should be repeated at periodic intervals. Mateo and Smith (2001) note that although significant fiscal and human resources are expended by organizations in diversity initiatives, there is a need to be more diligent in monitoring and evaluating outcomes. They recommend the development of a grid that articulates goals, diversity initiatives, and outcome measures.

Promoting Harmony in the Multicultural Workplace

After conducting a cultural assessment of the health care organization, institution, or agency, the nurse will have data about the strengths and weaknesses; fiscal, human, and community resources; areas in which to pursue change; and readiness of the staff to engage in change.

As indicated in Box 12-4, there are **facilitators** and **barriers** to promoting harmony in the multicultural workplace. Facilitators include identification of the cultural values of the organization, institution, or agency; clear articulation of the mission statement and policies about diversity; zero tolerance for discrimination; effective cross-cultural communication; skill with conflict resolution involving diversity; and commitment to multiculturalism at all levels of management. The barriers that must be overcome include hatred, prejudice, bigotry, racism, discrimination,

BOX 12-4

Promoting Harmony in the Multicultural Workplace

Facilitators

Identification of cultural values of the organization, institution, or agency

Mission statement and policies about diversity

Zero tolerance for discrimination

Effective cross-cultural communication

Skill with conflict resolution involving diversity

Commitment to multiculturalism at all levels of management

Barriers

Hatred

Prejudice

Bigotry

Racism

Discrimination

(Negative attitudes or behaviors based on race, ethnicity, religion, gender, sexual orientation, national origin, class, handicap/disability)

and ethnoviolence. Negative behaviors aimed at employees, patients, their families, others significant to them, and other visitors, based on race, ethnicity, religion, gender, sexual orientation, national origin, class, or handicap/disability should not be tolerated. All employees should be apprised that there will be zero tolerance for those who engage in negative behaviors, and management staff at all levels should be given the authority to impose sanctions when violations occur.

SUMMARY

Given the demographic composition of contemporary U.S. and Canadian societies, nurses will continue to find both challenges and opportunities as they practice nursing in multicultural health care settings. Microcosms of society at large, health care organizations, institutions, and agencies will consist of staff members from increasingly diverse backgrounds. It is important to

remember that culture influences the manner in which people perceive, identify, define, and solve problems in the workplace. Among the complex and interrelated factors that must be considered when workplace diversity is addressed are cultural perspectives on values, the meaning of work, interpersonal relationships, cross-cultural communication patterns (including etiquette, touch, space/distance), gender and sexual orientation, moral and religious beliefs, hygiene, and clothing. Characteristics of the staff member such as individual preferences, biases and prejudices for and against certain groups, educational background, and previous experiences living and working in culturally diverse settings also must be considered.

Understanding cultural differences in the workplace and developing skill in conflict resolution will continue to be needed in transcultural nursing administration in the new millennium. The successful transcultural nurse administrator will behave respectfully toward others from diverse backgrounds and will implement policies that promote cultural understanding, knowledge, and skill in the workplace. Nurses in leadership and management positions will apply the principles of transcultural nursing to the multicultural workplace, just as they have done in the past to provide culturally competent and congruent care for patients.

REVIEW QUESTIONS

1. Compare and contrast the concepts of hatred, prejudice, racism, discrimination, and ethnoviolence. Critically examine the manner in which they may manifest themselves in the health care workplace.

2. What is meant by transcultural nursing administration? How is transcultural nursing administration useful for nurses who hold leadership positions in multicultural health care settings?

3. How do the cultural meanings of work embraced by staff from diverse cultures influence the corporate culture and organizational climate of contemporary health care institutions, organizations, and agencies?

4. Identify strategies to promote effective cross-cultural communication in the multicultural workplace.

5. Critically analyze the cultural origins of conflict that may arise in the health care workplace.

6. Review the process and content of cultural self-assessment by organizations, institutions,

and agencies. What aspects of the change process must be considered during engagement in cultural self-assessment?

7. Identify facilitators and barriers to promoting harmony in the multicultural workplace.

CRITICAL THINKING ACTIVITIES

1. Using the guidelines in Box 12-3, conduct a cultural assessment of a health care organization, institution, or agency, or a specific unit or department within a larger facility.

2. Ask at least 10 nurses working at a health care organization, institution, or agency (hospital, long-term care facility, prison, home health care agency, or related facility) if they would be willing to respond to the items found in the instrument in Table 12-3, Individual Cultural Assessment Instrument. Average the numeric responses for each of the 20 items to identify trends. Write a 1-page summary of your findings that includes a critical analysis of the results. What do the responses tell you about the organizational climate and corporate culture that prevail within the health care facility?

3. Reflect on your personal experience with hatred, prejudice, bigotry, racism, discrimination, and/or ethnoviolence. Were you the victim or the perpetrator? How did you feel during the incident(s)? Discuss your

responses with another member of the class, preferably someone from a different cultural background from your own.

4. From a cultural perspective, critically examine the dress code or policy statement about clothing and accessories that are permitted for staff at a health care organization, agency, or institution. How effectively does the code or policy address the widespread diversity that characterizes our contemporary health care workforce? Identify the strengths and limitations of the dress code or policy statement. What modifications or changes would you recommend to accommodate the attire worn by staff from diverse cultures?

5. Choose two of the five case studies presented at the beginning of the chapter, and analyze them from the perspective of a nurse manager. For the purpose of analysis, assume the role of nurse manager, and critically examine approaches you might use to change the negative attitudes and behaviors of those mentioned in the case studies.

REFERENCES

Brown, I. C. (1973). *Understanding race relations.* Englewood Cliffs, NJ: Prentice-Hall.

Canadian Institute for Health Information. (2010). *Regulated nurses: Canadian trends, 2004 to 2008.* http://secure.cihi.ca/cihiweb/products/regulated_nurses_2004_2008_en.pdf. Accessed March 6, 2010.

Davis, P. D. (1995). Enhancing multicultural harmony. *Nursing Management, 26*(7), 32D–32E.

Henderson, G. (1994). *Cultural diversity in the workplace.* Westport, CT: Praeger.

Human Resources and Social Development Canada (2001). *Canadian citizen workforce population showing representation by employment equity occupational groups and unit groups (2001 NOC) for women, aboriginal peoples and visible minorities* (Table 14) [Data file]. Employment Equity Data Report. Retrieved December 29, 2006, from http://www.hrsdc.gc.ca/en/lp/lo/lswe/we/ee_tools/data/tables/annual/2001/Table14.pdf

Jung, C. A. (1968). In G. Adler (Ed.). *The collected works of Carl Jung* (Vol. 10). Princeton, NJ: University Press.

Mateo, M. A., & Smith, S. P. (2001). Workforce diversity: Challenges and strategies. *Journal of Multicultural Nursing & Health, 7*(2), 8–12.

Modern Language Association. (March 2006). Number and percentage of speakers per language in the entire U.S. http://www.mla.org/map_single. Accessed March 6, 2010.

Nixon, Y., & Bull, P. (2006). Cultural communication styles and accuracy in cross-cultural perception: A British and Japanese study. *Journal of Intercultural Communication, 12.* Available from http://www.immi.se/intercultural/

Parsons, L. C., & Reiss, P. L. (1999). Promoting collaborative practice with culturally diverse populations. *Seminars for Nurse Managers, 7*(1), 160–165.

Samovar, L. A., Porter, R. E., & McDaniel, E. R. (2006). *Intercultural communication: A reader.* Belmont, CA: Thomson/Wadsworth.

Statistics Canada. (November 2009). *2006 census: Immigration in Canada: A portrait of the foreign-born population, 2006 census findings.* http://www12.statcan.ca/census-recensement/2006/as-sa/97-557/index-eng.cfm. Accessed March 6, 2010.

Statistics Canada. (January 2010a). *Languages spoken most often at home (8), other language spoken regularly at home (9), immigrant status and period of immigration (9), age groups (17a) and sex (3) for the population of Canada, Provinces, territories and census metropolitan areas, 2006 census—20% sample data.* http://www12.statcan.ca/census-recensement/2006/dp-pd/tbt/Rp-eng.cfm?LANG=E&APATH=3&DETAIL=0&DIM=0&FL=A&FREE=0&GC=0&GID=837928&GK=0&GRP=1&PID=89187&PRID=0&PTYPE=88971,97154&S=0&SHOWALL=0&SUB=0&Temporal=2006&THE70&VID=0&VNAMEE=&VNAMEF=. Accessed March 6, 2010.

Statistics Canada. (January 2010b). *Selected language characteristics (165), registered Indian status (3), age groups (7) and sex (3) for the population of Canada, Provinces, territories and census metropolitan areas, 2006 census—20% sample data.* http://www12.statcan.ca/census-recensement/2006/dp-pd/tbt/Rp-eng.cfm?LANG=E&APATH=3&DETAIL=0&DIM=0&FL=A&FREE=0&GC=0&GID=843984&GK=0&GRP=1&PID=89152&PRID=0&PTYPE=88971,97154&S=0&SHOWALL=0&SUB=0&Temporal=2006&THE=73&VID=0&VNAMEE=&VNAMEF. Accessed March 6, 2010.

U.S. Census Bureau. (February 2007). Race and Ethnicity http://www.census.gov/population/www/pop-profile/files/dynamic/RACEHO.pdf

U.S. Census Bureau. (January 2010). Race and Hispanic Origin of Foreign-Born Population in the United States: 2007. http://www.census.gov/prod/2010pubs/acs-11.pdf. Accessed March 6, 2010.

U.S. Department of Health and Human Services. (March 2010). *The registered nurse population. Initial findings from the 2008 national sample survey of registered nurses.* http://bhpr.hrsa.gov/healthworkforce/rnsurvey. Accessed March 22, 2010.

U.S. Department of Health and Human Services. (2010). *HRSA news: HRSA study finds nursing workforce is growing more diverse.* http://newsroom.hrsa.gov/releases/2010/rnsurvey.htm. Accessed March 22, 2010.

Whittock, M., & Leonard, L. (2003). Stepping outside the stereotype. A pilot study of the motivations and experiences of males in the nursing profession. *Journal of Nursing Management, 11*, 242–249.

Williams, D. R., & Rucker, T. D. (2000). Understanding and addressing racial disparities in health care. *Minority Health, 2*(1), 30–39.

World Health Organization. (2009). *Global health atlas, human resources for health.* http://apps.who.int/globalatlas/dataQuery/reportData.asp?rptType=1. Accessed March 6, 2010.

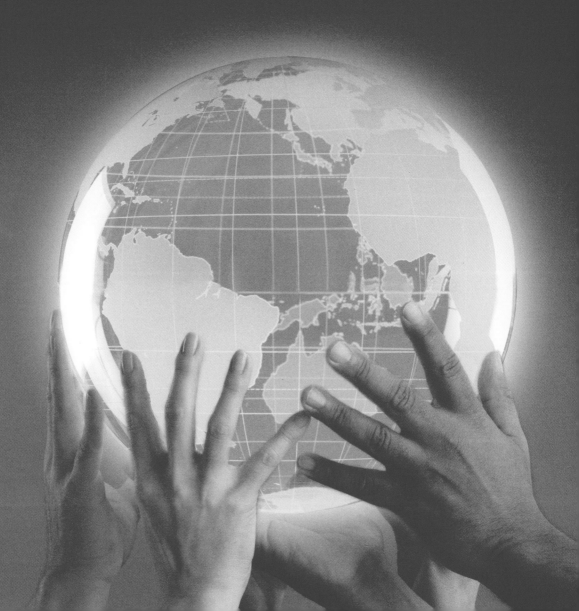

PART FOUR

Contemporary Challenges
in Transcultural Nursing

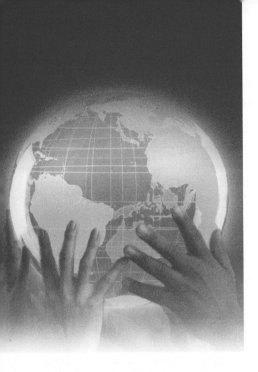

Religion, Culture, and Nursing

Patricia A. Hanson and
Margaret M. Andrews

KEY TERMS

Allah
Amish
Bad death
Baha'i International Community
Bereavement
Brahman
Brit milah
Buddha
Buddhism
Caste system
Catholic Charities USA
Catholicism
Christian Science
Church of Jesus Christ of Latter-Day
 Saints (Mormonism)
Curandero
Ethnoreligion
Eucharist
Faith healing
Fasting
Five core characteristics
 of the Amish
Five major dimensions of religion
Four Noble Truths
Friendscraft
Funeral
Garment

(key terms continue on page 352)

LEARNING OBJECTIVES

1. Explore the meaning of spirituality and religion in the lives of clients across the life span.
2. Identify the components of a spiritual needs assessment for clients from diverse cultural backgrounds.
3. Examine the ways in which spiritual and religious beliefs can be incorporated into the nursing care of clients from diverse cultures.
4. Discuss cultural considerations in the nursing care of dying for bereaved clients and families.
5. Describe the health-related beliefs and practices of selected religious groups in North America.

As an integral component of culture, religious and spiritual beliefs may influence a client's explanation of the cause(s) of illness, perception of its severity, decisions about healing intervention(s), and choice of healer(s). In times of crisis, such as serious illness and impending death, religion and spirituality are often a source of consolation for the client and family and may influence the course of action believed to be appropriate.

The first half of this chapter discusses dimensions of religion, religion and spiritual nursing care, religious trends in North America, and contributions of religious groups to the health care delivery system. The second half highlights the

K E Y   T E R M S *(continued)*

Good death
Grief
Hadith
Halal
Health Ministries
Hindu
Home going
Islam
Jehovah
Jehovah's Witnesses (Watch Tower
    Bible and Tract Society)
Judaism
Karma
Kosher
Mennonites
Mohel
Moslem/Muslim
Mourning
Native American Church
    (Peyote Religion)
Nirvana
Noble Eightfold Way
Ordinances
Pillars of Faith
Principle of totality
Protestantism
Qur'an (Koran)
Reincarnation
The Relief Society
Religion
Sacrament of the Sick
Seventh-Day Adventists
Shema
Shiva
Spiritual assessment
Spiritual concerns
Spiritual distress
Spiritual health
Spirituality
Spiritual nursing care
Talmud
Torah
Unitarian Universalist
Vedas
Wake (viewing, calling hours)
Word of Wisdom

health-related beliefs and practices of selected religions, which are presented in alphabetic order.

Dimensions of Religion

Religion is complex and multifaceted in both form and function. Religious faith and the institutions derived from that faith become a central focus in meeting the human needs of those who believe. The majority of faith traditions address the issues of illness and wellness, of disease and healing, of caring and curing (Ebersole, Hess, & Luggan, 2008; Fogel & Rivera, 2010; Leonard & Carlson, 2010).

Religious Factors Influencing Human Behavior

First, it is necessary to identify specific religious factors that may influence human behavior. No single religious factor operates in isolation, but rather exists in combination with other religious factors and the person's ethnic, racial, and cultural background. When religion and ethnicity combine to influence a person, the term **ethnoreligion** is sometimes used. Examples of ethnoreligious groups include the Amish, Russian Jews, Lebanese Muslims, Italian, Irish, or Polish Catholics, Tibetan Buddhists, American Samoan Mormons, and so forth.

Faulkner and DeJong (1966) have proposed **five major dimensions of religion** in their classic work on the subject: experiential, ritualistic, ideologic, intellectual, and consequential.

Experiential Dimension

The experiential dimension recognizes that all religions have expectations of members and that the religious person will at some point in life achieve direct knowledge of ultimate reality or will experience religious emotion. Every religion recognizes this subjective religious experience as a sign of religiosity.

Ritualistic Dimension

The ritualistic dimension pertains to religious practices expected of the followers and may include worship, prayer, participation in sacraments, and fasting.

Ideologic Dimension

The ideologic dimension refers to the set of beliefs to which its followers must adhere in order to call themselves members. Commitment to the group or movement as a social process results, and members experience a sense of belonging or affiliation.

Intellectual Dimension

The intellectual dimension refers to specific sets of beliefs or explanations or to the cognitive structuring of meaning. Members are expected to be informed about the basic tenets of the religion and to be familiar with sacred writings or scriptures. The intellectual and the ideologic are closely related because acceptance of a dimension presupposes knowledge of it.

Consequential Dimension

The consequential dimension refers to religiously defined standards of conduct and to prescriptions that specify what followers' attitudes and behaviors should be as a consequence of their religion. The consequential dimension governs people's relationships with others.

Religious Dimensions in Relation to Health and Illness

Obviously, each religious dimension has a different significance when related to matters of health and illness. Different religious cultures may emphasize one of the five dimensions to the relative exclusion of the others. Similarly, individuals may develop their own priorities related to the dimension of religion. This affects the nurse providing care to clients with different religious beliefs in several ways. First, it is the nurse's role to determine from the client, or from significant others, the dimension or combinations of dimensions that are important so that the client and nurse can have mutual goals and priorities.

Second, it is important to determine what a given member of a specific religious affiliation believes to be important. The only way to do this is to ask either the client or, if the client is unable to communicate this information personally, a close family member.

Third, the nurse's information must be accurate. Making assumptions about clients' religious belief systems on the basis of their cultural, ethnic, or even religious affiliation is imprudent and may lead to erroneous inferences. The following case example illustrates the importance of verifying assumptions with the client.

Observing that a patient was wearing a Star of David on a chain around his neck and had been accompanied by a rabbi upon admission, a nurse inquired whether he would like to order a kosher diet. The patient replied, "Oh, no. I'm a Christian. My father is a rabbi, and I know it would upset him to find out that I have converted. Even though I'm 40 years old, I hide it from him. This has been going on for 15 years now."

The key point in this anecdote is that the nurse validated an assumption with the patient before acting. Furthermore, not all Jewish persons follow a kosher diet nor wear a Star of David.

Fourth, even when individuals identify with a particular religion, they may accept the "official" beliefs and practices in varying degrees. It is not the nurse's role to judge the religious virtues of clients but rather to understand those aspects related to religion that are important to the client and family members. When religious beliefs are translated into practice, they may be manipulated by individuals in certain situations to serve particular ends; that is, traditional beliefs and practices are altered. Thus, it is possible for a Jewish person to eat pork or for a Catholic to take contraceptives to prevent pregnancy.

Although some find it necessary to label such occurrences as exceptional or accidental, such a point of view tends to ignore the fact that change can and does occur within individuals and within groups. Homogeneity among members of any religion cannot be assumed. Perhaps the individual once embraced the beliefs and practices of the religion but has since changed his or her views, or perhaps the individual never accepted the religious beliefs completely in the first place. It is important for the nurse to be open to variations in religious beliefs and practices and to allow for the possibility of change. Individual choices frequently arise from new situations, changing values and mores, and exposure to new ideas and beliefs. Few people live in total social isolation, surrounded by only those with similar religious backgrounds.

Fifth, ideal norms of conduct and actual behavior are not necessarily the same. The nurse is frequently faced with the challenge of understanding and helping clients cope with conflicting norms. Sometimes conflicting norms are manifested by guilt or by efforts to minimize or rationalize inconsistencies.

Sometimes norms are vaguely formulated and filled with discrepancies that allow for a variety of interpretations. In religions having a lay organization and structure, moral decision making may be left to the individual without the assistance of members of a church hierarchy. In religions having a clerical hierarchy, moral positions may be more clearly formulated and articulated for members. Individuals retain their right to choose regardless of official church-related guidelines, suggestions, or even religious laws; however, the individual who chooses to violate the norms may experience the consequences of that violation, including social ostracism, public removal from membership rolls, or other forms of censure. Social ostracism is especially problematic for those clients experiencing mental illness (Fayard, Harding, Murdoch, & Brunt, 2007; Fogel & Rivera, 2010; Matthew, 2008; Yurkovich & Lattergrass, 2008).

Religion and Spiritual Nursing Care

For many years, nursing has emphasized a holistic approach to care in which the needs of the total person are recognized. Most nursing textbooks emphasize the physical and psychosocial needs of clients rather than ways to address spiritual needs (Black, 2009; Ebersole et al., 2008; Fayard et al., 2007; Yurkovich & Lattergrass, 2008). Comparatively little has been written about guidelines for providing spiritual care to clients from diverse cultural backgrounds. Because nurses endeavor to provide holistic health care, addressing spiritual needs becomes essential.

Religious concerns evolve from and respond to the mysteries of life and death, good and evil, and pain and suffering. Although the religions of the world offer various interpretations of these phenomena, most people seek a personal understanding and interpretation at some time in their lives.

Ultimately, this personal search becomes a pursuit to discover a Supreme Being, God, gods, or some unifying truth that will give meaning, purpose, and integrity to existence (Ebersole et al., 2008; Keehl, 2009; Leonard & Carlson, 2010; Yurkovich & Lattergrass, 2008).

Before spiritual care for culturally diverse clients is discussed, an important distinction needs to be made between *religion* and *spirituality*. Derived from Latin roots, the term religion means to tie or hold together, to secure, bind, or fasten. It refers to the establishment of a system of attitudes and beliefs. **Religion** refers to an organized system of beliefs concerning the cause, nature, and purpose of the universe, especially belief in or the worship of a Supreme Being who is called by various names according to ethnoreligious traditions and beliefs. Among the important functions of religion is to create and nurture communal and individual spirituality. Religious activities often include reading scriptures or sacred writings (e.g., Qu'ran, Torah, Bible), praying, singing, and/or participating in individual or communal worship services (Leonard & Carlson, 2010).

Spirituality is born out of each person's unique life experience and his or her personal effort to find purpose and meaning in life. When people search for meaning or for a connection that transcends themselves, they are acting as spiritual beings. Spirituality exists in connections to others, the environment and the universe that lies beyond human experience. It refers to an ultimate reality. Present in all individuals, spirituality may be expressed as inner peace, and strength (Buck, 2006; Keehl, 2009; Narayanasamy, 2006; Yuen, 2007).

Spirituality encompasses "embracing, celebrating and voicing all the connections with the ultimate/mystery/divine, within me and beyond me, in experiences that give me meaning, purpose, direction, and values for my daily journey" (Leonard & Carlson, 2010; Spirituality in Healthcare Module, p. 1). While religion and spirituality have similarities and overlapping concepts, they are separate and distinct from one another (Black, 2009; Buck, 2006; Keehl, 2009). In general, religion addresses questions related to what is true and right and helps individuals determine where they belong in the scheme of their life's journey. Spirituality emphasizes the pursuit of meaning, purpose, direction, and values.

Spiritual Nursing Care

The goal of **spiritual nursing care** is to assist clients in integrating their own religious beliefs about a Supreme Being or a unifying truth into the ultimate reality that gives meaning to their lives. This is especially meaningful when people face a serious health challenges or crisis that precipitated the need for nursing care in the first place. Spiritual nursing care promotes clients' physical and emotional health as well as their **spiritual health**. When providing care, the nurse must remember that the goal of spiritual intervention is not, and should not be, to impose his or her religious beliefs and convictions on the client (Amos, 2007; Gordon, 2006; Hubbell, Woodard, Barksdale-Brown, & Parker, 2006; Keehl, 2009; Tzeng & Yin, 2006; Yuen, 2007).

Although spiritual needs are recognized by many nurses, spiritual care is often neglected. Among the reasons why nurses fail to provide spiritual care are the following: (1) they view religious and spiritual needs as a private matter concerning only an individual and his or her Creator; (2) they are uncomfortable about their own religious beliefs or deny having spiritual needs; (3) they lack knowledge about spirituality and the religious beliefs of others; (4) they mistake spiritual needs for psychosocial needs; and (5) they view meeting the spiritual needs of clients as a family or pastoral responsibility, not a nursing responsibility.

Spiritual intervention is as appropriate as any other form of nursing intervention and recognizes that the balance of physical, psychosocial, and spiritual aspects of life is essential to overall good health. Nursing is an intimate profession, and nurses routinely inquire without hesitation about very personal matters such as hygiene and sexual habits. The spiritual realm also requires a personal, intimate type of nursing intervention (Black, 2009; Gordon, 2006; Hubbell et al., 2006; Keehl, 2009; Tzeng & Yin, 2006; White, 2007).

In North America, efforts to integrate spiritual care and nursing have been under way for approximately four decades. In 1971 at the White House Conference on Aging, the spiritual dimension of care was defined as those aspects of individuals pertaining to their inner resources, especially their ultimate concern, the basic value around which all other values are focused, the central philosophy of life that guides their conduct, and the supernatural and nonmaterial dimensions of human nature. The spiritual dimension encompasses the person's need to find satisfactory answers to questions about the meaning of life, illness, or death (Ebersole et al., 2008; Jett & Touhy, 2010; Keehl, 2009; Moberg, 1971, 1981; Yuen, 2007).

In 1978, the Third National Conference on the Classification of Nursing Diagnoses recognized the importance of spirituality by including "**spiritual concerns**," "**spiritual distress**," and "**spiritual despair**" in the list of approved diagnoses. Because of practical difficulties, these three categories were combined at the 1980 National Conference into one category, spiritual distress, which is defined as disruption in the life principle that pervades a person's entire being and that integrates and transcends the person's biologic and psychosocial nature. Moberg (1981) acknowledges the multidimensional nature of spiritual concerns and defines them as the human need to deal with sociocultural deprivations, anxieties and fears, death and dying, personality integration, self-image, personal dignity, social alienation, and philosophy of life.

Assessment of Ethnoreligious and Spiritual Issues

As discussed in Chapter 3, cultural assessment includes assessment of the relationship between religious and spiritual issues as they relate to the health care status of clients. In the integration of health care and religious/spiritual beliefs, the focus of nursing intervention is to help the client maintain his or her own beliefs in the face of a serious health challenge or crisis and to use those beliefs to strengthen the client's coping patterns.

BOX 13-1

Assessing Spiritual Needs in Clients from Various Ethnoreligious Backgrounds

What do you notice about the client's surroundings?

- Does the person have religious objects, such as the Qur'an (Koran) Bible, prayer book, devotional literature, religious medals, rosary, or other type of beads, photographs of historic religious persons or contemporary religious leaders (e.g., Catholic Pope, Dalai Lama, or image of another religious figure), paintings of religious events or persons, religious sculptures, crucifixes, objects of religious significance at entrances to rooms (e.g., holy water founts, a mezuzah, or small parchment scroll inscribed with an excerpt from scripture), candles of religious significance (e.g., Paschal candle, menorah), shrine, or other item?
- Does the person wear clothing that has religious significance (e.g., head covering, undergarment, uniform)? Does the hair style connote affiliation with a certain ethnoreligious group, for example, earlocks worn by Hasidic Jewish men?
- Are get well greeting cards religious in nature or from a representative of the person's church, mosque, temple, synagogue, or other religious congregation?

How does the person act?

- Does the person appear to pray at certain times of the day or before meals?
- Does the person make special dietary requests (e.g., kosher diet, vegetarian diet, or refrain from caffeine, pork or pork derivatives such as gelatin or marshmallows, shellfish, or other specific food items)?
- Does the person read religious magazines or books?

What does the person say?

- Does the person talk about God (Allah, Buddha, Yahweh, Jehova), prayer, faith, or religious topics?
- Does the person ask for a visit by a clergy member or other religious representative?
- Does the person express anxiety or fear about pain, suffering, dying or death?

How does the person relate to others?

- Who visits? How does the person respond to visitors?
- Does a priest, rabbi, minister, elder, or other religious representative visit?
- Does the person ask the nursing staff to pray for or with him/her?
- Does the person prefer to interact with others or to remain alone?

If the religious beliefs are contributing to the overall health problem (e.g., guilt, remorse, expectations), you can conduct a **spiritual assessment**. To be therapeutic, begin by asking questions that clarify the problem, and nonjudgmentally support the client's problem solving (Buck, 2006; Hubbell et al., 2006; Keehl, 2009; Yhlen & Ashton, 2006; Yuen, 2007; Yurkovick & Lattergrass, 2008).

Summarized in Box 13-1 are guidelines for assessing spiritual needs in clients from diverse cultural backgrounds (Figure 13-1).

Spiritual Nursing Care for Ill Children and Their Families

In a broad sense, any hospitalization or serious illness can be viewed as stressful and therefore has the potential to develop into a crisis. You may find that religion plays an especially significant role when a child is seriously ill and in circumstances that include dying, death, or bereavement.

Illness during childhood may be an especially difficult clinical situation. Children as well as adults have spiritual needs that vary according to their developmental level and the relative importance of religion and spirituality in the lives of their primary providers of care. Parental perceptions about the illness of their child may be partially influenced by religious beliefs. For example, some parents may believe that a transgression against a religious law has caused a congenital anomaly in their offspring. Other parents may delay seeking medical care because they believe that prayer should be tried first.

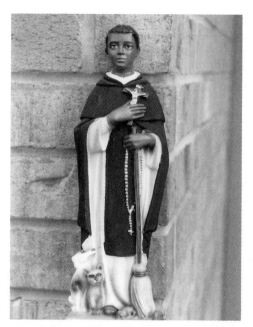

FIGURE 13-1 This statue commemorates the Roman Catholic Saint Martin De Porres. Born in Peru during the 16th century to a Spanish father and a Black mother, Martin De Porres studied medicine, which he later, as a member of the Dominican Order, put to use in helping the poor. He is honored by some Catholics as the patron saint of African Americans. When assessing the needs of clients from diverse backgrounds, nurses can observe for the presence of religious objects in the client's home or yard (© Copyright M. Andrews).

The nurse should be respectful of parents' preferences regarding the care of their child. When you believe that parental beliefs or practices threaten the child's well-being and health, you are obligated to discuss the matter with the parents. It may be possible to reach a compromise in which parental beliefs are respected and necessary care is provided. On rare occasions, it may become a legal matter (Fogel & Rivera, 2010; Matthew, 2008). Religion may be a source of consolation and support to parents, especially those facing the unanswerable questions associated with life-threatening illness in their children.

Spiritual Nursing Care for the Dying or Bereaved Client and Family

All people do not mourn alike. Mourning is a form of cultural behavior, and it is manifest in a multicultural society. Mourning customs help people cope with the loss of loved ones. Nurses inevitably focus on restoring health or on fostering environments in which the client returns to a previous state of health or adapts to physical, psychological, or emotional changes. However, one aspect of care that is often avoided or ignored, though every bit as crucial to clients and their families, is death and the accompanying dying and grieving processes.

Death is indeed a universal experience, but one that is highly individual and personal. Although each person must ultimately face death alone, rarely does a person's death fail to affect others. There are many rituals, serving many purposes, that people use to help them cope with death. These rituals are often determined by cultural and religious orientation. Situational factors, competing demands, and individual differences are also important in determining the dying, bereavement, and grieving behaviors that are considered socially acceptable (Amos, 2007).

The role of the nurse in dealing with dying clients and their families varies according to the needs and preferences of both the nurse and client, as well as the clinical setting in which the interaction occurs. By understanding some of the cultural and religious variations related to death, dying, and bereavement, the nurse can individualize the care given to clients and their families.

Nurses are often with the client through various stages of the dying process and at the actual moment of death, particularly when death occurs in a hospital, nursing home, extended care facility, or hospice. The nurse often determines when and whom to call as the impending death draws near. Knowing the religious, cultural, and familial heritage of a particular client as well as his or her devotion to the associated traditions and practices may help the nurse determine whom to call when the need arises.

Religious Beliefs Associated with Dying

Universally, people want to die with dignity. Historically this was not a problem when individuals died at home in the presence of their friends and families. Now, when more and more people are dying in institutions (hospitals, hospices, and extended care facilities) ensuring dignity throughout the dying process is more complex. Once death is seen as a problem for professional management, the hospital displaces the home, and specialists with different kinds and degrees of expertise take over for the family (Amos, 2007).

The way in which people commemorate death tells us much about their attitude and philosophy of life and death. Although it is beyond the scope of this book to explore the philosophic and psychological aspects of death in detail, some points will be made that relate to nursing care.

Preparation of the Body

A nurse may or may not actually participate in the rituals associated with death. When people die in the United States and Canada, they are usually transported to a mortuary, where the preparation for burial occurs.

In many cultural groups, preparation of the body has traditionally been very important. Whereas members of many cultural groups have now adopted the practice of letting the mortician prepare the body, there are some, particularly new immigrants, who want to retain their native and/ or religious customs. For example, for certain Asian immigrants it is customary for family and friends of the same sex to wash and prepare the body for burial or cremation. In other situations, the family or religious representatives may go to the funeral home to prepare the body for burial by dressing the person in special religious clothing.

If a person dies in an institution, it is common for the nursing staff to "prepare" the body according to standard procedure. Depending on the ethnoreligious practices of the family, this may be objectionable—the family members may view this washing as an infringement on a special task that belongs to them alone. If the family is present, you should ask family members about their preference. If ritual washings will eventually take place at the mortuary, you may carry out the routine procedures and reassure the family that the mortician will comply with their requests, if that has in fact been verified.

North American **funeral** customs have been the topic of lively discussion. The initial preparation of the body has been described in the following way:

"After delivery to the undertaker, the corpse is in short order sprayed, sliced, pierced, pickled, trussed, trimmed, creamed, waxed, painted, rouged and neatly dressed...transformed from a common corpse into a beautiful memory picture. This process is known in the trades as embalming and restorative art, and is so universally employed in North America that the funeral director does it routinely without consulting the corpse's family. He regards as eccentric those few who are hardy enough to suggest it might be dispensed with. Yet no law requires it, no religious doctrine commends it, nor is it dictated by considerations of health, sanitation or even personal daintiness. In no part of the world but in North America is it widely used. The purpose of embalming is to make the corpse presentable for viewing in a suitably costly container, and here too the funeral director routinely without first consulting the family prepares the body for public display" (Kalish & Reynolds, 1981, p. 65).

This extensive preparation and attempt to make the body look "alive," "just as he used to," or "just as if she were asleep" may reflect the fact that North Americans have come into contact with death and dying less than have other cultural groups.

Funeral Practices

By their very nature, people are social beings who need to develop social attachments. When these social attachments are broken by death, people need to bring closure to the relationships. The funeral is an appropriate and socially acceptable time for the expression of sorrow and grief. Although there are some mores that dictate acceptable behaviors associated with the expression of grief, such as crying and sobbing, the wake and funeral are generally viewed as times when members of the living social network can observe and comfort the grieving survivors in their mourning, and say a last goodbye to the dead person. It is important to keep in mind that even the terms used for the wake and the funeral may vary according to religious and cultural beliefs. What is called a **wake** in many North American religions may be called a **viewing** or **Home going** by others.

Customs for disposal of the body after death vary widely. Muslims have specific rituals for washing, dressing, and positioning the body. In traditional Judaism, cosmetic restoration is discouraged, as is any attempt to hasten or retard decomposition by artificial means. As part of their lifelong preparation for death, Amish women sew white burial garments for themselves and for their family members (Wenger, 1991). For the viewing and burial, faithful Mormons are dressed in white temple garments. Burial clothes and other religious or cultural symbols may be important items for the funeral ritual. If such items are present, you should ensure that they are taken by the family or sent to the funeral home.

Believing that the spirit or ghost of the deceased person is contaminated, some Navajos are afraid to touch the body after death. In preparation for burial, the body is dressed in fine apparel, adorned with expensive jewelry and money, and wrapped in new blankets. After death, some Navajos believe that the structure in which the person died must be burned. There are specific members of the culture whose role is to prepare the body and who must be ritually cleansed after contact with the dead.

Funeral arrangements vary from short, simple rituals to long, elaborate displays. Among the Amish, family members, neighbors, and friends are relied on for a short, quiet ceremony. Many Jewish families use unadorned coffins and stress simplicity in burial services. Some Jews fly the body to Jerusalem for burial in ground considered to be holy. Regardless of economic considerations, some groups believe in lavish and costly funerals.

Attitudes Toward Death

Taboos

In some cultures, people believe that particular omens, such as the appearance of an owl or a message in a dream, warn of approaching death. Breaking a taboo may be believed to cause death, and the nurse may be seen as the responsible agent! The literature contains numerous reports of incidents in which nurses have removed objects of religious and spiritual significance that are believed to have healing powers from clients and patients of all ages—rosaries from the cribs of infants, necklaces worn by elderly Native Americans, and so forth. In some cases, the intention of the nurse was benevolent, as when the nurse indicated that the item was removed to be kept in a safe place with other valuables.

Voodoo beliefs and practices are known to exist in North America. Incidents of sudden death or minor injuries after hexing have been attributed to the power of suggestion and to total social isolation, which have been thought to trigger fatal physiologic responses and sensitization of the autonomic nervous system.

Unexpected Death, Violent Death, and Suicide

Acceptance of sudden, violent death is difficult for family members in most societies. For example, suicide is strictly forbidden under Islamic law. In the Filipino culture, suicide brings shame to the individual and to the entire family. Many Christian religions prohibit suicide and may impose sanctions even after death for the "sin." For example, a Roman Catholic who commits suicide may be denied burial in blessed ground or in a Catholic cemetery. In some religions, a church funeral is not permitted for a suicide victim, requiring the family to make alternative arrangements. This imposition of religious law can further add to the grief of surviving family members and friends.

The Northern Cheyenne believe that suicide, or any death resulting from a violent accident, disturbs the individual's spiritual balance. This disharmony is termed **bad death** and is believed to render the spirit earthbound in its wanderings, thus preventing it from entering the spirit world.

A **good death** among the Tohono O'odham comes at the end of a full life, when a person is prepared for death. A bad death, by contrast, occurs unexpectedly and violently, leaving the victim without a chance to settle affairs or to say good-bye.

"A 'bad death' is 'bad' because evil caused it, which leaves the soul of the dead unrestful, unfulfilled, and desirous of returning to the living out of a longing for what has been taken away. The soul returns to the living, although not out of malevolence, to visit loved ones. It is on these visits, that the dead can bring a form of *ka:cim mumkidag* (staying–Indian–sickness), to the living—hence their dangerousness" (McIntyre, 2008).

The categories of "good" and "bad" deaths among the Tohono O'odham have implications for research on excess deaths. Accidents, homicide, and suicide produce bad deaths; in Tohono O'odham eyes, these are deaths that should not occur, deaths that should be avoided if possible. "Bad" deaths are excess deaths. If the medical community's concern is with eliminating excess deaths, it must also be concerned with the larger cultural, social, and economic context in which these deaths occur. Other causes of death, while still important, may affect a people to a much lesser degree. Diabetes mellitus, for example, most often affects people of more advanced years and, because of its slow progress, allows them to prepare for death. This is still an excess death by Western medical standards, but it is not a "bad" death (Kozak, 1991; Yurkovick & Lattergrass, 2008).

Death memorials provide a place for the dead to go without bringing harm to the living, and a place for the living to go to help the dead to a proper afterlife. Among the Tohono O'odham, there has been a notable increase in violent deaths, particularly for young males. The majority of these violent deaths are the result of motor vehicle accidents and are marked by roadside death memorials or shrines. Suicides and homicides are also sometimes commemorated with death memorials.

Deaths resulting from nonviolent but untimely causes can be equally difficult for the patient, family, and friends. Cancers and chronic diseases may give the patient and family time to "prepare" for the death, but the death still occurs and must receive attention.

The Death of a Child

Although a great deal has been written about children's conceptions of death, cross-cultural studies have not yet been reported. Children develop a concept of death through innate cognitive development, which has significant cultural variations, and through acquired notions conveyed by the family, which vary according to the family's cultural beliefs. Thus, it is unsafe to assume that all children, regardless of family culture, will develop parallel concepts of and reactions to death.

Most children's initial experiences with death occur with the loss of a pet rather than a person. Because of reduced childhood mortality and delayed adult mortality, Western children are much less exposed to death in family than they used to be, and they tend to be sheltered from the experience. The current lack of direct exposure of children to death is both a class phenomenon and a cultural phenomenon.

In many societies of the Western world, children are considered precious, valued, and vulnerable; they are protected and often the first to be saved in emergencies. In less developed societies, by contrast, parents are less likely to see most of their children grow into adulthood because of a very high infant mortality rate. As a result, a child's life may be viewed as less valued and precious than an adult's, but it is still viewed as valuable to the parents and other loved ones. Regardless of the sociocultural situation, each society has a special view of the significance of children and their death as it affects the bereaved family.

Bereavement, Grief, and Mourning

Bereavement is a sociologic term indicating the status and role of the survivors of a death. **Grief** is an affective response to a loss, whereas **mourning** is the culturally patterned behavioral response to a death. What differs between cultural groups is not so much the feelings of grief but their forms of expression or mourning.

Different family systems may alleviate or intensify the pain experienced by bereaved persons. In the typical nuclear North American family, the death of a member leaves a great void because the same few individuals fill most of the roles. By contrast, cultural groups in which several generations and extended family members commonly reside within a household may find that the acute trauma of bereavement is softened by the fact that the familial role of the deceased is easily filled by other relatives. It should be noted, however, that the loss is experienced and mourned irrespective of the person's cultural background.

Although nurses frequently encourage clients and their families to express their grief openly, many people are reluctant to do so in the institutional setting. The nurse often sees family members when they are still in shock over the death and are responding to the situation as a crisis rather than expressing their grief. When asked who would be sought for comfort and support in a time of bereavement, most frequently named were a family member or a member of the clergy. In an institutional setting, a nurse who has been with the patient and family throughout the dying process may be surprised at the time of death when the grieving persons turn to other family, and the nurse is "left out."

Summary of Beliefs Related to Death and Dying

Contemporary bereavement practices of various cultural and religious groups demonstrate the wide range of expressions of bereavement. Each group reflects practices that best meet its members' needs. Once you understand this, you can better appreciate their role in promoting a culturally appropriate grieving process, and to realize that hindering or interfering with practices that the client and family find meaningful can disrupt the grieving process. Bereaved people can experience physical and psychological symptoms, and they may succumb to serious physical illnesses, leading even to death. Although bereavement is regarded as a universal stressor, the magnitude of the stress and its meaning to the individual vary

significantly cross-culturally. For example, one Western misconception is that it is more stressful to mourn the death of a child than the death of an older or more distant relative. Yet, cross-cultural studies show that emotional attachments to relatives vary significantly and are not based on Western concepts of kinship.

Although traditional funeral and post-funeral rituals have benefited both bereaved persons and their social groups in their original settings, the influence of the contemporary Western urban setting is unknown. It is likely that in North America, most individuals have assimilated United States and Canadian practices in varying degrees. You should obtain information from individual clients in a caring manner, explaining that you wish to provide culturally appropriate nursing care.

Religious Trends in the United States and Canada

The United States and Canada are cosmopolitan nations to which all of the major and many of the minor faiths of Europe and other parts of the globe have been transplanted. Religious identification among people from different racial and ethnic groups is important because religion and culture are interwoven. Table 13-1 details the statistical breakdown of major religious affiliations of the United States and Canada (Figure 13-2). Selected religious groups and their respective memberships numbers in the United States and Canada are identified in Table 13-2.

As discussed, a wide range of beliefs frequently exists within religions—a factor that adds complexity. Some religions have a designated spokesperson or leader who articulates, interprets, and applies theological tenets to daily life experiences, including those of health and illness. These leaders include Jewish rabbis, Catholic priests, and Lutheran ministers. Some religions rely more heavily on individual conscience, whereas others entrust decisions to a group of individuals, or to a single person vested with ultimate authority within their religious tradition.

TABLE 13-1
Major Religious Affiliations of United States and Canada (%)

	USA	CANADA	WORLD
Christianity	76.5	77.1	32.9
Atheism, Agnosticism, no affiliation	13.2	17	12.5
Judaism	1.4	1.1	0.2
Islam	0.5	2.0	19.9
Buddhism	0.5	1	6
Hinduism	0.4	0.9	14
Major Christian Faith Groups			
Roman Catholic	24.5	50.8	32.3
Protestant	52	35	9.2

Source: www.religioustolerance.org, March 18, 2007.

Although it is impossible to address the health-related beliefs and practices of any religion adequately, this chapter offers a brief overview of selected groups. Some of the world's religions fall into major branches or divisions, such as Vaishnavite and Shaivite Hinduism; Theravada and Mahayana Buddhism; Orthodox, Reform, and Conservative Judaism; Roman Catholic, Orthodox, and Protestant Christianity; and Sunnite and Shi'ite Islam. There also are subdivisions into what are often called denominations, sects, or schools of thought and practice.

Contributions of Religious Groups to the Health Care Delivery System

In the United States and Canada, many denominations own and operate health care institutions and make significant fiscal contributions that help control health care costs. For example, the Roman Catholic Church, the largest single denomination in the United States, is also a major stakeholder in the health care field. The nation's

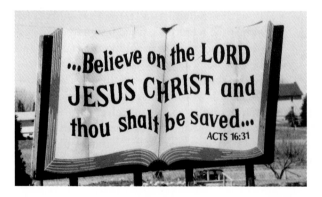

FIGURE 13-2 Eighty-five percent of North Americans report religious affiliation with a Christian church. Of the 60% affiliated with protestant groups in the United States, Baptists account for 21%; Methodists, 9%; Lutherans, 7%; Presbyterians, 5%; and Episcopalians, 2%. Catholics comprise 3%. Those belonging to non-Christian religions total 6% of the population, whereas those reporting no religious affiliation account for 9% (© Copyright M. Andrews).

TABLE 13-2
Membership for Selected Religious Bodies in the United States and Canada

RELIGIOUS BODY (YEAR REPORTED)	MEMBERSHIP
African Methodist Episcopal Church (2006)	2,500,000
African Methodist Episcopal Zion Church (2006)	1,432,795
American Baptist Churches in the U.S.A. (2006)	1,424,840
Assemblies of God (2006)	2,779,095
Baptist Bible Fellowship International (2006)	1,200,000
Buddhist (1990)	780,000
Christian Churches and Churches of Christ (2006)	1,071,615
Church of God in Christ (2006)	5,499,875
Church of Jesus Christ of Latter-Day Saints (2006)	5,999,177
Churches of Christ (2006)	1,500,000
Episcopal Church (2006)	2,284,233
Evangelical Lutheran Church of America (2006)	4,930,429
Greek Orthodox Diocese America (2006)	1,500,000
Hindu (1990)	227,000
Islam (2002)	6–7,000,000
Jehovah's Witnesses (1999)	1,029,902
Jewish (1998)	7,320,000
Lutheran Church—Missouri Synod (2006)	2,463,747
Muslim/Islamic (1990)	3,600,000
National Baptist Convention of America, Inc. (2006)	3,500,000
National Baptist Convention, U.S.A., Inc. (2006)	5,000,000
National Missionary Baptist Convention, U.S.A., Inc. (2006)	2,500,000
Orthodox Church in America (2006)	1,064,000
Pentecostal Assemblies of the World, Inc. (2006)	1,500,000
Presbyterian Church (U.S.A.) (2006)	3,189,573
Progressive National Baptist Convention, Inc. (2006)	2,500,000
Roman Catholic Church (2006)	67,820,833
Southern Baptist Convention (2006)	16,267,494
United Church of Christ (2006)	1,265,786
United Methodist Church (2006)	8,186,254

Yearbook of American and Canadian Churches (2006).

622 Catholic hospitals (Fogel & Rivera, 2010) treat more than 17 million patients annually and account for approximately 10% of all hospital beds. In addition, the Catholic Church is responsible for treating more than 6 million individuals at its 392 other health-related centers. Moreover, there are under direct Catholic auspices 79 non-residential schools for the handicapped; 14 facilities for the deaf and hearing impaired; 4 centers for the blind and visually impaired; 517 facilities for the aged; 72 facilities for abused, abandoned, neglected, and emotionally disturbed children; 116 centers for those with developmental disabilities; 2 residences for the orthopedically and physically handicapped; 8 cancer hospitals; and 11 substance abuse centers (accessed on March 1, 2010 at http://www.catholichealthcare.us/).

Catholic Charities USA, an umbrella agency that oversees nonhospital work, reports that its agencies serve more than 10 million people each year, often functioning as a centralized referral source for clients ultimately treated in non-Catholic agencies (accessed at http://www.catholiccharitiesusa.org/ on March 1, 2010). Similarly, there are many Jewish hospitals, day care centers, extended care facilities, and organizations to meet the health care needs of Jewish and non-Jewish persons in need. For example, the National Jewish Center for Immunology and Respiratory Medicine is a research and treatment center for respiratory, immunologic, allergic and infectious diseases, whereas the Council for Jewish Elderly provides a full range of social and health care services for seniors, including adult day care, care/

BOX 13-2

Internet Websites for Selected Religions

Religion	Website
Amish	www.800padutch.com/amish.shtml
Baha'i	www.Bahai.org
Buddhist	www.buddhanet.org
	www.buddhism.about.com
Catholicism (Roman Rite)	www.catholic.org
Christian Science	www.tfccs.com
	www.tfccs.com/aboutchristianscience
Church of Jesus Christ of Latter Day Saints (Mormonism)	www.lds.org
Hinduism	www.hindunet.org
Islam	www.islamicity.com
	www.islam101.com
	www.islamworld.net
Jehovah's Witnesses	www.watchtower.org
Judaism	www.judaism.about.com
Mennonite	www.mennoniteuse.org
Native American Churches	www.nativeamericanchurch.net
	www.americanindianchurch.net
A source for general information about many denominations	www.religioustolerance.org

case management, counseling, transportation, and advocacy.

According to the Pew Forum on Religion and Public Policy, many other denominations, including the Lutheran, Mennonite, Methodist, Muslim, and Seventh-Day Adventist groups, own and operate hospitals and health care organizations similar to those described previously (accessed on March 1, 2010 at http://pewforum.org/docs).

In Canada, hospital care, outpatient care, extended care, and medical services have been publicly funded and administered since the Medical Care Act of 1966. However, before the Medical Care Act and into the present, religious organizations have made important contributions to the health and well-being of Canadians at individual, community, and societal levels. For example, countless church-run agencies, charities, and facilities offer care and social support to individuals and families coping with such conditions as chronic illness, disability, poverty, and homelessness. At the national level, church-run organizations, such as the Catholic Health Association of Canada, are committed to addressing social justice issues that affect the health system and offer leadership through research and policy development regarding health care ethics, spiritual and religious care, and social justice.

The remainder of this chapter will provide an overview of selected religions and their health-related beliefs and practices. The religious groups have been listed in alphabetical order. For a quick online overview of religious beliefs and practices for various groups, refer to Box 13-2.

Amish

The term **Amish** refers to members of several ethnoreligious groups who choose to live separately from the modern world through manner of dress, language, family life, and selective use of technology. There are four major orders or affiliating groups of Amish: (1) *Old Order Amish*, the largest group, whose name is often used synonymously with "the Amish"; (2) the ultraconservative *Swartzentruber* and *Andy Weaver Amish*, both more conservative than the Old Order Amish in their restrictive use of technology and shunning of members who have dropped out or committed serious violations of the faith; (3) the less conservative *New Order Amish*, which emerged in the 1960s with more liberal views of technology but with an emphasis on high moral standards in restricting alcohol and tobacco use and in courtship practices; and (4) the *Liberal Beachy Amish*.

The total population of Amish is estimated at 160,000, spread throughout more than 220 settlements in 21 states and one Canadian province (about 1/20th of 1% of the total populations of the United States and Canada). In 1900, there were approximately 5,000 Amish, representing the number who immigrated to the United States during the 18th and 19th centuries. During the 20th century, however, the population grew as the Amish became less frequent targets for conversion and growing numbers of children (80–85%) chose, as adults, to be baptized Amish. As a result, the population grew to 85,000 by 1979 and has nearly doubled today. More than half are younger than age 18 (Donnermeyer, 1997).

General Beliefs and Religious Practices

The imperative to remain separate is the common theme of the nearly 500-year history of the Amish and is based on the following scripture passages:

"Be not conformed to this world, but be ye transformed by the renewing of your mind"

(Romans 12:2)

"Be ye not unequally yoked together with unbelievers; for what fellowship hath righteousness with unrighteousness? and what communion hath light with darkness?"

(II Corinthians 6:14)

The Amish are direct descendants of a branch of Anabaptists (which means "to be rebaptized") which emerged during the Protestant Reformation and resided in Switzerland, The Netherlands, Austria, France, and Germany. Anabaptists stressed adult baptism, separation from and nonassimilation with the dominant culture, conformity in dress and appearance, marriage to others within the group, nonproselytization, nonparticipation in military service, and a disciplined lifestyle with an emphasis on simple living. These basic tenets remain today.

A former Catholic priest from The Netherlands named Menno Simmons (1496–1561) wrote down the beliefs and practices of the Anabaptists, who became known as **Mennonites**. In 1693, under the leadership of a church elder named Jacob Ammann (1656–1730), a more conservative group broke away and formed the group currently known as the Amish.

Core Characteristics

According to Donnermeyer's (1997) classic study, there are **five core characteristics of the Amish**.

Subculture

First, the Amish are a subculture: a group with beliefs, values, and behaviors which are distinct from the greater culture of which the group is a part. The Amish maintain their separateness and distinctiveness from United States and Canadian societies in a variety of ways. Geographically, the Amish live close together in areas referred to as settlements and rely primarily on the horse and buggy or bicycles for transportation.

The Amish continue to practice their faith in the tradition of Anabaptism, which includes small church districts of a few dozen families led by a bishop, church services that rotate from house to house of each family (no church building), the practice of adult baptism, communion twice a year, and shunning. Church leaders are chosen through a process of nomination and drawing by lot, and they serve for life. All but a few Amish marry, extended family remains important, and divorce is rare. The Amish dress in distinctive clothing (plain colors and mostly without buttons and zippers). They speak a form of German among themselves known as Pennsylvania Dutch or High German, and they sometimes refer to non-Amish as the "English."

Ordung

The second core feature of the Amish is the *ordung*, which is used for passing on religious values and way of life from one generation to the next. Parts of the *ordung* are based on specific biblical passages, but much of it consists of rules for living the Amish way.

Meidung/Shunning

The third characteristic of the Amish is *meidung*, the practice of shunning members who have violated the *ordung*. After all members of the church district have discussed the case and agreed to impose *meidung*, the individual is separated from the rest of his or her community. It is the church's method of enforcing the *ordung*. *Meidung* is an important way of maintaining both a sense of community among Amish and a sense of separation from the rest of the world. Sanctions for violations against important values, beliefs, and behaviors that define distinctiveness from the majority culture enable the Amish to retain their religious and cultural identity. In most cases, when *meidung* is applied, it is for a limited time. *Meidung* applies only to Amish adults who have been baptized, not to their unbaptized children. Children of Amish who choose not to be baptized often become members of neighboring Mennonite congregations and maintain contact with their Amish relatives.

With less serious violations of the *ordung*, a member is visited privately by the deacon and a minister, and the matter is resolved quietly. For more serious offenses, the punishment is carried out publicly during a church service. A few offenses, such as adultery and divorce, are automatically conditions of excommunication. By displaying deep sorrow and repentance for an offense, excommunicated members can be allowed back, but this is not easily accomplished.

Selective Use of Technology

The fourth core characteristic is the selective use of technology. The Amish selectively use many modern technologies, but only if this does not threaten their ability to maintain a community of believers. Technologically, the Amish restrict the use of

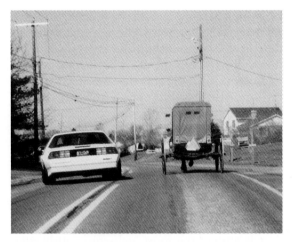

FIGURE 13-3 Although the Amish restrict their use of technology for reasons that are, in part, health-related, they ironically find themselves at a high risk for accidents that frequently result from the careless use of technologic developments by non-Amish neighbors.

electricity in their homes and farms, and they limit their use of telephones. Although they ride in automobiles, trains, and airplanes, they do not operate them. Tractors for farm field work might reduce the opportunity for sons and daughters to help parents with farm chores, and the farm would become larger, reducing the number available for future generations. Thus, technology is not inherently bad, but when its consequences result in destruction of family and community life, it is avoided (Figure 13-3).

Gelassenheit

The fifth and final core characteristic of the Amish is *gelassenheit*. This term means "submission," or yielding to a higher authority, and it represents a general guide for behavior among Amish members. *Gelassenheit* represents the high value that the Amish place on maintaining a sense of community, which is accomplished by not drawing too much attention to one's self. Amish cite *gelassenheit* as the reason they avoid having their photographs taken and prohibit mirrors in their homes.

Holy Days and Sacraments

Amish hold church services every other Sunday on a rotating basis in the homes or barns of church district members. The church services last several hours with hymns, scriptures, and services in High German or Pennsylvania Dutch. The family hosting the services is expected to provide a meal for all in attendance. Christmas celebrations include family dinners and exchange of gifts. Weddings last all day and include eating and singing. An important part of Amish life is informal visiting. Families often visit one another without advance notice, and it is common for unexpected visitors to stay for a meal. Amish observe adult baptism and communion twice a year.

Social Activities (Dating, Dancing)

The Amish strive for high standards of conduct in both their private and public lives. This includes chastity before marriage and humility in dress, language, and behavior. The function of dating is to afford individuals an opportunity to become acquainted with each other's character. Couples contemplating marriage may engage in a practice called bundling, in which they lie together in bed, fully clothed, without having sexual contact.

Substance Use

Alcoholic beverages and drugs are forbidden unless prescribed by a physician. Tobacco use is prohibited.

Health Care Practices

Illness is seen as the inability to perform daily chores; physical and mental illness are equally accepted. Health care practices within the Amish culture are varied and include folk, herbal, homeopathic, and Western biomedicine. Unlike the use of episodic biomedicine, however, preventive medicine may be seen as against God's will. The use of the Western biomedical health care system is largely episodic and crisis oriented. If Western biomedicine fails, there is no hesitancy in visiting an herb doctor, pow-wow doctor (a practitioner of a folk healing art, known as *brauche*, in which touch is used to heal), or a chiropractor. Folk, professional, and alternative care are often used simultaneously. Cost, access, transportation, and advice from family and friends are the major factors that influence healing choices (Wenger, 1990).

Medical and Surgical Interventions

The use of narcotic drugs is prohibited. There are no restrictions against the use of blood, blood products, or vaccines if advised by health care providers.

Practices Related to Reproduction

The Amish believe that the fundamental purpose of marriage is the procreation of children, and couples are encouraged to have large families. Children are an economic asset to the family because they assist their parents with housework, farm chores, gardening, and family business. Women are expected to have children until menopause. If situations arise that justify sterilization (e.g., removal of cancerous reproductive organs), those called upon to make the decisions would rely on the best medical advice available and the council of the church leaders. Although the Amish family structure is patriarchal, the grandmother is often a key decision maker concerning reproductive and other health-related issues.

Abortion is inconsistent with Amish values and beliefs. Artificial insemination, genetics, eugenics, and stem cell research are also inconsistent with Amish values and beliefs.

Religious Support System for the Sick

Visitors

Individual members of local and surrounding communities assist and support one another in time of need. From cradle to grave, each person knows that he or she will be cared for by those in the community. **Friendscraft** is a unique three-generational extended family support network inherent in the Amish community which provides informal support, emotional and financial assistance, and advice. The extended family consists of aunts, uncles, cousins, and grandparents, who usually live only a few miles away and can be counted on to assist in times of illness.

Title of Religious Representative

The Amish do not use religious titles. There are approximately 1,100 Amish church districts in the United States and Canada, each representing about 20 to 35 families, and a minimal hierarchy of church leaders (a bishop, deacon, and two ministers). The bishop is the spiritual head; the deacon assists the bishop and is responsible for donations to help members with medical bills and other expenses; and the ministers help the bishop with preaching at church services and providing spiritual direction for the church district and its members. Although bishops meet periodically, there is no church hierarchy above the level of the church district. Because the Amish are surrounded by American and Canadian societies, which continuously exert strong economic and cultural pressures that are incompatible with Amish values, the Amish represent a subculture that is among the most "self-consciously engineered of all societies" (Donnermeyer, 1997, p. 9).

Church Organizations to Assist the Sick

Individual members of local church districts look after the needs of the sick person and his or her family.

Practices Related to Death and Dying

Prolongation of life (right to die) and euthanasia are personal matters that may be discussed with the bishop, ministers, and/or family members. Autopsy is acceptable in the case of medical necessity or legal requirement but is seldom performed on the Amish. Although there is no specific prohibition, the Amish usually prefer to bury the intact body and generally do not donate body parts for medical research. Bodies are buried in small cemeteries in Amish communities on private property.

Addendum: Meeting Health Expenses

The Amish beliefs in self-sufficiency, separation from the world, and mutual aid have resulted in their rejection of formal assistance that comes from outside the Amish community. For example, the Amish obtained exemption for self-employed workers from Social Security, including Medicare, in 1965 on religious grounds and received exemption for all Amish workers from these programs in 1988. Amish seldom purchase commercial health insurance; instead, they have traditionally relied on personal savings and various methods of mutual assistance within the immediate and larger Amish community to meet their medical expenses. It is expected that each family has planned for future health care needs (e.g., childbirth and minor illness), but it is recognized that catastrophic illnesses resulting in extensive medical expenses do sometimes occur. In these instances, the Amish community provides assistance, usually through participation in one of the Amish Hospital Aid plans.

Changing occupational patterns among the Amish have resulted in shifting views toward commercial health insurance. According to Donnermeyer (1997), in Holmes County, Ohio, only 32.9% of Amish breadwinners earn their living as farmers: 24.5% are active farmers, 4% are retired farmers, and 3.4% hold dual occupations (both farm and nonfarm). Similar trends have been reported among other Amish settlements, where 30 to 80% of adult men work in nonfarm wage labor jobs in construction, factories, and home-based shops (e.g., cabinetmaking, harness making, blacksmithing, and so forth). The underlying reasons for the change are attributed to two factors: population growth and difficulty finding sufficient farmland for the growing numbers of Amish.

Baha'i International Community

The Baha'i Faith is an independent world religion. It has members in approximately 340 countries and localities and represents 1,900 ethnic groups and tribes. North American membership is 161,366, and worldwide membership is 7,666,000.

General Beliefs and Religious Practices

The writings that guide the life of the **Baha'i International Community** comprise numerous works by Baha'u'llah, prophet-founder of the Baha'i Faith. Central teachings are the oneness of God, the oneness of religion, and the oneness of humanity. Baha'u'llah proclaimed that religious truth is not absolute but relative, that Divine Revelation is a continuous and progressive process, that all the great religions of the world are divine in origin, and

that their missions represent successive stages in the spiritual evolution of human society.

For Baha'is, the basic purpose of human life is to know and worship God and to carry forward an ever-advancing civilization. To achieve these goals, they strive to fulfill certain principles:

1. Fostering of good character and the development of spiritual qualities, such as honesty, trustworthiness, compassion, and justice.
2. Eradication of prejudices of race, creed, class, nationality, and sex.
3. Elimination of all forms of superstitions that hamper human progress, and achievement of a balance between the material and spiritual aspects of life. An unfettered search for truth, and belief in the essential harmony of science and religion, are two aspects of this principle.
4. Development of the unique talents and abilities of every individual through the pursuit of knowledge and the acquisition of skills for the practice of a trade or profession.
5. Full participation of both sexes in all aspects of community life, including the elective, administrative, and decision-making processes, along with equality of opportunities, rights, and privileges of men and women.
6. Fostering of the principle of universal compulsory education.

Baha'is may not be members of any political party, but they may accept nonpartisan government posts and appointments. They are expected to obey the government in their respective countries and, without political affiliation, may vote in general elections and participate in the civic life of their communities.

The Baha'i administrative order has neither priesthood nor ritual; it relies on a pattern of local, national, and international governance, created by Baha'u'llah. Institutions and programs are supported exclusively by voluntary contributions from members.

The Baha'i International Community has consultative status with the United Nations Economic and Social Council and with the United Nations Children's Fund. It is also affiliated with the

United Nations Environment Program and with the United Nations Office of Public Information.

The World Center of the Baha'i Faith is in Israel, established in the two cities of Haifa and 'Akka. The affairs of the Baha'i world community are administered by the Universal House of Justice, the supreme elected council, in Haifa.

Holy Days and Sacraments

Extending from sunset to sunset are Baha'i holy days, feast days, and days of fasting. These holy days are not contraindications to medical care or surgery.

Although the Baha'i faith does not have sacraments in the same sense that Christian churches do, it does have practices that have similar meanings to members. These practices include the recitation of obligatory prayers and participation in the observance of holy days and the Nineteen-Day Fast, which is mandatory for all Baha'is between the ages of 15 and 70 years. Exceptions are made for illness, travel away from home, and pregnancy. **Fasting** occurs from sunrise to sunset for an entire Baha'i month, which consists of 19 days.

Social Activities (Dating, Dancing)

Baha'is strive for high standards of conduct in both their private and public lives; this includes chastity before marriage; moderation in dress, language, and amusements; and complete freedom from prejudice in their dealings with peoples of different races, classes, creeds, and orders.

The Baha'i Faith forbids monastic celibacy, noting that marriage is fundamental to the growth and continuation of civilization. The function of dating is to afford individuals an opportunity to become acquainted with each other's character. Those contemplating marriage are encouraged to engage in some form of work and service together—a practice intended to promote assessment of their own maturity and readiness for marriage as well as to improve their knowledge of the character and values of the prospective marriage partner.

Substance Use

Alcoholic beverages and drugs are forbidden unless prescribed by a physician. Tobacco use is strongly discouraged.

Health Care Practices

With an attitude of harmony between religion and science, Baha'is are encouraged to seek out competent medical care, to follow the advice of those in whom they have confidence, and to pray.

Medical and Surgical Interventions

The use of narcotic drugs is prohibited except by prescription. There are no restrictions against the use of blood, blood products, or vaccines if advised by health care providers. Amputations, organ transplantation, biopsies, and circumcision are permitted if advised by health care providers.

Practices Related to Reproduction

Birth Control
Baha'is believe that the fundamental purpose of marriage is the procreation of children. Individuals are encouraged to exercise their discretion in choosing a method of family planning. Baha'u'llah taught that to beget children is the highest physical fruit of man's existence. The Baha'i teachings imply that birth control constitutes a real danger to the foundations of social life. It is against the spirit of Baha'i law, which defines the primary purpose of marriage to be the rearing of children and their spiritual training. It is left to each husband and wife to decide how many children they will have. Baha'i teachings state that the soul appears at conception. Therefore, it is improper to use a method that produces an abortion after conception has taken place (e.g., intrauterine device). Methods that result in permanent sterility are not permissible under normal circumstances. If situations arise that justify sterilization (e.g., removal of cancerous reproductive organs), those called upon to make the decision would rely on the best medical advice available and their own consciences.

Amniocentesis
Amniocentesis is permitted if advised by health care providers.

Abortion
Members are discouraged from using methods of contraception that produce abortion after conception has taken place (e.g., intrauterine

device). A surgical operation for the purpose of preventing the birth of an unwanted child is strictly forbidden.

Baha'i teachings state that the human soul comes into being at conception. Abortion and surgical operations for the purpose of preventing the birth of unwanted children are forbidden unless circumstances justify such actions on medical grounds. In this case, the decision is left to the consciences of those concerned, who must carefully weigh the medical advice they receive in the light of the general guidance given in the Baha'i writings.

Artificial Insemination

Although there are no specific Baha'i writings on artificial insemination, Baha'is are guided by the understanding that marriage is the proper spiritual and physical context in which the bearing of children must occur. Couples who are unable to bear children are not excluded from marriage, because marriage has other purposes besides the bearing of children. The adoption of children is encouraged.

Eugenics and Genetics

The Baha'is view scientific advancement as a noble and praiseworthy endeavor of humankind. Baha'i writings do not specifically address these two branches of science.

Religious Support System for the Sick

Individual members of local and surrounding communities assist and support one another in time of need. Religious titles are not used. Individual members of local communities look after the needs of the sick.

Practices Related to Death and Dying

Because human life is the vehicle for the development of the soul, Baha'is believe that life is unique and precious. The destruction of a human life at any stage, from conception to natural death, is rarely permissible. The question of when natural death has occurred is considered in the light of current medical science and legal rulings on the matter.

Autopsy is acceptable in the case of medical necessity or legal requirement. Baha'is are permitted to donate their bodies for medical research and for restorative purposes. Local burial laws are followed. Unless required by state law, Baha'i law states that the body is not to be embalmed. Cremation is forbidden. The place of burial must be within 1 hour's travel from the place of death. This regulation is always carried out in consultation with the family, and exceptions are possible.

Buddhist Churches of America

Buddhism is a general term that indicates a belief in Buddha and encompasses many individual churches. There are approximately 900,000 Buddhists in North America, and the worldwide membership is greater than 600 million.

The Buddhist Churches of America is the largest Buddhist organization in mainland United States. This group belongs to the largest subsect of Jodo Shinshu Buddhism (Shin Buddhism), Honpa Hongwanji, which is the largest traditional sect of Buddhism in Japan. The Jodo Shinshu sect was started in Japan and its headquarters are in Kyoto, Japan. The group of churches in Hawaii is a different organization of Shin Buddhism, called Honpa Hongwanji Mission of Hawaii. There are numerous Buddhist sects in the United States and Canada, including Indian, Sri Lankan, Vietnamese, Thai, Chinese, Japanese, Tibetan, and so on.

Buddhism was founded in the 6th century B.C. in northern India by Gautama Buddha. In the 3rd century B.C., Buddhism became the state religion of India and spread from there to most of the other Eastern nations. The term **Buddha** means "enlightened one."

At the beginning of the Christian era, Buddhism split into two main groups: Hinayana, or southern Buddhism, and Mahayana, or northern Buddhism. Hinayana retained more of the original teachings of Buddha and survived in Sri Lanka (formerly Ceylon) and southern Asia. Mahayana, a more social and polytheistic Buddhism, is strong in the Himalayas, Tibet, Mongolia, China, Korea, and Japan.

General Beliefs and Religious Practices

Buddha's original teachings included **Four Noble Truths** and the **Noble Eightfold Way**, the philosophies of which affect Buddhist responses to health and illness. The Four Noble Truths expound on suffering and constitute the foundation of Buddhism. The truths consist of (1) the truth of suffering, (2) the truth of the origin of suffering, (3) the truth that suffering can be destroyed, and (4) the way that leads to the cessation of pain.

The Noble Eightfold Way gives the rule of practical Buddhism, which consists of (1) right views, (2) right intention, (3) right speech, (4) right action, (5) right livelihood, (6) right effort, (7) right mindfulness, and (8) right concentration. **Nirvana**, a state of greater inner freedom and spontaneity, is the goal of all existence. When one achieves Nirvana, the mind has supreme tranquility, purity, and stability.

Although the ultimate goals of Buddhism are clear, the means of obtaining those goals are not religiously prescribed. Buddhism is not a dogmatic religion, nor does it dictate any specific practices. Individual differences are expected, acknowledged, and respected. Each individual is responsible for finding his or her own answers through awareness of the total situation.

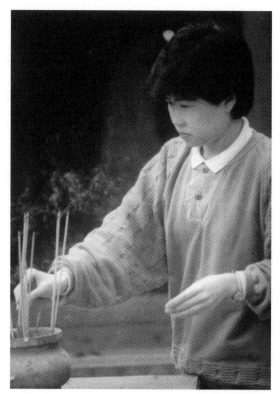

FIGURE 13-4 A Buddhist woman lights incense in remembrance of deceased ancestors during the Chinese New Year celebration (© Copyright M. Andrews).

Holy Days

"The major Buddhist holy day is Saga Dawa (or Vesak) which is the observance of Sakyamuni Buddha's birth, enlightenment and parinirvana. This holiday falls during the months of May or June. It is based on a Lunar calendar, and therefore the actual date varies from year to year." (Figure 13-4). Although there is no religious restriction for therapy on those days, they can be highly emotional, and a Buddhist patient should be consulted about his or her desires for medical or surgical intervention. Some Buddhists may fast for all or part of this day.

Sacraments

Buddhism does not have any sacraments. A ritual that symbolizes one's entry into the Buddhist faith is the expression of faith in the Three Treasures (Buddha, Dharma, and Sangha).

Diet

Moderation in diet is encouraged. Specific dietary practices are usually interconnected with ethnic practices. Some branches of Buddhism have strict dietary regulations, for example, vegetarianism, while others do not. It is important to inquire the patient's preferences.

Health Care Practices

Buddhists do not believe in healing through a faith or through faith itself. However, Buddhists do believe that spiritual peace, and liberation from anxiety by adherence to and achievement of awakening to Buddha's wisdom, can be important factors in promoting healing and recovery.

Medical and Surgical Interventions

There are no restrictions in Buddhism for nutritional therapies, medications, vaccines, and other therapeutic interventions, but some individuals may refrain from alcohol, stimulants, and other drugs that adversely affect mental clarity. Buddha's teaching on the Middle Path may apply here; he taught that extremes should be avoided. What may be medicine to one may be poison to another, so generalizations are to be avoided. Medications should be used in accordance with the nature of the illness and the capacity of the individual. Whatever will contribute to the attainment of Enlightenment is encouraged. Treatments such as amputations, organ transplants, biopsies, and other procedures that may prolong life and allow the individual to attain Enlightenment are encouraged.

Practices Related to Reproduction

The immediate emphasis is on the person living now and the attainment of Enlightenment. If practicing birth control or having an amniocentesis or sterility test will help the individual attain Enlightenment, it is acceptable.

Buddhism does not condone the taking of a life. The first of Buddha's Five Precepts is abstention from taking lives. Life in all forms is to be respected. Existence by itself often contradicts this principle (e.g., drugs that kill bacteria are given to spare a patient's life). With this in mind, it is the conditions and circumstances surrounding the patient that determine whether abortion, therapeutic or on demand, may be undertaken.

Religious Support System for the Sick

Support of the sick is an individual practice in keeping with the philosophy of Buddhism, but Buddhist priests often render assistance to those who become ill.

Practices Related to Death and Dying

If there is hope for recovery and continuation of the pursuit of Enlightenment, all available means of support are encouraged. If life cannot be prolonged so that the person can continue to search for Enlightenment, conditions might permit euthanasia. If the donation of a body part will help another continue the quest for Enlightenment, it might be an act of mercy and is encouraged. The body is considered but a shell; therefore, autopsy and disposal of the body are matters of individual practice rather than of religious prescription. Burials are usually a brief graveside service after a funeral at the temple. Cremations are common.

Religious Objects

Prayer beads and images of Sakyamuni Buddha and other Buddhist deities may be utilized for specific prayer or meditation practices.

Addendum

The headquarters of the Buddhist Churches of America is at 1710 Octavia Street, San Francisco, California 94109 (Telephone: [415] 776-5600). Additional material is available at the Buddhist Bookstore of the Buddhist Churches of America Headquarters. Information on Buddhism and temple locations in Canada can be found at http://buddhismcanada.com/

Catholicism (According to the Roman Rite)

With a North American membership of approximately 97 million and a worldwide membership of more than 1 billion, some 32 rites exist within **Catholicism**. Of these, the Roman Rite is the major body.

General Beliefs and Religious Practices

The Roman Catholic Church traces its beginnings to about A.D. 30, when Jesus Christ is believed to have founded the church. Catholic teachings, based on the Bible, are found in declarations of church councils and Popes and in short statements of faith called creeds. The oldest and most authoritative of these creeds are the Apostle's Creed and the Nicene

Creed, the latter being recited during the central act of worship, called the Eucharistic Liturgy, or Mass. The creeds summarize Catholic beliefs concerning the Trinity and creation, sin and salvation, the nature of the church, and life after death.

Holy Days

Catholics are expected to observe all Sundays (including Easter Sunday) as holy days. Sunday or holy day worship services may be conducted any time from 4:00 pm on Saturday until Sunday evening. Other days set aside for special liturgical observance are: Christmas (December 25th), Solemnity of Mary, Mother of God (January 1st), Ascension Thursday (the Lord's ascension bodily into Heaven, observed 40 days after Easter), Feast of the Assumption (August 15th), All Saints Day (November 1st), and the Feast of the Immaculate Conception (December 8th).

Sacraments

The Roman Catholic Church recognizes seven sacraments: Baptism, Reconciliation (formerly Penance or Confession), Holy Communion or the **Eucharist** (Figure 13-5), Confirmation, Matrimony, Holy Orders, and Anointing of the Sick (formerly Extreme Unction).

Religious Objects

Rosaries, prayer books, and holy cards are often present and are of great comfort to the patient and their family. They should be left in place and within the reach of the patient whenever possible (Accessed on March 1, 2010 at http://www.catholichealthcare.us/).

Diet (Foods and Beverages)

The goods of the world have been given for use and benefit. The primary obligation people have toward foods and beverages is to use them in moderation and in such a way that they are not injurious to health. Fasting in moderation is recommended as a valued discipline. There are a few days of the year when Catholics have an obligation to fast, which means to abstain from meat and meat products. Catholics fast and abstain on Ash Wednesday

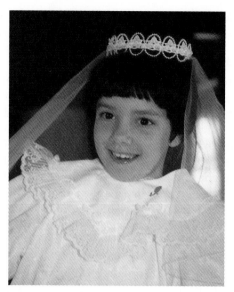

FIGURE 13-5   In the Roman Catholic tradition, when children reach the age of reason (about 7 years), they continue the ongoing initiation into their religion by making their First Communion. In addition to the religious ritual, there are sometimes cultural traditions surrounding this event, many of which involve a family celebration after the religious services have concluded (© Copyright M. Andrews).

and Good Friday, and abstinence is required on all of the Fridays of Lent. The sick are never bound by this prescription of the law. Healthy persons between the ages of 18 and 62 are encouraged to engage in fasting and abstinence as described.

Social Activities (Dating, Dancing)

The major principle is that Sunday is a day of rest; therefore, unnecessary servile work is prohibited. The seven holy days are also considered days of rest, although many persons must engage in routine work-related activities on some of these days.

Substance Use

Alcohol and tobacco are not evil per se. They are to be used in moderation and not in a way that would be injurious to one's health or that of another party. The misuse of any substance is not only harmful to the body but also sinful.

Health Care Practices

In time of illness, the basic rite is the **Sacrament of the Sick**, which includes anointing of the sick, communion if possible, and a blessing by a priest. Prayers are frequently offered for the sick person and for members of the family. The Eucharistic wafer (a small unleavened wafer made of flour and water) is often given to the sick as the food of healing and health. Other family members may participate if they wish to do so.

Medical and Surgical Interventions

As long as the benefits outweigh the risk to the individuals, judicious use of medications is permissible and morally acceptable. A major concern is the risk of mutilation. The Church has traditionally cited the **principle of totality**, which states that medications are allowed as long as they are used for the good of the whole person. Blood, blood products, and amputations are acceptable if consistent with the principle of totality. Biopsies and circumcision are also permissible.

The transplantation of organs from living donors is morally permissible when the anticipated benefit to the recipient is proportionate to the harm done to the donor, provided that the loss of such an organ does not deprive the donor of life itself or of the functional integrity of his or her body.

Practices Related to Reproduction

Birth Control
The basic principle is that the conjugal act should be one that is love-giving and potentially life-giving. Only natural means of contraception, such as abstinence, the temperature method, and the ovulation method are acceptable. Ordinarily, artificial aids and procedures for permanent sterilization are forbidden. Birth control (anovulants) may be used therapeutically to assist in regulating the menstrual cycle.

Amniocentesis
The procedure in and of itself is not objectionable. However, it is morally objectionable if the findings of the amniocentesis are used to lead the couple to decide on termination of the pregnancy or if the procedure injures the fetus.

Abortion
Direct abortion is always morally wrong. Indirect abortion may be morally justified by some circumstances (e.g., treatment of a cancerous uterus in a pregnant woman). Abortion on demand is prohibited. The Roman Catholic Church teaches the sanctity of all human life, even of the unborn, from the time of conception.

Sterility Tests and Artificial Insemination
The use of sterility tests for the purpose of promoting conception, not misusing sexuality, is permitted. Although artificial insemination has been debated heavily, traditionally it has been looked on as illicit, even between husband and wife.

Eugenics, Genetics, and Stem Cell Research
Research in the fields of eugenics and genetics is objectionable. This violates the moral right of the individual to be free from experimentation and also interferes with God's right as the master of life and human beings' stewardship of their lives. Some genetic investigations to help determine genetic diseases may be used, depending on their ends and means. There is support for research using adult stem cells, but opposition for the use of embryonic stem cells.

Religious Support System for the Sick

Visitors
Although a priest, deacon, or lay minister usually visits a sick person alone, the family or other significant people may be invited to join in prayer. In fact, that is most desirable, since they too need support.

The priest, deacon, or lay minister will usually bring the necessary supplies for administration of the Eucharist or administration of the Sacrament of the Sick (in the case of a priest). The nursing staff can facilitate these rites by ensuring an atmosphere of prayer and quiet and by having a glass of water on hand (in case the patient is unable to swallow the small wafer-like host). Consecrated wine can be made available but is usually not given in the hospital or home. The nurse may wish to join in the prayer. Candles may be used if the patient is not receiving oxygen. The priest, deacon, or lay minister will usually appreciate any information pertaining to the patient's ability to swallow. Any other information the nurse believes may help the priest or deacon respond to the patient with more care and effectiveness would be appreciated, but HIPPA laws must be remembered and information that violates privacy not divulged.

Catholic lay persons of either gender may visit hospitalized or homebound elderly or sick persons. Although they may not administer the Sacrament of the Sick or the Sacrament of Reconciliation, they may bring Holy Communion (the Eucharist).

Title of Religious Representative
The titles of religious representatives include Father (priest), Mr. or Deacon (deacon), Sister (Catholic woman who has taken religious vows), and Brother (Catholic man who has taken religious vows).

Environment During Visit by Religious Representative
Privacy is most conducive to prayer and the administration of the sacraments. In emergencies, such as cardiac or respiratory arrest, medical personnel will need to be present. The priest will use an abbreviated form of the rite and will not interfere with the activities of the health care team.

Church Organizations to Assist the Sick
Most major cities have outreach programs for the sick, handicapped, and elderly. More serious needs are usually handled by Catholic Charities and other agencies in the community or at the local parish level. Organizations such as the St. Vincent DePaul Society may provide material support for the poor and needy as well as some counseling services, depending on the location. In the United States, the Catholic Church owns and operates hospitals, extended care facilities, orphanages, maternity homes, hospices, and other health care facilities. Although the majority of tertiary care facilities in Canada are publicly owned, many such institutions are strongly influenced

by the leadership of the Catholic Church and its members. It is usually best to consult the pastor or chaplain in specific cases for local resources.

Practices Related to Death and Dying
Prolongation of Life (Right to Die)
Members are obligated to take ordinary means of preserving life (e.g., intravenous medication) but are not obligated to take extraordinary means. What constitutes extraordinary means may vary with biomedical and technologic advances and with the availability of these advances to the average citizen. Other factors that must be considered include the degree of pain associated with the procedure, the potential outcome, the condition of the patient, economic factors, and the patient's or family's preferences.

Euthanasia
Direct action to end the life of patients is not permitted. Extraordinary means may be withheld, allowing the patient to die of natural causes.

Autopsy and Donation of Body
This is permissible as long as the corpse is shown proper respect and there is sufficient reason for doing the autopsy. The principle of totality suggests that this is justifiable, being for the betterment of the person who does the giving.

Disposal of Body and Burial
Ordinarily, bodies are buried. Cremation is acceptable in certain circumstances, such as to avoid spreading a contagious disease. Because life is considered sacred, the body should be treated with respect. Any disposal of the body should be done in a respectful and honorable way.

Christian Science (Church of Christ, Scientist)

Christian Science accepts physical and moral healing as a natural part of the Christian experience. Members believe that God acts through universal, immutable, spiritual law. They hold that genuine spiritual or Christian healing through prayer differs radically from the use of suggestion, willpower, and all forms of psychotherapy, which are based on the use of the human mind as a curative agent. In emphasizing the practical importance of a fuller understanding of Jesus' works and teachings, Christian Science believes healing to be a natural result of drawing closer to God in one's thinking and living. The church does not keep membership data; there are 3,000 congregations worldwide.

General Beliefs and Religious Practices

Holy Days

Besides the usual weekly day of worship (Sunday), other traditional Christian holidays are observed on an individual basis. Worldwide, Wednesday evenings are observed as times for members to gather for testimony meetings.

Sacraments

Although sacraments in a strictly spiritual sense have deep meaning for Christian Scientists, there are no outward observances or ceremonies. Baptism and holy communion are not outward observances but deeply meaningful inner experiences. Baptism is the daily purification and spiritualization of thought, and communion is finding one's conscious unity with God through prayer.

Social Activities (Dating, Dancing) and Substance Use

Members are encouraged to be honest, truthful, and moral in their behavior. Although every effort is made to preserve marriages, divorce is recognized. The Christian Science Sunday School teaches young people how to make their religion practical in daily life as related to school studies, social life, sports, and family relationships. Members abstain from alcohol and tobacco; some abstain from tea and coffee.

Health Care Practices

Viewed as a by-product of drawing closer to God, healing is considered proof of God's care and one element in the full salvation at which Christianity aims. Christian Science teaches that faith must rest not on blind belief but on an understanding of the present perfection of God's spiritual creation. This is one of the crucial differences between Christian Science and **faith healing**. The practice of Christian Science healing starts from the Biblical basis that God created the universe and human beings "and made them perfect." Christian Science holds that human imperfection, including physical illness and sin, reflects a fundamental misunderstanding of creation and is therefore subject to healing through prayer and spiritual regeneration.

An individual who is seeking healing may turn to Christian Science practitioners, members of the denomination who devote their full time to the healing ministry in the broadest sense. In cases requiring continued care, nurses grounded in the Christian Science faith provide care in facilities accredited by the mother church, the First Church of Christ, Scientist, in Boston, Massachusetts. Individuals may also receive such care in their own homes. Christian Science nurses are trained to perform the practical duties a patient may need while also providing an atmosphere of warmth and love that supports the healing process. No medication is given, and physical application is limited to the normal measures associated with hygiene. The *Christian Science Journal*, a monthly publication, contains a directory of qualified Christian Science practitioners and nurses throughout the world.

Before they can be recognized and advertised in *The Christian Science Journal*, practitioners must have instruction from an authorized teacher of Christian Science and provide substantial evidence of their experience in healing. There are approximately 4,000 Christian Science practitioners throughout the world. Practitioners who speak other languages may also be listed in appropriate editions of *The Herald of Christian Science*, which is published in 12 languages.

The denomination has no clergy. Practitioners are thus lay members of the Church of Christ, Scientist, and do not conduct public worship services or rituals. Their ministry is not an office within the church structure but is carried out on an individual basis with those who seek their help through prayer. Both members and nonmembers are welcome to contact practitioners by telephone, by letter, or in person for help or for information.

Christian Science practitioners are supported not by the church but by payments from their patients. Their ministry is not restricted to local congregations but extends worldwide. Many insurance companies include coverage of payments to practitioners and Christian Science nursing facilities in their policies. In spite of such superficial resemblances to the health care professions, the work of Christian Science practitioners involves a deeply religious vocation, not simply alternative health care. Practitioners do not use medical or psychologic techniques.

The term *healing* applies to the entire spectrum of human fears, grief, wants, and sin as well as to physical ills. Practitioners are called upon to give Christian Science treatment not only in cases of physical disease and emotional disturbance but also in family and financial difficulties, business problems, questions of employment, schooling problems, theological confusion, and so forth. The purpose of prayer, or Christian Science treatment, is to deal with these interrelated and complex problems of establishing God's law of harmony in every aspect of life. When healings are accomplished through perception and living of spiritual truth, they are effective and permanent. Physical healing is often the manifestation of a moral and spiritual change (Christian Science Publishing Society, 1978, 1994).

Ordinarily, a Christian Science practitioner and a physician are not employed in the same case, because the two approaches to healing differ so radically. During childbirth, however, an obstetrician or qualified midwife is involved. Since bone setting may be accomplished without medication, a physician is also employed for repair of fractures if the patient requests this medical intervention. In cases of contagious or infectious disease, Christian Scientists observe the legal requirements for reporting and quarantining affected individuals. The denomination recognizes public health concerns and has a long history of responsible cooperation with public health officials.

Christian Scientists are not arbitrarily opposed to doctors. They are always free to make their own decisions regarding treatment in any given situation. They generally choose to rely on spiritual healing because they have seen its effectiveness in the experience of their own families and fellow church members—experience that goes back over 100 years and in many families for three or four generations. Where medical treatment for minor children is required by law, Christian Scientists strictly adhere to the requirement. At the same time, they maintain that their substantial healing record needs to be seriously considered in determining the rights of Christian Scientists to rely on spiritual healing for themselves and their children. They do not ignore or neglect disease, but they seek to heal it by the means they believe to be most efficacious.

Medical and Surgical Procedures

Christian Scientists ordinarily do not use medications. Immunizations and vaccines are acceptable only when required by law. Ordinarily, members do not use blood or blood components. A Christian Scientist who has lost a limb might seek to have it replaced with a prosthesis. Christian Scientists are unlikely to seek transplants and are unlikely to act as donors. Christian Scientists do not normally seek biopsies or any sort of physical examination. Circumcision is considered an individual matter.

Practices Related to Reproduction

Matters of family planning (i.e., birth control) are left to individual judgment. Because abortion involves medication and surgical intervention, it is normally considered incompatible with Christian Science. Artificial insemination is unusual among Christian Scientists. Christian Scientists are opposed to programs in the field of eugenics and genetics.

Religious Support System for the Sick

As discussed previously, Christian Scientists have their own nurses and practitioners. No special religious titles are used. Although each branch church elects two Readers for Sunday and Wednesday services, Christian Scientists are a church of laymen and laywomen. Organizations to assist the sick include Benevolent Homes staffed by Christian Science nurses, and visiting home nurse services.

Practices Related to Death and Dying

A Christian Science family is unlikely to seek medical means to prolong life indefinitely. Family members pray earnestly for the recovery of a person as long as the person remains alive.

Euthanasia is contrary to the teachings of Christian Science. Most Christian Scientists believe that they can make their particular contribution to the health of society and of their loved ones in ways other than donation of the body. Disposal of the body is left to the individual family to decide. The individual family decides the form of burial and burial service.

Addendum

A wide variety of books and journals are published by the Christian Science Publishing Society, Boston, Massachusetts. Most major cities have Christian Science Reading Rooms, which carry these publications and are staffed by church members, who are available to provide additional information (accessed on March 1, 2010 at http://www.tfccs.com/aboutchristianscience/).

The Church of Jesus Christ of Latter-Day Saints (Mormonism)

The **Church of Jesus Christ of Latter-Day Saints**, commonly known as **Mormonism**, is a Christian religion established in the United States in the early 1800s. North American membership is approximately 6 million, and the worldwide membership was approximately 13.5 million.

General Beliefs and Religious Practices

Holy Days/Special Days

Sunday is the day observed as the Sabbath in the United States. In other parts of the world the Sabbath may be observed on a different day; in Israel, for example, members observe the Sabbath on Saturday.

Sacraments

Sacraments are commonly called **ordinances**.

Ordinances of Salvation
1. Baptism at the age of accountability (8 years or after); never performed in infancy or at death; always by immersion.
2. Confirmation at the time of baptism to receive the gift of the Holy Ghost.
3. Partaking of the sacrament of the Lord's Supper at weekly Sunday sacrament meetings.
4. Endowments*
5. Celestial Marriage*
6. Vicarious ordinances*

Ordinances of Comfort, Consolation, and Encouragement
1. Blessing of babies
2. Blessing of the sick
3. Consecration of oil for use in blessing of the sick
4. Patriarchal blessings
5. Dedication of graves

After being deemed worthy to go to a temple, a member of the Church of Jesus Christ of Latter Day Saints will wear a special type of underclothing, called a **garment**. In a health care setting, the garment may be removed to facilitate care. As soon as the individual is well, he or she is likely to want to wear the garment again. An elderly person may not wish to part with the garment in the hospital. The garment has special significance to the person, symbolizing covenants or promises the person has made to God.

Diet

Members of this church have a strict dietary code called the **Word of Wisdom**. This code prohibits

*These ordinances occur in temples. Temples are sacred places of worship that are accessible only to observant Mormons, who are "worthy" to enter them as deemed by their local religious leaders.

all alcoholic beverages (including beer and wine), hot drinks (i.e., tea and coffee, although not herbal tea), tobacco in any form, and any illegal or recreational drugs.

Fasting to a member means no food or drink (including water), usually for 24 hours. Fasting is required once a month on the designated fast Sunday. Pregnant women, the very young, the very old, and the ill are not required to fast. The purpose of fasting is to bring oneself closer to God by controlling physical needs. The person is expected to donate the price of what has not been eaten to the church to be used to care for the poor.

Social Activities (Dating, Dancing)

The Church of Jesus Christ of Latter Day Saints has a wide variety of activities for its youth and encourages group activities until young people are at least 16. Young men are highly encouraged to perform missions for the church for 2 years at their own expense, beginning at the age of 19 years. Women may go on missions when they are 21, but marriage is more strongly emphasized for them.

Substance Use

Alcohol, caffeinated beverages (such as tea, coffee, and soda), and tobacco are forbidden. In recent years, "recreational drugs" and nonmedically indicated sedatives and narcotics have also been considered forbidden substances.

Health Care Practices

The members of the Church of Jesus Christ of Latter Day Saints believe that the power of God can be exercised on their behalf to bring about healing at the time of illness. The ritual of blessing the sick consists of one member (Elder) of the priesthood (male) anointing the ill person with oil and a second Elder "sealing the anointing with a prayer and a blessing." Commonly, both Elders place their hands on the individual's head. Faith in Jesus Christ and in the power of the priesthood to heal, requisite to the healing use of priesthood, does not preclude medical intervention but is seen as an adjunct to it. Mormons believe that medical intervention is one of God's ways of using humans in the healing process.

Medical and Surgical Procedures

There is no restriction on the use of medications or vaccines. It is not uncommon to find many members using herbal folk remedies, and it is wise to explore in detail what an individual may already have done or taken. There is no restriction on the use of blood or blood components.

Surgical intervention is a matter of individual decision in cases of amputations, transplants, and organ donations (of both donor and recipient). Biopsies and resultant surgical procedures are also a matter of individual choice. The circumcision of infants is viewed as a medical health-promotion measure and is not a religious ritual.

Practices Related to Reproduction

Birth Control
According to church doctrine, one of the major purposes of life is procreation; therefore, any form of prevention of the birth of children is contrary to church teachings. Exceptions to this policy include ill health of the mother or father and genetic defects that could be passed on to offspring.

Amniocentesis
Amniocentesis is a matter of individual choice. However, even if the fetus is found to be deformed, abortion is not an option unless the mother's life is in danger.

Abortion
Abortion is forbidden in all cases except when the mother's life is in danger. Even in these circumstances, abortion is looked upon favorably only if the local priesthood authorities, after fasting and prayer, receive divine confirmation that the abortion is acceptable.

In the event of pregnancy resulting from rape, the church states that the child should be born and put up for adoption if necessary, rather than be aborted. The final decision rests with the mother. No official church sanction is used if she chooses to abort the child. Abortion on demand is strictly forbidden.

Sterility/Fertility Testing and Artificial Insemination

Because bearing children is so important, all measures that can be taken to promote having children are acceptable. Artificial insemination is acceptable if the semen is from the husband.

Religious Objects

Copies of scriptures are often found at the bedside of members of this church. Reading these scriptures often brings comfort during times of illness. Scriptures sacred to members of the Church of Jesus Christ of Latter Day Saints include: the Bible (Old and New Testament), the Book of Mormon, Doctrine and Covenants, and Pearl of Great Price.

Religious Support System for the Sick

Visitors

The Church of Jesus Christ of Latter Day Saints has a highly organized network, and many church representatives are likely to visit a hospitalized member, including the bishop and two counselors (leaders of the local congregation), home teachers (two men assigned to visit the family each month), and visiting teachers (two women assigned to visit the female head of household each month). Friends within the local congregation can also be expected to visit.

Title of Religious Representative

Various titles are used for members of this church's hierarchy. The term *Elder* is generally acceptable regardless of a man's position, and the term Sister is acceptable for women.

Environment Needed for Health-Related Rituals

To perform a blessing of the sick, the Elders performing the blessing need privacy and, if possible, quiet. They generally bring a vial of consecrated oil with which to anoint the person. If they plan to perform a Sacrament of the Lord's Supper, they usually bring what they need with them. Bread and water are used for this ordinance.

Church Organizations to Assist the Sick

The Relief Society is the organization for helping members. It is organized by the women of the church, who work closely with priesthood leaders to determine the general needs of members, including use of the church-run welfare organization. Church members who are in need may receive local help, such as child care when parents are ill or hospitalized and money for medical expenses.

Practices Related to Death and Dying

Whenever possible, medical science and faith healing are used to reverse conditions that threaten life. When death is inevitable, the effort is to promote a peaceful and dignified death. Members of this church firmly believe that life continues beyond death and that the dead are reunited with loved ones; therefore, the belief is that death is another step in eternal progression.

Euthanasia is not acceptable because members hold the belief that life and death are in the hands of God, and humans must not interfere in any way. Autopsy is permitted with the consent of the next of kin and within local laws. Organ donation is permitted; it is an individual decision. Cremation is discouraged but not forbidden; burial is customary. A local priesthood member dedicates the graves.

Hinduism

The **Hindu** religion may be the oldest religion in the world. There are over 1.4 billion Hindus worldwide, with a North American following of approximately 1.3 million members.

General Beliefs and Religious Practices

Although no common creed or doctrine binds Hindus together, many refrain from eating beef (ElGindy, 2008. Hindu dietary practices: Feeding the body, mind, and spirit. *Minority Nurse.com*. Retrieved December 15, 2008).

http://www.minoritynurse.com/dietic/hindu-dietary-practices-feedding-body-mind-and-soul.

Hindus may be monotheistic, polytheistic, or atheistic; however the basis of Hindu belief is the unity of everything. The major distinguishing characteristic is the social caste system.

The religion of Hinduism is founded on sacred, written scripture called the **Vedas**.

Brahman is the principle and source of the universe and the center from which all things proceed and to which all things return. **Reincarnation** is a central belief in Hinduism. The law of **karma** determines life. According to karma, rebirth is dependent on moral behavior in a previous stage of existence. Life on earth is transient and a burden. The goal of existence is liberation from the cycle of rebirth and redeath and entrance into what in Buddhism is called nirvana (a state of extinction of passion).

The practice of Hinduism consists of roles and ceremonies performed within the framework of the **caste system**. These rituals focus on the main ethnoreligious events of birth, marriage, and death. Hindu temples are dwelling places for deities to which people bring offerings. There are numerous places for religious pilgrimage.

Holy Days (Based on a Lunar Calendar)

1. Purnima (day of full moon)
2. Janamasthtmi (birthday of Lord Krishna)
3. Ramnavmi (birthday of Rama)
4. Shivratri (birth of Lord **Shiva**)
5. Naurate (nine holy days occurring twice a year; in about April and October)
6. Dussehra
7. Diwali
8. Holi

Diet, Social Activities (Dating, Dancing), and Substance Use

The eating of meat is forbidden because it involves harming a living creature. Social activities are strictly limited by the caste system. Substance use is not restricted.

Health Care Practices

Some Hindus believe in faith healing; others believe illness is God's way of punishing people for their sins.

Medical and Surgical Procedures

The use of medications, blood, and blood components is acceptable. Persons who lose a limb are not outcasts from society. Loss of a limb is considered to be caused by "sins of a previous life." Organ transplantations are acceptable for both donors and recipients.

Practices Related to Reproduction

All types of birth control are acceptable. Amniocentesis is acceptable, although not often available. No Hindu policy exists on abortion, either therapeutic or on demand. Artificial insemination is not restricted, but it is not often practiced because of lack of availability.

Noting the exact time of a baby's birth is very important, because it is used to determine the baby's horoscope. Males are not circumcised. Breast feeding is expected. The infant is traditionally given a name on the 10th day following the birth, although in American hospitals the child is sometimes named at birth.

Religious Objects

A small picture of a deity may be found at the bedside. Prayer is often accompanied by the use of a "mala" (prayer beads) and a mantram (a sound representing an aspect of the divine). Facing North or East during prayer is preferable, but not required.

Religious Support System for the Sick

Religious representatives use the title of priest. Church organizations to assist the sick do not exist; family and friends within the caste provide help.

Practices Related to Death and Dying

No religious customs or restrictions related to the prolongation of life exist. Life is seen as a perpetual cycle, and death is considered as just one more step toward nirvana. Euthanasia is not practiced. Autopsy is acceptable. The donation of body or parts is also acceptable.

Cremation is the most common form of body disposal. Ashes are collected and disposed of in holy rivers. The fetus or newborn is sometimes buried.

Islam

Islam is a monotheistic religion founded between 610 and 632 A.D. by the prophet Muhammad. Derived from an Arabic word meaning "submission," Islam literally translated means "submission to the will of God." A follower of Islam is called **Moslem** or **Muslim**, which means "one who submits." The current North American membership is approximately 6–7 million, and the worldwide membership ranges between 2 and 3 billion (Nimer, 2002).

Muhammad, revered as the prophet of **Allah** (God), is seen as succeeding and completing both Judaism and Christianity. Good deeds will be rewarded at the last Judgment, whereas evil deeds will be punished in hell.

General Beliefs and Religious Practices

Pillars of Faith

Islam has five essential practices, or **Pillars of Faith**. These are (1) the profession of faith (*Shahada*), which requires bearing witness to one true God and acknowledging Muhammad as his messenger; (2) ritual prayer five times daily at dawn, noon, afternoon, sunset, and night, facing Mecca, Saudi Arabia, Islam's holiest city (*salat*); (3) almsgiving (*zakat*) to the needy, reflecting the Koran's admonition to share what one has with those less fortunate, including widows, orphans, homeless persons, and the poor; (4) fasting from dawn until sunset throughout Ramadan during the ninth month of the Islamic lunar calendar; and (5) making a pilgrimage to Mecca at least once during one's lifetime (*Hajj*).

Sources of Faith

The sources of the Islamic faith are the **Qur'an (Koran)**, which is regarded as the uncreated and eternal Word of God, and **Hadith** (tradition), regarded as sayings and deeds of the prophet Muhammad. All Muslims recognize the existence of the sharia and the five categories into which it divides human conduct: required, encouraged, permissible, discouraged, and prohibited.

Sects of Islam

Various sects of Islam have developed. When Muhammad died, a dispute arose over the leadership of the Muslim community. One faction, the *Sunni*, derived from the Arabic word for "tradition," felt that the caliph, or successor of Muhammad, should be chosen as Arab chiefs customarily are: by election. Therefore, they supported the succession of the first four (the "rightly guided") caliphs who had been Muhammad's companions. The other group maintained that Muhammad chose his cousin and son-in-law, Ali, as his spiritual and secular heir and that succession should be through his bloodline. In 680 A.D., one of Ali's sons, Hussein, led a band of rebels against the ruling caliph. In the course of the battle Hussein was killed, and with his death began the *Shi'a*, sometimes called the *Shi'ite* movement, whose name comes from the word meaning "partisans of Ali." The Shi'a and the Sunni are the two major branches of Muslims; the Sunni constitute about 85% of the total. The Sunni are found in Lebanon, the West Bank, Jordan, and throughout Africa, whereas the Shi'a are in Iran, Iraq, Yemen, Afghanistan, and Pakistan. The Shi'a and the Sunni also have different rituals, practices, and structural and political orientations.

Holidays, Special Observances, and Sacraments

Days of observance in Islam are not "holy" days but days of celebration or observance. The Muslims follow a lunar calendar, so the days of observance change yearly.

Each Muslim observance has its own significance. They are listed here in the same order in which they occur in the Muslim lunar calendar, and their standard Arabic names are used. However, the Arabic spellings for the names of the holidays may vary, or local names may be used.

Muharam 1 Rasal-Sana (or New Year): The first day of the first month, celebrated much the same as the first day of the year is celebrated throughout the world.

Muharam 10 Ashura (the 10th of the first month): A religious holiday through which pious Muslims may fast from dawn to sunset. For Shi'ite Muslims, this is a special day of sorrow commemorating the assassination of the prophet's grandson, Hussein.

Rabi'i 12 Maulid al-Nabi: The birthday of the prophet Muhammad. In some regions this holiday goes on for many days; it is a time of festivities and exchanging of gifts.

Rajab 27 Lailat al-Isra wa al Miraj (literally, "The Night of the Journey and Ascent"): Commemorates Muhammad's night journey from Mecca to the al-Aqsa mosque in Jerusalem and his ascent to heaven and return on the same night.

Sh'ban 14: This is the 14th night of the 8th month of Sh'ban. It is widely celebrated by pious Muslims and is sometimes called the Night of Repentance. It is treated in many parts of the Muslim world as a New Year's celebration.

Ramadan (the ninth month of the Muslim year): This entire month is devoted to meditation and spiritual purification through self-discipline. It is a period of abstinence from eating, drinking, smoking, and sexual relations. The fast is an obligation practiced by Muslims throughout the world unless they are old, infirm, traveling, or pregnant. The fast is from sunup to sundown, at which time a meal (*Iftar*) is taken (Bazy, 2006; Wehbe-Alamah, 2005).

Ramadan 27 Lailat al-Qadir (next to the last night of the fasting month): This is simply called the Night of Power and Greatness, and it is by custom a very special holy time. It commemorates the time when revelation was first given to Muhammad.

Shawwal 1 "Id ad-Fitr": This is called the Lesser Feast because it begins immediately after the month-long Ramadan feast. It is perhaps Islam's most joyous festival, marking as it does the month of abstinence and the cleansing of the believer. It usually lasts for 2 or 3 days. Families and friends visit one another's homes, new clothes and presents are exchanged, and sweet pastries are a favorite treat.

Dhu al-Hijjah 1–10: Muslims, if they are able, are obliged to undertake a pilgrimage to Mecca at least once in their lifetime. This journey, called the Hajj, is performed during the last month of the Muslim calendar, Dhu al-Hijjah.

Dhu al-Hijjah 10: All Muslims, whether they are on the pilgrimage or at home, participate in the feast of the sacrifice, Id al-Adha, which marks the end of the Hajj on the tenth of Dhu al-Hijjah. The feast is the Feast of the Sacrifice, called the Greater Feast, and is observed by the slaughtering of animals and the distribution of the meat. In some places this is done individually. The meat is shared equally among the family and the poor. Sometimes the slaughtering takes place in public areas, and the meat is then distributed.

Sacraments are not observed.

Diet and Substance Use

Eating pork and drinking alcoholic or other intoxicating beverages are strictly prohibited. In all cases, moderation in one's life is expected. Some Muslims consume meat that has been ritually slaughtered by the process called **halal**, which means "the lawful or that which is permitted by Allah."

Fasting during the month of Ramadan is one of the pillars of Islam. Children (boys 7 years old, girls 9 years old) and adults are required to fast. Pregnant women, nursing mothers, the elderly, and anyone whose physical condition is so fragile that a physician recommends not fasting, are exempt from fasting but are expected to fast later in the year or to feed a poor person to make up for the unfasted Ramadan days (Wehbe-Alamah, 2005).

Religious Objects

A prayer rug and the Koran are often present with a Muslim patient and should not be handled or touched by anyone who is ritually unclean. Nothing should be placed on top of these items. Some Muslims may wear an amulet, which is a black string or a silver or gold chain, on which sections of the Koran are attached. If worn by the patient it should not be removed and should remain dry.

Health Care Practices

Muslim women typically prefer to have female physicians and health care providers while men prefer male physicians and health care providers (Wehbe-Alamah, 2005, 2008). Faith healing is not acceptable unless the psychological health and morale of the patient are deteriorating. At that time, faith healing may be used to supplement the physician's efforts (Khan, 2008; Lyvers, Barling, & Harding-Cook, 2006).

Medical and Surgical Procedures

There are no restrictions on medications. Even items normally forbidden (e.g., pork derivatives) are permitted if prescribed as medicine. The use of blood and blood components is not restricted. Amputations are not restricted. Organ transplantations are acceptable for both donor and recipient. Biopsies are acceptable. No age limit is fixed, but circumcision is practiced on boys at an early age. For adult converts, it is not obligatory, although it is sometimes practiced.

Practices Related to Reproduction

Birth Control

All types of birth control are generally acceptable in accordance with the law of "what is harmful to the body is prohibited." The family physician's advice on method of contraception is required. The husband and wife should agree on the method.

Amniocentesis

Amniocentesis is available in many Islamic countries. "Progressive" doctors and expectant parents use amniocentesis only to determine the status of the fetus, not the sex of the child; this is left in the hands of God.

Abortion

No official policy on abortion, either therapeutic or on demand, exists. There is a strong religious objection to abortion, which is based on Muhammad's condemnation of the ancient Arabian practice of burying unwanted newborn girls alive.

Artificial Insemination, Eugenics, and Genetics

Artificial insemination is permitted only if from the husband to his own wife. No official policy exists on practices in the fields of eugenics and genetics. Different Islamic schools of thought accept differing opinions.

Religious Support System for the Sick

In Islam, care of the physical body is not regarded highly. In many wealthy, oil-rich Middle Eastern nations, expatriates are hired to staff hospitals and provide for health care. Even in the United States, care of the sick does not resemble the Catholic corporal work of mercy or the Jewish mitzvah. Islamic clerics, called imams, may provide guidance that could be helpful for emotional and psychological disorders. Formal, organized support systems to assist the sick do not exist; family and friends provide emotional and financial support.

Practices Related to Death and Dying

The right to die is not recognized in Islam. Any attempt to shorten one's life or terminate it (suicide or otherwise) is prohibited. Euthanasia is thus not acceptable. Autopsy is permitted only for medical and legal purposes. The donation of body parts or body is acceptable, without restrictions.

Burial of the dead, including fetuses, is compulsory. It is important in Islam to follow prescribed burial procedures. Under conditions that cause fragmentation of the body, sections of the burial ritual may be omitted. The burial procedure consists of five steps:

1. Ghasl El Mayyet: Rinsing and washing of the dead body according to Muslim tradition. Muslim women cleanse a woman's body; Muslim men, a man's body.
2. Muslin: After being washed three times, the body is wrapped in three pieces of clean white cloth. The Muslim word for "coffin" is the same as that for "muslin."
3. Salat El Mayyet: Special prayers for the dead are required.
4. The body should be processed and buried as soon as possible. The body should always be buried so that the head faces toward Mecca.

5. Burial of a fetus: Before a gestational age of 130 days, a fetus is treated like any other discarded tissue. After 130 days, the fetus is considered a fully developed human being and must be treated as such.

Thanks to Dr. Hiba Wehbe-Alamah, University of Michigan-Flint for her review of this section on Islam.

Jehovah's Witnesses

North American membership of the **Jehovah's Witnesses** is 1,029,902; worldwide membership is approximately 6,035,564.

General Beliefs and Religious Practices

Many North Americans have at one time or another encountered ministers of the **Watch Tower Bible and Tract Society**, known as Jehovah's Witnesses. The name Jehovah's Witnesses (the name that members prefer) is derived from the Hebrew name for God (**Jehovah**) according to the King James Bible. Thus, Jehovah's Witnesses is a descriptive name, indicating that members profess to bear witness concerning Jehovah, his Godship, and his purposes. Every Bible student devotes approximately 10 hours or more each month to proselytizing activities.

Holy Days and Sacraments

Although Witnesses do not celebrate Christmas, Easter, or other traditional Christian holy days, a special observance of the Lord's Supper is held. Witnesses and others may attend this important meeting, but only those numbered among the 144,000 chosen members (Revelation 7:4) may partake of the bread and wine as a symbol of the death of Christ and the dedication to God. This memorial of Christ's death should take place on the day corresponding to Nisa 14 of the Jewish calendar, which occurs some time in March or April. These elite members will be raised with spiritual bodies (without flesh, bones, or blood) and will assist Christ in ruling the universe. Others who benefit from Christ's ransom will be resurrected with healthy, perfected physical bodies (bodies of flesh, bones, and blood) and will inhabit this earth after the world has been restored to a paradisiacal state. Sacraments are not observed.

Social Activities (Dating, Dancing) and Substance Use

Youth are encouraged to socialize with members of their own religious background. Members abstain from the use of tobacco and hold that drunkenness is a serious sin. Alcohol used in moderation, however, is acceptable.

Health Care Practices

The practice of faith healing is forbidden. However, it is believed that reading the scriptures can comfort the individual and lead to mental and spiritual healing.

Medical and Surgical Procedures

Medications
To the extent that they are necessary, medications are acceptable.

Blood and Blood Products
Blood in any form, and agents in which blood is an ingredient, are not acceptable. Blood volume expanders are acceptable if they are not derivatives of blood. Mechanical devices for circulating the blood are acceptable as long as they are not primed with blood initially. In some cases, children have been made wards of the court so that they could receive blood when a medical condition mandating blood transfusion was life threatening. This can threaten the standing of the child in the community and must be approached with great care.

The determination of Jehovah's Witnesses to abstain from blood is based on scriptural references and precedents in the history of Christianity. Courts of justice have often upheld the principle that each individual has a right to bodily integrity, yet some physicians and hospital administrators have turned to the courts for legal authorization to force blood to be used as a medical treatment for an individual whose religious convictions prohibit the use of blood.

Surgical Procedures

Although surgical procedures are not in and of themselves opposed, the administration of blood during surgery is strictly prohibited (Jehovah's Witness Official Web Site, 2010). There is no church rule pertaining to the loss of limbs or the amputation of body parts. If they are a violation of the principle of bodily mutilation, transplants are forbidden. However, this is usually an individual decision. Blood may not be used in this or any surgical procedure. Biopsies are acceptable. Circumcision is an individual decision.

Practices Related to Reproduction

Sterilization is prohibited because it is viewed as a form of bodily mutilation. Other forms of birth control are left to the individual. Amniocentesis is acceptable. Both therapeutic and on-demand abortions are forbidden. Sterility testing is an individual decision. Artificial insemination is forbidden both for donors and for recipients. Jehovah's Witnesses do not condone any activities in the areas of eugenics and genetics; they are considered to interfere with nature and therefore are unacceptable.

Religious Support System for the Sick

Individual members of congregation, including elders, visit the ill. Visitors pray with the sick person and read scriptures. Because members do not smoke, it is preferred that patients be placed in rooms where no smoking is allowed. If a man, the religious representative is referred to as "Mr." or "Elder"; if female, as "Ms." or "Mrs." Religious titles are not generally used. Individuals and members of the congregation look after the needs of the sick.

Practices Related to Death and Dying

The right to die or the use of extraordinary methods to prolong life is a matter of individual conscience. Euthanasia is forbidden. An autopsy is acceptable only if it is required by law. No parts are to be removed from the body. The human spirit and the body are never separated. The donation of a body is forbidden. Disposal of the body is a matter of individual preference. Burial practices are determined by local custom. Cremation is permitted if the individual chooses it.

Addendum

Jehovah's Witnesses are opposed to saluting the flag, serving in the armed forces, voting in civil elections, and holding public office. These prohibitions are related to belief in a theocracy that is in harmony with their understanding of New Testament Christianity. Governed by a body of individuals, members united with the theocracy are to dissociate themselves from all activities of the political state and give full allegiance to "Jehovah's organization." This practice is related to the belief that Jesus Christ is King and Priest and that there is no need to hold citizenship in more than one kingdom. Members also refrain from gambling.

A pamphlet entitled *Jehovah's Witnesses and the Question of Blood* may be obtained free of charge from the World Headquarters for the Jehovah's Witnesses at 117 Adams Street, Brooklyn, NY, 11201.

Judaism

Judaism is an Old Testament religion that dates back to the time of the prophet Abraham. Worldwide, there are approximately 18 million Jews. Membership includes approximately 7 million members in the United States and 371,000 members in Canada.

General Beliefs and Religious Practices

Judaism is a monotheistic religion. Jewish life historically has been based on interpretation of the laws of God as contained in the **Torah** and explained in the **Talmud** and in oral tradition. Ancient Jewish law prescribed most of the daily actions of the people. Diet, clothing, activities, occupation, and ceremonial activities throughout the life cycle are all part of Jewish daily life.

Today there are at least three schools of theological thought and social practice in Judaism. The three main divisions include Orthodox, Conservative, and Reform. There is also a fundamentalist sect, called Hasidism. Hasidic Jews cluster in metropolitan areas and live and work only within their Jewish communities.

Any person born of a Jewish mother or anyone converted to Judaism is considered a Jew. All Jews are united by the core theme of Judaism, which is expressed in the **Shema**, a prayer that professes a single God.

Holy Days

The Sabbath is the holiest of all holy days. The Sabbath begins each Friday 18 minutes before sunset and ends on Saturday, 42 minutes after sunset, or when three stars can be seen in the sky with the naked eye.

Other Holy Days are as follows:

1. Rosh Hashanah (Jewish New Year)
2. Yom Kippur (Day of Atonement, a fast day)
3. Succot (Feast of Tabernacles)
4. Shmini Atzeret (8th Day of Assembly)
5. Simchat Torah
6. Chanukah (Festival of Lights, or Rededication of the Temple in Jerusalem)
7. Asara B'Tevet (Fast of the 10th of Tevet)*
8. Fast of Esther
9. Purim
10. Passover
11. Shavuot (Festival of the Giving of the Torah)
12. Fast of the 17th of Tammuz
13. Fast of the 9th of Ave (Commemoration of the Destruction of the Temple)

Holy days are very special to practicing Jews. If a condition is not life-threatening, medical and surgical procedures should not be performed on the Sabbath or on holy days. Preservation of life is of greatest priority and is the major criterion for determining activity on holy days and the Sabbath. If a Jewish patient is hesitant to receive urgent and necessary treatment because of religious restrictions, a rabbi should be consulted.

Sacraments/Rituals

Brit milah, the covenant of circumcision, is performed on all Jewish male children on the 8th day after birth (Figure 13-6). Although circumcision is a surgical procedure, for Jews it is a fundamental reli-

*Not observed by liberal or Reform Jews.

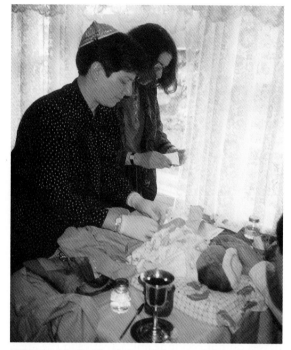

FIGURE 13-6 The *brit milah*, or covenant of circumcision, is being performed in the home of this 8-day-old Jewish infant by two mohels, one of whom is a Jewish pediatrician.

gious obligation. Circumcision is usually performed by a **mohel**, a pious Jew with special training, or by the child's father. Because the severing of the foreskin constitutes the essence of the ritual, the practice of having a non-Jewish or nonobservant physician perform the circumcision in the presence of a rabbi or other person who pronounces the blessing is not acceptable according to Jewish law. Circumcision may be delayed if medically contraindicated. For example, if the child has hypospadias, a congenital defect of the urethral wall for which surgical repair usually occurs at age 3 years and requires the use of the foreskin in reconstructive plastic surgery, the circumcision may be delayed. At times, Jewish law requires postponement of circumcision, though contemporary medical science recognizes no potential threat to the health of the baby (e.g., for physiologic jaundice). As soon as the jaundice disappears, the brit milah may be performed. In Reform and

Conservative traditions, girls mark the eighth day of life with a dedication ceremony in which prayers and blessings are invoked on her behalf.

The bar mitzvah (meaning "son of the commandment") is a confirmation ceremony for boys at age 13 that has been preceded by extensive religious study, including mastery of key Torah passages in Hebrew. In Reform and Conservative traditions, the bas (or bat) mitzvah (meaning "daughter of the commandment") is the equivalent ceremony for girls.

Diet

The dietary laws of Judaism are very strict; the degree to which they are observed varies according to the individual. Strictly observant Jews never eat pork, never eat predatory fowl, and never mix milk dishes and meat dishes. Only fish with fins and scales are permissible; shellfish and other water creatures are prohibited.

The word **kosher** comes from a Hebrew word *kashrut* that means "proper." All animals must be ritually slaughtered to be kosher. This means that the animal is to be killed by a specially qualified person, quickly, with the least possible pain. More colloquially, many people think that "kosher" refers to a type of food. If a patient asks for kosher food, it is important to determine what he or she means.

Religious Objects

On the Sabbath and on holidays it is customary to light two candles in candleholders. Many Jewish men and some women wear *kipot* or *yarmulkes* (small head coverings) and *tallit* (prayer shawls) when praying. A *siddur* (prayer book) may also be present. (Accessed on March 18, 2007 at http://www.healthsystem.virginia.edu/internet/chaplaincy/jewish.cfm).

Social Activities (Dating, Dancing)

Like all ethnic groups, Jews tend toward endogamy. Social activities that might lead to marriage outside the faith are discouraged. However, it is recognized that a significant number of individuals in Jewish society will seek partners outside of the Jewish faith. When this occurs, every effort is made to bring the non-Jewish partner into Judaism and to keep the Jewish partner a member and part of Jewish society.

Substance Use

The guideline is moderation. Wine is a part of religious observance and used as such. Drunkenness is not a sign of a good Jew. Historically, Jews well connected with their faith have had a low incidence of alcoholism.

Health Care Practices

Medical care from a physician in the case of illness is expected according to Jewish law. There are many prayers for the sick in Jewish liturgy. Such prayers and hope for recovery are encouraged.

Medical and Surgical Procedures

There are no restrictions when medications are used as part of a therapeutic process. There is a prohibition in Judaism against ingesting blood (e.g., blood sausage, raw meat). However, this does not apply to receiving blood transfusions. Beliefs and practices related to body mutilation (e.g., organ transplantation, amputations) vary widely among Jews. Individual beliefs should be explored with the client before any procedure that involves body mutilation.

Practices Related to Reproduction

Birth Control

It is said in the Torah that Jews should be fruitful and multiply; therefore, it is a *mitzvah* (a good deed) to have at least two children. Since the Holocaust of World War II, it has been increasingly acceptable to have more children to replace those that were lost. It is permissible to practice birth control in traditional and liberal homes (Forsythe, 1991).

In the past, contraception was limited to the woman; vasectomy was prohibited. Currently, Judaism permits contraception by either partner, although Hasidic and Orthodox Jews rarely use vasectomy.

Abortion

Although therapeutic abortion is always permitted if the health of the mother is jeopardized, traditional Judaism regards the killing of an unborn child to be a serious moral offense, whereas liberal Judaism permits it with strong moral admonitions (i.e., it is not to be used as a means of birth control). The fetus, although not imbued with the full sanctity of life, is a potential human being and is acknowledged as such.

Sterility Testing and Artificial Insemination
Sterility testing is permissible when the goal is to enable the couple to have children. Artificial insemination is permitted under certain circumstances. A rabbi should be consulted in each individual case.

Eugenics and Genetics
Jews have an understandable aversion to genetic engineering because of the experimentation carried on during the Nazi era. At the same time, eugenic practices are permitted under a limited range of circumstances. The Jewish belief in the sanctity of life is a guiding factor in rabbinical counseling.

Religious Support System for the Sick

Visitors
The most likely visitors will be family and friends from the synagogue. To visit the sick is a mitzvah of service (an obligation, a responsibility, and a blessing). There are often many Jewish social service agencies to help those in need. The Jewish Federation and Jewish Community Service are two large organizations that provide services to fulfill a variety of needs.

Title of Religious Representative
The formal religious representative from a synagogue is the rabbi. A visit from the rabbi may be spent talking, or the rabbi may pray with the person alone or in a minyan, a group of 10 adults 13 years or older. If the patient is male and strictly observant, he may wish to have a prayer shawl (*tallit*), a cap (*kippah*), and *tefillin* (special symbols tied onto the arms and forehead). If the patient's own materials are not at the hospital, it may be necessary to ask that they be brought. Prayers are often chanted. If possible, privacy should be provided.

Practices Related to Death and Dying

Prolongation of Life (Right to Die)
A person has the right to die with dignity. If a physician sees that death is inevitable, no new therapeutic measures that would artificially extend life need to be initiated. It is important to know the precise time of death for the purpose of honoring the deceased after the first year has passed.

Euthanasia
Euthanasia is prohibited under any circumstances. It is regarded as murder. However, in the administration of palliative medications that carry the calculated risk of overdose, the amelioration of pain is paramount.

Autopsy
Any unjustified alteration in a corpse is considered a desecration of the dead, to be avoided in normal circumstances. When postmortem examinations are justified, they must be limited to essential organs or systems. Needle biopsy is preferred. All body parts must be returned for burial. Jewish family members may ask to consult with a rabbinical authority before signing an autopsy consent form.

Donation of Body Parts
This is a complex matter according to Jewish law. If it seems necessary, consultation with a rabbi should be encouraged (Weiss, 1988).

Burial
The body is ritually washed at a funeral home after death, if possible by members of the Chevra Kadisha (Ritual Burial Society). The body is then clothed in a simple white burial shroud. Embalming, a process wherein the blood of the deceased is replaced by an embalming fluid, and cosmetic treatment of the body are forbidden. Public viewing of the body is considered a humiliation of the dead. Relatives are forbidden to touch or embrace the deceased, except when involved in preparation for interment. The exact time of burial is significant for sitting shiva, the mourning period. After death in an institution, a nurse may wash the body for transport to the funeral home. Ritual washing then occurs later. Human remains, including a fetus at any stage of gestation, are to be buried as soon as possible. Cremation is not in keeping with Jewish law.

Addendum

Additional information can be obtained from Synagogue Council of America, 432 Park Avenue South, New York, NY 10016; phone (212) 686-8670; or the Canadian Jewish Congress, 100 Sparks Street Suite 650, Ottawa, Ontario, K1P 5B7, phone (613) 233-8703, fax (613) 233-8748, e-mail canadianjewishcongress@cjc.ca.

Mennonite Church

Membership in the United States is 122,545; in Canada: 207,970; and worldwide: 1,250,000.

Mennonites take their name from Menno Simons, an Anabaptist bishop who united a fragmented group of Anabaptists in the early 1500s. Menno had been a Catholic priest in Holland but left the church over theological differences after his brother was killed as an Anabaptist. The word "Anabaptist" comes from the doctrine that baptism to be valid must be upon confessed faith.

General Beliefs and Religious Practices

Mennonites believe that each person is responsible before God to make decisions based on his or her understanding of the Bible. For this reason, there are a minimum of official statements or regulations. Even when these are to be found, for example, the Mennonite Confession of Faith, they are perceived by members as guidelines rather than proclamations to supplant individual responsibility. It should also be noted that the Mennonite faith encompasses a wide spectrum of cultural circumstances, which are more responsible for variations among individual Mennonites than is the basic theology, which is relatively uniform. It is therefore necessary to ascertain individual preferences and to work with patients on a one-to-one basis rather than stereotyping according to religious affiliation.

Holy Days and Sacraments

Mennonites observe the religious days of the traditional Christian churches. Observance places no restrictions on health-related procedures on these days. Mennonites observe Baptism and Holy Communion as official church sacraments. Patients will request sacraments as necessary. Neither sacrament is believed necessary for salvation.

Social Activities (Dating, Dancing)

No restrictions are placed on social activities.

Health Care Practices

Healing is believed to be a part of God's work in the human body through whatever means he chooses to use, whether medical science or healing that comes in answer to specific prayer. There is no religious ritual to be applied unless the patient asks for one in whatever way is personally meaningful. Sometimes anointing of oil is practiced.

Medical and Surgical Procedures

No specific guidelines or restrictions exist for the administration of medications, blood and blood components, or surgical procedures.

Practices Related to Reproduction

Birth Control

All types of contraception are acceptable. The choice is left to the individual.

Abortion

Therapeutic abortions are acceptable. Mennonites generally believe that on-demand abortion must be decided according to the specifics of individual cases. The church has chosen to avoid making a ruling that must be followed unquestionably. The individual must follow her own conscience and learn to live with the consequences. Some parts of the Mennonite Church have adopted statements opposing abortion on demand.

Artificial Insemination

The church does not have regulations regarding artificial insemination. The individual conscience and point of view of the patient need to be respected. Usually, artificial insemination is sought only if husband and wife are donor and recipient, respectively.

Eugenics and Genetics

The church accepts scientific endeavor as a valid activity that needs to respect all of God's creation. The concerns of eugenics and genetics in its future potential have not been fully confronted. Mennonites believe that God and human beings work together in caring for and improving the world.

Practices Related to Death and Dying

The church does not believe that life must be continued at all cost. Health care professionals should decide whether to take heroic measures on the basis of the patient's individual circumstances and the emotional condition of the family. When life has lost its purpose and meaning beyond hope of meaningful recovery, most Mennonites feel that relatives should not be censured for allowing life-sustaining measures to be withheld.

Euthanasia as the termination of life by an overt act of the physician is not condoned. Autopsy and the donation of the body are acceptable, without restrictions. Procedures for disposal of body and burial follow local customs and legal requirements.

Native North American Churches

Differentiating Native North American health care practices from their religious and cultural beliefs is much more difficult than with the other religions presented in this chapter. Native North Americans represent 2 million people and approximately 600 tribal units within North America. Each group has individual beliefs and practices, yet they maintain a similar nonprescriptive attitude toward health care.

There is in the United States and Canada today a specific religion called the **Native American Church** or **Peyote Religion**. Encompassing members of many tribes, its focus is on the revival of Native North American culture, beliefs, and spirituality.

When trying to support a Native American in physical or psychological crisis, the nurse needs to remember several seemingly unrelated facts. First, the non-Westernized Native North American belief about disease is not necessarily based on symptoms. Disease may be attributed to intrusive objects, soul loss, spirit intrusion, breach of taboo, or sorcery. Disease may also be attributed to natural or supernatural causes. Second, the Native North American may embrace an organized, usually Christian religion and still be a member of a particular Native North American tribe. Native North Americans also balance "modern theories of disease" with long-standing tribal beliefs or customs. Therefore, during illness and particularly hospitalization, Native North Americans may ask to see a priest or minister as well as a tribal "medicine man" or **curandero**. Visits from these persons will likely be spiritually supportive, although the form of the support may vary greatly.

The spiritual basis for much of Native North American belief and action is symbolized by the number four. This number, which pervades much of North American Indian thought, is seen in the extended hand, which means life, unity, equality, and eternity. The clasped hand symbolizes unity, the spiritual law that binds the universe.

It is this unity on which decisions should be made. Questions about abortion, the use of drugs, giving and receiving blood, the right to life, euthanasia, and so on do not have dogmatic "yes" or "no" answers; rather, answers are based on the situation and the ultimate unity or disunity that a decision would produce.

To the Native North American, everything is cyclical. Communication is the key to learning and understanding; understanding brings peace of mind; peace of mind leads to happiness; and happiness is communicating. Other guidelines also function in groups of four.

Four guidelines toward self-development are

1. Am I happy with what I am doing?
2. What am I doing to add to the confusion?
3. What am I doing to bring about peace and contentment?
4. How will I be remembered when I am gone, in absence and in death?

The four requirements of good health are

1. Food
2. Sleep
3. Cleanliness
4. Good thoughts

The four divisions of nature are

1. Spirit
2. Mind
3. Body
4. Life

The four divisions of goals are

1. Faith
2. Love
3. Work
4. Pleasure

The four ages of development are the

1. Learning age
2. Age of adoption
3. Age of improvement
4. Age of wisdom

The four expressions of sharing are

1. Making others feel you care
2. An expression of interest
3. An expression of friendship
4. An expression of belonging

Unity, the great spiritual law, also can be expressed in four parts

1. Going into the silence in spirit, mind, and body
2. The union through which all spirituality flows
3. A goal toward communicating with all things in nature
4. Recognized through sense, emotions, and impressions.

In concert with the belief in the interconnectedness of all things, natural remedies in the form of herbal medicine are often used. (It is interesting to note that Native North American folk medicine and herbal remedies provided the forerunners of many of today's pharmaceutical remedies.) Herbal treatments are still used today and may be requested by Native North American patients in a Western medical setting.

A nurse caring for a Native North American client should be careful to obtain a careful and complete history, including a list of whatever native remedies have been tried. The patient may not know the names of herbs used in treatment, and the tribal medicine man or woman may need to be consulted.

Respecting the concept that religion, medicine, and healing are inseparable to the Native North American, one must be sensitive to the fact that asking for the names of native medicines or descriptions of healing practices tried in an attempt to cure the person before his or her entrance into the Western medical system is not just simply obtaining a history, but also entering into the realm of what might be not only private but also very sacred. The nurse must use care and sensitivity and show deep respect for the information received.

Protestantism

In its broadest meaning, **Protestantism** denotes the whole movement within Christianity that originated in the 16th century with Martin Luther and the Protestant Reformation. Historically and traditionally, the chief characteristics of Protestantism are the acceptance of the Bible as the only source of infallible revealed truth, the belief in the universal priesthood of believers, and the doctrine that Christians are justified in their relationship to God by faith alone, not by good works or dispensations of the church.

It is difficult to accurately categorize Protestant churches and impossible to mention them all, because there are more than 30,000 denominations. Protestantism is basically non-Roman Western Christianity, and it can be divided into four major forms: Lutheran, Anglican, Reformed, and free (or independent) church.

Lutheranism

The oldest and second largest Protestant religion, Lutheranism began in 1517 with Martin Luther's split from the Roman Catholic Church. Lutherans emphasize theological doctrine and spirituality. Many North American Lutherans are of German or Scandinavian heritage.

Anglicanism

Anglicanism is represented by the established Church of England and similar churches. Unlike most other Protestant churches, they have an episcopal system of government in which each church or parish is served by a priest who is supervised by a bishop. A bishop supervises a group of churches called a diocese. A bishop, in turn, is responsible to a council of bishops. Anglican churches allow their clergy to marry. The Methodist church was established by followers of John Wesley, an 18th-century Anglican who sought to bring reform to the Church of England. Wesley's movement spread to the United States and Canada in the 18th century.

Reformed Denominations

The Reformed denominations include Presbyterianism and are based on the teachings of John Calvin and his followers. These churches are distinguished from Lutheranism and Anglicanism, which maintain symbolic and sacramental traditions that originated before the Protestant Reformation.

Free or Independent Churches

Free or independent churches, including the Baptists, Congregationalists, Adventists, and Churches of Christ exercise congregational government. Each local denomination is an independent autonomous unit and there is no official doctrine.

With 27 million members, the Baptist church makes up more than 10% of the population of the United States. Black and White Baptist church denominations exist separately. The largely White Southern Baptist Convention has about 12 million members, whereas 9 million Blacks (30% of all Blacks in the United States) are members of the National Baptist Conventions.

Health Care Practices

Given the wide diversity that exists within Protestant denominations, it is beyond the scope of this text to identify health-related beliefs and practices for each group. Selected Protestant denominations (e.g., Adventists, Jehovah's Witnesses) have been included in this section largely because they have significant health-related practices. For further information about specific Protestant churches, you are encouraged to visit www.adherents.com or the official web pages of the various groups for a synopsis of their beliefs.

Seventh-Day Adventists

North American membership of **Seventh-Day Adventists** is approaching 1,000,000; worldwide membership now exceeds 10.65 million.

Doctrinally, Seventh-Day Adventists are heirs of the interfaith Millerite movement of the late 1840s, although the movement officially adopted the name Seventh-Day Adventist in 1863. Between 1831 and 1844, William Miller, a Baptist preacher and former army captain in the War of 1812, launched the "great second advent awakening," which eventually spread throughout most of the Christian world. At first, the work was largely confined to North America, but it quickly spread to Switzerland, Africa, Italy, Egypt, and many other nations.

General Beliefs and Religious Practices

Seventh-Day Adventists accept the Bible as their only creed and hold certain fundamental beliefs to be the teaching of the Holy Scriptures. The official statements by the General Conference of the Seventh-Day Adventists concerning the scriptures, the trinity, creation, nature of man, the great controversy (Christ versus Satan), life, death, resurrection, and other topics may be found at www.adventist.org.

Holy Days

The seventh day (Saturday) is observed as the Sabbath, from Friday sundown to Saturday sundown. The Sabbath is the day that God blessed and sanctified. It is a sacred day of worship and rest. Saturday worship services are held, as are weekly evening prayer meetings (usually midweek).

Sacraments/Rituals

There are three church ordinances: (1) baptism by immersion, (2) the Ordinance of Humility, and (3) the Lord's Supper or Communion. There are no rituals at the time of birth. There is no requirement for a final sacrament at death. If requested by the individual or family member, the dying person might be anointed with oil.

Diet

Seventh-Day Adventists believe that because the body is the temple of God, it is appropriate to abstain from any food or beverage that could prove harmful to the body. Because the first human diet consisted of fruits and grains, the Church encourages a vegetarian diet. Nevertheless, some members prefer to eat meat and poultry. Based on a passage in Leviticus 11:3, nonvegetarian members refrain from eating foods derived from any animal having a cloven hoof that chews its cud (e.g., meat derived from pigs, rabbits, or similar animals). Although fish with fins and scales are acceptable (e.g., salmon), shellfish are prohibited. Consumption of some birds is prohibited, but common poultry such as chicken and turkey are acceptable. Fermented beverages are prohibited. Fasting is practiced, but only when members of a specific church elect to do so. Practiced in degrees, fasting may involve abstention from food or liquids. Fasting is not encouraged if it is likely to have adverse effects on the individual.

Social Activities (Dating, Dancing) and Substance Use

Dancing is not encouraged as a form of recreation or social activity. Members are encouraged to date other members or persons holding similar beliefs and values. Members should abstain from the use of fermented beverages and tobacco products.

Health Care Practices

The church believes in divine healing and practices anointing with oil and prayer. This is in addition to healing brought about by medical intervention. Since 1865, the church has maintained chaplains and physicians as inseparable in its institutions.

Medical and Surgical Procedures

Adventists operate one of the world's largest religiously operated health systems, including a medical school. The **Health Ministries** include 166 hospitals and sanitariums, 117 nursing homes and retirement centers, 371 clinics and dispensaries, 30 orphanages and children's homes, and 12 airplanes and medical launches. Physical medicine and rehabilitation are emphasized and recommended, along with therapeutic diets. There are no restrictions on the use of vaccines. Similarly, there are no restrictions on the use of blood and blood products, amputations, organ transplants, donation of organs, biopsies, and circumcisions.

Practices Related to Reproduction

The use of birth control is an individual decision; the church prohibits cohabitation except between husband and wife. There are no restrictions on amniocentesis. Therapeutic abortion is acceptable if the mother's life is in danger and in cases of rape and incest. On-demand abortion is unacceptable because Adventists believe in the sanctity of life. Artificial insemination between husband and wife is acceptable. Although the church views practices in the fields of eugenics and genetics as an individual decision, it upholds the principle of responsibility in dealing with children.

Religious Support System for the Sick

At the request of the sick person or the family, the pastor and elders of the church will come together to pray and anoint the sick person with oil. The religious representative is referred to as Doctor,

Pastor, or Elder. There is a worldwide Seventh-Day Adventist health system, which includes hospitals and clinics.

Practices Related to Death and Dying

Although there is no official position, the church has traditionally followed the medical ethics of prolonging life and euthanasia. Autopsy and the donation of the entire body or parts are acceptable. No directives or recommendations exist regarding disposal of the body. No specific directives concerning burial exist; this is an individual decision.

Addendum

The Seventh-Day Adventist church is opposed to the use of hypnotism in the practice of medicine or under any other circumstance. Clinical implications for psychotherapy from the Seventh-day Adventist tradition has been addressed by faculty from Loma Linda University School of Medicine (Fayard et al., 2007).

Unitarian Universalist Church

Worldwide, Unitarian Universalist membership is 800,000, with a North American membership of 221,760.

General Beliefs and Religious Practices

Unitarianism was officially organized in 1774 in England. This organization occurred after a long history of debate and dissension regarding the nature of God, particularly regarding the Trinitarian concept, which existed in various forms in the Catholic and Protestant religions. The Unitarian Universalist Association is the modern institutional embodiment of two separate denominations that grew out of movements and faith traditions extending back to the Christian Reformation era (14–16th century C.E.). Universalist convictions include the belief that all creation will ultimately be drawn back to its divine source and that no person or thing would be ultimately and forever excluded.

The Unitarian conviction is reflected in the belief that God is ultimately and absolutely one.

Holy Days and Sacraments

No religious holy days are celebrated. Members come from various cultural and religious backgrounds and observe special days according to their own heritage and desire.

Normal milestones of life (birth, marriage, death) may be celebrated religiously. Although it is uncommon, puberty and divorce may include religious observances.

Unitarian Universalism does not believe in a need for sacraments. Baptism of infants and occasionally of adults is sometimes performed as a symbolic act of dedication. The Lord's Supper is administered in some congregations.

Diet and Substance Use

No restrictions on diet exist. Substances should be used according to reason.

Health Care Practices

Faith healing is considered largely superstitious and wishful thinking. Members believe in the use of the empirical method, reason, and science to facilitate healing.

Medical and Surgical Procedures

The use of medications is not restricted. The use of blood and blood products is similarly not restricted. Amputations, organ transplants, biopsies are not restricted. Circumcision is viewed as a health practice, not a religious one.

Practices Related to Reproduction

Unitarian Universalists strongly favor all types of birth control as a human right. Both therapeutic and on-demand abortion are acceptable. Members strongly favor the right of the mother to decide. Amniocentesis is not restricted and is encouraged if medical evaluation deems it necessary. Sterility testing is acceptable; in fact, more research is encouraged. Both donation and receipt of artificial insemination are acceptable and strongly favored as a human right.

Practices Related to Death and Dying

Members favor the right to die with dignity. Personhood is sacred, not the spark of life. Members tend to favor nonaction, including withdrawal of technical aids when death is imminent or when the patient has made a written request in advance. Autopsy is recommended. The donation of the body is acceptable. Cremation is most common. Donation to a medical school for study is not uncommon. Burial of a fetus is rare. A memorial service in the church or at home without the body present is customary.

SUMMARY

Religious and cultural beliefs are interwoven and influence a client's understanding of illness and health care practices. In times of serious illness

and death, religion may be a source of consolation for the client. Five dimensions of religion influence human behavior, including health-related practices. The goal of spiritual nursing care is to assist clients in integrating their own religious beliefs about God or a unifying truth into the ultimate reality that gives meaning to their lives in relationship to the health care crisis that has precipitated the need for nursing care. For the nurse providing spiritual nursing care, issues related to death and dying are of particular importance. Health-related beliefs and practices of select religions are important to understand, especially considering the diverse religious groups in the United States and Canada. Evidence-Based Practice 13-1 provides information regarding other research done on this topic, and Box 13-3 summarizes some of the religious and nonreligious holidays covered in this chapter.

EVIDENCE-BASED PRACTICE 13-1

Spirituality, Religion, Culture, and Health

There is considerable scientific research analyzing the potential connection between and among spiritual and religious practices, culture, and health. A metasynthesis of findings involving more than 7,000 participants in 25 research studies pertaining to spirituality, religion, intercessory prayer, culture, and health reveals the following:

- Regular participation in spiritual or religious practices lowers the overall mortality rate of the population by 12–46% per year; in 11 studies;
- Mortality for African Americans who participate in religious services at least weekly decreases by 10% for women and 17% for men in one study;
- For the elderly regular attendance at religious services improve physical health and psychological well-being in two studies;
- People with high levels of religious beliefs or spirituality have lower levels of the cortisol, cholesterol, and cardiac arrhythmias in response to stress in three studies;
- Positive thinking that is associated with spirituality and religion produces nearly a 30% drop in perception of pain in one study;

- Religious experience such as meditation lowered blood pressure in 14 studies;
- Spirituality is connected to immune and endocrine functioning in three studies;
- Spirituality and religion are associated with a slower progression of Alzheimer's Disease in two studies;
- People who pray before surgery have better surgical outcomes and report feeling less anxious before and after surgery in one study [another study found the opposite outcome, i.e., more complications after surgery];
- Women who attended weekly religious services were more successful in cigarette smoking cessation in three studies;
- Men and women who attended weekly religious services were more successful in adhering to a cardiac rehabilitation program after being diagnosed with coronary artery disease in one study;
- Intercessory prayer increased the success of women undergoing *in vitro* fertilization in one study;
- Faster recovery from depression, anxiety, and bereavement was reported for Christian, Muslim, and Buddhist patients in one study;

(Evidence-Based Practice continues on page 398)

EVIDENCE-BASED PRACTICE 13-1

Spirituality, Religion, Culture, and Health (*continued*)

- Some people undergoing surgery may not wish to know that others are offering prayers on their behalf in one study;
- Hispanic men with HIV did not report religion as being helpful in coping with their disease in one study.

Clinical Application

While some of the studies have methodological limitations and most are epidemiological investigations, this growing body of research supports nurses' encouragement of patients who find daily or weekly prayer and other religious or spiritual practices to be meaningful. The best clinical practices demonstrated by nurses would include the following:

- Taking a spiritual and religious history of each patient;
- Asking, "Do spiritual or religious beliefs or practices provide comfort or cause distress?";

- Encouraging patients to engage in spiritual and religious practices that they find satisfying and meaningful without imposing your own beliefs or practices on others;
- Refraining from implying that religion is good or bad, only that it can provide comfort or cause stress;
- Recognizing that, in times of physical or emotional stress such as hospitalization, people who do not regularly participate in spiritual or religious practices might turn to these practices for comfort, support, and hope;
- Respecting that spiritual and religious practices can influence the patient's coping by providing
  - an optimistic world view
  - a hopeful perspective on life even in the face of serious or terminal diagnoses
  - a sense of empowerment and control

BOX 13-3

Religious and Nonreligious Holidays in the United States and Canada

This calendar is a guide to religious and nonreligious holidays that are celebrated in the United States and Canada. The list is not exhaustive but is given to encourage the reader to be aware of the many holidays and festivals that are reflective of the great mixture of religious and ethnic groups in North America.

B = Buddhist	I = Islam	O = Eastern Orthodox Christian
Ba = Baha'i	J = Jewish	
C = Christian (general)	Ja = Jain	P = Protestant
Ci = Civic holiday	M = Mormon	RC = Roman Catholic
H = Hindu		S = Sikh

January

1 New Year's Day Ci
1 Feast of St. Basil O
6 Epiphany C
7 Nativity of Jesus Christ O
3rd Monday Martin Luther King, Jr. Birthday Observance Ci

February

Black History Month (U.S.)
8 Scout Day Ci
14 Valentine's Day Ci
Mid-month President's Day (U.S.) Ci
Other holidays that often fall in February according to the lunar calendar

BOX 13-3 (*continued*)

Chinese New Year
Ramadan (30 days) I
Nehan-e (Death of Buddha) B
Vasant Panchami (Advent of Spring)
H, Ja
Ash Wednesday RC, P
Purim J

March

Women's History Month (U.S.)
17 St. Patrick's Day C
25 Annunciation C
Other holidays that often occur in March according to the lunar calendar
Eastern Orthodox Lent begins O
Higan-e (First Day of Spring) B
Naw-Ruz (Baha'i and Iranian New Year)
Palm Sunday RC, P
First Day of Passover (8 days) J
Holi (Spring Festival) H, Ja
Maundy Thursday RC, P
Good Friday RC, P
Easter C, RC, P, M
Mahavir Jayanti (Birth of Mahavir) Ja

April

16 Yom Ha'atzmaut (Israel Independence Day) J
Holidays that often occur in April according to the lunar calendar
Hanamatsuri (Birth of Buddha) B
Yom Hashoah (Holocaust Remembrance Day) J, Ci
Baisakhi (Brotherhood) S
Huguenot Day P
Ramavani (Birth of Rama) H
Palm Sunday O
Holy Friday O
Easter O

May

5 Cinco de Mayo Ci
23 Victoria Day (Canada)
30 Memorial Day Ci
Holidays that often occur in May according to the lunar calendar
Shavuot J

Idul-Adha (Day of Sacrifice) I
Ascension Day RC, P
Pentecost RC, P

June

12 Anne Frank Day
14 Flag Day (U.S.) Ci
24 Nativity of St. John the Baptist RC, P, O
Holidays that often occur in June according to the lunar calendar
Ratha-yatra
Ascension Day O
Muharam (I)
Pentecost O
Islamic New Year I
Hindu New Year H

July

1 Canada Day (Canada) Ci
4 Independence Day (U.S.) Ci
24 Pioneer Day M
Holidays that often occur in July according to the lunar calendar
Obon-e B

August

6 Transfiguration C
15 Feast of the Blessed Virgin Mary RC, O

September

1st Monday Labor Day (U.S.) Ci
15 National Hispanic Heritage Month (30 days) Ci
17 Citizenship (U.S. Constitution) Ci
19 San Gennaro Day RC
25 Native American Day Ci
Holidays that often occur in September according to the lunar calendar
Higan-e (First Day of Fall) B
Rosh Hashanah (Jewish New Year: 2 days) J

October

12 Columbus Day (U.S.) Ci
Thanksgiving Day (Canada) Ci
24 United Nations Day Ci
31 Reformation Day P
31 Halloween RC, P, Ci

(box continues on page 400)

BOX 13-3

Religious and Nonreligious Holidays in the United States and Canada (continued)

Holidays that often occur in October according to the lunar calendar
Dusserah (Good over Evil) H, JA
Yom Kippur (Atonement) J
Sukkot (Tabernacles) J
Shemini 'Azeret (end of Sukkot)
Diwali, or Dipavali (Festival of Lights) H, Ja

November

1 All Saints Day RC, P
11 Veterans Day Ci
25 Religious Liberty Day Ci
1st Tuesday Election Day (U.S.) Ci
4th Thursday Thanksgiving Day (U.S.) Ci
Holidays that often occur in November according to the lunar calendar

Baha'u'llah Birthday Ba
Guru Nanak Birthday S

December

6 St. Nicholas Day C
8 Feast of the Immaculate Conception RC
10 Human Rights Day Ci
12 Festival of Our Lady of Guadalupe (Mexico-Hispanic)
25 Christmas C, RC, P, M, Ci
Holidays that often occur in December according to the lunar calendar
Bodhi Day (Enlightenment) B
Hanukkah (Jewish Festival of Lights: 8 days) J
Kwanzaa (7 days)

REVIEW QUESTIONS

1. When assessing the spiritual needs of clients from diverse cultural backgrounds, what key components should you consider?
2. In providing nursing care for the dying or bereaved client and family, what cultural considerations should the nurse include in the plan?
3. Compare and contrast the religious beliefs and practices concerning diet, medications, and procedures for five of the religious groups discussed in this chapter.
4. Analyze the contributions of religious organizations to the United States (and/or Canadian)

health care delivery system. What effect do health care facilities that are owned and operated by religious groups have on the overall cost and quality of health care in the United States and Canada? Critically analyze concerns about these religiously operated facilities in terms of philosophical, ethical, and legal aspects pertaining to types of services offered to patients.
5. What religious rituals mark significant developmental milestones for children and adolescents? Identify the ritual or ceremony, the approximate age at which the child or adolescent participates in it, and the name of the religion(s) associated with it.

CRITICAL THINKING ACTIVITIES

1. Visit a church or worship center not of your own belief system and interview a member of the clergy or an official representative about the health-related beliefs of that religion. Discuss with him or her the implications of those beliefs for someone hospitalized for an acute or chronic illness. Inquire about the ways in which nurses can

be of most help to hospitalized members of this religion.

2. Interview members of various religions concerning their beliefs about health and illness. Compare these interviews with the published beliefs or official statements from these religions. Discuss the implications of the differences (if any) that you found.

3. Interview fellow students, classmates, or co-workers (if you are employed) about what they know of the health beliefs of various religions, especially those religions most often encountered among the patients with whom you work. Make a poster or prepare a presentation comparing the results of your interviews with the official beliefs of those religions. Share this information with your classmates.

4. Interview four or more members of the same religious group who are of various ages (i.e., children, teenagers, young adults, middle-aged, and elderly). Ask them about their religious beliefs and how they affect their health. Compare the results, commenting on similarities and differences.

5. Explore the meaning of various unique items of clothing worn by members of different religions. These may be in the form of items worn on the head or body. When are shoes removed? For which religious groups?

6. If you have thought about the above exercises in terms of physical health, consider each of the questions from the perspective of mental health and spiritual health.

REFERENCES

Amos, A. (2007). Death in hospital: Place of religion in the care of the patient. *Islam and Christian–Muslim Relations, 18*(3), 325–331.

Bazy, N. (2008). *Beauty of Ramadan: Guide to the Muslim month of prayer and fasting for Muslims and non-Muslims* (3rd ed.). Canton, MI: Read The Spirit Books.

Black, P. (2009). Cultural and religious beliefs in stoma care nursing. *British Journal of Nursing, 18*(I3), 790–793.

Buck, G. H. (2006). Spirituality concept analysis and model development. *Holistic Nursing Practice, 20*(6), 288–297.

Christian Science Publishing Society (1978). *What is a Christian Science practitioner?* Boston: Christian Science Publishing Society.

Christian Science Publishing Society (1994). *Science and health.* Boston: Christian Science Publishing Society.

Donnermeyer, J. F. (1997). Amish society: An overview. *The Journal of Multicultural Nursing and Health, 3*(2), 6–12.

Ebersole, P., Hess, P., & Luggan, A. S. (2008) *Toward healthy aging* (6th ed.). St. Louis, MO: C. V. Mosby.

ElGindy, G. (2008). Hindu dietary practices: Feeding the body, mind and spirit. *Minority Nurse.com.* Retrieved December 15, 2008 at http://www.minoritynurse.com/dietic/hindu-dietary-practices-feedding-body-mind-and-soul.

Faulkner, J. E., & DeJong, C. F. (1966). Religiosity in 5 D: An empirical analysis. *Social Forces, 45,* 246–254.

Fayard, C., Harding, G., Murdoch, W., & Brunt, J. (2007). Clinical implications for psychotherapy from the Seventh-day Adventist tradition. *Journal of Psychology and Christianity, 26*(2), 207–217.

Fogel, S. B., & Rivera, L. A. Accessed on February 17, 2010 at www.abanet.org. Religious beliefs and healthcare necessities: Can they coexist? *Human Rights Magazine,* American Bar Association.

Gordon, S. (2006). *Spirituality can soothe body and soul.* Accessed on March 18, 2007 at www.healthfinder.gov.

Hubbell, L. S., Woodard, E., Barksdale-Brown, D., & Parker, J. (2006). Spiritual care: Practices of nurse practitioners in federally designated non-metropolitan areas of North Carolina. *Journal of the American Academy of Nurse Practitioners, 18,* 379–385.

Jehovah's Witness official Web site. (2010). *How can blood save your life?* Accessed at http://www.watchtower.org/e/hb/article_00.htm.

Jett, K., & Touhy, T. (2010). *Ebersole and Hess' gerontological nursing and healthy aging.* St. Louis: Mosby.

Kalish, R. A., & Reynolds, D. K. (1981). *Death and ethnicity: A psychocultural study.* New York: Baywood.

Keehl, M.S. (2009). *Spirituality: A qualitative study of perceptions of student nurse practitioners concerned with spiritual care for themselves and their patients.* PhD Thesis. Flint, Michigan: University of Michigan-Flint.

Khan, F. (2008). An Islamic appraisal of minding the gap: Psycho-spiritual dynamics in the doctor–patient relationship. *Journal of Religious Ethics, 36,* 77–96.

Leonard, B., & Carlson, D. (2010). *Spirituality in health care.* Accessed on February 17, 2010 at www.csh.umn.edu/modules/spirituality.

Lyvers, M., Barling, N., & Harding-Cook, J. (2006). Effect of belief in "psychic healing" on self-reported pain in chronic pain suffers. *Journal of Psychosomatic Research, 60*(1), 59–61.

Matthew, D. B. (2008). Race, religion, and informed consent—Lessons from social science. *Journal of Law, Medicine, and Ethics, 35,* 150–173.

McIntyre, A. J. (2008). *The Tohono O'odham and Pimeria Alta.* Chicago: Arcadia Publishing.

Moberg, D. (1971). *Spiritual well-being.* Washington, DC: White House Conference on Aging.

Moberg, D. (1981). Religion and the aging family. In: P. Ebersole & P. Hess (Eds.), *Toward healthy aging* (pp. 349–351). St. Louis, MO: C.V. Mosby.

Narayanasamy, A. (2006). The impact of empirical studies of spirituality and culture on nurse education. *The Journal of Clinical Nursing, 15*(7), 840–851.

Nimer, M. (2002). *The North American Muslim Resource Guide to Community Life in the United States and Canada.* New York, NY: Routledge.

Stolley, J. M. & Koenig, H. (1997). Religion/spirituality and health among elderly African Americans and Hispanics. *Journal of Psychosocial Nursing, 35*(11), 32–38.

Tzeng, H., & Yin, C. (2006). Learning to respect a patient's spiritual needs concerning an unknown infectious disease. *Nursing Ethics, 13*(1), 17–28.

Wehbe-Alamah, H. (2005). *Generic and professional health care beliefs, expression and practices of Syrian Muslims living in the Midwestern United States.* (Unpublished doctoral dissertation). Duquesne University: Pittsburgh, PA.

Wehbe-Alamah (2008). Bridging generic and professional care practices for Muslim patients through use of Leininger's culture care modes. *Contemporary Nurse, 1–2,* 83–97.

Weiss, D. W. (1988). Organ transplantation, medical ethics and Jewish law. *Transplantation Proceedings, 20*(1), 1071–1075.

Wenger, A. F. (1990). The culture care theory and the Old Order Amish. In: M. M. Leininger (Ed.). *Culture care diversity and universality: A theory of nursing* (pp. 147–178). New York: National League for Nursing Press.

Wenger, A. F. (1991). Culture specific care and the Old Order Amish. *Imprint, 38*(2), 80–85.

White, K.A. *Crisis of conscience: Reconciling religious health care providers' beliefs and patients' rights. http://www3.baylor.edu/-Charles_Kemp/Hispanic_health.htm.* Accessed on March 14, 2007.

Woods, T. E., & Ironson, G. H. (1999). Religion and spirituality in the face of illness. *Journal of Health Psychology, 4*(3), 393–412.

Yearbook of American and Canadian Churches, Annual. (2006). New York: National Council of the Churches of Christ in the United States of America.

Yhlen, K., & Ashton, K. (2006). Bloodless care: When blood transfusion is not an option. *Journal of Legal Nurse Consulting, 17*(2), 3–5.

Yuen, E. J. (2007). Spirituality, religion, and health. *American Journal of Medical Quality, 22*(77), 77–79.

Yurkovick, E. E., & Lattergrass, I. (2008). Defining health and unhealthiness: Perceptions held by Native Americans with persistent mental illness. *Mental Health, Religion and Culture, 11*(5), 437–459.

2000 census of the population and housing data paper listing (CPH-L-133). Washington, DC: U.S. Government Printing Office.

Cultural Competence in **Ethical Decision Making**

Dula F. Pacquiao

KEY TERMS

Advance directives
Advocacy
American Nurses Association Code
   of Ethics
Autonomy
Beneficence
Categorical imperatives
Community empowerment and
   partnership
Compassion
Cultural competence
Deontological theory of ethics
Distributive justice
Ethic of care
Ethics
Fidelity
Health disparity/inequity
Health Insurance Portability and
   Accountability Act
Informed consent
Nonmaleficence
Normative ethics
Patient Self-Determination Act
Patients' Bill of Rights
Positive and negative rights
Principle-based ethics
Social justice

(key terms continue on page 404)

LEARNING OBJECTIVES

1. Analyze the moral dilemma underlying health and care disparities.
2. Describe how moral philosophies are socially and culturally constituted.
3. Discuss ethical principles and theories supporting human rights.
4. Differentiate social justice from distributive justice.
5. Describe the Model of Cultural Competent Ethical Decision Making.
6. Use research findings relevant to ethical decision making.

In 2000, the U.S. Department of Health and Human Services (DHHS) established the national goal of eliminating health disparities by launching its Healthy People 2010 initiative. The DHHS and the National Institutes of Health defined **health disparity** as population-specific differences in the burden of disease (incidence, prevalence, and mortality), health outcomes, and access to care (Fink, 2009). Health disparities according to the Institute of Medicine (2002) are "racial or ethnic differences in the quality of health care that are not due to clinical-access factors or clinical needs, preferences or appropriateness of intervention" (p. 32).

Carter-Porras and Baquet (2002) defined health disparity as a "chain of events signified by a difference in: 1) environment, 2) access to, utilization of and quality of care, and 3) health status

K E Y   T E R M S (*continued*)

Truth telling
Universal Declaration of Human Rights
Utilitarianism
Veracity

or a particular health outcome" (p. 427). There is a growing consciousness that differential health status across populations is linked with unequal life conditions external to the individual. Whitehead's (1991) definition of **health inequities** was adopted by the EURO/WHO to mean differences in health, which are not only unnecessary and avoidable but also unfair and unjust. Canada considers 12 factors as determinants of health inclusive of social, cultural, and biologic factors: (1) income and social status, (2) social support networks, (3) education, (4) employment and working conditions, (5) social environments, physical environments, (7) personal health practices and coping skills, (8) healthy child development, (9) biology and genetic endowment, (10) health services, (11) gender, and (12) culture (Federal, Provincial and Territorial Advisory Committee on Population Health, 1999).

Globalization has intensified the awareness that wealthy countries are healthier than poor countries. This is not true, however, with the United States, which is considered the richest country in the world and spends the most on health care at $6,350 per person in 2005. Compared to the 30 developed countries that comprise the Organization of Economic Cooperation and Development (OECD), the United States ranks near the bottom on most standard measures of health status in 2005 (Marmot & Bell, 2009). Among 192 countries in 2004, the United States ranked 46th in average life expectancy and 42nd in infant mortality. One exception was the better life expectancy of individuals from 65 years of age, which possibly reflects access to comprehensive health services through Medicare starting at age 65. The United States is the only developed country without universal health access for all its citizens (Schroeder, 2007).

Pogge (2002) noted that past and present policies of wealthy nations have created and maintained poverty and ill health and, therefore, wealthy nations bear a commensurate responsibility to alleviate these problems. An example is the massive recruitment of health care professionals from third world countries creating a "brain drain" in the sending countries because of the loss of experienced health care practitioners and educators.

Krieger (2008) has argued that societal patterns of disease represent the biologic consequences of life and work conditions of different social groups produced by each society's economic and political priorities. Human beings according to Krieger embody or "incorporate biologically their social and material world throughout their life course from utero to death" (p. 225). The Health Care Reform bill signed by President

Obama excludes payment for abortion except under specific circumstances such as rape, incest, and the like. This exception unduly disadvantages the poor because of their inability to afford this service, which can further place them in poverty because of the caring demands of a growing child preventing gainful employment of the parent, and the burden of supporting an additional family member. Pregnancy during teenage can interfere with educational achievement and earning potential in adulthood.

Studies of racial residential isolation concentrating poor blacks in neighborhoods with overcrowded housing, low-quality health services and schools, violent and polluted environments, and limited availability of affordable healthy foods create cumulative health risks and limited opportunities for economic mobility that perpetuate social and environmental injustices resulting in poor health. Class and racial inequality differentially affect the living standards, working conditions, and environmental exposures of the dominant and subordinated classes, creating class and racial/ethnic health differences. A society's economic, political, and social relationships affect both how the people live and their environment, and shape patterns of disease distribution. Societal distribution of health and illness cannot be separated from a society's political economy and political ecology.

Studies of chronic stress from unrelenting experiences with discrimination, marginalization, and lack of control over one's life circumstances are linked with sustained high levels of cortisol and other stress hormones that increase one's susceptibility to chronic diseases such as hypertension, cardiac disease, diabetes, cancer, and increased incidence of preterm births (Barker, 2007; Shuey & Wilson, 2008; Williams, Costa, Odunlami, & Mohammed, 2008). Poor intrauterine conditions such as increased levels of maternal stress hormones and malnutrition have been correlated with coronary disease in adulthood (Barker). Williams and his associates stressed the importance of addressing upstream factors or social determinants as more significant in improving health than downstream or physical pathologies alone.

Understanding the fundamental causes of poor health facilitates accurate assignment of responsibility and identification of measures to rectify the problem.

The Commission on Social Determinants of Health (CSDH, 2008) recommended these actions to promote health equity: (1) improve the circumstances in which people live throughout their life course, (2) address inequities in distribution of power, wealth, and resources in local and global contexts, and (3) measure the problem, evaluate the action, and expand the knowledge base.

Population-based health and globalization heightened the awareness of existing social inequities that impact on health and fueled the growing mandate for development of cultural competence of health care professionals. **Cultural competence** has a moral agenda to understand the impact of culture on people's lives, respect these cultural differences, and minimize the negative consequences of cultural differences (Pacquiao, 2008). Elimination of health disparities could not occur without culturally competent practitioners but cultural competence alone is not enough in eliminating health inequalities. It requires practice within the framework of social justice and human rights.

Ethics and Health Disparities

The ethos of a free market economy dominates the U.S. health care system where physicians function primarily as free agents, selling their services to patient/consumers, who cushion the potential impact of serious illness by purchasing health insurance through their employers or from out-of-pocket. Catastrophic illness can destroy gainful employment and place patients and their families in poverty. Some 37 million Americans, mostly working people and members of families, have no health insurance and earn just enough to be disqualified from receiving publicly funded medical care (Loewy, 2007). Health care is distributed unevenly and cuts certain groups from accessing preventive and early intervention care they cannot afford that ultimately drives them to the Emergency Room needing extraordinary and exceedingly expensive treatments. The recent health care reform attempts to ameliorate this problem but there are other considerations central to accessing quality and timely health services. Racism, residential segregation, and environmental injustices need to be addressed squarely in order to identify, anticipate, prevent, manage, and remedy their consequences in health and quality of life (Johnstone & Kanisaki, 2008).

A central question is whether there is a right to health for all Americans. Unlike other rights such as the right of speech and religion categorized as negative rights, right to health is a **positive right** or an entitlement that is dependent on a society's willingness and ability to provide. **Negative rights**, on the other hand, protect individuals from interference in their exercise of personal activities or liberties (Loewy, 2007).

The **Universal Declaration of Human Rights** (UDHR, 1948) was based on Kant's work, which emphasized treating every human being with dignity as an end by itself. Human rights aimed to protect the inherent dignity, and equal and inalienable rights of all people. The UDHR was especially focused on the poor, vulnerable, and marginalized populations who are routinely excluded from the benefits and opportunities of the political, economic, and social mainstream. Every individual has a right to a standard of living adequate for health and well-being that includes medical care and other basic necessities like food, clothing, and housing. The right to health is a free-standing human right that is closely linked to many other human rights protection contained in international treaties and domestic constitutions including right to life, nondiscrimination, privacy and freedoms of associations, assembly, and movement. Thus, human rights are universal and indivisible.

Kirch and Vernon (2009) assert that there is a neglect of justice and a lack of a unified theory of justice in the U.S. health care. Although the traditional ethos of medicine has focused on the fundamentals of beneficence, nonmaleficence, individual autonomy, and justice, in the United States, nonmaleficence and autonomy are front and center. Nonmaleficence emphasizes patient safety and autonomy has taken-for-granted respect for individual patient and physician autonomy. Physician autonomy has been aligned with fiscal independence. The American concept of autonomy is based on John Stuart Mill's work on liberty, which is construed as negative freedom, freedom from restraint, to do what everyone wants as long as it does not harm others. By contrast, autonomy according to Kant is based on the integration of freedom and responsibility. Autonomous individuals can adopt moral constraints, and willingly submit to norms to which they have given their consent.

Social justice according to Rawls (Beauchamp & Childress, 2008) has two major requirements. First, people have maximal liberty compatible with same degree of liberty for everyone, thus defining the limits of individual liberty. Second, deliberate inequalities are unjust unless they work to the advantage of the least well-off. Social justice focuses on social consequence and responsibility for actions by the society or the government. The United States, however, is a market-driven economy emphasizing the culture of individualism, entrepreneurial capitalism, and individual responsibility.

Distributive justice is not social justice (Shanley & Asch, 2009). There is a difference between giving all persons equal rights and opportunity within a system of inequity (i.e., distributive justice), and altering the conditions under which inequality or oppression arises (social justice). According to Hofrichter (2003), social justice is "an opposition to inequality and demands an equitable distribution of collective goods, institutional resources and life opportunities. Achieving equality requires not merely redressing or ameliorating inequitable outcomes but creating a society that does not produce material inequality" (p. 12).

Ethical Concepts

A moral philosophy consists of beliefs and assumptions about what is right and wrong. This is the basis of ethics, which prescribes the proper action to take in a given situation. **Ethics** translates moral philosophies into action. **Normative ethics** defines actions that are morally right or wrong. The **American Nurses Association Code of Ethics** and the Canadian Nurses Association Code of Ethics are sets of principles or standards guiding professional nursing practice. They reflect the norms of valued beliefs and ideals in mainstream American and Canadian societies.

The **ethic of care** is drawn from psychologic and feminist theories that emphasizes actions promoting positive relationships with and full understanding of the individual in his or her situational context. Under the ethic of care, practitioners need to develop empathy, compassion, and relationships that promote trust, growth, and well-being. This relationship is significant in caring for the frail and vulnerable individuals who are unable to advocate for themselves. Decisions about withdrawal of life support should take into consideration the individual's particular life context, (e.g., previous life, current situation, and relationships with significant others).

The **deontological theory of ethics** is derived from the work of Immanuel Kant, upholding reason as the basis for morality. Deontologists believe that human beings are duty bound to use reason. Reason yields universally applicable **categorical imperatives** that can be clearly, consistently, and practically used in all situations. Truth telling and respect for individual autonomy are considered intrinsically moral acts.

In contrast, **utilitarianism** is grounded in the belief that the utility or consequence of an action is the only relevant consideration in judging behaviors. Utilitarians believe in the idea of the greatest good for the greatest number. Proponents of utilitarianism such as Jeremy Bentham and John Stuart Mill argued that no action should be judged by itself but rather by its usefulness or end results (Bloch & Green, 2006).

The contrasting perspective between deontology and utilitarianism is illustrated by debate on the use of public funds for abortion. Deontologists believe that preserving human life including that of an embryo/fetus is morally right. Hence, funding abortion that kills the unborn fetus is not ethical. On the other hand, utilitarians believe abortion may be funded in cases of rape or incest to improve the well-being of the woman and prevent psychosocial harm to an unwanted child. Abortion may be mandated to control population growth.

Principle-based ethics or principlism was introduced by Beauchamp and Childress (2001) in an attempt to reconcile the divergence between teleological and deontological models. It links moral decision making on scientific findings rather than universal rules. Principlism is based on the philosophical pragmatism of William James. The principles of **beneficence** and **nonmaleficence** require that care providers act in ways that benefit and cause no harm to consumers of their care. Focusing on patient safety emphasizes prevention of harm. Use of evidence-based practice is aimed to promote the most effective and safe interventions for patients. Some authors believe that beneficence is a much higher level principle as it does not only address prevention of harm but also acting to benefit the patient. A nurse working in the Emergency Room notes increased numbers of patients coming in for diabetic complications. She observes the principle of beneficence by not only addressing their immediate care needs but also contacting the local public health office, churches, and visiting nursing services to organize community programs to prevent and manage diabetes.

The principle of **autonomy** is closely linked with respect for an individual's free will and includes the right to make choices about issues affecting one's being. Autonomous persons should be allowed to determine their own actions or delegate decision making to others when they become incapable of making such decisions. The **Patient Self-Determination Act** of 1991 is a legal protection of a person's autonomy or self-determination in these situations through advance directives. An individual's autonomy is ensured when a nurse provides appropriate information that could enhance the person's ability to make informed decisions about his or her care.

The principle of justice is discussed previously. It relates to the fair, equitable, and appropriate treatment or use of resources in light of what a person needs, weighed against the needs of others. The documents Healthy People 2010 (U.S. Department of Health and Human Services, 2000) and Achieving Health for All: A Framework for Health Promotion (Health Canada, 1986) describe existing disparities in access to health care services and health outcomes among population groups in the United States and Canada.

The principle of **fidelity** is the obligation to remain faithful to one's commitments. Nurses have an obligation to maintain standards of professional practice as a condition of continuing licensure. The principle of **veracity** upholds the virtues of being honest and telling the truth. **Truth telling** is recognized as a prerequisite to a trusting relationship. **Informed consent** requires veracity of information presented to clients and fidelity of practitioners to professional standards.

Contrasting Social Construction of Morality

Morals and philosophic beliefs are constituted within the social, historical, and cultural experiences of a society. These beliefs evolve as normative patterns of assumptions that serve as an implicit framework guiding the actions and thoughts of group members, which may or may not be shared by persons outside of the cultural group.

One of the most common sources of ethical conflicts in health care is rooted in the contrasting conceptualization of human beings in the Western and non-Western cultures. In Western cultures, there is a pervasive belief that human beings are endowed with the capacity for reason and action. Because reason is a universal capacity for all humans, it is through reason that humans can be expected to make valid and truthful judgments in any situations. The philosophic traditions of universalism and rationalism have shaped the Western concept of the person as the focus of moral reasoning. The person is the basic unit imbued with universal capacity for reason and action. Differences are attributed to deficits in cognitive skills, motivation, information, and/or linguistic tools. Approaches to ethical dilemmas, therefore, are based on the belief that by compensating for these deficits, a person can be expected to make a rational decision that is universally regarded as logical and morally acceptable.

However, not all human behaviors can be classified as simply rational or irrational. Culture can be arbitrary, and human beings create their own distinctive, symbolic realities. Many of our ideas and practices are beyond logic and experience. In some groups, religious and spiritual dimensions highly influence behaviors. Among such ethnoreligious groups as devout Muslims, Hindus, and Jews, religion is embedded in everyday life. Decisions about euthanasia, for example, may not be acceptable to an Orthodox Jew whose beliefs uphold the sanctity of life. Jews generally consult their rabbi regarding matters pertaining to life and death decisions (see Figure 14-1). Religion increases the awareness of the power and benevolence of God over humans; hence, earthly decisions are left to God, and the attitude is one of acceptance of fate rather than control over one's destiny.

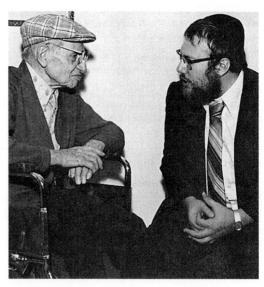

FIGURE 14-1 Consultation with a rabbi.

Members of Jehovah's Witnesses oppose blood transfusion as a lifesaving measure, contradicting the logic of scientific reasoning. Similarly, Christian Scientists may prefer their own religious and spiritually based practices of healing to those of scientific medicine.

Organ donation may be considered heroic in the biomedical profession and mainstream American culture. Religious, historical, and cultural influences may prevent other groups from becoming an organ donor. African Americans may be hesitant to become an organ donor because of past and present experiences that built a collective sense of mistrust of the health care system and health professionals (see Evidence-Based Practice 14-1). Cultural practices such as female circumcision, body piercing and tattooing, and taking home a newborn's afterbirth appear illogical and without any scientific basis. Yet these practices are supported by value–belief

systems that are deeply entrenched in religious, philosophical, and social structure of certain groups. To professional practitioners, resistance to valid and scientifically proven measures belies common sense, but cultural traditions of some groups transcend rationality and logic. Indeed, common sense is not common after all; it is uniquely constructed within the social and cultural life contexts of human groups.

Another common source of moral conflict stems from contrasting views of a person between Western and non-Western cultures. In the West, individualism is the norm; the person is viewed as a self-contained entity, fully integrated and self-motivating, independent of social roles and relationships, and distinct from all others. In contrast, among collectivistic cultures there is greater continuity and mutuality among group members. The Xhosa tribe in South Africa emphasizes collective decisions where tribal elders make major

EVIDENCE-BASED PRACTICE 14-1

Trust, Mistrust, and Satisfaction of Care Among African American Patients

A descriptive-correlational study of a convenience sample of 100 middle-aged and older community-dwelling adults to analyze the relationships between cultural mistrust, medical mistrust, and racial identity, and predict patient satisfaction with care by nurse practitioners. The study used five instruments: *Cultural Mistrust Inventory, Group based Medical Mistrust Scale, Black Racial Identity Attitude Scale, Trust in Provider Scale,* and the *Michigan Consortium Patient Satisfaction Questionnaire.* Correlations and stepwise multiple regressions were used to analyze the data. Findings included moderate cultural mistrust of European American providers and mistrust of the health care system, and high levels of trust and satisfaction with their nurse

practitioners. Study showed strong potential for nurse practitioners to overcome cultural mistrust among African American adults.

Clinical Application

1. Identify the factors that contributed to the mistrust of Euro-American practitioners by African American patients.
2. Describe ways by which non-African American nurses can establish trust and promote satisfaction with care by their African American patients.
3. Identify the ethical principles violated when a Euro-American nurse interprets the preference for racially concordant practitioners by African American patients as discriminatory.

Reference: Benkert, R., Hollie, B., Nordstrom, C. K., Wickson, B., & Bins-Emerick, L. (2009). Trust, mistrust, racial identity and patient satisfaction in urban African-American primary care patients of nurse practitioners. *Journal of Nursing Scholarship, 41*(2), 211–219.

decisions about the distribution of human and material resources to provide care for their members (see Figure 14-2). Members of collective cultures expect physical presence of family members who are dying or seriously ill (see Evidence-Based Practice 14-2). Numbers of family members present generally exceed the norm for visitation in most hospitals.

Family and kinship patterns assign different roles, status, and power among group members. The social hierarchy governs decision making, interactions, roles, and obligations of members. Whereas Western health care providers value the individual's autonomy in decision making, filial piety and respect for the authority of one's elders are the guiding principles among traditional Asian cultures in making decisions about care. Influenced by the Confucian ethic, the Korean culture accepts inherent social inequality among family members as a condition for achieving collective harmony. By contrast, the Western value of instrumental individualism prizes the ability of individuals to make choices and rely upon themselves to achieve their purpose in life. Although a traditional Chinese adult relies upon family members and the physician to make decisions, a typical American or Canadian adult expects to be given information so he or she can make a decision.

Respect for patient autonomy has become the focal context for health care decisions in the

---

EVIDENCE-BASED PRACTICE 14-2

Perception by Critical Care Unit Nurses of Family Presence During Resuscitation

This study used a descriptive, qualitative online survey of Canadian critical care nurses to identify issues regarding family presence during resuscitation (FPDR) of adult family members. Two hundred and forty-two of the total 450 nurses who completed the online survey responded to the qualitative portion of the survey regarding FPDR. Content analysis and constant comparison techniques were used to analyze the data and derive the following themes. Nurses perceived both benefits and risks of FPDR for family members and the health care team. Presence afforded family members to see that everything possible was done; they are able to provide emotional support and say good-bye to their family members. Potential psychological trauma and physical harm to family members during the procedure were identified as risks. FPDR provides health team members the opportunity to see the patient as part of a family and facilitates family acceptance of decision to discontinue resuscitation. However, nurses were concerned that family members may view the health team as inadequate with consequent professional liabilities; they also feel that family members may constrain them from using humor to defuse their anxiety. Family members unable to cope with the crisis can distract health team members from their job in order to attend to the family members' needs.

Clinical Application

1. Identify ethical and legal issues that can arise when health care professionals do not allow FPDR.
2. Describe policies and organizational arrangements that could enhance effective of FPDR.
3. Identify cultural groups that can benefit from an FPDR policy.

Reference: McClement, S. E., Fallis, W. M., & Pereira, A. (2009). Family presence during resuscitation: Canadian critical care nurses' perspectives. *Journal of Nursing Scholarship, 41*(3), 233–240.

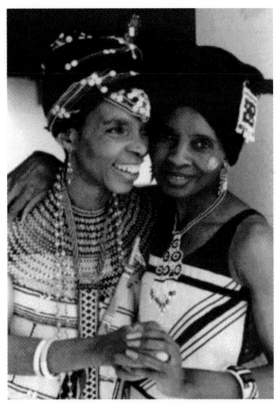

FIGURE 14-2 Women of the South African Xhosa tribe at a wedding of a family member. (Courtesy of Beatrice Mabutho)

United States and Canada. Ethical principles are applied to ensure and maximize individual autonomy. The autonomy paradigm, which has been institutionalized in health care, underlines interactions with and expectations of patients and families by practitioners. The Patient Self Determination Act of 1991 mandates health care practitioners to provide clients with information about advance directives. **Advance directives** are intended to assure patients' autonomy in situations when they can no longer make a decision. Individuals' choices are presumably carried out on their behalf in the event that they cannot consciously and competently represent their own will. Although the intent of advance directives is laudable within the Western ethos of self-determination, other cultures subscribe

to the belief that the fate of human beings is beyond their control.

The **Health Insurance Portability and Accountability Act** ensures confidentiality of an individual's health information. Health care practitioners are required to seek the patient's informed consent before any information is shared with others, including family members. This poses difficulty for collectivistic groups where family members decide which information is shared with the patient and other family members. The tension between managed care and individual rights to choose and seek redress for infractions of these rights created a long-drawn-out debate on the **Patients' Bill of Rights** in the U.S. Congress. It struck the core of individual rights versus limiting these rights to give cost-effective care to more people.

The concept of individual autonomy brings an associated expectation of individual responsibility and accountability. This creates a predilection to reward self-care and label those individuals as noncompliant when they do not adhere to prescribed biomedical regimen. Health professionals tend to ignore social factors that hinder an individual patient's ability to act on health teaching and prescribed regimen (see Evidence-Based Practice 14-3). Because the focus of care is on individual responsibility and accountability, vulnerable groups tend to avoid seeking medical help unless they are desperately ill or selectively act on parts of the regimen that they have the capacity and resources to implement.

Model for Culturally Competent Ethical Care

Globalization has heightened the need for health professionals to have a worldwide perspective and assume an ethical–moral obligation to enter and function in a worldwide community (Leininger & McFarland, 2006). Health professionals need to have world citizenship skills (Pacquiao, 2008) such as the ability to critically evaluate one's self and one's own cultural traditions. Critical self-reflection

EVIDENCE-BASED PRACTICE 14-3

Political and Economic Contexts of Self-Management of Diabetes Mellitus Among Mexican Americans

This is a study of the political and economic dimensions of diabetes self-management among low-income Mexican adults, using critical ethnographic analysis of focus group data from forty participants (20 caregivers at home and 20 diabetic patients) in one community health center clinic. Thematic findings included (1) self-management involved management of physical, mental, and emotional symptoms as well as food control; other life stresses compounded problems of disease management; (2) family and neighborhood environments posed barriers to self-management of diabetes mellitus; the home environment and access to basic necessities as food and shelter compounded difficulty in disease-management; (3) hassles of the health care environment such as access to medications, Medicaid protocols, and the like were stressful to participants.

Clinical Application

1. Analyze why the paradigm of self-care and self-reliance fails to address the problem of these patients.
2. Describe the features of an effective plan to enhance self-management of diabetes by poor Mexican Americans.
3. Identify the ethical principles violated when nurses focus solely on disease and ignore the sociopolitical contexts in teaching patients in self-management of their chronic condition.

Reference: Clark, L., Vincent, D., Zimmer, L., & Sanchez, J. (2009). Cultural values and political economic contexts of diabetes among low-income Mexican Americans. *Journal of Transcultural Nursing, 20*(4), 382–394.

examines one's own beliefs and practices to determine reasonable support for personal beliefs rather than accept them as absolute truths. Another skill is the ability to see the equality of humanity in order to develop a genuine concern and commitment to the welfare of all persons. Lastly, one needs to have the ability to see the world from the point of view of the other. Understanding and feeling the distress of another provides the impetus for the desire to help.

Figure 14-3 presents the model for culturally competent ethical decisions. The model emphasizes the universal core ethical principles of advocacy for social justice and protection of human rights. Social justice is doing what is best for a person or group based on their needs and the fundamental principle that human beings have inalienable rights. Social justice implies that because of certain conditions that increase risks to a person or group compromising their capacity to self-advocate and access to life with

quality, actions of health care professionals should not only be non-malevolent (doing no harm), but most significantly do what benefits the care recipients (beneficent). Social justice is central to advocating for elimination of health disparities by ensuring the basic human right

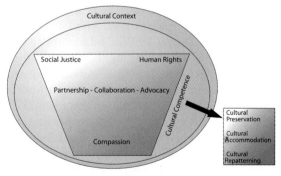

FIGURE 14-3 Model for cultural competent ethical decision.

to access quality health care. Social justice and human rights principles are necessary conditions for each other thus, fundamentally complementary. The human rights principle shifts accountability and responsibility to the government and society and do not rest solely on the individual. Right to health is a right of citizenship and is a shared responsibility by the society and the individual. Assuring the right to health care becomes a moral obligation of society and not just the individual and/or his/her family alone.

Cultural competent care for vulnerable populations is achieved by commitment to both principles. Cultural competence imposes attention to the contextual reality in which social justice and human rights protection are pursued. For example, if the right to health is guaranteed, how much health care is equitable and just? The United States being a rich country can certainly provide much more quality health care for its citizens than a third world country. Cultural competence also builds the assurance that actions are informed by the valued premises of society and the situated environment of the people. The pursuit of social justice and human rights protection should not endanger the lives of the people one is advocating for. People's rights may be compromised during wars, famine, etc. Advocacy should take into consideration the social and environmental realities of time and space. Although the principle of social justice and human rights are universal, these concepts evolve from human conditions in specific contexts. Hence, there is need to apply these concepts in a culturally competent fashion.

Advocacy for social justice and human rights, require collaborative partnerships with individuals, families and communities. It involves partnership between the national and local government, health care workers, local communities and nongovernmental organizations. It is a multisectoral partnership that attends to the whole spectrum of keeping people healthy from preventive to rehabilitative services. It promotes maximum **community empowerment** and individual self-reliance and participation in the planning, organization, operation, and control. It involves

people locally, empowering them to advocate for themselves by influencing policies and programs and monitoring that social justice is applied. The community becomes a real partner in health achievement by building community solidarity and social cohesion for effective networks (Gargioni & Raviglione, 2009).

Community partnership for social justice and human rights protection can be achieved at so many levels. Entry-level nurses can develop a comprehensive knowledge of the communities in which they live and work. Assessing the strengths and challenges of these communities is important in focusing the partnership between the health care organizations in which they work and their communities. All nurses can make referrals to other organizations and services. Participation in organizational committees targeted towards community development and partnership building is a good vehicle for involvement. Nurses can also participate in influencing health and social policies impacting on the community through their professional organizations, churches, parent-teacher organizations and municipal boards. Communicating with legislators and political leaders is another venue for advocacy.

The force that moves individuals and groups towards advocacy for social justice and human rights protection is compassion. **Compassion** is the critical motivation that compels people to act on behalf of others which emerges from an affective and cognitive understanding and identification with others' experiences. It is the fire that ignites the energy to take on actions on problems involving enormous risks, complexities and resources. Compassion requires the ability to distinguish the oppressed from the oppressor, victims from perpetuators, and the disadvantaged from the powerful. Compassion is the commitment to go beyond the purview of one's own perspectives and affiliations. It is beyond cultural desire (Campinha-Bacote, 2007) as it moves the person to action.

Compassionate actions need to be culturally congruent and competent otherwise advocating social justice for one group may bring consequent disenfranchisement of others. Culturally competent compassion is immersed in balancing the rights of the vulnerable with those of others. Culturally competent action modes according to Leininger (2002) are embedded in cultural preservation, accommodation, and repatterning. One or all three modes of action may be used simultaneously or in a continuum of actions.

Cultural preservation maintains the core values, beliefs, and practices significant to the individual or group. Cultural accommodations negotiates with existing cultural differences in order to find a meaningful existence of one's cultural life ways with those of others. Cultural repatterning attempts to help individuals and groups change their way of life to achieve a healthy, safe and meaningful existence.

Model Applications

Case I: The recent mandate for all health care workers to be vaccinated against the H1N1 virus has created uproar in some who claimed that they will expose themselves and their families to unnecessary risks. Some questioned the effectiveness of the vaccine against the virus. The dilemma demonstrated an ethical conflict between individual rights and public health protection. Childress et al. (2002) proposed certain conditions when public health mandate can superimpose individual right to autonomy. First is the concept of effectiveness of the measure. Second, is the proportionality of the mandate in terms of public good versus individual right. Third is the concept of necessity that was prompted by the threat of an epidemic and mounting deaths. Fourth is whether the mandate creates least infringement so policies regarding availability and accessibility of services to be provided if the individual gets sick should be arranged. Fifth is the public justification such as existence of the threat in the locality and lack of more efficacious treatment available.

The application of cultural maintenance and preservation of individual rights can be fostered by building consensus (Buchanan, 2008). This is extremely important in the United States, which is a country steeped in individual autonomy. Cultural negotiation and repatterning can be applied by using the media, health experts, and patients in disseminating information to build consensus. Organizations can build consensus by conducting town meetings with their employees to address concerns and focus on building common ground.

Public health ethics can contribute to human rights by: (a) reinforcing the normative claims of international human rights law, (b) strengthening advocacy for human rights, and (c) bridging the divide between public health practitioners and human rights advocates in contemporary health sectors. Human rights can also contribute to public health ethics by contributing to the discourse on determinants of health through: (a) definitions of the right to health and the notion of the indivisibility of rights, (b) emphasis on duties of states to progressively realize the health of citizens, and (c) recognition of the protection of human rights as itself a determinant of health (Nixon & Forman, 2008).

Case II: A 19-year-old Black Caribbean male is admitted for abdominal and back pain secondary to a sickle cell crisis. He has had a history of frequent hospitalizations for pain relief. The physician ordered intravenous fluids and Demerol 100 mg every 4 hours for pain prn. The patient has been complaining that what the doctor ordered was not enough and nurses ignored his complaints. He uses abusive language with the nursing staff. Most of the nurses believe he is addicted to narcotics and will not give any pain medication before the fourth hour. They also refuse to call the physician because he also believes that the patient is drug-dependent and consistently ignores the patient's request for change of medication.

The paternalistic attitudes of the nurses and the physician create additional suffering on the part of the patient. Assumptions that need to be uncovered are the health professionals' attitudes towards race, age, and narcotics. Racial stereotypes can lead to discriminatory and unfair treatment of the patient. In this situation, the patient needs pain relief, not rehabilitation from drug dependence. The history of frequent admission could be attributed to factors external to the individual such as frequent infections due to overcrowded environment, chronic stress from absenteeism and inability to participate in normal developmental activities, lack of knowledge of disease management, and lack of access to preventive care, and so on. Without a comprehensive understanding of the social, personal, and individual behavioral factors that contribute to frequent hospitalization, nurses hold the individual solely responsible for his disease exacerbations. Advocacy for social justice and individual right to pain relief should move caregivers toward bracketing their own personal attributions of the patient's condition. Partnering with the patient and his family, the school and employer can provide some insights that can make a difference to his health and chronic disease management. Health professionals need to repattern their thinking, and use accommodation by working with the patient and his family along with the physician in creating an effective care service delivery in and out of the hospital. Cultural preservation can occur when there is a full appreciation of the patient's personhood and suffering. Advocacy requires compassionate understanding of his situation by listening to his lived experience.

SUMMARY

Strategies in facilitating the transformation of the individual's compassion to action are centered on collaboration, partnership, and advocacy. Collaborative partnership with patients/families and communities is built on mutual understanding and empathy. Listening to the stories of patients and families and knowing their social and environmental contexts can sensitize caregivers to the subjective and highly personal construction of their experiences. This encounter develops empathy for the person's suffering and facilitates a full understanding of the person as a human being.

Repeated cultural encounters enhance the health care professionals' ability in demonstrating attentiveness, genuine concern, presence, warmth, and empathy. Clinical encounters with diversity are found to be significant in developing cultural proficiency and effectiveness (Pacquiao, 2007). Community involvement and immersion in diverse communities create the appropriate context for partnership, collaboration, and compassionate understanding.

Health care providers need experience in caring especially for vulnerable populations locally or abroad. Experience with organizations and advocacy groups such as local churches, the Red Cross, homeless shelters, Doctors without Borders, and other opportunities can build the skills for culturally competent ethical thinking. Awareness of resources locally, nationally, and globally promote access to and development of more comprehensive services. Building collaborative partnerships with organizations and communities is important as vulnerable populations have complex, multiple needs that are both simultaneous and evolving.

Partnerships allow sharing of resources, services, and best practices across local, national, and global contexts. Service learning is an excellent opportunity for nursing students to learn about organizations and the communities they serve. Strengthening the community health nursing experience in the curriculum sensitizes students to public health issues and social inequities affecting population health.

REVIEW QUESTIONS

1. Describe ethical dilemmas associated with the current state of population health and care disparities.
2. Discuss the cultural underpinnings supporting pros and cons of health care reform in the United States.
3. Analyze the reasoning behind the differences in health access and outcomes between the populations of the United States and Canada.
4. Explain how the principles of social justice and human rights protection reduce health disparities.

CRITICAL THINKING ACTIVITIES

Identify an example of an ethical dilemma that you have encountered at work. Note that ethical dilemmas occur more frequently in clinical situations. For some of them, you may need some time to think before making a decision on your own, whereas other decisions are more complex and need referral to the ethics committee of the organization.

Identify the particulars of the situation:

1. Who are the people involved?
2. What is the setting?
3. How do different individuals or groups perceive the problem?
4. Identify conflicting values and beliefs at the individual, organizational, and societal levels that influence perceptions.
5. What assessment data about the situation are missing?
6. How can additional information be obtained?
7. Using the Model of Cultural Competent Ethical Decision Making, how would you redefine the problem?
8. What culturally congruent strategies do you recommend?

BIOETHICS RESOURCES

1. **Biomedical Ethics Unit**
   McGill University General Information
   James Administration Building
   845 Sherbrooke Street West
   Montreal, Quebec H3A 2T5
   Phone: (514) 398-6980
   Fax: (514) 398-8349
   http://www.mcgill.ca

2. **Boston University School of Public Health**
   Department of Health Law, Bioethics and Human Rights
   715 Albany Street
   Boston, MA 02118
   Phone: (617) 638-5300
   http://www.bumc.bu.edu

3. **Center for Medical Ethics and Health Policy**
   Baylor College of Medicine
   One Baylor Plaza
   Houston, TX 77030
   Phone: (713) 798-4951
   Fax: (713) 798-5678
   http://www.bcm.edu/ethics

4. **Cleveland State University**
   The Bioethics Center
   College of Liberal Arts & Social Sciences
   2121 Euclid Avenue, RT 1655
   Cleveland, OH 44115-2214
   Phone: (216) 687-9255
   Fax: (216) 523-7482
   http://www.csuohio.edu/class/bioethics/

5. **Columbia University**
   Center for Bioethics
   College of Physicians and Surgeons
   630 West 168th Street, 3rd Floor,
       Suite 3-470
   New York, NY 10032
   Phone: (212) 342-0452
   Fax: (212) 342-0451
   http://www.bioethicscolumbia.org

6. **Dalhousie University**
   Health Law Institute
   6061 University Avenue
   Halifax, Nova Scotia B3H 4H9
   Phone: (902) 494-6881
   Fax: (902) 494-6879
   http://hli.law.dal.ca

7. **Emory University**
   Emory Center for Ethics

1531 Dickey Drive
Atlanta, GA 30322
Phone: (404) 727-4954
http://ethics.emory.edu

8. **Georgetown University**
Joseph and Rose Kennedy Institute of Ethics
Healy, 4th Floor
Washington, DC 20057
Phone: (202) 687-8099
Fax: (202) 687-8089
http://kennedyinstitute.georgetown.edu

9. **Harvard University**
The Harvard University Program in Ethics and
    Health
641 Huntington Avenue
Boston, MA 02115
Phone: (617) 432-5950
Fax: (617) 432-3721
http://peh.harvard.edu

10. **Indiana University**
Center for Bioethics
410 W 10th Street-Suite 3100
Indianapolis, IN 46202
Phone: (317) 278-4034
Fax: (317) 278-4050
http://www.bioethics.iu.edu

11. **Indiana University**
Association for Practical and
    Professional Ethics
618 East Third Street
Bloomington, IN 47405-3602
Phone: (812) 855-6450
Fax: (812) 856-4969
http://www.indiana.edu

12. **Indiana University Bloomington**
Poynter Center for the Study of Ethics and
    American Institutions
618 East Third Street
Bloomington, IN 47405-3862
Phone: (812) 855-0261
Fax: (812) 855-3315
http://poynter.indiana.edu

13. **Johns Hopkins**
Berman Institute of Bioethics Seminar Series
201 North Charles–Suite 1701
Baltimore, MD 21201
Phone: (410) 625-7865

Fax: (410) 625-7877
http://www.bioethicsinstitute.org

14. **Loyola University Chicago Stritch School of
Medicine**
The Neiswanger Institute for Bioethics and
    Health Policy
2160 S. First Avenue
Bldg. 120, Room 280
Maywood, IL 60153
Phone: (708) 327-9200
Fax: (708) 327-9209
http://bioethics.lumc.edu

15. **Michigan State University**
Center for Ethics and Humanities in the Life
    Sciences
C-208 East Fee Hall
East Lansing, MI 48824-1316
Phone: (517) 355-7550
Fax: (517) 353-3289
http://www.bioethics.msu.edu

16. **National Institutes of Health**
Department of Bioethics
10 Center Drive
Building 10, Room 1C118
Bethesda, MD 20892-1156
Phone: (301) 496-2429
Fax: (301) 496-0760
http://www.bioethics.nih.gov/home/
    index.shtml

17. **Stanford School of Medicine**
Stanford University Center for Biomedical Ethics
701 Welch Road
Building A, Suite 1105
Palo Alto, CA 94304
Phone: (650) 723-5760
Fax: (650) 725-6131
http://bioethics.stanford.edu

18. **State University of New York**
SUNY Upstate Medical University
Center for Bioethics and Humanities
618 Irving Avenue
Syracuse, NY 13210
Phone: (315) 464-5404
http://www.upstate.edu/bioethics

19. **The University of Texas Southwestern Medical
Center at Dallas**
The Program in Ethics in Science & Medicine

5323 Harry Hines Boulevard
Dallas, TX 75390
Phone: (214) 648-3111
http://www8.utsouthwestern.edu/utsw/cda

20. **University of British Columbia**
The W. Maurice Young Centre for Applied Ethics
227–6356 Agricultural Road
Vancouver, BC V6T 1Z2
Phone: (604) 822-8625
Fax: (604) 822-8627
http://www.ethics.ubc.ca

21. **University of Buffalo**
Center for Clinical Ethics and Humanities in
    Health Care
Veteran's Affairs Medical Center
3495 Bailey Avenue
Buffalo, NY 14215
Phone: (716) 862-8530
Fax: (716) 862-8533
http://wings.buffalo.edu/faculty/research/bioethics/

22. **University of Chicago**
MacLean Center for Clinical Medical Ethics
5841 S. Maryland Avenue
MC 6098
Chicago, IL 60637
Phone: (773) 702-1453
Fax: (773) 702-0090
http://medicine.uchicago.edu/centers

23. **University of Houston**
Health Law & Policy Institute
100 Law Center Houston
Houston, TX 77204-6060
Phone: (713) 743-2101
http://www.law.uh.edu/healthlaw

24. **University of Miami**
UM Ethics Programs
P.O. Box 016960
(M-825)
Miami, FL 33101
Phone: (305) 243-5723
Fax: (305) 243-6416
http://www6.miami.edu/ethics

25. **University of Michigan Medical School**
Bioethics Program
300 North Ingalls Street
7D20
Ann Arbor, MI 48109-5429

Phone: (734) 936-5222
Fax: (734) 936-8944
http://www.med.umich.edu/bioethics

26. **University .of Minnesota**
Center for Bioethics
N504 Boynton
410 Church St. SE
Minneapolis, MN 55455
Phone: (612) 624-9440
Fax: (612) 624-9108
http://www.ahc.umn.edu/bioethics

27. **University of North Carolina of Chapel Hill**
Parr Center for Ethics
Department of Philosophy
207 Caldwell Hall
Chapel Hill, NC 27599-3125
Phone: (919) 843-5641
Fax: (919) 962-3329
http://parrcenter.unc.edu

28. **University of Pennsylvania**
Center for Bioethics
3401 Market Street
Suite 320
Philadelphia, PA 19104-3308
Phone: (215) 898-7136
Fax: (215) 573-3036
http://www.bioethics.upenn.edu

29. **University of Pittsburgh**
Center for Bioethics and Health Law
3708 Fifth Avenue
Medical Arts Building, Ste 300
Pittsburgh, PA 15213-3405
Phone: (412) 647-5700
Fax: (412) 647-5877
http://www.bioethics.pitt.edu

30. **University of Toronto**
Joint Centre for Bioethics
155 College Street
Suite 754
Toronto, ON M5T 1P8
Phone: (416) 978-2709
Fax: (416) 978-1911
http://www.jointcentreforbioethics.ca

31. **University of Utah School of Medicine**
Division of Medical Ethics and Humanities
75 South 2000 East #108
Salt Lake City, UT 84132

Phone: (801) 587-7170
Fax: (801) 587-5884
http://medicine.utah.edu/internalmedicine/medi-
calethics

32. **University of Washington School of Medicine**
Department of Bioethics and Humanities
UW Mailbox 357120
Seattle, WA 98195
Phone: (206) 685-7515
http://depts.washington.edu/bioethx

33. **Center for Practical Bioethics**
Harzfeld Building
1111 Main Street
Suite 500
Kansas City, MO 64105-2116
Phone: (800) 344-3829
Fax: (816) 221-2002
http://www.practicalbioethics.org

34. **Medical College of Wisconsin**
Center for the Study of Bioethics
8701 Watertown Plank Road
Milwaukee, WI 53226
Phone: (414) 456-8498
Fax: (414) 456-6511
http://www.mcw.edu/bioethics

35. **Case Western Reserve University**
Department of Bioethics
School of Medicine, TA200
10900 Euclid Avenue
Cleveland, OH 44106-4976
Phone: (216) 368-6196
Fax: (216) 368-8713
http://www.case.edu/med/bioethics

36. **Cleveland Clinic**
Department of Bioethics
9500 Euclid Avenue
Cleveland, OH 44195
Phone: (216) 444-8720
Fax: (216) 444-9275
http://www.clevelandclinic.org./bioethics

37. **The National Catholic Bioethics Center**
6399 Drexel Road
Philadelphia, PA 19151
Phone: (215) 877-2660
Fax: (215) 877-2688
http://www.ncbcenter.org

38. **Tuskegee University National Center for**
Bioethics in Research & Health Care
Tuskegee University
44-107 John A. Andrew Building
Tuskegee, AL 36088
Phone: (334) 724-4554
Fax: (334) 727-7221
http://www.tuskegee.edu

39. **East Carolina University**
The Bioethics Center
University Health Systems of East Carolina
East Fifth Street
Greenville, NC 27858-4354
Phone: (252) 328-6131
http://www.ecu.edu/bioethics

40. **The Hastings Center**
21 Malcolm Gordon Road
Garrison, NY 10524-4125
Phone: (845) 424-4040
Fax: (845) 424-4545
http://www.thehastingscenter.org

REFERENCES

Barker, D. J. P. (2007). The origins of the developmental origins theory. *Journal of Internal Medicine, 261*, 412–417.

Beauchamp, T., & Childress, J. (2001). *Principles of biomedical ethics* (5th ed.). New York: Oxford University Press.

Beauchamp, T. L., & Childress, I. F. (2008). *Principles of biomedical ethics* (6th ed). New York: Oxford University Press.

Benkert, R., Hollie, B., Nordstrom, C. K., Wickson, B., & Bins-Emerick, L. (2009). Trust, mistrust, racial identity and patient satisfaction in urban African-American primary care patients of nurse practitioners. *Journal of Nursing Scholarship, 41*(2), 211–219.

Bloch, S., & Green, S. A. (2006). An ethical framework for psychiatry. *British Journal of Psychiatry, 188*(1), 7–12.

Buchanan, D. R. (2008). Autonomy, paternalism, and justice: Ethical priorities in public health. *American Journal of Public Health, 98*(1), 15–21.

Campinha-Bacote, J. (2007). *The process of cultural competence in the delivery of healthcare services* (5th ed.). Ohio: Transcultural C.A.R.E. Associates Press. http://www.transculturalcare.net/Resources.htm. Accessed July 22, 2007.

Carter-Porras, O., & Baquet, C. (September–October 2002). What is a health disparity? *Public Health Reports, 117*, 426–434.

Childress, J. R., Faden, R. R, Gaare, R. D., Gostin, L. O., Kahn, J., Bonnie, R. J., et al. (2002). Public health ethics: Mapping the terrain. *Journal of Law and Medical Ethics, 30*, 170–178.

Clark, L., Vincent, D., Zimmer, L., & Sanchez, J. (2009). Cultural values and political economic contexts of diabetes among low-income Mexican Americans. *Journal of Transcultural Nursing, 20*(4), 382–394.

Commission on Social Determinants of Health. (2008). *Final report: Closing the gap in a generation: Equity through action on social determinants of health.* Geneva, Switzerland: WHO.

Department of Health and Human Services, HRSA. (2000). *Eliminating health disparities in the U.S.* Rockville, MD: Author.

Federal, Provincial and Territorial Advisory Committee on Population Health. (1999). *Towards a healthy future: Second report on health of Canadians.* Ministry of Public Works and Government Services, Canada.

Fink, A. M. (2009). Toward a definition of health disparity: A concept analysis. *Journal of Transcultural Nursing, 20*(4), 349–357.

Gargioni, I., & Raviglione, M. (2009). The principles of primary health care and social justice. *Journal of Medical Perspectives, 7*, 103–105.

Health Canada. (1986). *Achieving health for all: A framework for health promotion.* Retrieved on April 19, 2011, from http://www.hc-sc.gc.ca

Hofrichter, R. (2003). The politics of health inequalities. In R. Hofrichter (Ed.). *Health and social justice* (pp. 1–53). San Francisco, CA: Jossey-Bass.

Institute of Medicine. (2002). *Unequal treatment: Confronting racial and ethnic disparities in health care.* Washington, DC: National Academies Press.

Johnstone, M. J., & Kanisaki, O. (November 18, 2008). The neglect of racism as an ethical issue in health care. *Journal of Immigrant and Minority Health.* Retrieved on March 26, 2007, from http://www.springerlink.com/content/e7x52214r3172021/fulltext.pdf

Kirch, D. G., & Vernon, D. J. (2009). The ethical foundation of American medicine: In search of social justice. *Journal of American Medical Association, 301* (14), 1482–1484.

Krieger, N. (2008). Proximal, distal, and the politics of causation: What's level got to do with it? *American Journal of Public Health, 98*(2), 221–230.

Leininger, M. (2002). Transcultural nursing and globalization of healthcare: Importance, focus and historical aspects. In M. Leininger and M. McFarland, *Transcultural nursing concepts, theories, research and practice* (3rd ed., pp. 3–44). New York: McGraw Hill.

Leininger, M. M., & McFarland, M. R. (2006). *Culture care diversity and universality, a worldwide nursing theory* (2nd ed.). Boston, MA: Jones and Bartlett.

Loewy, E. H. (2007). Ethics and evidence-based medicine Is there a conflict? *Medscape General Medicine, 9*(3), 30–43.

Marmot, M. G., & Bell, R. (2009). Action on health disparities in the U.S.: Commission on Social Determinants of Health. *The Journal of the American Medical Association, 301*(11), 1169–1171.

McClement, S. E., Fallis, W. M., & Pereira, A. (2009). Family presence during resuscitation: Canadian critical care nurses' perspectives. *Journal of Nursing Scholarship, 41*(3), 233–240.

Nixon, S., & Forman, L. (2008). Exploring synergies between human rights and public health ethics. *BMC International Health and Human Rights, 8*, 2–11.

Pacquiao, D. F. (2007). The relationship between cultural competence education and increasing diversity in nursing schools and practice settings. *Journal of Transcultural Nursing, 18*(1), 28S–37S.

Pacquiao, D. F. (March 2008). Nursing care for vulnerable populations using a framework of cultural competence, social justice and human rights. *Contemporary Nurse, 28*(1–2), 189–197.

Pogge, T. W. (2002). Responsibilities for poverty-related ill health. *Ethics and International Affairs, 16*, 71–79.

Schroeder, S. A. (2007). We can do better—Improving the health of the American people. *New England Journal of Medicine, 357*, 1221–1228.

Shanley, M. L., & Asch, A. (2009). Involuntary childlessness, reproductive technology, and social justice: The medical mask on social illness. *Journal of Women in Culture and Society, 34*(4), 851–874.

Shuey, K. M., & Wilson, A. E. (2008). Cumulative disadvantages and black-white disparities in life-course health trajectories. *Research on Aging, 30*(2), 200–225.

Universal Declaration of Human Rights. (1948). *Universal declaration of human rights* (Vol. 71). Rep. No. GA RES 217(III). UN GAOR, 3rd Session, Suppl. No. 13 UN Doc A/910.

Whitehead, M. (1991). *The concepts and principles of equity and health.* Copenhagen: WHO/EURO.

Williams, D. R., Costa, M. V., Odunlami, A. O., & Mohammed, S. A. (November 2008). Moving upstream: How interventions that address social determinants of health can improve health and reduce disparities. *Journal of Public Health Management Practice, 14*(Suppl.), S8–S17.

Perspectives on International Nursing

Paula Herberg

KEY TERMS

Development aid
Development aid organizations
International Council of Nurses
International health
International nursing
Millennium Development Goals
Nongovernmental organizations
(NGOs)
Pan American Health Organization
(PAHO)
UN High Commissioner for
Refugees
United Nations Development
Program
World Health Organization (WHO)

LEARNING OBJECTIVES

1. Identify health issues from a global perspective (Millennium Development Goals).
2. Outline the services provided by international health/development aid organizations.
3. Discuss the role of international nursing and midwifery services.
4. Identify the parameters and challenges of international nursing as a career specialty.
5. Identify ways that nurses can prepare for international nursing.
6. Explore criteria for nurses to consider when choosing an international "sending" agency.
7. Identify selected health care agencies that send U.S. and Canadian nurses abroad.

Throughout this text, the emphasis has been largely on U.S. and Canadian cultures and subcultures. This chapter will provide a more global perspective and focus on the work that is done in the international arena to promote human development and health. The chapter will highlight the field of international nursing and the ways in which nurses from the United States and Canada can contribute to the global efforts to improve the health status of the world's peoples.

Health as a Global Concern

According to the International Council of Nurses (ICN, 2003), 30,000 children die each day from preventable diseases. The global toll from infectious diseases, malnutrition, and other effects of poverty and environmental pollutants is staggering. New forms of deadly viruses are discovered with seeming regularity, and health workers are not immune from contagion. (See Research Application 15-1 for a study on African nurses who cared for Ebola victims.)

Health and illness statistics can only show a cross section of the real magnitude of the global disease burden. These statistics are readily available from reliable sources such as the United Nations (UN) (http://www.UN.org), the Centers for Disease Control and Prevention (CDC) (http://www.cdc.gov), the World Health Organization (WHO) (http://www.who.org), and others. Using current WHO (2006, 2009a, 2009b, 2009b) data, the following is a snapshot of global health concerns:

- Approximately 5 million people die from AIDS-related causes, including tuberculosis (TB), every year. By some estimates, 11 of every 1,000 adults age 15 to 49 worldwide are HIV infected. Globally, an estimated 13 million children under age 15 have lost one or both parents to AIDS.
- More than 150 million children under age 5 in the developing world are malnourished, including almost half the children in southern Asia.
- In 2002, there were 815 million hungry people in the developing world.
- More than 10 million children under age 5 die annually from six major causes: pneumonia, diarrhea, malaria, measles, neonatal pneumonia, preterm delivery, and asphyxia at birth.
- More than 500,000 women die each year from pregnancy-related causes. In 2002, 50% of the deaths in Africa, 45% in Asia, 4% in Latin America, and less than 1% in more developed areas.
- Estimates of the number of cases of acute malaria are as high as 500 million. Young children living in sub-Saharan Africa account for 80% of malaria deaths (1–2 million annually).
- TB kills more than 1.7 million people a year. An estimated 8.8 million new cases were identified in 2003.

RESEARCH APPLICATION 15-1

Nursing During an Ebola Outbreak in Central Africa

Hewlett, B. L., & Hewlett, B. S. (2005). Providing care and facing death: Nursing during an Ebola outbreak in Central Africa. *Journal of Transcultural Nursing*, 16(4), 289–297.

Little research has been done to examine the experiences of nurses who work during outbreaks of deadly epidemics. In 1995, 2000, and again in 2003, outbreaks of Ebola hemorrhagic fever (EHF), one of the deadliest known viruses on Earth, occurred in Central Africa (Republic of the Congo and Uganda). Some of the earliest victims of Ebola were nurses. In the Democratic Republic of the Congo, approximately 20% of those who died were health care professionals. In Uganda, of the 224 victims, 14 were nurses.

This study used open-ended and semistructured interviews with individual nurses and small groups during the outbreaks in Uganda and the Republic of Congo in 2003. Three key themes emerged: (1) lack of protective gear, basic equipment, and other resources needed to provide care; (2) stigmatization by family, coworkers, and community; and (3) exceptional commitment to the nursing profession, even in the context of placing their own lives in jeopardy:

> My children were afraid of me, they were afraid to touch me. I wanted to quit, but I knew that if I quit all the others would want to quit. My husband was afraid and feared me. . . . We ate on separate plates and used separate silverware.
>
> —*Ugandan Nurse (Hewlett & Hewlett, 2005, p. 289)*

RESEARCH APPLICATION 15-1 *(continued)*

Clinical Application

The major themes identified by nurses in this study are present, to some degree, at all times when nurses work in areas where communicable diseases run rampant and unknown dangers in the environment exist, whether that is in rural villages or urban slums. Resources are generally always lacking. Stigmatization, discrimination, and folk beliefs and attitudes are prevalent, not only concerning Ebola, but also HIV and other infectious disease processes. During times of epidemics, health care workers, including nurses, often risk their own lives to provide care. This study provides insights into the experiences of nurses during such times. It highlights the need to understand the cultural models of illness: "Often health educators, and local, national, and international medical personnel were not aware or did not consider the possibility that existing traditional beliefs and practices actually contribute to EHF control efforts" (Hewlett & Hewlett, 2005, pp. 292–293).

This research demonstrates the potential benefit of indigenous cultural models and asks that international teams listen more closely to local nurses and communities. It points out the reality of permeable national and international borders with regard to newly emerging infectious diseases (Severe Acute Respiratory Syndrome [SARS] and swine flu, to name just two) and the globalization of diseases. What happens in a remote African village or Asian town cannot be ignored. The study provides some valuable lessons in how to deal more effectively with infection control.

- In 2002, 1.1 billion people (one-sixth of the world's population) lacked access to safe drinking water. Sharp disparities are seen in access to sanitation between urban and rural areas.

Millennium Development Goals

World leaders met at the Millennium Summit and adopted the *UN Millennium Declaration*, endorsed by 189 countries (UN, 2006). The intent of the declaration was outlined in the identification of **Millennium Development Goals** (MDGs), to be reached by 2015. The MDGs represent commitments from governments to tackle and reduce poverty, hunger, ill health, and other inequalities.

The MDGs were set out as realistic, attainable goals aimed at relieving the worst of human suffering, including the overarching goal of cutting poverty in half. The MDGs served as a catalyst for change and began a process focused on improving living conditions for millions of people around the globe. The MDGs were based on the recognition that nations could assist each other through trade, **development aid**, debt relief, access to essential drugs, and technology transfer. Box 15-1 shows eight individual goals that were identified.

One important aspect of the MDGs is that they are not mutually exclusive. The MDGs emphasize that positive global development relies as much on health and education as on economic growth. Each of the MDGs has identified targets

---

BOX 15-1

Millennium Development Goals

MDG 1	Eradicate Extreme Poverty and Hunger
MDG 2	Achieve Universal Primary Education
MDG 3	Promote Gender Equity and Empower Women
MDG 4	Reduce Child Mortality
MDG 5	Improve Maternal Health
MDG 6	Combat HIV/AIDS, Malaria, and Other Diseases
MDG 7	Ensure Environmental Sustainability
MDG 8	Develop a Global Partnership for Development

TABLE 15-1
Health in the Millennium Development Goals

MDG	HEALTH TARGETS (BY 2015)	HEALTH INDICATORS
1. Eradicate poverty and hunger	1. Halve the proportion of people whose income is less than U.S. $1.00/day;	• Prevalence of underweight children (<5 years old)
	2. Halve the proportion of people who suffer from hunger	• Proportion of population below minimum level of dietary energy consumption
4. Reduce child mortality	5. Reduce the under-5 mortality rate by two-thirds	• Under-5 mortality rate • Infant mortality rate • Proportion of 1-year-olds immunized against measles
5 Improve maternal health	6. Reduce the maternal mortality ratio by three-quarters	• Maternal mortality ratio • Proportion of births attended by skilled health personnel
6. Combat HIV/AIDS, malaria, and other diseases	7. Have halted and begun to reverse the spread of HIV/AIDS	• HIV prevalence among young pregnant women (15–24 years old) • Condom use rate of contraceptive prevalence rate • Ratio of school attendance by orphans vs. nonorphans aged 10–14 years
	8. Have halted and begun to reverse the incidence of malaria and other major diseases	• Prevalence and death rates associated with malaria • Proportion of population using effective antimalaria prevention/treatment measures • TB prevalence and mortality rates • Proportion of TB cases detected and cured under DOTS (directly observed treatment short-course)
7. Ensure environmental sustainability	10. Halve the proportion of people without sustainable access to safe drinking water and sanitation	• Proportion of population with sustainable access to improved water source, urban and rural
	11. By 2020, achieve a significant improvement in the lives of at least 100-million slum dwellers	• Proportion of population with access to improved sanitation, urban and rural
8. Global partnership for development	17. In cooperation with pharmaceutical companies, provide access to affordable, essential drugs in developing countries	• Proportion of population with sustainable access to affordable essential drugs

Modified from the World Health Organization. (2009a, 2009b, 2009b). *Health in the millennium development goals.* Retrieved April 23, 2009, from http://www.who.int/mdg/goals/en/print.html

(16 in total) and indicators (48) that can be measured over time. As such, they serve as a blueprint for sustainable development and provide concrete measures of success and failure in each area. Of the MDGs, six focus specifically on health areas, and this includes nine targets and 17 indicators directly measuring health-related outcomes (Table 15-1).

In 2002, the UN secretary-general commissioned the Millennium Project to develop an action plan to achieve the MDGs. This was headed by Professor Jeffrey Sachs and culminated in the 2005 report *Investing in Development: A Practical Plan to Achieve the Millennium Development Goals.* Work is now underway to provide needs assessments and identify baseline measures for each indicator in all countries, rich and poor. Millennium Project personnel, in conjunction with the UN, selected "pilot countries" to help identify best practices for incorporating MDG targets and time lines into national strategies for poverty reduction. These pilot countries (Dominican Republic, Ethiopia, Ghana, Kenya, Senegal, Tajikistan, and Yemen) will serve as models for other developing countries throughout the world (UN, 2006).

Five years after the identification of the MDGs, the World Economic Forum (2005) published a progress report on the success and failures of the world body to implement needed changes to reach MDG targets. This report card, based on a 10-point scale (10 = target achieved), indicated the following:

Peace and security	3/10
Poverty	5/10
Hunger	4/10
Education	4/10
Health	5/10
Environment	2/10
Human rights	2/10

Reporting specifically on health, the report stated that "although the world did marginally better in 2005 than in 2004, moving from a score of 4 to 5, it remains far off the track on all its health goals" (p. 22).

Responding to Global Needs for Health, Development, and Humanitarian Assistance

Governments around the globe take the responsibility for meeting the needs of their citizens and responding to the best of their abilities. In some cases, however, outside assistance is beneficial to support or enhance the efforts of individual governments and to coordinate a global response to common concerns when needed. This has been the case in fields such as health, education, and humanitarian assistance.

In many instances, nurses participate in emergency relief work following natural disasters or volunteer their time for direct patient care services (operating room, clinics, etc.). See Krommenhoek (2009) for an example of volunteer work in Chad. These tend to be short-term or intermittent assignments, not taking the place of the nurses' usual employment. In other cases, nurses are involved in long-term "development" work at the systems level (sometimes referred to as *capacity building*), which often involves needs assessments, strategic planning, mentoring and education, policy discussions, financial analysis, and work with professional bodies inside the country to strengthen the ability of that sector (health care delivery, nursing education, regulatory bodies, for example) to perform. This is often a career choice that demands learning a new, development-oriented vocabulary and set of skills.

There are several ways to categorize external assistance efforts. In this chapter, we will look at four categories. The first category, and one of the most widely used, is the *international* or *intergovernmental organizations* category. This is sometimes referred to as "multilateral aid." The second category contains the numerous **nongovernmental organizations (NGOs)** that work at international, national, and local levels around the globe. The third category represents *national government aid agencies* (also called "bilateral agencies") that provide humanitarian aid and assistance (such as the United States Agency for International Development [USAID]). The fourth category

BOX 15-2

List of Development Aid Organizations

Major Government Aid/Donor Agencies

- Australia—Australian Agency for International Development (AusAID)
- Canada—Canadian International Development Agency (CIDA) and International Development Research Centre (IDRC)
- Denmark—Ministry of Foreign Affairs: Development Policy Section
- European Union—European Commission: Development Directorate-General
- France—Department for International Cooperation and French Development Agency (AfD)
- Germany—Deutsche Gesellschaft für Technische Zusammenarbeit (GTZ)
- Italy—Ministry of Foreign Affairs: Italian Development Cooperation Program
- Japan—Japan International Cooperation Agency (JICA)
- New Zealand—New Zealand Agency for International Development (NZAid)
- Norway—Ministry of Foreign Affairs: International Development Program and Norwegian Agency for Development Cooperation (NORAD)
- Spain—Spanish Agency for International Cooperation (AECI)
- Sweden—Sida
- Switzerland—Swiss Agency for Development Cooperation (SDC)
- United Kingdom—Department for International Development (DFID)
- United States—United States Agency for International Development (USAID) and the Peace Corps

Major Intergovernmental Organizations

- African Development Bank
- Asian Development Bank (ADB)
- European Bank for Reconstruction and Development
- Inter-American Development Bank
- International Bank for Reconstruction and Development (IBRD: The World Bank)

- International Fund for Agricultural Development (IFAD)
- International Monetary Fund (IMF)
- International Organization for Migration (IOM)
- Organization for Economic Cooperation and Development (OECD)
- United Nations (UN)
  - United Nations Children's Fund (UNICEF)
  - United Nations Development Program (UNDP)
  - United Nations Environment Programme (UNEP)
  - United Nations High Commissioner for Refugees (UNHCR)
  - World Food Program (WFP)
- World Health Organization (WHO)
  - Pan American Health Organization (PAHO)
- World Trade Organization (WTO)

Major Nongovernmental Organizations (NGOs)

- Amnesty, International
- CARE, Inc.
- Catholic Relief Services
- Council of World Churches
- Inter*Action*
- International Committee of the Red Cross (ICRC)
- International Rescue Committee (IRC)
- Joint Commission International
- Médécins Sans Frontières/Doctors Without Borders
- Mercy Corps
- Oxfam International
- Project HOPE (Health Opportunities for People Everywhere)
- Relief International
- Save the Children
- Voluntary Services Overseas
- World Vision

Professional Organizations

- International Council of Nurses
- Sigma Theta Tau International Honor Society of Nursing

includes *professional organizations* that are international in scope. A list of major **development aid organizations** is shown in Box 15-2.

Intergovernmental Organizations

Some organizations, which espouse common aims of international significance, are formed by member states (governments) through treaties or charters. Such treaties allow the organization to establish its own operating systems and governing mechanisms. Probably the best-known international organizations are the UN and the North Atlantic Treaty Organization (NATO).

The United Nations

In 1945, representatives of 50 countries met in San Francisco to develop a UN Charter. The UN was initiated on October 24, 1945, when the charter was ratified by a majority of countries, including China, France, the Soviet Union, the United Kingdom, and the United States. The purposes of the UN are to (1) maintain international peace and security, (2) develop friendly relations among nations, (3) cooperate in solving international economic, social, cultural, and humanitarian problems, (4) promote respect for human rights and fundamental freedoms, and (5) serve as a center for harmonizing the actions of nations in attaining these ends (UN, 2009a).

The UN is made up of six principal units: the General Assembly, Security Council, Economic and Social Council, Trusteeship Council, International Court of Justice, and Secretariat. The total UN institution, however, is much larger and contains 15 separate agencies and other individual programs or bodies. UN agencies offer several types of assistance.

Emergency Relief

The UN began relief operations in Europe following World War II (WWII) and continues to be a major provider of humanitarian relief operations worldwide. The UN has been recognized internationally as taking a lead role in responding to natural and man-made disasters by providing emergency relief and assistance where needed. In the last decade, civil wars have become a major cause of emergency situations. When natural disasters (floods, droughts, earthquakes) are added to the equation, emergencies affect millions of people and cause billions of dollars of damage. Unfortunately more than 90% (UN, 2006) of all disaster victims live in developing countries, where poverty and poorly developed infrastructures compound the problems.

Humanitarian Assistance

When needed, the UN is often among the first to offer humanitarian assistance. In 1 year alone, the UN raised more than $1.4 billion to assist 35 million people in 16 countries and regions (UN, 2006). The **UN High Commissioner for Refugees** (UNHCR) provides international assistance to more than 22 million refugees and displaced persons. The World Food Program delivers one-third of the world's emergency food assistance.

Prevention

The role of prevention in reducing the vulnerability of nations to disasters is another important activity of the UN. This includes developing early warning and detection systems and assisting disaster-prone countries to carry out contingency planning and preparedness measures. The **United Nations Development Program** (UNDP) is the primary agency for this activity. Headquartered in New York City, the UNDP is the UN's global development network. It publishes an annual Human Development Report available from the UNDP Web site (UNDP, 2006).

UN Volunteers

In 1970 the General Assembly created the UN Volunteers program to help implement development work requested by various member states.

The UN Volunteers program reports to the UNDP through country offices worldwide. More than 30,000 UN volunteers have supported humanitarian peace, relief, and development operations in more than 166 countries since 1971 (UN, 2009b). If you are interested in more information about becoming a UN volunteer, check the Web site at http://www.unvolunteers.org/

The World Health Organization

The **World Health Organization (WHO)** is a part of the UN family and serves as the specialized agency for health. It was established in 1948 with the goal of promoting the attainment of the highest possible level of health by all peoples. In 1978, WHO changed the nature of the debate about "health" when it issued its now classic Alma-Ata declaration, defining health as "a state of complete physical, mental and social well-being and not merely the absence of disease or infirmity" (WHO, Regional Office for Europe, 2006). WHO is governed through the World Health Assembly (WHA), which convenes annually in Geneva, Switzerland, and contains 192 member states.

WHO has numerous branches and services. Its headquarters are in Geneva, Switzerland, and it convenes the WHA annually to discuss policy and other matters. Official delegations from around the world gather in Geneva for deliberations. Global nursing issues are often on the agenda. In fact, there is a dedicated WHO branch for Nursing and Midwifery Services (WHO, 2009b).

Nursing and Midwifery Services

The nursing and midwifery team at WHO headquarters is responsible for coordinating efforts across member countries. It links across WHO technical programs worldwide and coordinates common efforts with WHO regional and country offices, where WHO nurse advisors often reside. WHO has long focused its attention on the global status of nursing and midwifery. It has been a major agenda item throughout the 1990s and into the new millennium. WHO recognizes that nursing and midwifery services are vital to obtaining desired health outcomes and urges member states to give them priority attention. To this end, WHO has issued several resolutions on strengthening nursing and midwifery services to member states by (1) providing policy and technical advice, (2) facilitating capacity building and collaboration, and (3) supporting the enhancement of systems that generate evidence for decision making.

A WHO (2002) publication, *Nursing and Midwifery Services: Strategic Directions 2002–2008*, identifies five key areas for intervention: (1) human resource planning, (2) management of personnel, (3) evidence-based practice, (4) education, and (5) stewardship. The document addresses WHA Resolution 54.12, *Strengthening Nursing and Midwifery* (WHO, 2001), which promotes the achievement of WHO's health objectives as well as the UN MDGs.

The Pan American Health Organization

The **Pan American Health Organization (PAHO)** (2009) is a member of the UN system and serves as the Regional Office for the Americas of the WHO. PAHO has worked for more than 100 years as an international public health agency, improving the health and living standards of the countries of the Americas (includes the Caribbean, Central and South America, and the United States).

United Nations Children's Fund

The United Nations Children's Fund (UNICEF, 2009) works in more than 157 countries and employs more than 7,000 people. Its primary aim is to promote the rights of children and to overcome obstacles such as poverty, violence, disease, and discrimination (UNICEF, 2009). UNICEF focuses on (1) girls' education; (2) immunizations; (3) prevention and treatment of HIV/AIDS among young children and their families;

(4) creation of protective environments for children to avoid abuse, violence, and exploitation; and (5) prevention of discrimination, against women and girls in particular.

Nongovernmental Organizations

NGOs are usually established by groups of individuals or associations as private enterprises. NGOs may be professional associations, foundations, multinational businesses, or simply groups with a common interest in humanitarian assistance activities (development and relief). They are not mandated by government agreements or charters. Many NGOs play an important role in the international health and development arena by virtue of the services they provide. However, they are not usually given any official governmental status. NGOs can be established at the local, regional, national, or international level. They can have secular or religious affiliations. The best-known NGO (actually an NGO hybrid) is probably the International Committee of the Red Cross (ICRC). Other well-known examples include Médécins Sans Frontières, Amnesty International, Save the Children, World Vision, and CARE, Inc. The following section contains a sampling of well-known NGOs.

International Committee of the Red Cross and International Federation of Red Cross and Red Crescent Societies

The ICRC was established in 1863 as a humanitarian organization whose mission was to aid the victims of war and other internal violence. Today it is recognized as a major international relief organization. The ICRC includes the International Federation of Red Cross and Red Crescent Societies (2009), with 183 member states. The ICRC is a private association formed under the Swiss Civil Code but not mandated by governments. It is based on international law, specifically the Geneva Conventions and is recognized as having an "international legal status" (ICRC, 2009) unlike other NGOs. Therefore, it enjoys certain privileges and immunities similar to those of UN agencies.

The federation's mission is *to improve the lives of vulnerable people* and focuses on four core areas: promoting humanitarian values, disaster relief, disaster preparedness, and community health. ICRC often deals with victims of natural disasters, poverty brought about by socioeconomic crises, and refugees.

Catholic Relief Services

Catholic Relief Services (CRS) was founded in 1943 by the Catholic bishops of the United States. They work in more than 90 countries to assist the poor and disadvantaged, alleviate suffering, and foster charity and justice as part of their faith-based mission. As the official international relief and development agency of the U.S. Catholic community, CRS is also committed to educating U.S. citizens to fulfill their moral responsibilities toward their global neighbors by helping the poor, working to remove the causes of poverty, and promoting social justice (CRS, 2009).

CARE, Inc.

CARE works with poor communities in more than 70 countries around the world to find lasting solutions to poverty. With a broad range of programs based on empowerment, equity, and sustainability, CARE seeks to facilitate change through (1) strengthening capacity for self-help, (2) providing economic opportunities, (3) delivering emergency relief, (4) influencing policy decisions at national and local levels, and (5) addressing discrimination in all its forms (CARE, 2009). CARE is one of the world's largest private international humanitarian organizations, which was founded in 1945 to provide relief to survivors of WWII. CARE programs are community based in areas such as education, health care, and economic development and use a combination of skills training, provision of resources, and knowledge building. Program areas include the following:

- Agriculture and natural resources
- Education
- Emergency relief
- Health
- HIV/AIDS
- Nutrition
- Small economic activity development
- Water, sanitation, and environmental health

Project HOPE

The name Health Opportunities for People Everywhere (HOPE) is reflected in its mission: to achieve sustainable advances in health care around the world by implementing health education programs and providing humanitarian assistance in areas of need (Project HOPE, 2009). Initiated in 1958 as the S.S. HOPE, the world's first peacetime hospital ship, Project HOPE now conducts land-based training and health care education programs on five continents, including North America. More than 5,000 health care professionals and volunteer educators have worked for HOPE. It now provides approximately 100 million worth of resources to 20 to 30 countries each year. Project HOPE programs focus on

- Infectious disease: AIDS and TB
- Women's and children's health
- Health professional education (training of trainers)
- Health systems and facilities
- Humanitarian assistance

Oxfam International

Oxfam was founded in 1995 by a group of like-minded independent NGOs that wanted to work together internationally to achieve greater impact in reducing poverty by their collective efforts (Oxfam, 2009). The name "Oxfam" comes from the Oxford Committee for Famine Relief, founded in Britain during WWII. Oxfam International is a confederation of 12 organizations based in Australia, Belgium, Canada, Germany, Great Britain, Hong Kong, Ireland, the Netherlands, New Zealand, Spain, and the United States who work together with over 3,000 partners in more than 100 countries to find lasting solutions to poverty, suffering, and injustice. Oxfam programs undertake

- Long-term development
- Emergency work
- Research and lobbying
- Campaigning, alliance building, and media work

Save the Children

Save the Children was formed in 1932 by a group of concerned U.S. citizens reacting to the plight of Appalachia during the Depression. Today it is one of the leading international relief and development organizations (an alliance composed of 27 national Save the Children organizations) promoting the well-being of children and works in more than 100 countries. Save the Children works on the principle of self-sufficiency and helps families define and solve problems faced by children in their communities (Save the Children, 2009).

Doctors Without Borders/Médécins Sans Frontières (MSF)

MSF works in more than 70 countries to deliver emergency aid to those affected by armed conflict, disease, disasters, and other forms of exclusion from health care. It is an independent medical humanitarian organization founded in 1971. MSF consists of an international network with sections in 19 countries (MSF, 2009).

MSF is often one of the first to respond at the scene of an emergency (Lau, 2005). MSF volunteers (doctors, nurses, logisticians, water-and-sanitation experts, administrators, and other medical and nonmedical professionals) often work in very remote and/or dangerous parts of the world (Nestrell, 2004). They are available on short notice, usually dedicating 6 to 12 months to each assignment. MSF teams are composed of international volunteers and skilled local staff. Together, they work closely with national medical professionals, cooperate with other aid organizations, and carry out more than 3,800 aid missions annually.

Mercy Corps

Since 1979, Mercy Corps has provided more than $1 billion in assistance to people in 81 nations. Mercy Corps is a nonprofit organization with headquarters in Portland; Seattle; Cambridge; Washington, DC; and Edinburgh, Scotland. The agency's programs currently reach 7 million people in more than 35 countries (Mercy Corps, 2009). The organization was founded as Save the Refugees Fund, in response to the plight of Cambodian refugees fleeing the famine, war, and genocide of the "Killing Fields."

Mercy Corps pursues its mission through emergency relief services, sustainable economic development, and civil society initiatives. Mercy Corps has played an important role in responding to the massive tragedy of the Indian Ocean tsunami, war in Afghanistan, massive food shortages in North Korea, ethnic conflict in the Balkans, and economic transitions in Central Asia and the Caucasus.

World Vision

World Vision (2009) is a Christian relief and development organization dedicated to helping children and their communities worldwide by tackling the causes of poverty. The organization began in the 1950s working with orphaned children in the Korean War.

The program expanded into other Asian countries and eventually into Latin America, Africa, Eastern Europe, and the Middle East. In the 1960s, World Vision expanded its global relief efforts to people suffering from natural disasters. By the 1970s, the organization had incorporated vocational and agricultural training for families into its efforts to promote self-sustainable change.

In 1990, World Vision began addressing the urgent needs of children orphaned by AIDS in Uganda and quickly expanded operations to other hard-hit African countries. By 2004, nearly 300,000 orphans and vulnerable children had been sponsored in AIDS-affected communities.

International Rescue Committee

Founded in 1933, the International Rescue Committee (IRC, 2009) is at work in 25 countries and is a global leader in emergency relief, rehabilitation, postconflict development, and resettlement services. The IRC delivers lifesaving aid in emergencies, helps those uprooted by war and fleeing from persecution, cares for war-traumatized children, and rehabilitates environmental and health care systems. IRC supports capacity building endeavors with local schools, organizations, and civil governments.

IRC is known for its work with refugees, providing emergency assistance: water, food, shelter, sanitation, and medical care in the immediate crisis, and then working with people to rebuild their lives by providing education, training, and economic assistance. IRC also helps thousands of refugees in the resettlement process in the United States.

Governmental Organizations

United States Agency for International Development

In 1961, President John F. Kennedy signed into law the Foreign Assistance Act and thereby created the USAID. The United States has a long history of assisting others around the globe to overcome the effects of poverty, natural disasters, and oppression. USAID has its roots in the Marshall Plan reconstruction of Europe following WWII and in President Harry Truman's Point Four Program. U.S. foreign assistance serves two purposes: furthering America's foreign policy and improving the lives of peoples in the developing world (USAID, 2009).

USAID is an independent agency of the federal government that receives guidance from the secretary of state. Spending less than one-half of 1% of the federal budget, USAID works around the world to achieve its goals in three areas: (1) economic growth, agriculture, and trade; (2) global health; and (3) democracy, conflict prevention, and humanitarian assistance. Assistance support is carried out in four global regions: sub-Saharan Africa, Asia and the Near East, Latin America and the Caribbean, and Europe and Eurasia.

USAID is located in Washington, DC, with field offices around the globe. The agency works in close partnerships with more than 300 U.S.-based private voluntary organizations, indigenous associations, colleges, and universities, more than 3,500 American business companies, international NGOs, other governments, and other U.S. government bodies.

The Peace Corps

The Peace Corps was initiated in 1960, when then-Senator John F. Kennedy, in a speech to University of Michigan students, challenged them to spend 2 years serving their country in the cause of peace by living and working in developing countries. From that inspiration emerged the Peace Corps (Peace Corps, 2009). Since that time, more than 182,000 Peace Corps volunteers have worked in over 138 host countries on issues ranging from AIDS education, information technology, and environmental preservation.

The Peace Corps' mission is threefold: (1) helping interested countries meet their needs for trained personnel, (2) helping promote better understanding of Americans by others; and (3) helping to promote a better understanding of other peoples by all Americans. Today the Peace Corp continues to expand into new countries, such as East Timor, and into new fields, such as information technology. In 2003, more than 1,000 new volunteers were included in President Bush's HIV/AIDS Act.

The Centers for Disease Control and Prevention

The CDC started in 1946 as a malaria control agency. Today it is one of 13 major branches of the U.S. Department of Health and Human Services (CDC, 2009). The U.S. Department of Health and Human Services is the agency responsible for protecting the health and safety of all Americans and providing essential human services where needed. CDC is at the forefront of the nation's public health efforts. The CDC's work is often carried out in the field, involving national and international travel, collecting data, and developing strategic plans for intervention. It is recognized globally for its role in researching and investigating outbreaks of infectious disease and its action-oriented approach to control. The CDC also carries out educational campaigns on health and safety measures for the general public.

Canadian International Development Agency (CIDA)

The CIDA is a part of the Canadian government and administers foreign aid programs in developing countries (CIDA, 2009). It reports to the Canadian Parliament through the Minister for International Cooperation. CIDA's mission is to support sustainable development and reduce poverty in developing countries in order to promote a more equitable and prosperous world. CIDA works with other Canadian organizations, public and private, as well as other international organizations. Priorities identified focus on social development programs such as the treatment of sexually transmitted infections (STIs) in third world countries; basic education and child protection, especially for girls; economic and environmental sustainability;

programs that benefit women directly; and systems of good governance.

Professional Organizations

The International Council of Nurses

The **International Council of Nurses** (ICN) is an independent, nongovernmental federation of national nurses' associations representing more than 128 countries. Its headquarters are in Geneva, Switzerland. Founded in 1899, ICN is the oldest international professional organization in the health care field. The ICN works either through its own projects or in collaboration with other international organizations to promote health services. It encourages efforts by national nurses' associations to develop nursing standards and advance the economic position of nurses (ICN, 2009). ICN promotes its objectives through standard-setting programs, seminars, publications, and meetings. The official publication of the ICN is the *International Nursing Review*.

International organizations, notably WHO and UNICEF, work closely with the ICN on matters affecting health in all parts of the world. For example, ICN and WHO have issued a joint declaration on AIDS, dealing with the rights and responsibilities of nurses worldwide in caring for people infected with this disease. ICN also has worked with WHO to increase nurses' awareness and knowledge of the problems related to substance abuse and help nurses provide care for patients with addictions. The organization is active in such UN initiatives as Safe Motherhood and Occupational Health. ICN is involved with the UN Millennium Project and issued a comprehensive report, *Tackling the UN Millennium Development Goals* in 2003.

ICN advances the cause of nursing and nurses worldwide. It is particularly effective in the areas of professional practice, regulation, education, and socioeconomic welfare. ICN has pioneered an international classification of nursing practice—ICNP and the Leadership for Change Program. The ICN *Code for Nurses* has shaped the ethical practice of nursing in many countries throughout the world. ICN also provides a series of fact sheets for quick reference on a number of topics of interest to current health and social matters. Readers are encouraged to visit the ICN Web site at http://www.icn.ch.

The World's Nurses

Although there is little global statistical information on nursing or midwifery personnel because of classification problems and lack of established information systems, it is widely accepted that there are insufficient nurses to care for the world's population. What is known is that the majority of nurses work in the developed world, and approximately one-quarter are in the United States. Although accepted benchmarks for nursing personnel (four to five nurses per one physician) are reached in most Western countries, the ratio flattens in the developing world. In Pakistan, the nurse-to-physician ratio is reversed: four to five physicians for every nurse.

In addition to a lack of uniformity in classifying nursing and midwifery personnel, there are significant discrepancies in roles and functions, standards of performance, and quality of care by nurses in various parts of the world. The scope of practice for nurses varies widely from country to country. In parts of Africa and Asia, nurses may prescribe medications, perform some surgeries, suture wounds, and set fractured bones. In other places, they may not be allowed to take blood pressures or dress wounds. In yet other situations, nurses may consider bedside care (bathing and assisting with bedpans, for example) to be outside their realm of practice. In some cases apprenticeship training occurs, with on-the-job skill development and clinical instruction being supervised by staff nurses working on the unit.

Educational Preparation for Nurses

Each country has its own system of nursing education and career mobility. Curricula vary widely in content, length, standards, and evaluation criteria. General education required to enter the nursing program ranges from 6 to 13 years, and the length of the program varies from 1 to 4 years. There are general and specialty programs at the basic level of education. Specialization usually requires post-basic education. In some countries midwifery is a specialized field at the master's level; in others, it is the most basic level of preparation and is a stand-alone field, not connected to nursing.

Nurse Migration

Given the high demand for nursing services and the scarcity of nurses to meet that demand, it is not surprising that nurses are a mobile population. The important topic of foreign nurses migrating to the United States, United Kingdom, Australia, and Canada requires its own in-depth study and will not be covered in this chapter. The focus here is on U.S. and Canadian nurses who venture away from home.

Since the days of Florence Nightingale, highly trained nurses have traveled to all parts of the globe to practice their profession. Many young English-women traveled to Germany for formal education as nurses. During the Crimean War, nurses traveled with Nightingale to Scutari to care for soldiers with battle wounds as well as infectious diseases such as cholera. Nightingale's hospital reforms reached from Europe to India (Nightingale, 1859). As early as 1867, graduates of the Saint Thomas Hospital Nursing School were found in Australia, Canada, Sweden, Germany, and most large hospitals in the United Kingdom and the United States.

North American Nurses Abroad

Early in the development of U.S. and Canadian nursing history, nurses prepared in the Night-ingale tradition traveled abroad. In 1885 Linda Richards became the first U.S. nurse on record to engage in international nursing when she went to Japan under the auspices of the American Board of Missions to establish a school of nursing. Records from the Presbyterian Mission Board of Canada indicate that nurses were sent abroad more than 100 years ago, mainly to Taiwan, China, and India. The life of one exemplary missionary nurse, Ruth Harnar, is illustrated in Box 15-3.

Nurses in both the United States and Canada served in WWI and WWII. The MASH units of the Korean War are familiar to many through movies and television. With the creation of WHO in 1948

BOX 15-3

Spotlight on Ruth May Harnar (1919–2004)

Dr. Ruth May Harnar[1], the daughter of missionaries, was born and reared in India. She knew at an early age she wanted to be a medical missionary and at age 12 began studying the Hindi language in earnest. She pursued her goal by completing her basic nursing education at Johns Hopkins University before returning to India in 1944, amid the chaos of WWII. She worked for the Division of Overseas Ministries of the Christian Church (Disciples of Christ). She returned to the United States to do her master's degree at the Frances Payne Bolton School of Nursing at Case Western Reserve University, graduating in 1952. In 1974 she completed her PhD in nursing education from Columbia University with a dissertation on the contributions made by church-based schools of nursing on nursing education in India.

Dr. Harnar devoted her life's work to helping educate Indian nurses and village health workers to serve community-based populations and in mission hospitals. She worked as nursing superintendent and acting director at Jackman Memorial Hospital in Bilaspur, India; as director of the graduate school for nurses at Indore, India; and in community health positions responsible for health assessments and immunization programs of approximately 1,200 school children annually. In 1947, Dr. Harnar and three Indian nurse colleagues served in the refugee camps that resulted from the partitioning of India and Pakistan when British rule ended.

Throughout her career, Dr. Harnar was known as a nurse educator. She developed a Hindi postgraduate syllabus approved by the India Nursing Council. She

BOX 15-3 *(continued)*

wrote curricula for nurses in training and administered final examinations throughout central India. She taught science and other subjects and helped organize a program of visual aids in the nursing schools and hospitals. In 1955 she made an extended trip to Nepal, where she worked in the medical and evangelistic programs of the United Church of Nepal. In the early 1970s, Dr. Harnar worked with the Voluntary Health Association of India in New Delhi, where she coauthored a curriculum for training village health workers and traveled throughout India to conduct training sessions. This curriculum is still widely used throughout India and elsewhere in the region.

In the early 1980s, after retiring from the mission field, Dr. Harnar served as a visiting professor at the University of California, San Francisco (UCSF), School of Nursing, developing and teaching a new course in international nursing. In 1985 she moved to Geneva, Switzerland, to serve with the Christian Medical Commission of the World Council of Churches. In 1987, Dr. Harnar joined the faculty of the Aga Khan University in Karachi, Pakistan, to help develop a village health worker program and to assist in the startup of the Community Health Sciences (CHS) Department of the Medical College. She was responsible for the development and training of community health nurses and female health visitors for community-based health

care programs in the poverty-stricken areas of Karachi in the rural Sindh province. Dr. Harnar's familiarity with South Asian culture and her fluency in Hindi/Urdu were of special importance in her work with staff, students, and community members. She also was a member of the initial planning team for the new RN to BSN program in the School of Nursing.

From 1992 until her death in November 2004, Dr. Harnar lived in a retirement community in Indianapolis, Indiana. She continued to be an active member of her church and shared her wealth of knowledge and experiences with the Nursing School at Indiana University. In 2002, the newly renovated nursing school building at Jackman Hospital in Bilaspur, India, was renamed the Jarvis and Harnar Nursing School.

In tribute to Dr. Harnar, John Bryant, former dean of the School of Public Health at Columbia University and a colleague at the Aga Khan University, said, "In the professional careers of those who work in the various corners of international health, one of the rich rewards is coming to know others who have dedicated their lives to enhancing the well-being of people who live in poverty and despair, to give them a chance for a life of health and dignity. Ruth Harnar was one of those precious persons who inspired us all and did so in joyful humility" (J. Bryant, personal communications, 2005).

[1]Thanks to the family and friends of Dr. Harnar for providing this information. Also, the Global Ministries (2004) News article on Dr. Harnar, retrieved August 4, 2005, from http://www.globalministries.org/news/harnar.htm

and the proliferation of technical assistance programs, nurses have become increasingly involved in international health. The ICRC has employed nurses as members of its relief teams for many years. In the 1960s with the establishment of USAID and CIDA, more funds became available for development, which expanded the number of health-related projects carried out. The demand for international nurses increased dramatically as agencies responded to the urgent health needs around the world. Today nurses have many opportunities to go abroad for the purposes of travel, research, education, consultation, and service in virtually all clinical practice specialty areas and administrative/management roles, as well

as to assist in times of disaster relief. See Case Study 15-1 for a look at the realities of establishing and working in a refugee camp.

Working in a Refugee Camp: A Personal Journey

In early 1979 Cambodia's Khmer Rouge regime was overthrown, and amid the battles, hundreds of thousands of Cambodian citizens fled westwards toward the borders with Thailand and Laos. Before the end of the crisis, numerous camps and detention centers were established along these

(case study continues on page 436)

borders with the assistance of local governments, the UN High Commissioner for Refugees (UNHCR) and various international relief agencies.

By December, more than 150,000 refugees were being housed in Thailand. One of the first camps to open was Sa Kaeo, with an estimated population of about 30,000. These people arrived with only the clothes on their backs and handheld belongings. They were literally driven by truck from the border and dumped into the muddy fields of Sa Kaeo. The camp grew up around them. Many of these people were critically ill with malaria, diarrhea, kwashiorkor and other nutritional problems associated with months of starvation, respiratory diseases including TB and pneumonia, and infections caused by a variety of wounds. Pregnant women were numerous.

I arrived in Sa Kaeo at the beginning of November 1979 as part of a team of three nurses "loaned" by CARE, Inc., to the IRC to help establish the field hospital. I left by December 5th that same year. However, that 1 month at Sa Kaeo was one of the most grueling and rewarding experiences of my life.

The first night we were housed on the Thai border, and we slept on the floor of someone's house. We could hear the gun battles going on through the night. We made the 1-hour drive to the camp at sunrise the next morning and began what would become the customary process of checking in at the gate (as a military detention center, we all carried ID and had to cross a barbed-wire fence to enter the camp). Later we would find an apartment in Sa Kaeo. By now our IRC group had grown to three nurses and two physicians. Our team of five would be responsible for the care of all the patients in our charge—24/7. It rained just about every day; it was hot and humid, and the mosquitoes thrived. We were given Fansidar tablets to take (before it was known they were not a safe medication for malaria). We worked every day and occasionally round the clock. There were few breaks, no real times for meals, and very little food available, especially in the beginning. There were only primitive latrines.

Gradually the camp began to take shape. The hilly area became "residential"; tents and tarps were provided along with buckets and basins. The flat area became the "mess hall," and the field

hospital grew beyond that, starting with a kind of "tent city."

Various aid agencies took on specific roles: The Israelis handled triage and ER/OR, the French and Germans handled maternity and pediatrics, the Thai Red Cross took on general medical patients, and the IRC was given the role of "ICU/acute med/surg." Each NGO had its own mandate. The UNHCR and CDC coordinated supplies and equipment, as well as rudimentary mortality and morbidity reports and other epidemiological studies. The engineers began to build water towers, outhouses, and more permanent wardlike structures (at least they had partial walls and a thatch roof). A quasipermanent group of Thai food vendors took up residence just outside the barbed wire, providing the only "fast food" available to aid workers.

Around it all, we had to care for our patients. Our "ward" was designed with 120 cots—60 per side with a middle walkway. Most cots had more than one patient (especially if the patient were a mother or a child). The cots were about 2½ feet from ground level, which made it hard on our backs. The ground was covered with small pebbles (certainly the engineers who designed it were not nurses!). All our patients were very ill. Many had cerebral malaria and were only semiconscious. Most were dehydrated and needed IVs. Many had diarrhea. There were wounds to be dressed. None of our patients spoke English, nor did our ward "helpers"—teenage girls who were well enough to work. We had no "systems" in place, but we knew they were needed.

So how did we cope? I like to think we did a great job because we were creative and we improvised, we were able to zero in on the basic essentials and not worry about much else, and we were willing to keep working even when exhausted:

- We divided the patients into two cohorts of 60 each (plus bedmates). Each patient was given an armband with a cot number and letter. We referred to our patients as "1A" or perhaps "3B," and we knew who we were talking about.
- We implemented a team task approach. Each half of the ward had a doctor–nurse team. We used 4 × 6 cards as charts. The doctor saw each patient and wrote orders on the cards (medications, IVs, dressings). Any other "comfort" measures were left to the ward helpers. They carried and emptied bedpans (mainly plastic

buckets that required the patient to get out of the cot and use), changed sheets, gave sponge baths, provided drinks of water, and helped with running errands.

- We began each day at the "nurses' station," filling up syringes with set amounts of injectables, based on the ones we knew we needed: Imferon, penicillin, quinine, etc. We kept filled syringes in cups (we labeled the cups but not the syringes). We did the same with standard pills and tablets. This became our stock medication supply. The nurse took her set of cards, prepared her medication cart (a plastic laundry basket) with needed medications and supplies (by putting each item into small plastic cups), and carried a large water bottle. Each patient had his or her own cup at the bedside. In my month at Sa Kaeo, I learned three Cambodian phrases: "where's your cup?," "swallow this," and "please or thank you."

- The two team nurses spent the day giving out meds and doing treatments to a minimum of 60 patients each.

- The third nurse was called the "IV nurse." She started and monitored all IVs in the ward (up to 100 of them on any given day). As we could not keep fluids going overnight because of lack of staff, each IV had to be started over again each morning.

- We worked very long days and carried flashlights to see in the dark. We did not take breaks except when absolutely necessary (luckily the new outhouses were close to our ward).

- On a rotation basis set up by UNHCR/CDC, each NGO took turns being the "night shift" for camp. This meant a doctor–nurse team worked a full 24 hours straight—the usual "day shift" plus being on call all night for the entire field hospital (about 1,000 patients). On those nights, we would be called out to deliver babies or see dying patients. We made two rounds of the entire field hospital, checking on especially sick patients. Otherwise we catnapped on the floor of the ward or in the supply tent. I remember the night the doctor and I each delivered a baby at the same time on two adjoining delivery tables! I had never delivered a baby before.

Over the course of a month, our patient population stabilized. We had many deaths in the first week, but it gradually tapered off. We were able to discharge patients. I saw sad, dirty, and hungry children begin to smile. We made sense of our workload and actually got to have breaks. IRC began hiring more permanent nurses to take our places. When we left in December, our ICU had been converted to the TB ward.

Some nurses work abroad because job prospects are better than in their home countries. Some do so as a means to an end: to allow them to travel and experience other cultures. Some want to compare nursing practices in other countries with their own. Military nurses are given foreign postings but care primarily for their own countrymen and women. Some nurses join overseas missionary groups in order to participate in faith-based activities, and others volunteer with emergency relief agencies because they "want to help" in times of disasters.

One image that comes to mind for many is that of traveling to an exotic locale, living in "primitive" conditions, having exciting and even dangerous encounters with locals, and working selflessly and tirelessly to aid the sick and injured. In fact, nurses have a broad range of options for working outside their home countries. These can be categorized as shown in Box 15-4.

Nurses can apply directly to public and private facilities (service and education) in host countries as long as they are able to work out visa and

---

BOX 15-4

International Job Options for Nurses

Working for or in the host country directly
    Government or public facility
    Private facility

Working for an Intergovernmental Organization

Working for an International, National, or Local NGO

Working for a Bilateral Aid Agency and its Subcontractors

Working on a Grant-funded University or Research Project

Working for a Mission Group

Working for the Military

BOX 15-5

Characteristics of International Nursing

1. Understanding the organizational structures, including communication and decision-making bodies, for health care policy and procedures at national, provincial or state, and local levels

2. Understanding the organizational structures, including communication and decision-making bodies, for nursing policy and procedures (regulations, practice standards, education, evaluation) at national, provincial or state, and local levels

3. Understanding and appreciating the status of nursing within the country and within specific health care systems (doctor–nurse relationships, decision making, authority, image, scope of practice)

4. Understanding and using concepts of development and capacity building

5. Assessing population health parameters in comparison with other countries

6. Experiencing challenges related to understanding and working within new or different systems of health care delivery and nurse practice regulations in other countries

7. Learning about the nursing role and clients' expectations of nurses

8. Working with counterparts who ultimately bear responsibility for nursing practice, education, and research in their nations

9. Functioning safely with unfamiliar equipment, supplies, and medications

10. Confronting ethical dilemmas having complex transnational components

11. Working with limited or unfamiliar health care resources

12. Collaborating with health care team members representing categories that may not exist in the United States or Canada

13. Learning about tropical illnesses and other health care problems unfamiliar in the nurse's home country (including cultural definitions of health, illness, and culture-bound syndromes)

14. Understanding and effectively working with political, social, economic, and cultural systems unlike those in the nurse's home country

15. Identifying and effectively using health care resources in the host country

16. Solving problems related to visas, immunizations, licenses, insurance, and other necessities of living in a foreign country

---

other requirements. Young graduates often seek employment in the United Kingdom or Europe as a means of paying for extended stays there. Nurses have also had a long tradition of working in the hospitals of the Middle East, especially Saudi Arabia, as employees of large U.S. or multinational oil companies. Other nurses take part in short-term health-related projects run by universities and/or church groups either as volunteers or paid staff. Many nurses volunteer to serve in times of disaster but do not intend to make long-term stays in the countries they serve. Embassies and consulates employ nurses abroad to care for their expatriate communities.

Although all these situations are legitimately international experiences, they do not define the field of international nursing in itself. The field of international nursing, as discussed in the following section is a career option for nurses interested in more long-term commitments to an international health career. Some of the issues discussed, however, such as preparing to go abroad, are useful for all nurses who work outside their home country.

The Field of International Nursing

International nursing is a specialty because it consists of a unique body of knowledge with specific problems and domains of practice not shared by other recognized nursing specialties. International nursing is concerned with finding long-term sustainable solutions to problems of global importance to nursing. It is involved with development of individual nurses and capacity building of professional nursing systems at local and state levels. The unique characteristics of international nursing are listed in Box 15-5.

International nursing requires nurses to operate outside their own familiar comfort zones and to understand and function outside their own cultural base (language, interpersonal relationships, customs, and belief systems to name a few). Case Study 15-2 describes a child's situation that stems from a conflict of traditional religious beliers and modern health care measures.

CASE STUDY 15-2

Traditional Beliefs Versus Modern Medicine: AK's Story

Twelve-year-old AK lives with his parents in Malindi District in Kenya. He is currently in the Malindi District hospital waiting to have both feet amputated above the ankles to stop the spread of a jigger infestation (parasitic fleas) and subsequent gangrene infection. Without the amputation of his feet, the gangrene will continue spreading and he will lose his legs and ultimately his life.

Jiggers are common in the Malindi district, but infestation can be prevented by wearing closed toe shoes. The infestation/infection can be cured if treatment is started early when the parasitic fleas are newly burrowed into the skin. The District Medical Officer noted that the jigger menace is high in the area but compounded by parents whose "retrogressive" beliefs keep them from seeking medical attention or taking needed medications.

AK is in acute pain as his lies in his hospital bed, but he is more shocked to learn that his parents are in jail. He says he wishes the world would come to an end. AK's parents are currently in jail because they refused to seek medical help based on their religious beliefs. His father, the head of the Imani Moja Church, stated that "healing comes from God and death is natural. I believe the child would recover by God's grace" (p. 2). He and his wife have been praying for a miracle cure for AK for the last 2 years, while he remained bedridden, unable to stand or go to school. The magistrate charged AK's father with neglecting his parental responsibility by refusing to take his son for medical treatment; and, sentenced him to 2 years in prison. The magistrate felt that his beliefs were "totally unacceptable" in modern society.

Gitau, P. (2009). My parents' faith will cost me my feet or my life. *The Standard*. Published August 20, 2009. Nairobi, Kenya.

There are many reasons for incorporating international nursing content into the curriculum and providing clinical learning opportunities whereby nurses and nursing students can experience other parts of the world. The globalization of nursing is a known fact. Political alignments and technology encourage mobility and an interchange of ideas so that national borders are less obvious and obscure. Nurses must increasingly see themselves as part of a global community in which problems, solutions, resources, and opportunities are shared [see for example Rassin, Klug, Nathanzon, Kan, & Silner. (2009); Lee, Y, K., Lee, D., & Woo, J. (2009)].

International nursing is not the same as transcultural nursing, although the two share many of the same tenets and philosophical underpinnings. However, the focus of international nursing extends beyond those areas of concern in transcultural nursing. The world is made up of many cultures, and the processes of learning how to deliver culturally sensitive high-quality nursing or health care to a diverse population is the realm of transcultural nursing. International nursing uses all the skills of transcultural nursing within a broader context of "development" or "capacity building."

International Nursing as a Career

The total number of persons whose primary professional focus is **international health** is unknown despite efforts to gather data. An estimated 9,000 U.S. health professionals are working in the international health field. Of these, 3,800 are considered long term or employed for 1 year or more; 1,700 are short term, usually consultants; and 3,200 are volunteers. Of the total, the largest category is nurses, followed by physicians and administrators. Of the long-term professionals, many work on 2- or 3-year contracts; however, a core of international health professionals (educators, administrators, consultants, and researchers) work their entire careers in the field.

As with other careers, international nursing has benefits and drawbacks. Travel is stimulating,

RESEARCH APPLICATION 15-2
Becoming a Foreign Nurse

Magnusdottir, H. (2005). Overcoming strangeness and communication barriers: A phenomenological study of becoming a foreign nurse. *International Nursing Review, 52,* 263–269.

Icelandic society has seen a shift in demographics in the last 10 to 15 years from a basically homogeneous population to an increasingly multicultural one because of the influx of foreign residents. In the health field, this has been largely caused by an increase in foreign nurses seeking employment. In 2003, foreign nurses at the largest hospital in Iceland accounted for 4.5% of the employed nurses and overall accounted for approximately 2.5% of all nurses working in Iceland.

This study used a phenomenological approach to explore the experience of foreign nurses working at three hospitals in Iceland. Based on the Vancouver school of phenomenological research, the participants were seen as coresearchers. Purposeful sampling was used to identify 11 registered nurses from seven countries who participated in unstructured interviews (dialogues) about the topic. The participants were asked to describe and reflect on their experiences of ". . . being a foreign nurse working at a hospital in Iceland." Thematic analysis was applied to the data.

The overriding theme emerging from the data was one of "growing through overcoming strangeness and communication barriers." Five key themes identified included (1) tackling the initial, multiple challenges; (2) becoming an outsider and the need to be included; (3) struggling with the language barrier; (4) adjusting to a different work culture; and (5) overcoming challenges to succeed. Working in a foreign country displaces people from their own culture and puts them in unfamiliar surroundings. This can result in powerful disorientation and feelings of conflict, frustration, and struggle. The author notes that one interesting finding was that experiences of nurses from neighboring countries that were linguistically and culturally close to Iceland (for example, Canada and the United States) were initially as strenuous as the experiences of others from more distant lands.

Clinical Application
This study confirmed that the process of acculturation can be stressful and overwhelming, even painful and destabilizing, yet the end result is often positive. Being a "stranger" is a well-known phenomenon, and instances of racism and dislike of "the other" are realities to be addressed. Coworkers and supervisors may be more important than personal support systems when adjusting on the job. Language barriers are central to adjustment (as an instrument of communication and a vehicle of thought). Losing one's language was a major contributor to the nurses' loss of a sense of belonging. Nurses thinking about working overseas can use the insights in this study to help meet the challenges of a new working environment.

but not all travel experiences are positive. Living abroad has many challenges. Interpersonal skills can be challenging when many health projects have multinational teams with nurses, physicians, and others from dozens of different countries. As shown in Research Application 15-2, the process of adjusting to nursing in another country is often stressful. Bolton (2004b) warns would-be international aid workers that this is not a traditional career path. It requires the ability to adapt to what he calls "intensely challenging" situations and to withstand periods of emotional strain. Case Study 15-3 highlights the emotional roller coaster of working in a health care environment in which the "norms" of behavior are not familiar.

CASE STUDY 15-3

Two Afghan Girls: A Study in Contrasts

Parween was admitted to the intensive care unit of a local hospital in Kabul, Afghanistan, during the morning hours of a cold winter day. She was 13 years old, dark haired, fair skinned, and pale. Her brown eyes were wide in both pain and fear. Pain due to her condition, which was vaginal bleeding of unknown origin. Fear because she had been admitted to a hospital—in and of itself a frightening experience but compounded by the fact that this hospital was known to have "foreigners" on the staff (a team of Canadian and U.S. nurses and doctors working for CARE, Inc.).

The ICU was referred to as the "model ward" in the hospital because it was intended to serve as a model of excellent patient care with up-to-date equipment. The unit was staffed by a female head nurse and four staff nurses (two men, two women) plus one "nana/bacha" team of housekeepers who functioned as nurse's aides. A female CARE nurse worked as counterpart to the head nurse. The model ward had four beds and very few high-tech features beyond the only defibrillator in the country at that time. There were basic supplies, linens, and medications.

Parween came to the model ward with her family, three older brothers. They had brought her from her village to the city for treatment. The bleeding had started at home and progressed to the point where the family realized some form of

medical treatment was needed. However, she had not yet been examined by any physician, having been admitted from the ER directly to the unit. She was awake and alert but bleeding profusely. Her vital signs were taken, and a male laboratory technician drew blood to type and cross-match. Her three brothers stood guard around her bed. The head nurse started an IV. Blood was ordered and eventually started (by the CARE nurse).

Then the doctor entered the unit. The doctor was both male and foreign. The brothers would not let him near their sister. Following much discussion between the brothers and the head nurse, it was clear that the brothers were hesitant to let anyone examine their sister, given her age and the location of the bleeding. However, they agreed to let a female physician do the examination.

Unfortunately, most of the doctors in this hospital were male. As an adult medical/surgical facility, it was not seen as either a "women's or a maternity" hospital, where the majority of female physicians practiced. It took some time to find an appropriate physician. When she finally came, the brothers had a change of heart and would not let her examine their sister. They refused to consider any surgical procedures. Although they understood that without treatment their sister would most likely not survive, they choose comfort measures only over any form of "invasion of privacy" as they saw it. The brothers were not cold and unfeeling; they wept and demonstrated the depth of their sadness over their sister's condition. They sat at her bedside constantly. They held her hand. They believed it was their duty to protect her honor. Parween died the next morning.

Gulalai was only 10 years old. She lived in northern Afghanistan, far from any real towns. One day she cut her foot while playing, and it became infected. As the infection spread, so did the pain. Her family knew she needed medical attention. There were no health posts or clinics anywhere near their home. They decided to bring her to the "big city," Kabul, for treatment. Her father and brother began the arduous trek, literally carrying Gulalai on their backs over the mountains to the nearest big town, where they hitched a ride in a truck to Kabul.

When they arrived at the CARE hospital days later, Gulalai had gangrene and was dangerously

(case study continues on page 442)

CASE STUDY 15-3 *(continued)*

ill. After an examination, her family was told she needed immediate surgery if she was to have any chance to live. The doctors explained that they would need to amputate her left leg just above the knee. This was a major blow to the father and brother, not only because Gulalai was so near death, but because of the major implications of her losing a leg. The father worried about her ability to contribute to the family income if she could not work in the fields as she had before; he worried about how she would cope with the household chores that were part of her daily life, and how his wife would cope, caring for the other children, the chores, and a handicapped daughter. He wondered if she would be able to navigate the rough terrain on crutches. But most of all, the father and the brother worried about Gulalai's marriage prospects if she lost a leg. Would the families in their village shun her as a potential bride? Would she be destined to remain a spinster all her life? These were heavy concerns that needed to be weighed as they made the decision for Gulalai's treatment.

In the end, the father agreed to allow the surgery. He did not have all the answers, but he put his faith in Allah and said they would find a way to manage. Gulalai lost her leg and spent many months in the hospital recuperating. She became a familiar site walking the hallways with her crutches, her hair lightly covered with a shawl. She was shy but liked to smile. Her father and brother returned home but came back when she was discharged. They were so happy to see her healthy and mobile—they bought her a new pair of crutches, and then they all left the hospital.

In order to be successful in the international arena, the nurse needs a high degree of dedication, exceptional technical knowledge, and facility in informal diplomacy. Based on 16 years of personal experience, the author believes the following characteristics are critical for successful international nursing careers:

- High frustration tolerance and acceptance of ambiguity
- Resourcefulness
- Sense of adventure
- Open mind, flexible attitude
- Sense of humor
- Hardiness
- Cultural sensitivity and willingness to learn
- Enjoyment of diversity
- Language facility
- Ability to take criticism and intense scrutiny

When reflecting on their international experiences, most nurses who have spent substantial periods of time abroad indicate that they have learned from the exchange as well as contributed to improved health in the host country. Research on this subject reveals that nurses identify gaining increased knowledge in the following areas: cultural awareness, alternative health care delivery models, ways to include family members in nursing care, conservation of resources, nonbiomedical nursing interventions, and increased political awareness.

Preparation for International Nursing

Nurses often ask about academic qualifications and experience needed for international health work. There is in fact no identified standard set of educational or experiential requirements. All nurses who work overseas need to be clinically competent. Without earning the respect of the host country nurses, not much will happen. Local nurses expect you to be an expert in your field.

International nurses work with intelligent, skilled, and well-motivated professionals from all over the world. They are exposed to differing ideologies, methodologies, lifestyles, and languages. It is important that nurses have the skills, knowledge, and abilities needed to work with an international team. As Bolton (2004a) states, "Ideals cannot feed people." In addition to the obvious technical skills, nurses need good organizational management skills, people skills, oral presentation skills, teaching skills, research skills (most projects have built-in performance indicators that require quantitative and qualitative research methods), and writing abilities (projects require documentation and written reports; many require grant proposals and grant updates). Intergovernmental agencies and NGOs look for employees with a proven track record. Experience with a range of cultures and contexts is preferred. Employers want to gauge if you are likely to have an easy time learning a new language and adapting to new customs. In some cases, the first step is to gain experience by volunteering or serving as an intern on a project.

Internship Experiences

Another type of overseas experience involves an international internship in which students are given the opportunity to see firsthand if they are truly suited to international work. Many internships are academic in nature and can be taken for college credits toward a degree. Some internships require the student to pay academic and living costs as well as a program fee (Rubin, 2009). An example of an internship programs is Global Volunteers. Global Volunteers (2009) is a private, nonprofit international development organization working in close collaboration with local people worldwide. Service: direct service-learning programs: short-term volunteer teams in long-term service projects on six continents. United Nations Economic and Social Council (ECOSOC) status enables them to work with UN agencies and other NGOs to help achieve UN goals, especially as they relate to children. Tax deductible fees are paid directly to Global Volunteers. Contact: http://www.globalvolunteers.org.

The Peace Corps, Volunteer Services Overseas (VSO), and UN Volunteers are other good places to look for volunteer experiences. Many universities offer courses in humanitarian assistance and international development, with or without internship experiences.

Academic Preparation

With increasing frequency U.S. and Canadian nurse educators are recognizing the importance of incorporating international nursing into the curriculum of baccalaureate, master's, and doctoral programs and in providing continuing-education courses with an international focus. Nurses and nursing students are expressing an increased interest in international nursing and are traveling, studying, and working abroad in greater numbers. Nursing students are seeking information about the appropriate ways in which to become prepared for the practice of nursing in other countries and are choosing programs that have internationalized their curriculum.

As nurses prepare for international work, they may ask, "How can I ever learn all I need to know about this culture so I won't appear foolish or alienate people?" First of all, recognize that it is impossible to learn all there is to know about another culture, regardless of how many years spent living in the country. By definition, the nurse will always be perceived as an outsider, stranger, or foreigner to some extent. See Case Study 15-4 for one nurse's experience preparing for an international position.

CASE STUDY 15-4

Preparing for an International Nursing Assignment

In 1974 Brenda Jones, age 27, had 2 years of pediatric nursing experience, a master's degree in pediatric nursing, and 2 years of experience teaching pediatrics in a large university school of nursing. She had always wanted to "do something" internationally, so she applied to several development aid agencies (NGOs) to see what was available. She was ready to commit to a multiyear assignment and was excited about the prospects of traveling and doing something useful in a developing country.

Two major NGOs interviewed Brenda. She was prepared to discuss her clinical skills and what she felt she had to offer but was surprised by how much of the interview was focused on (1) her health status, (2) her motivations for going abroad, and (3) her coping and adjusting skills in new environments, including her "hardiness tolerance" for things like lack of plumbing or toilet facilities, presence of scorpions and other insects, and living in a group or dormlike situation with other women. Both agencies wanted to know if she spoke a foreign language (even with 6 years of Spanish in school, she had to answer "no" to that question).

Brenda was faced with really examining her motivations for taking on this type of work.

(case study continues on page 444)

Bolton (2004a) reports that the ICRC sometimes asks applicants, "What are you running away from?" He points out that one needs strong motivations to leave one's home, family, and comfortable surroundings to go live and work in war zones or in impoverished environments. Citing Helen Fielding's novel *Cause Celeb*, he refers to a character wearing an "aide T-shirt questionnaire" that reads: (a) Missionary? (b) Mercenary? (c) Misfit? (d) Broken Heart? This tongue-in-cheek message points out the need to examine one's own motives carefully and to think about how they might impact performance.

Two weeks after the first interview, Brenda was offered a nursing position in Saigon, Vietnam, at a major NGO field hospital. Although excited at first, she was forced to decline the position after her parents' strong reaction to her serving in a war zone (a reaction she had not thought about sufficiently). In hindsight she realized preparing her family for the change was as important as preparing herself. She was later offered a position in an established NGO hospital in south Asia, in a country she knew next to nothing about; she accepted the position as a "nurse educator."

The human resources director at the NGO told Brenda she would be working in an adult, 100-bed medical/surgical hospital in the capital city. She would work with the nurses to ensure quality care in support of the NGO's physician internship training program. In addition, she would interface with the students who came to the hospital for clinical practice. She would be joining a team of U.S. and Canadian physicians, nurses, laboratory technicians, and medical records personnel. She was told that none of the local nurses spoke English and that she would be expected to learn the local language.

Brenda had 1 month to prepare herself. The NGO stressed the importance of getting to know the country and sent her bulk documents to read containing information about the country: history, geography, politics, culture, ethnic groups, economy, and health care system. They included a large orientation manual for new employees with tips on how to pack (only two suitcases allowed), essential items to bring, what not to bring, and what to consider about dress in the country, norms of behavior, and dos and don'ts.

The NGO sent bibliography lists with suggested readings, and Brenda scoured the library looking for titles. She checked the university library for government documents on the country. She read all the *National Geographic* magazine stories and even whatever novels she could find.

Finally, she thought about the language. Living in the Washington, DC area, she was able to connect with the Foreign Service Institute and ask for assistance. Although she was not eligible for training, they put her in contact with the language instructor. He was willing to give her private lessons. So, twice a week, after work, Brenda drove to Alexandria, Virginia, and met with her language instructor—for a total of eight lessons. He agreed to provide the lessons for free, stating, "If you are going to help my people, I am willing to help you." The encounter with a native speaker was invaluable. Beyond the basics of pronunciation, grammar, reading, and writing, Brenda learned firsthand about the land and its peoples, customs, and traditions. She even got to sample some local foods!

When Brenda arrived in country, she felt she had a start in getting to know the people. At least she could say "hello." She surprised the local driver, who took her from the airport to the city, with her ability to read road signs and bits of billboards in the local language. She was fortunate that her employer believed language training was crucial to success. On arrival, Brenda was told she would not start working at the hospital right away. Instead, she spent the first month in full-time language study (provided by the Peace Corps). The second month she had half-day lessons. Then she hired a private tutor (provided by the NGO) who continued her lessons during her entire 2-year stay in country.

Research on international health care indicates that most U.S. and Canadian nurses work with more than one culture, often rotating back and forth between an international assignment and a position in North America. Skills and attitudes that nurses can develop have been identified by the Peace Corps (2009) and include

1. Listening skills, including awareness of nonverbal cues
2. Careful observation

3. Patience, not always expecting "them" to take the lead in adjusting
4. Ability to take risks, try new things
5. Awareness of one's own values and cultural assumptions
6. Ability to identify culture resources in the community
7. Recognition that the reasons for one's feelings of frustration may be cultural in origin

Summarized in Box 15-6 are ways in which U.S. and Canadian nurses can prepare in advance and orient themselves to their host country, in addition to formal academic study.

Patterns of Cultural Adjustment

Whenever people are immersed in another culture, they will go through a period of cultural adjustment. One of the more well-known patterns

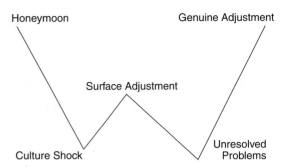

FIGURE 15-1 The W model of cultural adjustment.

of cultural adjustment is the W model. Many variations on this theory exist, but the general pattern has been well documented in intercultural communications research. It is one of the few concepts agreed on by most professionals involved in cross-cultural education. Figure 15-1 illustrates the theory.

Cultural Adjustment

Five stages of cultural adaptation are illustrated as the points on W; this pattern may depend on the length of stay and the purpose of being in the other culture. The five stages are

1. Excitement, or the honeymoon period, which is characterized by enthusiasm resulting from the newness and sense of adventure.
2. Culture shock. The excitement is gone. Things are not "like back home"; social cues and relationships are difficult; there are feelings of alienation and homesickness and a temporary dislike of the host culture.
3. Surface adjustment. During this stage, the nurse is beginning to catch on; things are starting to make sense; rudimentary language (more accurate communication) skills are acquired, and the nurse is able to communicate some basic ideas and feelings, making some relationships in the local culture; the nurse begins to feel more comfortable.
4. Frustration and a deeper level of unresolved problems; the assignment period in the

---

BOX 15-6

Preparations and Orientation for International Assignments

- Reading about the culture, politics, economics, religions, and health care systems; try to find out about the specific work environment
- Getting information from the employing agency about what to bring, including specialized equipment, textbooks, or other materials
- Reviewing with the employing agency the nature of the work and any specific job performance expectations
- Reviewing scholarly and popular literature about the culture
- Talking with host nationals living in the United States or Canada
- Eating foods from the host country
- Contacting the consulate or embassy of the country to be visited
- Contacting U.S. or Canadian government offices for information about travel, passports, and visas
- Studying the language
- Watching documentaries or travel films
- Visiting the country as a tourist prior to taking a professional position

culture may seem very long, and the nurse may experience feelings of boredom, frustration, and isolation.

5. Genuine adjustment, which is characterized by acceptance of the new culture as just another way of living; the nurse may not always approve of cultural practices but understands the differences and begins to peel back some of the rich layers of the culture. The nurse has established genuine, real relationships with people in the host country.

All nurses experience the components identified in the cultural pattern when living in an unfamiliar culture. Some may decide that trying to adjust is too difficult and return home at the early "cultural shock" stage. Being aware that there is a pattern to feelings and reactions to the new culture is one step in making the nurse more effective in the international setting. Clients from other nations experience similar cultural patterns when they enter the United States or Canada. Shorter in duration, a phenomenon know as *reentry shock* can be expected when the nurse returns home. Reentry shock consists of feelings of general dissatisfaction, criticism for lifeways of his or her home country, and free-floating anxiety.

Going Abroad

In the next section, you will be given guidelines for making decisions about going abroad and choosing sending agencies that are congruent with your philosophical beliefs.

Motivation

Before choosing a sending agency, it is essential to examine one's motivation for going abroad. In studies of U.S. nurses engaging in international consultation, several reasons motivating nurses have been identified, including enjoyment of people from other cultures, interest in travel, moral convictions, religious beliefs, financial rewards, personal invitation by host country counterparts, cross-cultural exchange of ideas, professional commitment, and service to those in need. Identifying motivation and determining the goals and purposes for the international experience will facilitate selection of the appropriate type of position and sending agency.

Length of Time Abroad

Related to the motivation for going abroad is the length of time that you plan to spend overseas. Before contacting potential sending agencies, it is important to determine a time commitment, stated in terms of days, weeks, months, or years. Opportunities for short-term international experiences (less than 6 months) vary widely and are likely to require trade-offs in benefits provided by the agency. Travel study programs usually assume that the applicant is willing to pay part or all of the expenses for the trip. Long-term international experiences offer a wide variety of opportunities, with contracts varying according to the agency's needs and resources.

Geographic Region

If a particular region is preferred, this must be matched with the sending agency's activities and projects. Some agencies specialize in a particular region, whereas others have programs on virtually every continent. The following reasons may motivate the nurse to choose a particular region or country: (1) political stability of the country, (2) personal or emotional reasons such as a significant other living in the area or familiarity with the language, and/or (3) matching host country needs with the expertise of the nurse.

Although global politics may shift rapidly, the Middle East, South Africa, and certain parts of Central and South America have a reputation for volatile politics including anti-American demonstrations. Personal safety is a concern, and careful research should be conducted before accepting an assignment in a politically unstable area. U.S. Department of State reports, information provided by the sending agency, informal discussions with recently returned visitors to the county, and current news sources may provide the necessary information to determine the safety of an area.

Reasonable Expectations of Sending Agencies

Although specific details will vary according to the sending agency, Box 15-7 is intended to

provide guidelines for asking questions. Sending agencies expect questions and recognize that interviewing is a two-way process.

Negotiating a Contract

The preceding discussion has focused on some aspects that are reasonable to expect in a

---

BOX 15-7

Guidelines for Choosing an Intternational Sending Agency

Salary or Stipend

- What is the salary or stipend in U.S. or Canadian dollars?
- If any portion is paid in local currency, what is the exchange rate?
- What has been the history of fluctuation in the exchange rate during the past 2 years?
- What is the cost of living compared with the salary or stipend?
- What is the average cost for housing, food, transportation, and utilities in the host country? Will the sending agency cover any of these costs?
- Can local currency be exchanged for U.S. dollars? Can U.S. or Canadian dollars be used to purchase local currency?
- Can salary earned in the country be taken out of the country? If so, by what means? Bank transfer? Cashier's check? Cash and carry?
- What length of time is usually required for bank transactions? International transfers? Local banking needs?
- To which governments are taxes owed? What is the rate of taxation? How, when, and where should tax statements be processed or filed?

Travel to Host Country Assignment

- Is round-trip airfare paid by the agency? Are spouses and/or dependents sent or eligible for discounted fares?
- Is there a payback clause for early contract termination?
- Who makes travel arrangements? Is a confirmation by the ticket holder required?
- How frequently are return trips to the United States or Canada allowed and/or paid for by the agency?

Housing and Moving

- Does the agency provide housing? Is it in an expatriate community or in a local neighborhood?
- What is the type of housing provided? Are accommodations shared?
- Are there toilet and bathing facilities, central heating and/or air conditioning, running water, and window screens?
- What type of energy is used? What is the average monthly cost?
- Is there a reliable source of electricity available? If not, is there a generator?
- Is the housing furnished or unfurnished?
- What are the conditions of the move? By what means (air, land, sea)? Are travel and household insurance included? Amount of coverage provided? Who is responsible for packing?
- What household goods and commodities are reasonable to expect locally? At what cost?
- Does the agency have special arrangements for shipping items such as regular mail pouch service, agency deliveries, etc?
- If housing allowance is given, are family members included?
- Who is responsible for daily maintenance (housecleaning, cooking, gardening, upkeep)?
- What are the security arrangements?

Local Transportation

- Are vehicles available to staff for job-related travel? For personal use after hours and on weekends?
- What is the cost of gasoline? Maintenance of a vehicle? Does the agency employ a mechanic? Are reliable local mechanics available? Are replacement parts for vehicles available?

(box continues on page 448)

BOX 15-7

Guidelines for Choosing an Intternational Sending Agency (*continued*)

- Does the agency provide car loans? What are the terms? Is there a waiting list for vehicle purchases? If so, how long? What is the average price for a vehicle?
- What are the local regulations on drivers' licenses and automobile insurance?
- If vehicles are not available, what methods of local transportation are used by agency staff? Cost? Availability? Safety?
- Are employees expected to drive? Does the agency hire drivers? Are women permitted to drive vehicles? If not, when are drivers available? Costs?

Insurance Benefits

- What types of health, life, disability, and retirement insurance are available? Are family members included?
- In case of illness, what is the agency policy concerning treatment? What health care facilities may be accessed for personal and family health care?
- If local hospitals are used, what is the quality of care compared with the United States or Canada? What type of pediatric care is available locally for dependent children?
- Is paid leave and/or airfare to the United States granted for health care emergencies? For compassionate leave?

Vacations and Holidays

- What U.S., Canadian, and/or local holidays does the agency recognize?
- What is the length and frequency of vacation or holiday absences? Are there limitations to travel during vacation?
- In politically volatile areas, are more frequent vacations or designated leaves (R&R) permitted and/or encouraged?
- Does the agency have an informal or formal network allowing for staff to vacation at a reduced cost?

- Do staff members offer hospitality to other agency members while traveling? Is it expected that all staff reciprocate by housing agency members during vacations and/or job-related travel?

Orientation Program

- What are the length, location, and nature of the agency orientation?
- Are language studies required? Where do language studies occur? Who pays for classes?
- Are local interpreters available? Are there any gender-related or age-related factors to consider when using an interpreter?
- Does the orientation include study of the political, economic, social, cultural, religious, and health-related aspects of the host country?
- Who is the U.S./Canadian ambassador to the host country? Where is the U.S./Canadian embassy/ consulate located? Does the agency enjoy any special "privileges" (movies, commissary shopping, and access to information)?
- In case of natural disaster or political unrest, what is the emergency evacuation plan for expatriates? How are expatriates linked to their embassy/ consulate emergency communication systems?

Other

- Are local and private schools available for children? In English? How hard are they to get into? Do they meet U.S./Canadian/international educational standards?
- Does the agency provide an educational stipend for dependent children? In country only?
- Does the agency provide employment opportunities for spouses? How easy is it to find work in the local economy? Are there special rules and regulations about spouses working in country?
- Does the agency provide advice about U.S./Canadian income tax laws and filing returns while overseas?

---

contractual agreement with a sending agency. Before signing the contract, it is important to study the details carefully and to discuss any unclear matters with the agency representative. A written job description should accompany the contract along with a statement detailing the conditions surrounding contract termination by either the nurse or the sending agency.

Choosing an International Sending Agency

Because there are many agencies that send nurses abroad, it is impossible to provide an exhaustive list. The ones discussed in this chapter provide an overview of agencies that use nurses for health-related projects abroad. Not included were universities, foundations, private industries, study or travel groups, and the U.S. and Canadian military organizations. One Web site that can assist in the search for the right agency is InterAction (2009).

Nurses may affiliate themselves with a variety of sponsoring agencies. Sponsorship may be through a U.S. or Canadian organization or through the host country (ministry of health, university, hospital, school of nursing, public health agency, or private enterprise). Joint sponsorships, though relatively rare, also may occur. For example, some religious groups have both international and national organizations that may elect joint sponsorship.

SUMMARY

With increasing frequency, U.S. and Canadian nurses are traveling, studying, researching, consulting, teaching, administering, and practicing nursing abroad. The decision to engage in an international interchange requires much thought and planning. Philosophical congruence with the sending agency or organization, selection of geographic area of interest, length of time available, and matching background with host-country needs are factors that interplay with the desire to go abroad.

Many U.S. and Canadian nurses are relatively naive about negotiating a contract with a sending agency. An overview of reasonable questions to pursue with the agency has been provided, including discussions of salary or stipend, travel to the assignment site, housing and moving expenses, local transportation, insurance coverage, vacation and holiday leave, and orientation policies.

REFERENCES

Bolton, M. (2004a). *Aid agencies prefer professionals to inexperienced volunteers.* Retrieved April 1, 2009, from http://www.transitionsabroad.com/publications/magazine/0501/aid_agencies_prefer_professionals_to_volunteers.shtml

Bolton, M. (2004b). *Becoming an aid worker: An experienced professional explains how it's done.* Retrieved March 29, 2009, from http://www.transitionsabroad.com/publications/magazine/0409/becoming_an_international_aid_worker.shtml

Canadian International Development Agency. (2009). Homepage at http://www.acdi-cida.gc.ca/index-e.htm

CARE, Inc. (2009). Homepage at http://www.care.org/

Catholic Relief Services. (2009). Homepage at http://crs.org/

Centers for Disease Control and Prevention. (2009). Homepage at http://www.cdc.gov/

Gitau, P. (2009). My parents' faith will cost me my feet or my life. *The Standard.* Published August 20, 2009. Nairobi, Kenya

Global Ministries. (2004). *News: Ruth May Harnar.* Retrieved August 4, 2005, from http://www.globalministries.org/news/harnar.htm

Global Volunteers. (2009). Homepage at http://www.globalvolunteers.org/

Hewlett, B. L., & Hewlett, B. S. (2005). Providing care and facing death: Nursing during an Ebola outbreak in Central Africa. *Journal of Transcultural Nursing, 16*(4), 289–297.

InterAction. (2009). Homepage at http://www.interaction.org

International Committee of the Red Cross. (2009). Homepage in English at http://www.icrc.org/eng

International Council of Nurses. (2003). *Tackling the UN millennium development goals. 2002–2003 biennial report.* Geneva, Switzerland: Author. Retrieved April 1, 2009, from http://www.icn.ch/02-03BiennialReport.pdf

International Council of Nurses. (2009). Homepage at http://www.icn.ch/

International Federation of Red Cross and Red Crescent Societies. (2009). Homepage at http://www.ifrc.org/

International Rescue Committee. (2009). Homepage at http://www.theirc.org/

Krommenhoek, L. (2009). Vaccinating against measles in Chad: Battered trucks and donkey tracks, *Médecins Sans Frontières Voices from the field.* Retrieved June 1, 2009, from http://www.doctorswithoutborders.org/news/article_print.cfm?id=3525

Lau, E., Médecins Sans Frontières. (2005). *Voices from the field: Aceh is completely smashed.* Retrieved December 2006, from http://www.doctorswithoutborders.org/news/voices/2005/01-2005_aceh.cfm/

Lee, Y. K., Lee, D., & Woo, J. (2009). Tai chi and health-related quality of life in nursing home residents. *Journal of Nursing Scholarship, 41*(1), 35–43.

Magnusdottir, H. (2005). Overcoming strangeness and communication barriers: A phenomenological study of becoming a foreign nurse. *International Nursing Review, 52,* 263–269.

Médecins Sans Frontières/Doctors Without Borders. (2009). Homepage at http://www.doctorswithoutborders.org/aboutus/index.cfm

Mercy Corps. (2009). Homepage at http://www.mercycorps.org/

Nestrell, J., Médecins Sans Frontières. (2004). *Voices from the field: Nurse Jessica Nestrell. Going upriver: MSF aid worker battles measles in Congo.* Retrieved December 2006, from http://www.doctorswithoutborders.org/news/voices/2004/10-2004_drc.cfm

Nightingale. (1859, 2007). *Notes on nursing.* Gloucestershire, UK: Tempus Publishing Group.

Oxfam. (2009). Homepage at http://www.oxfam.org.uk/

Pan American Health Organization. (2009). Homepage at http://www.paho.org/

Peace Corps. (2009). Homepage at http://www.peacecorps.gov/index.cfm

Project HOPE. (2009). Homepage at http://www.projecthope.org/

Rassin, M., Klug, E., Nathanzon, H., Kan, A., & Silner, D. (2009). Cultural differences in child delivery: Comparisons between Jewish and Arab women in Israel. *International Nursing Review, 56,* 123–130.

Rubin, K. (2009). Overseas internships: Jumpstart careers. *International Educator, 18*(3), 58–70.

Sachs, J. (2005). *Investing in development: A practical plan to achieve the Millennium Development Goals.* New York: UN Publications.

Save the Children. (2009). Homepage at http://www.savethechildren.org/

UNICEF. (2009). Homepage at http://www.unicef.org/

United Nations. (2006). *UN Millennium Project.* Accessed December 8, 2006, at www.unmillenniumproject.org

United Nations. (2009a). Homepage in English at http://www.un.org/english/

United Nations. (2009b). Volunteers' homepage at http://www.unv.org/

United Nations Development Program. (2006). *Human development report 2006: Beyond scarcity: Power, poverty and the global water crisis.* Retrieved from http://hdr.undp.org/hdr2006/pdfs/report/HDR06-complete.pdf

United States Agency for International Development. (2009). Homepage at http://www.usaid.gov/

World Economic Forum. (2005). *Global governance initiative. Annual Report 2006.* Washington, DC: Communications Development, Incorporated. Retrieved April 1, 2007, from http://www.weforum.org/pdf/Initiatives/GGI_Report06.pdf

World Health Organization. (2001). *Strengthening nursing and midwifery* (WHA 54.12). Geneva, Switzerland: Author.

World Health Organization. (2002). *Strategic directions for strengthening nursing and midwifery services.* Geneva, Switzerland: Author. Accessed June 2006 from http://whqlibdoc.who.int/publications/2002/924156217X.pdf

World Health Organization. (2006). *The Nursing and Midwifery programme at WHO: What Nursing and Midwifery services mean to health.* Retrieved March 1, 2009 from http://www.paho.org/English/DPM/SHD/HR/midwives-nurses-leafletWHA06-eng.pdf

World Health Organization. (2009a). Homepage at www.who.org

World Health Organization. (2009b). Homepage for Nursing and Midwifery. Retrieved, from http://www.who.int/hrh/nursing_midwifery/en/

World Health Organization. (2009c). *Health and the Millennium Development Goals.* Retrieved March 1, 2009, from http://www.who.int/mdg/en/

World Health Organization, Regional Office for Europe. (2006). *Declaration of Alma Ata.* Retrieved April 23, 2009, from http://www.euro.who.int/AboutWHO/Policy/20010827_1

World Vision. (2009). Homepage at http://www.worldvision.org

Andrews/Boyle Transcultural Nursing Assessment Guide for Individuals and Families

Joyceen S. Boyle
and Margaret M. Andrews

Biocultural Variations and Cultural Aspects of the Incidence of Disease

Does the client and/or family members relate a health history associated with genetic or acquired conditions that are more prevalent for a specific cultural group (e.g., diabetes, hypertension, cardiovascular disease, sickle cell anemia, Tay-Sachs disease, G-6-PD deficiency, lactose intolerance)? Does the client's family relate such a history?

Are there socioenvironmental conditions more prevalent among a specific cultural group that can be observed in the client or family members (e.g., lead poisoning, alcoholism, HIV/AIDS, drug abuse, ear infections, family violence, fetal alcohol spectrum disorder [FASD], obesity, respiratory diseases)?

Are there diseases against which the client has an increased resistance (e.g., skin cancer in darkly pigmented individuals, malaria for those with sickle cell anemia)?

Does the client have distinctive features characteristic of a particular ethnic or cultural group (e.g., skin color, hair texture)? Do his or her family members have such features? Within the family group, are there variations in anatomy characteristic of a particular ethnic or cultural group (e.g., body structure, height, weight, facial shape and structure [nose, eye shape, facial contour], upper and lower extremities)?

How do anatomic, racial, and ethnic variations affect the physical and mental examination?

Communication

What language does the client speak at home with family members? In what language would the client prefer to communicate with you? What other languages does the client speak or read? What other languages do the client's family members speak or read?

What is the fluency level of the client in English—both written and spoken? What is the fluency level of the client's family members?

Does the client need an interpreter? Do his or her family members need an interpreter? Does the health care setting provide interpreters? Who would the client and his or her family members prefer to assist with interpretation? Is there anyone whom the client would prefer not to serve as an interpreter (e.g., member of the opposite sex, person younger or older than the client, member of a rival tribe, ethnic group, or nationality)?

What are the rules and style (formal or informal) of communication? How does the client prefer to be addressed? What do his or her family members prefer? What are the preferred terms for greeting?

How is it necessary to vary the technique and style of communication during the relationship with the client to accommodate his or her cultural background (e.g., tempo of conversation, eye contact, sensitivity to topical taboos, norms of confidentiality, and style of explanation)? How do these factors vary with family members, if at all?

What are the styles of individual and family members' nonverbal communication?

How does the client's nonverbal communication compare with that of individuals from other cultural groups? How does the client's style of nonverbal communication differ from the health care provider's style? How does it affect the client's relationships with you and with other members of the health care team? How does communication with the family influence the care environment?

How do the client and family members feel about health care providers who are not of the same cultural or religious background (e.g., Black, middle-class nurse; Hispanic of a different social class; Muslim or Jewish care provider)? Does the client prefer to receive care from a nurse of the same cultural background, gender, and/or age? How do family members react to care providers of different cultural backgrounds, age, and gender?

Cultural Affiliations

With what cultural group(s) does the client report affiliation (e.g., American, Hispanic, Irish, Black, Navajo, American Indian, or combination)? It is becoming increasingly common for Americans to identify with two or more groups, such as Native American and African American. Tiger Woods, for example, has identified himself as being of Thai and African American heritage. Equally important, to what degree does the client identify with the cultural group (e.g., "we" concept of solidarity or as a fringe member)?

How do the views of other family members coincide or differ from the client regarding cultural affiliations?

What is the preferred term that the cultural group chooses for itself? What term does the client choose?

Where was client born? Where were his or her parents born? What are the generational similarities and differences in regards to cultural identification, language, customs, values, and so on?

Where has the client lived (country, city, or area within a country) and when (during what years of his or her life)? If the client has recently immigrated to the United States or another country, knowledge of prevalent diseases in his or her country of origin as well as sociopolitical history may be helpful. If the client is a recent immigrant, did he or she live in countries of transit? For how long? Current residence? Occupation? Occupation in home country?

Cultural Sanctions and Restrictions

How does the client's cultural group regard expression of emotion and feelings, spirituality, and religious beliefs? How are feelings related to dying, death, and grieving expressed in a culturally appropriate manner?

How do men and women express modesty? Are there culturally defined expectations about male–female relationships, including the nurse–client relationship?

Does the client or family express any restrictions related to sexuality, exposure of various parts of the body, or certain types of surgery (e.g., vasectomy, hysterectomy, abortion)?

Are there restrictions against discussion of dead relatives or fears related to the unknown?

Developmental Considerations

Are there any distinct growth and development characteristics that vary with the cultural background of the client and family (e.g., bone density, psychomotor patterns of development, fat folds)?

What factors are significant in assessing children of various ages from the newborn period through adolescence (e.g., male and female circumcision, expected growth on standards grid, culturally acceptable age for toilet training, duration of breast-feeding, introduction of various types of foods, gender differences, discipline, and socialization to adult roles)?

What are the beliefs and practices associated with developmental life events such as pregnancy, birth, marriage, and death?

What is the cultural perception of aging (e.g., is youthfulness or the wisdom of old age more valued)?

How are elderly persons cared for within the cultural group (e.g., cared for in the home of adult children, placed in institutions for care)? What are culturally accepted roles for the elderly?

Economics

Who is the principal wage earner in the family and what is the income level? Is there more than one wage earner? Are there other sources of financial support? (*Note:* These may be potentially sensitive questions.)

What insurance coverage (health, dental, vision, pregnancy, cancer, or special conditions) does the client and his or her family have?

What impact does the economic status have on the client and his or her family's lifestyle and living conditions?

What has been the client and family's experience with the health care system in terms of reimbursement, costs, and insurance coverage?

Educational Background

What is the client's highest educational level obtained? What values do the family members express regarding educational achievements?

Does the client's educational level affect his or her knowledge level concerning his or her health literacy—how to obtain the needed care, teaching related to or learning about health care, and any written material that he or she is given in the health care setting (e.g., insurance forms, educational literature, information about diagnostic procedures and laboratory tests, admissions forms, etc.)? Does the client's educational level affect health behavior? As an example, in the United States, cigarette smoking and obesity have been linked to socioeconomic levels.

Can the client read and write English, or is another language preferred? If English is the client's second language, are health-related materials available in the client's primary language? Are all family members fluent in English?

What learning style is most comfortable and familiar? Does the client prefer to learn through written materials, oral explanations, videos, and/or demonstrations?

Does the client access health information via the Internet?

Do the client and family members prefer intervention settings away from hospitals and other clients which may have negative connotations for them? Are community sites such as churches, schools, or adult day-care centers a good alternate choice for the client and his or her family, considering they are informal settings that may be more conducive for open discussion, demonstrations, and reinforcement of information and skills? Are the client and family more comfortable in their home setting?

Health-Related Beliefs and Practices

To what cause does the client attribute illness and disease or what factors influence the acquisition of illness and disease (e.g., divine wrath, imbalance in hot/cold, yin/yang, punishment for moral transgressions, a hex, soul loss, pathogenic organism, past behavior, growing older)? Is there congruence within the family on these beliefs?

What are the client's cultural beliefs about ideal body size and shape? What is the client's self-image in relation to the ideal?

How does the client describe his or her health-related condition? What names or terms are used? How does the client express pain, discomfort, or anxiety?

What do the client and family members believe promotes health (e.g., eating certain foods, wearing amulets to bring good luck, sleeping, resting, getting good nutrition, reducing stress, exercising, praying or performing rituals to ancestors, saints, or other deities)?

What is the client's religious affiliation? How is the client actively involved in the practice of religion? Do other family members have the same religious beliefs and practices? Do the client and/or family members incorporate religious practices, such as healing ceremonies or prayer, into health/illness care?

Does the client and his or her family rely on cultural healers (e.g., curandero, shaman, spiritualist, priest, medicine man or woman, minister)? Who determines when the client is sick and when he or she is healthy? Who influences the choice or type of healer and treatment that should be sought?

In what types of cultural healing or health promoting practices does the client engage (e.g., use of herbal remedies, potions, or massage; wearing of talismans, copper bracelets, or chains to discourage evil spirits; healing rituals; incantations; or prayers)? Do family members share these beliefs and practices?

How are biomedical or scientific health care providers perceived? How do the client and his or her family perceive nurses? What are the expectations of nurses and nursing care workers?

Who will care for the client at home? What accommodations will family members make to provide caregiving?

How does the client's family and cultural group view mental disorders? Are there differences in acceptable behaviors for physical versus psychological illnesses?

Kinship and Social Networks

What is the composition of a "typical family" within the kinship network? What is the composition of the client's family?

Who makes up the client's social network (family, friends, peers, neighbors)? How do they influence the client's health or illness status?

How do members of the client's social support network define caring or caregiving? What is the role of various family members during health and illness episodes? Who makes decisions about health and health care?

How does the client's family participate in the promotion of health (e.g., lifestyle changes in diet, activity level, etc.) and nursing care (e.g., bathing, feeding, touching, being present) of the client?

Does the cultural family structure influence the client's response to health or illness (e.g., beliefs, strengths, weaknesses, and social class)?

What influence do ethnic, cultural, and/or religious organizations have on the lifestyle and quality of life of the client (e.g., the National Association for the Advancement of Colored People [NAACP], churches [such as African American Muslim, Jewish, Catholic, and others]) that may provide schools, classes, and/or community-based health care programs.

Are there special gender issues within this cultural group? Do the client and family members conform to traditional roles (e.g., women may be viewed as the caretakers of home and children, while men work outside the home and have primary decision-making responsibilities)?

Nutrition

What nutritional factors are influenced by the client's cultural background? What is the meaning of food and eating to the client and his or her family?

Does the client have any eating or nutritional disorders (e.g., anorexia, bulimia, obesity, lactose intolerance)? Do the client's family members have any similar disorders? How do the client and family view these conditions?

With whom does the client usually eat? What types of foods are eaten? What is the timing and sequencing of meals? What are the usual meal patterns?

What does the client define as food? What does the client believe constitutes a "healthy" versus an "unhealthy" diet? Are these beliefs congruent with what the client actually eats?

Who shops for and chooses food? Where are the foodstuffs purchased? Who prepares the actual meals? How are the family members involved in nutritional choices, values, and choices about food?

How are the foods prepared at home (type of food preparation, cooking oil[s] used, length of time foods are cooked [especially vegetables], amount and type of seasoning added to various foods during preparation)? Who does the food preparation?

Has the client chosen a particular nutritional practice such as vegetarianism or abstinence from red meat or from alcoholic or fermented beverages? Do other family members adhere to these beliefs and practices?

Do religious beliefs and practices influence the client's or family's diet (e.g., amount, type, preparation, or delineation of acceptable food combinations, [e.g., kosher diets])? Does the client or client's family abstain from certain foods at regular intervals, on specific dates determined by the religious calendar, or at other times? Are there other food prohibitions or prescriptions?

If the client or client's family's religion mandates or encourages fasting, what does the term *fast* mean (e.g., refraining from certain types of foods, eating only during certain times of the day, skipping certain meals)? For what period of time are family members expected to fast? Are there exceptions to fasting (e.g., are pregnant women or children excluded from fasting)?

Are special utensils used (e.g., chopsticks, cookware, kosher restrictions)?

Does the client or client's family use home and folk remedies to treat illnesses (e.g., herbal remedies, acupuncture, cupping, or other healing rituals often involving eggs, lemons, candles)? Which over-the-counter medications are used?

Religion and Spirituality

How does the client or family's religious affiliation affect health and illness (e.g., life events such as death, chronic illness, body image alteration, cause and effect of illness)?

What is the role of religious beliefs and practices during health and illness? Are there special rites or blessings for those with serious or terminal illnesses?

Are there healing rituals or practices that the client and family believe can promote well-being or hasten recovery from illness? If so, who performs these? What materials or arrangements are necessary for the nurse to have available for the practice of these rituals?

What is the role of significant religious representatives during health and illness? Are there recognized religious healers (e.g., Islamic Imans, Christian Scientist practitioners or nurses, Catholic priests, Mormon elders, Buddhist monks)?

Values Orientation

What are the client's attitudes, values, and beliefs about his or her health and illness status? Do family members have similar values and beliefs?

How do these influence behavior in terms of promotion of health and treatment of disease? What are the client's or family's attitudes, values, and beliefs about health care providers?

Does culture affect the manner in which the client relates to body image change resulting from illness or surgery (e.g., importance of appearance, beauty, strength, and roles in the cultural group)? Is there a cultural stigma associated with the client's illness (i.e., how is the illness or the manner in which it was contracted viewed by the family and larger culture)?

How do the client and his or her family view work, leisure, and education?

How does the client perceive and react to change?

How do the client and his or her family perceive changes in lifestyle related to current illness or surgery?

How do the client and his/her family view biomedical care or scientific health care (e.g., suspiciously, fearfully, acceptingly, unquestioningly, with awe)?

How does the client value privacy, courtesy, touch, and relationships with others?

How does the client relate to persons outside of his or her cultural group (e.g., withdrawal, suspicion, curiosity, openness)?

Andrews/Boyle Transcultural Nursing Assessment Guide for Groups and Communities

Joyceen S. Boyle
and Margaret M. Andrews

Family and Kinship Systems

Are the families nuclear, extended, or blended? Do family members live in close proximity? What are communication patterns within the distinct community groups? What is the role and status of individual family members? By age and gender?

How does the family and/or group members relate to the larger community or groups?

Are there distinct ethnic neighborhoods or areas of the community where distinct cultural groups, refugees, or immigrants live?

If working with a refugee community, ask about names of tribes and/or clans.

What place do the "ancestors" have in the worldview of the group? How is the belief in the power of the ancestors incorporated in the daily life and rituals of the group?

Is the group now or has it traditionally been matriarchal or patriarchal? Is there a preference for first cousins to marry?

Social Life and Networks

What are the daily routines of the group? What are the important life cycle events such as birth, marriage, death? How are they celebrated or observed?

How are the educational systems organized? How do they receive and accept input from the community? How do they assist students from new immigrants or refugees?

What are the social problems experienced by the group or within the community?

Are there special concerns with a particular ethnic or cultural group such as abuse of alcohol, FASD, gang membership, polygamy? How does the group view what we label as domestic violence and corporal punishment?

Are newly arrived groups, such as immigrants or refugees included within the local community or isolated? Who are the group's local leaders?

Are there centers or organizations that reach out to special groups within the community?

What activities or opportunities are available to community members? For example, are GED courses, English as a second language classes and/or work training available to newcomers?

How does the social environment contribute to a sense of belonging? Do all members of the group belong to a distinct religious group? What are the ways that the group practices its religion? What are the dominant religious groups within a community.

What are the group's social interaction patterns? Do all members of the group speak a common language?

Are ethnic grocery stores, restaurants, and churches located within the community? What foods do members of the cultural group commonly eat? What foods/substances do they commonly avoid (i.e., alcohol, pork products)?

Are members of the group comfortable moving away from the larger group?

Where are ethnic groups, immigrants, or refugees located within the larger community?

Political or Government Systems

Which factors in the political system influence the ways in which the group perceives its status vis-à-vis the dominant culture, that is, laws, justice, and cultural heroes?

How does the economic system influence control of resources such as land, water, housing, jobs, and opportunities?

What is the legal status of the group members? Refugee or immigrant visas? Temporary worker permits? Documented or undocumented?

How does the local government respond to the ethnic and cultural make-up of the community? What are the ways that the local community "embraces its diversity"?

Language and Traditions

Are there differences in dialects or languages spoken between health care professionals and local groups within the community?

What is the literacy level of members of the group? Can they read or write in any language?

Do health care facilities provide educational materials in diverse languages?

In what ways do the major cultural traditions of history, art, drama, and so on, influence the cultural identity of the group?

How are local cultures or ethnic traditions embraced during holidays or special celebrations?

Worldviews, Value Orientations, and Cultural Norms

What are the major cultural values about the relationships of cultural groups to nature and to one another? How can the group's ethical beliefs be described?

What are the norms and standards of behavior (authority, responsibility, dependability, and competition)?

Is the group communal versus individualistic? How different is their worldview from the dominant worldview of the larger society or culture?

What are the cultural attitudes about time, work, and leisure?

What are the common values of the group, such as education, work, and so on.

Are there unique cultural practices within the group that might bring wider community censure such as the role of women, discipline of children, relationships between husband and wife?

Religious Beliefs and Practices

What are the major religious beliefs and practices within the community?

How do they influence daily life? How do they relate to health practices? What are the practices surrounding major life events such as birth, marriage, death?

Does the cultural group have particular practices related to grieving or mourning?

Health Beliefs and Practices

What are the group's attitudes and beliefs regarding health and illness? Does the cultural group seek care from indigenous (folk) practitioners? Where do group members go to seek care? What makes the decisions about seeking health care? Accepting treatments? Are there biologic variations that are important to the health of this group? What are the group's expressed health concerns? Are there cultural or ethnic stores in neighborhoods selling medicinal herbs?

What are the primary health concerns and/ or illnesses in this population/cultural group? Examples might be: malaria, HIV/AIDS, female circumcision, malnutrition, tuberculosis. How do the group's concerns align with those of the local and state health care systems.

Health Care Systems

Do community health care facilities provide interpreters? Do physicians offices and other health care facilities offer educational materials in languages other than English? Are health facilities located in accessible locations, that is, in ethnic neighborhoods? Do health care providers incorporate aspects of other medical systems, that is, acupuncture and referrals to traditional healers?

Do members of the group have access to health care? Do they have adequate transportation? Are the hours of operation of health care facilities and availability of appointment times appropriate for members of the group?

Andrews/Boyle Transcultural Nursing Assessment Guide for Health Care Organizations and Facilities

Joyceen S. Boyle, Margaret M. Andrews, and Patti Ludwig-Beymer

Environmental Context

What is the general environment of the community that surrounds the health care organization? Where is the facility located in proximity to the population that it serves?

What is the socioeconomic status of the adjacent community? What are race/ethnicity characteristics of residents? What are the identified health disparities?

What are the community's views on health and illness?

Is there appropriate and easy access to the facility? Is the signage to the facility easy to understand and follow? Are there adequate parking facilities? Are bus routes nearby?

Is there access to social services? Where are residential and business districts located? What are the sources of employment near the facility?

What is the proximity to other health care facilities.

Language and Ethnohistory

What languages are spoken within the institution? By employees? By patients?

How formal or informal are the lines of communication within the organization?

Is the organizational governance hierarchical? What communication strategies are used within the organization?

What is the history of the organization? What was the original mission of the organization? How does the history influence the current organization? How has it traditionally responded to change?

Technology

How is technology used in the organization? Who uses it? Do all work stations have access to computers? Do all employees have access to email? Are electronic medical records being used? Is new technology in place in the emergency department, critical care areas, labor and delivery, laboratory, and X-ray departments?

Religious/Philosophical

Does the institution have a religious affiliation? How is this shown in the décor of the institution? How does the religious affiliation influence the philosophy, values, and norms of the agency?

Is the institution public or private? For profit or not-for-profit?

Are such documents such as The Patient's Bill of Rights prominently displayed within the institution. Are such documents displayed in languages other than English, that is, in Spanish?

Social Factors

What are the working relationships within nursing? Between nursing and ancillary services? Within each nursing unit? Between physicians and nurses? How closely are staff members aligned throughout the organization?

Is the environment initially "warm and loving"? How do volunteers or staff members at the information desk behave? Do employees get together outside of work?

Is there a hierarchal distance between ancillary staff, nurses and administrators?

How are family members welcomed (or not welcomed) to the unit? Is the waiting room comfortable? Reading materials? Are they appropriate for the visitors?

Are there public telephones available? Vending machines?

Is the signage adequate within the institution? Is the signage in languages other than English? Can visitors easily find their way to a specific unit or room?

What ways has the institution taken to be inclusive to visitors or patients?

Cultural Values

Are values explicitly stated? What is valued within the institution? What is valued as "good" and "bad"? Is there a gap between stated values and what actually happens on a daily basis?

Are interpreter services readily available? Translated medical literature and educational materials?

How does the institution value and institutionalize culturally competent care?

How does the institution recruit and retain minority staff members? How are personnel trained in cultural competencies?

Is there coordination with traditional healers, use of community health workers?

How does the organization respond to the community it serves? (clinic hours, locations, physical environment, network memberships, and written materials).

How does the interior design, decor and art work reflect the cultural values of the institution and community at large?

Political/Legal

Where does the power rest within the institution? With the administration? With the physicians? With the business office? With nursing? Is power shared? How is power divided among competing groups? Is there an active Board of Directors? What are their responsibilities? What types of legal actions have been taken against the institution? On behalf of the institution?

How do employees or staff have input? How does the institution encourage or value suggestions or contributions from staff?

Economic

What is the financial viability of the institution? Has this changed over the past 10 years? Who makes financial decisions? What values are the basis of financial decisions? How do the salaries and benefits compare with those of competitors in the immediate environment?

Education

How is education valued within the institution? What type of assistance (financial, scheduling, flexibility) is provided for staff seeking advanced training or degrees? What opportunities are offered those staff who are earning advanced degrees? Does the institution pay baccalaureate prepared nurses more than associate degree nurses?

Does the institution provide clinical learning experiences for medicine, nursing, and other health professionals. How does the institution demonstrate that it values students?

Are advanced practice nurses utilized? What is the educational background of staff nurses? Nurse managers? Nursing leaders? How does this compare with the educational levels of staff in competing institutions?

Components of a Cultural Assessment: Traditional Native American Healing

Joyceen S. Boyle

Worldview, Value Orientations, and Cultural Norms

In all Native American cultures, interactions on all levels contain the fundamental element of respect. Respect is how a person presents himself or herself to the world and how a person acts, and it is tied to being Native American. Respect is an essential element of the relationship between the healer and the client.

- Nature is more powerful than human beings.
- Individual success is not valued as highly as providing security and care to the extended family.
- The integrity of the individual must be respected. There is a respect for the decisions of others. There is also pressure for an individual to consider the extended family's welfare when making decisions.

Family and Kinship Systems

- Native Americans often have an extended family. Many are "matriarchal" in nature and consist of an older woman and her husband and unmarried children, together with married daughters and their husbands and children.
- Many Native Americans, including the Navajo, have unique categories of relatives.
- Descent is traced through the mother. The Navajo have a clan system of kinship.
- Head of household is the husband although the wife has a voice in decision making.
- Children are highly valued and are given responsibility early in life for making decisions about themselves.
- There is a prestige with aging as the elderly are seen as wise and experienced.
- Tribal and family ties are strong. Ties to the reservation remain for the younger generation

of Native Americans, drawing them back to the reservation frequently to visit family members.

- It is the extended families who provide care, comfort and assistance to elderly family members or those who are ill.

Religious Ideology or Philosophical Beliefs

- Religion enters every phase of the traditional American Indian life. It has an important emphasis in curing illness.
- Many important Native American ceremonies (prayers, purification ceremonies, sweat lodge) are used with illness. Theology and medicine are difficult to separate in traditional Native American culture.
- Earth and nature are part of traditional cosmology and health is viewed as harmony with nature, not just the curing of disease.
- Herbs are often used in Native American healing rituals. These herbs are often potent and can be dangerous if used by unskilled persons. Herbs such as peyote and the sacred datura may be used. The Tohono O'Odham have a saying about the sacred datura: If you have white skin and blue eyes, do not use it as you do not have the appropriate relationship with the earth.
- There may be certain individuals who are able to cause sickness in others by practicing witchcraft.

Traditional Beliefs and Practices of Healing

- Health is a reflection of a correct relationship between human beings and the environment. Health is associated with the mind, spirit, and connections with the creation and the creator.

- Illness is not an isolated episode in one's life. To make meaning of the illness, you must ask: How do I understand this illness in the trajectory of my life?
- The traditional healer is not technically a healer. Individuals heal themselves. The true healer is a facilitator as the responsibility for healing rests with the patient. The patient must take knowledge and incorporate that knowledge to heal himself/herself. Remember, healing does not equate with "cure".
- Harmony and balance in one's life are the ultimate goals of healing.
- Many Native Americans use both their traditional health care system, including traditional health care practices and the modern health care system.
- Different kinds of ceremonies may be used for healing. Sweat lodge, traditional herbs, songs, dances. and prayers are common. The traditional healer may fast before performing ceremonies. Unique ceremonies (for childbirth, for strength, for blessings) are common. The rituals (songs, prayers, dances) create a "healing environment".

Components of Traditional Healing

- An important component of traditional healing is unconditional love that encompasses the body, mind, and spirit as well as the individual's relations with the creator.
- Responsibility for healing rests with the patient. The traditional medicine practitioner is a facilitator. The true healer is the patient. The patient must take the knowledge, incorporate it into his or her life and heal themselves.
- The patient must seek or ask for assistance and play an active role in his or her recovery.
- Every illness is a learning experience for the patient and for the healer. Every healing situation

presents an opportunity for teaching or a cultural interpretation to help the patient understand his illness within the context of his or her life.

- There are no accidents in healing. An accident might be the spirits talking to you–to get your attention and make you change your ways.

Use of Herbal Remedies

- Fifty percent of the drugs that are commonly used in western medicine come from plants.
- Respect Mother Earth and the plants that have healing qualities. Express appreciation to the creator. Do not "strip" the plant. Take only what you need.
- Know your plants and know your patients. Traditional healers often remind us that there is a saying that individuals with white skin and blue eyes do not have the same relationships as a native does with Mother Earth. Many herbs are powerful and can be extremely dangerous.

- Many herbs require commitment on the part of the healer and the patient as the effect may disappear quickly and then a little more is given. Western medicine uses the active ingredient in the herb to produce the significant effects. Many herbs "nudge" you along.
- While many plants have healing qualities they cannot heal the individual without prayers and ceremonies.

What the mind cannot deal with
The body will manifest.
Therefore, to look for the cause
of Disease or disharmony (life
out of balance), look to the Spirit
for the Spirit cannot lie.

Edgar Monetathchi, Jr., 1987
Commanche Medicine Man*

*From the Traditional Indian Medicine Workshop presented by the University of Arizona Indians into Medicine Program and the Stoklos Native American Health Education Fund.

INDEX

Key to page references: *b* refers to material located in a box; *c* refers to a case study; *e* refers to evidence-based practice; *f* refers to a figure; *r* refers to a research application; *t* refers to a table

A

Abortion, 94
  Baha'i international community, 370–371
  Catholicism, 375
  Church of Jesus Christ of Latter-Day Saints, 380
  Islam, 385
  payment for, 405
Acculturation, 296
  concept of, 252
  stress of, 191, 252
Adolescents
  cultural backgrounds, 144
  culturally competent nursing care for
    extended family, 149
    family belief systems, 147–149
    family, nursing assessment of, 147
    nursing interventions, 149–151
  culture and development, 143–146
  girls
    female health care providers, 29
  health care needs of, 146
  with minority groups, 144
  unprotected intercourse of, 145*e*
Adulthood, 158, 160, 162
  cultural influences, overview of
    adult behavior, chronologic standards for, 159–160
    developmental tasks, 160–162
    developmental transition, 162–166
    physiologic development, 158
    psychosocial development, 158–159
  health-related situational crises
    African American women, 167–168
    caregiving, 167
    culturally competent nursing care, 171–178
    HIV/AIDS, context of, 168
    HIV preventive efforts, barriers, 170–171
    prevention challenges, 168–170
Adulthood transitions, 157
Advanced practice nurse specialty, non-white and
    non-Hispanic/Latino nurses by, 319*f*
Advocacy, for social justice, 413
Afghan girls, 441*c*–442*c*

African American patients, trust, mistrust and satisfaction
    of care, 409*e*
Agency for Healthcare Research and Quality (AHRQ), 218
Alcoholic Anonymous (AA), 261
Allah, 383
Allopathic medicine, 83
Alms-giving (zakat), 383
Alternative medical systems, 83
Alternative therapies, 84*b*–85*b*
American Organization of Nurse Execuitves (AONE), 212*b*
American women, HIV/AIDS cases, 169
Amish, use of technology, 367*f*
Andrews, Margaret, 9*f*
Anthropology, 4
Anxiety, 174
Arab Muslim culture, 266
Asian Americans' core cultural values, 263
Assess organizational culture, magnet model to, 226*b*–228*b*
Asylees, 285
Attitude change, 328
Ayurvedic healing, 51*f*

B

Beneficence, principles of, 407
Bigotry, 325
Biocultural aspects, of disease, 42*t*–44*t*
Biocultural variations, 54
  blood pressure, 55
  in body secretions, 59
  client's hygiene, 56
  and clinical significance, 67*t*–69*t*
  ears, 60
  eskimos, 59
  in ethnic group, 64*t*–66*t*
  eyes, 60
  hair, 59–60
  in height, 56*t*
  in illness, 67
  leukoedema, 61
  in mammary venous plexus, 61
  in measurements, 55

465

Biocultural variations (*Continued*)
  mouth, 60–61
  in musculoskeletal system, 61–67, 62*t*–63*t*
  physical appearance, 55
  in skin, 56
    age-related changes, 59
    cyanosis, 57
    ecchymoses, 58–59
    erythema, 58
    hyperpigmentation, 57
    jaundice, 57–58
    melanin, 56
    mongolian spots, 56–57
    pallor, 58
    petechiae, 58
    vitiligo, 57
  teeth, 61
  in vital signs, 55
Biomedical model, 76
Birth/culture
  birth positions, 109–110
  home birth, traditional, 106–107
  infant gender/multiple births, 110
  labor pain, cultural expression of, 109
  support during childbirth, 107–109
Black children, 149
Black church, 260
Black community, 258
Breast-feeding
  practices, 114
  promotion, 308
Brit milah, 388*f*
Buchholz's study, 100
Buddhist adolescent
  end-of-life care for, 154*c*
Buddhist family, 151
Buddhist woman, 372*f*

C

Caida de la mollera (fallen fontanel), 139
Cardiovascular disease (CVD) affects, 184
Caregiving, 167
Caring hospital, 237*c*–238*c*
Catholic Relief Services (CRS), 429
Center for Mental Health Services (CMHS), 246
Centers for Disease Control and Prevention (CDC)
  refugee reproductive health activities goals, 95*b*
Certified transcultural nurse-advanced (CTN-A), 14
Challenge of recovery for African American
    women, 258*e*–259*e*
Chief complaint, 40
Childbearing, 91, 161
  cultural belief systems, overview of, 92–94
  culture influences, 91

experiences, of lesbian families, 100*e*
  practices, 92–94
  practices, for Filipino women, 101
Childbirth
  birth positions, 109–110
  breast-feeding mother, 114
  cultural preparation for, 105
  dietary prescriptions, 112
  labor pain, 109
  postpartum vulnerability, 112
  support, 107–109
  traditional home birth, 106–107
  Western customs, 106
Childbirth practices, 92
Childhood obesity, 130*f*
Child poverty, in United States, 125
Child rearing
  model depicting cultural perspectives of, 127*f*
  practices, model of, 124*f*
Children
  African American and Hispanic, 138*f*
  childhood disorders, biocultural influences
    ethnicity, 140
    hereditary predisposition, 141
    immunity, 140
    intermarriage, 140
    race, 141
  chronic illness, 141–143
  common developmental, 126*f*
  culturally competent nursing care for
    extended family, 149
    family belief systems, 147–149
    family, nursing assessment of, 147
    nursing interventions, 149–151
  in culturally diverse society, 123–125
  culture-universal/culture-specific child rearing
    child abuse *vs.* folk healing, 136–137
    cosleeping, 132
    cradleboard, 132, 133*f*
    elimination, 133–134
    gender differences, 137
    menstruation, 134–135
    nutrition, 129–131
    obesity, 130*f*
    pandanus mat, 132
    parent–child relationship, 135–136
    premasticate, 129
    values, attitudes, beliefs, and practices of, 128
  die from, 132
  disability in, 141–143
  earthquake, Haitian, 134*f*
  health promotion
    culture-bound syndromes, 138–140
    health belief systems, 138–140
    illness, 137–138

overweight/obesity, prevention, 131e
with physical disabilities, 142f
as population
  child health status, 125–126
  crying, 128
  growth and development, 126–127
  height and weight, 127–128
  infant attachment, 128
  poverty, 125
  racial/ethnic composition, 125
Children's health, impact of poverty on, 125
Christian church
  North Americans report religious affiliation
    eighty-five percent of, 362f
Churches. See Black church; Christian church
  African American, 271, 279f
  Buddhist, 271
  European American, 271
  Native North American, 392
Civic responsibilities, 178
Client's care knowledge, 70
Clients of Asian heritage, 35
Clinical decision making/nursing actions, 69
  cultural care, 69–70
  cultural preservation, 69
  evaluation of, 70
  modes to guide, 69
CNM
  assessing mom and baby, 92f
  family-oriented pregnancy care, 93f
Collateral relationships, 27
Collectivism, 323
Commission on Social Determinants
    of Health (CSDH), 405
Communication, 451–452
  cross-cultural, 25f
  different cultures, 285f
Communication networks, 287
Community assessment example, 236b
Community-based nursing, 278
Community-based participatory research, 236
Community-based services, 186
Community-based settings, 277
Community empowerment, 413
Community health nursing, 278
Community health, psychiatric, and
    pediatric nurses, 132
Community health representatives (CHRs), 301
Community nursing interventions
  cultural competence
    coping behaviors, 303
    family systems, 302–303
    in health maintenance and health promotion, 300–302
    lifestyle practices, 303–305
    in prevention programs, 305–313

Community nursing practice
  cultural factors within, 283
    cultural diversity within, 284
    demographics and health care, 283–284
    Dinka culture, 288–294
    diverse cultural groups, access to, 297–300
    refugee, 284–288
    refugee families, planning nursing care for, 294–296
    traditional cultural values, maintenance of, 296–297
    United States, subcultures, 284
  cultural influences, 282–283
  cultural issues in, 281
Community partnership, for social justice, 413
Community settings
  culturally competent nursing care, overview of, 279–280
  transcultural framework, 280
    components, identifying and analyzing, 280–281
    subcultures identification, 280
    values and cultural norms of, 281
Compassion, 413
Complementary and alternative medicine (CAM), 82–84
  alternative medical systems, 83
  biologically based therapies, 83–84
  energy therapies, 84
  manipulative and body-based methods, 84
  mind–body medicine, 83
Complementary therapies, 84b–85b
Computer-based tools, 11
Consultation, with rabbi, 408f
Consumers, 247
  of mental health care, 247
  role of, 247, 248e
Continuing care retirement communities, 202
Contraception, 94
Corporate culture, 212, 324
  determining of, 324b
  training, 212
Cosleeping, 132
Cradleboard, 132, 133f
Critical care unit nurses
  of family presence, 410e
  nuclear family members, 224
Cross-cultural communication, 24, 25f, 332, 333f
  majority of conflicts, 332
multicultural workplace, strategies to
    promote effective, 334b
Cross-cultural perspectives, on proverbs and conflict, 329t
Cultural adjustment, W model of, 445f
Cultural affiliations, 452
Cultural assessment, 298
  basic principles of, 299t
  components of, 300t
  content of, 39
  goal of, 38
  of organization, institution, or agency, 342b–343b

Cultural belief systems, 74
  metaphor, 74
  worldview, 74
Cultural blind spot, 268
Cultural care
  assessment tools, 228
  competency-based, 268
  for substance-dependent African American women, 302e
Cultural code, 30
Cultural competence, 10, 213, 268, 283b, 405
Cultural competent ethical decision, model for, 412f
Cultural congruence, 10
Cultural differences, in response to drugs, 52t–53t
Cultural feeding practices, 129
Cultural groups honor life stages, in diverse ways, 250f
Culturally and linguistically appropriate health care
        services (CLAS), 18, 216b–217b
  minority health standards for, 19b
  Standards, 218
Culturally competent care, 278
  Campinha-Bacote model of, 8
  community for, 278
  ethical care
    model for, 411–414
      applications, 414–415
  foundation of, 278
  models of, 267
Culturally competent initiatives, 237
  development of, 237–238
Culturally competent nursing care, 17–36
  categories
    individual cultural competence, 17, 18
    organizational cultural competence, 17
  categories of, 17
  cross-cultural communication, 23–36
    cultural perspectives on intimacy, 27–28
    eye contact, 28–29
    with family members, 25–27
    interpreters, use of, 31
    language, 30–31
    non–english-speaking patients, 31–33
    nonverbal communication, 28
    proxemics, 30
    psychomotor skills, 24
    sex and gender, 30
    sick role behavior, 33–36
    silence, 28
    space and distance, 29–30
    touch, 29
  cultural assessment, 23
  culturally and linguistically appropriate health care
        services (CLAS), 18, 19
  cultural self-assessment, 20–23
  linguistic competence, 18
  skills needed for, 23

Culturally competent organizations, 212–218
  barriers to, 232–234
  definition of, 212
  individual health care providers, role of, 239
  need for, 218–220
  vision and values, 223t–224t
Culturally congruent care, 6, 18, 267
Culturally diverse women
  health beliefs, 256
  intrapartum nursing care for, 110b
  literature, 212
  mental health for, 245
Cultural norms
  behavior of, 458
  concept of, 244
Cultural pain, 249
Cultural sanctions, 452–453
Cultural self-assessment, 20, 338
Cultural values, 461
  beliefs, or practices, 252
  culture care model, 231
Culture-bound syndromes, 41, 253–255
Culture shock, 252
Culture-specific nursing care, 4
Culture-specific syndromes, 253
Culture-universal nursing care, 4
Culturologic nursing assessment, 38
Cumulative Index to Nursing and Allied
        Health Literature (CINAHL), 11
Curandero, 139, 392
Cyanosis, 23

D

Daughters food shopping, African fathers, 136f
Dayahs, 101
Death
  bad, 359
  good, 360
Deontological theory of ethics, 407
Depression, 40
Development aid organizations, list of, 426b
Developmental considerations, 453
Developmental crises, 160
Developmental tasks, 160
Developmental transitions, 167
The Diagnostic and Statistical Manual, 4th edition (DSMIV), 246
    American Psychiatric Association (APA)
        mental disorders, 246
Dietary supplements, 78
  decisions and evaluating information, 80b
Dinka culture, 289
Dinka family, 290–291
Dinka refugee family, 293c–294c
Dinka women's roles, 291–293

Discrimination, 325
Disease, incidence of
   biocultural variations and cultural aspects of, 451
Distributive justice, 406
Diverse cultural backgrounds, 11
Diverse cultural communities, access to, 297–300
Doctor of osteopathy (DO), 83
Douluer de Corps (pain in the body), 272
Dress code, 334
Dynamic hospital, 221

E

Economics, 453, 461–462
Education, 462
Educational background, 453
Educational Resources Information Center (ERIC), 11
Elderly ethnic Vietnamese, 191
Elderly individuals, 272
Emic (insider), 344
Emic & Etic patient perspectives, 249e
Empathy, 269, 270
Empty nest syndrome, 159
Enhancing the Rights of Adolescent Girls, 136
Environmental context, 18, 460
Epidemiologic model, 280
Ethical concepts, 406–411
Ethnicity, 185
Ethnic nursing care, 4
Ethnocentric, 10
Ethnohistory, 40, 460
Ethnoreligion, 352
Ethnoviolence, 327
Etic (outsider), 344
Etiquette, 333
Eucharist, 374
Evil eye (mal ojo), 75, 139
Expectations, conflicting role
   staff educated abroad, 337–338
Extended American family, 165f
Extended family, 149, 152
Eye contact, use of, 28

F

Facilitators, 345
Faith healing, 377
Family obligations, 331
Family planning services, 97
Family systems, 457, 463–464
Fast-food restaurants, popularity of, 130
Fasting, 380
Female health care providers, adolescent girls, 29
Fertility controls, and culture, 94–97
Fertility practices, 95
Folk healers, 80
Folk healing system, 79

Folk illnesses, 253
Foreign nurse, becoming, 440r
Formal attitude change approach, 328
Francophone community, 280
Friendscraft, 149

G

Garment, 379
Gelassenheit, 367
Gender-specific tasks
   differentiation of, 129f
Generativity, 160
Gestational diabetes
   baby's risk, 98
Ghost illness, 139
Giger and Davidhizar transcultural assessment model, 6
Ginseng, 45
Girls
   menstrual periods, 134
   mother, developmental stage, 135f
God's law of harmony, 378

H

Halal, 384
Healers
   scope of practice, 81t–82t
Healing practices, 464
Healing systems, 78
   types of
      complementary and alternative
         medicine (CAM), 82–84
      folk healing system, 79–82
      professional care systems, 78–79
      self-care, 78
Health, 397c–398c
   as global concern, 422–423
   global needs, 425–427
   governmental organizations
      Canadian International Development
         Agency (CIDA), 432–433
      CDC, 432
      Peace Corps, 432
      USAID, 431–432
   intergovernmental organizations
      humanitarian assistance, 427
      Pan American Health Organization (PAHO), 428
      prevention, 427
      United Nations Children's Fund (UNICEF), 428–429
      UN volunteers, 427–428
      World Health Organization (WHO), 428
   nongovernmental organizations
      CARE, 429–430
      Catholic Relief Services (CRS), 429
      Doctors Without Borders/Médécins Sans Frontières
         (MSF), 430–431

Health *(Continued)*
   Health Opportunities for People
      Everywhere (HOPE), 430
   ICRC, 429
   International Rescue Committee, 431
   Mercy Corps, 431
   Oxfam, 430
   Save the Children, 430
   World Vision, 431
  professional organizations
   International Council of Nurses (ICN), 433
   North American Nurses Abroad, 434–438
   World's Nurses, 433–434
Health behavior, 78
Health belief systems, 74, 459
  holistic paradigm, 76–77
  magico-religious paradigm, 75
  scientific paradigm, 75–76
Health care, 251*e*
  Storefront Church Resist Oppression, 176*e*
Health care institutions, 295
Health care organizations
  community resources, 345
  cultural self-assessment, 339–344
  demographic and descriptive data, 344
   multicultural workplace, promoting
    harmony, 345–346
   need and readiness for, 344–345
   strengths and limitations, 344
Health care provider decisions
  clash with parental preference, 148*e*
Health care settings
  form/checklist, 39
Health care systems, 459
Health care workforce
  advanced practice nurses (APNs), 319
  corporate cultures and subcultures, 323–325
  cultural assessment
   in multicultural workplace, 338–346
  cultural diversity, 316, 321
  cultural perspectives in, 323, 328
   on clothing and accessories, 334–335
   conflict, cultural origins of, 330–331
   conflict, cultural perspectives on, 329–330
   cross-cultural communication, 332–333
   on etiquette, 333–334
   family obligations, 331–332
   on gender and sexual orientation, 336–337
   on interpersonal relationships, 335–336
   long-standing historic rivalries, 336
   on moral and religious beliefs, 337
   on time orientation, 335
   on touch, 333
   multicultural population, challenges and opportunities
    of, 321–323

  multicultural workforce, 320
  multicultural workplace, 320
  negative attitudes and behaviors
   changing attitudes, 328
   formation of attitudes, 328
   hatred, 325
   prejudice, bigotry, and discrimination, 325–326
   racism, 326–327
   violence in, 327
  U.S. Department of Health and Human
   Services, 318
Health disparity, 218, 403
Health education, 295
Health-illness
  behaviors, 77–78
  transitions, 164
Health inequities
  definition of, 404
Health Ministries, 395
Health-related beliefs, and practices, 453–454
Healthy communities, 235
Herbal remedies, 46*t*–51*t*
  ayurvedic healing, 51*f*
  Chinese Americans, 51
  Mexican Americans, 53
  use of, 465
High blood, 174
Hijab, 266
Hispanic families, 197
Hispanic immigrants, 265
Historical Unresolved Grief, 262*e*
HIV/AIDS care, 173
HIV/AIDS prevention, 169*e*–170*e*
HIV/AIDS treatment, 172*c*
  economic resources, lack of, 174
HIV disease, individuals, 175
HIV-positive mothers, 101
HIV-positive women, reproductive decisions, 96*e*
Holistic, 77
  paradigm, 76
Homophobia, 171
Hot/cold theory of disease, 77
Human resource frame, 221
Human rights barriers
  for displaced persons, in Southern Sudan, 287
Hygiene, 332

         I

Illness behavior, 78, 185
  Mechanic's determinants of, 79*t*
Immigrant populations. *See* refugee
Immigrants, 284
  birth for, 312*t*
Individual cultural assessment instrument, 340*t*–341*t*

Individuals residing, in country, 287*t*
Infant attachment, 128
Infant relinquishment, 98
Infants, low birth weight, 143*f*
Informal social support, 194
Institutional racism, definition of, 232
International assignments
    preparations and orientation for, 445*b*
International Council of Nurses (ICN), 422, 433
International health, 440
International job options, for nurses, 437*b*
International legal status (ICRC), 429
International nursing
    agency, choosing, 449
    assignment, preparing for, 443*c*–444*c*
    as a career, 440–442
    characteristics of, 438*b*
    contract, negotiation, 447–448
    cultural adjustment, patterns of, 445–446
    field of, 439–440
    geographic region, 446–447
    going abroad, 446
    internship experiences, 443–445
    length of time abroad, 446
    motivation, 446
    preparation for, 442–443
    reasonable expectations of sending agency, 447
International sending agency
    choosing, guidelines, 447*b*–448*b*
International Society for the Prevention of Child Abuse
        and Neglect (ISPCAN), 136
Interpersonal communication, 268
Interpersonal relationships, cultural
        perspectives on, 335*f*
Interpreters, 33*e*–35*e*, 213
    health care, national council for, 35*b*
Intrauterine devices (IUDs), 94
Islamic law, blood, 135
Islam religious, 266
Islam's holiest city (salat), 383

J

Jehovah's Witnesses and the Question of Blood, 387
Joint commission standards
    address culture, 214*b*–215*b*

K

Kinship, 290
    network, 454, 457–458
    systems, 457, 463–464
Kosher, 389

L

Labor practices, 108
Language, 460

Languages spoken, 458
    barriers, 32*b*
    at home, 31*t*
Leininger, Madeleine, 9*f*
Leininger's culture care model, 228
    example of, 229*t*–232*t*
Leininger's Sunrise model, 8*f*
Leininger's theory
    of culture care diversity and universality, 6
Limited english proficiency (LEP), 213

M

Machismo, male, 265
Magico-religious paradigm, 75
Magnet designation, 224
Magnet research, forces of magnetism, 225*e*
Malnutrition, 130
Market economy, 405
Maternal morbidity, 93
Maternal mortality, 93
Maternal role attainment, 100–101
Medications, 41
    plant-derived, 44
    traditional Chinese medicine, 45
Mennonites, 366
Menopause, perception of, 158
Mental health care, 244, 253
    cultural competence
        process of, 267–268
    cultural values, beliefs, and practices, 256
        African Americans, 257–260
        Arab muslim cultural groups, 265–266
        Asian/Pacific Islander cultural groups, 262–263
        Hispanic/Latino cultural groups, 263–265
        Native Americans, 260–262
    culture-bound syndromes, 252–256
    decision making, consumers role, 247
    disparities in, 247–251
    immigration policy, 251–252
    intrapersonal reflection, 271–272
    patient's experience of pain, 272
    population trends, 246
    transcultural perspectives in, 243
        definition of, 244–246
Mental health nurses, 271
    working, 252
Mental health patients, cross-cultural
        communication skills, 269*f*
Metaphors, 74, 77
Mexican American pregnant women, practices, 104
Microorganisms attack, 76
Middle adult, 160
Midlife crisis, 159
Millennium development goals
    health in, 424*t*

Millennium development goals (MDGs), 423–425
Mitzvah (a good deed), 389
Mohel, 388
Moral beliefs, 337
Mortality, in United States and Canada, 235*b*
Mother–child relationships, 128
Mothers premasticate, 129
Muhammad's companions, 383
Multicultural health care setting
    origins of conflict, 331*f*
Multicultural workplace
    influence of cultural values, 340*f*
    promoting harmony, 346*b*

N

Names, guidelines for, 166*t*
National Association for the Advancement
    of Colored People [NAACP], 454
National Center for Complementary and Alternative
    Medicine (NCCAM), 83
National Center on Minority Health and Health
    Disparities (NCMHD), 236
The National Institute of Nursing Research
    (NINR), 247, 278
National Standards for Culturally and Linguistically
    Appropriate Services (CLAS),
    in health care, 216*b*–217*b*, 218
Native American culture believes, 260
Native American cultures, 463
Native Americans
    beliefs and practices related to diabetes, 310*b*
Naturalistic healing, 80
Nerves, 174
Nirvana, 372
Non–English-speaking patients, 233
Non–English-speaking patients, 33
Nongovernmental organizations (NGOs), 425
Non–insulin-dependent diabetes (NIDD), 309
Nonmaleficence, principles of, 407
Nonverbal communication, 28
Nonverbal expressions, 151
Normative ethics, 407
North American funeral customs, 358
North Atlantic Treaty Organization (NATO), 427
Nurse educators, 11
Nurse-patient interactions
    cultural influences, conceptual model for, 26*f*
Nurses providing care, to clients, 173
Nursing actions, 69
Nursing care
    application of cultural concepts to, 151–154
    factors to consider, 298*b*
    hospitalization of an Amish child, 152*b*–153*b*
    religion and spiritual, 351–401

    routine postpartum, 111
    transcultural perspectives
        of adults, 157
        of older adults, 182
Nursing during ebola outbreak
    in Central Africa, 422*r*–423*r*
Nursing interventions, 147
Nursing profession, motivations
    and experiences, 320*e*–321*e*
Nutrition, 454–455

O

Obesity, prevention, 131*e*
Older adults
    activity theory, 187
    age in place, 186
    challenge, 203
    client—ethnic/learn, 190*b*
    continuity theory, 187
    creative expression stimulates discussion, 204*f*
    disengagement theory, 187
    formal support, 194
    immigrant parent, 193*c*
    income level, 185
    long-term care, cost of, 185
    membership, in cultural group, 193
    needs for care, 186
    nonbiologic or social theories of, 187*b*
    nursing studies, 192*t*
    opportunities to recall and share life experiences, 204
    pain in elbows and knees, 190*c*
    pain management in, 199*e*
    responses in health care, 183*b*
    social networks, 196*t*
    traditional medicine or practices, 189
Older adults. *See* Elderly
    in contemporary society
        aging, social theories of, 187
        changing demographics, 184–185
        economic factors, 185–187
    cultural diversity, community level
        culture change, understanding, 191–194
        in different ethnic and cultural contexts, 188–191
        family members, caregiving of, 194–195
        members, variations, 197–198
        social support, dimensions of, 195–197
    culture influences, 183
    individual level, integrating social/cultural factors
        community-based services for, 201–204
        decisions on continuum of care, 200–201
        delivery of care, 204–205
        faith and spirituality, 199–200
        purpose of, 198
    in nursing care, 182

Organizational climate, 324
Organizational cultures, 211, 219
  assessment of, 224–232
  behavior, 220
  community context, 234–237
  and employees, 222–224
  physical environment of care, 234
  self-assessment, 339
  theories of, 221–222
Orthodox Jewish contraception, 96

P

Panethnic minority groups, 4
Papanicolaou (Pap), 295
Parent Teacher Association (PTA), 163
Participatory action research, 236
Patients' Bill of Rights, 411
Patient Self-Determination Act of 1991, 407
Peyote religion, 392
Phenylketonuria (PKU), 140
Physiologic development, 158
Political frame, 221
Political/government systems, 458
Political/legal, 461
Postpartum care, Jewish laws, customs, 161e
Postpartum period
  and culture
    African American pregnant women, 117–118
    American Indian pregnant women, 118–119
    on breast-feeding, 113–115
    dietary prescriptions, 112
    domestic violence during pregnancy, 115–116
    hispanic pregnant women, 116–117
    hot/cold theory, 111–112
    postpartum depression (PPD), 110–111
    postpartum seclusion, 112–113
Potential demographic, cultural, and health system barriers, 220
Poverty, in rural African American communities, 312
Pregnancy, 101
  abused pregnant woman, 115
  abuse within Indian culture, 118–119
  African American, 117
  beliefs and practices of, 307t
  cultural beliefs, 102b, 103
    activity, 103
    alternative lifestyle choices, 98–100
    biologic variations, 97–98
    food taboos and cravings, 103–104
    infant relinquishment, 98
    maternal role attainment alterations, 100–101
    nontraditional support systems, 101–103
    obstetric testing, 105

    prenatal care, 104–105
    preparation for childbirth, 105
  domestic violence, 115
  Hispanic culture, 117
  legacy of patriarchy, 116
  prevention of, 97
Premasticate, 130
Prenatal care, 116e
Principle of totality, 375
Production-oriented hospital, 221
Professional care systems, 78–79
Program of All-Inclusive Care for the Elderly (PACE), 203
Promotora model, 203
Promotoras (health workers), 306
Protestantism, 393
Proxemics, 30
Psychological Abstracts (PsycINFO), 11
Psychosocial development, 158
Pujos (grunting), 139
Purnell model, for cultural competence, 6

Q

Quality of care, largest disparities in, 219b

R

Refugees, 284–288
  camp, working in, 435c–437c
  families
    characteristics of, 163b
  Sudanese women, 288
  women, 295
Registered nurses (RNs), 316
  distribution of, 318f
Reincarnation, 382
Religions, 397c–398c, 455
  Amish
    addendum, 368–369
    beliefs and religious practices, 365–366
    gelassenheit, 367
    health care practices, 367–369
    holy days and sacraments, 367
    meidung/shunning, 366
    ordung, 366
    social activities, 367
    use of technology, 366–367
  Baha'i international community
    abortion, 370–371
    amniocentesis, 370
    artificial insemination, 371
    beliefs and religious practices, 369–370
    birth control, 370
    to death and dying, 371
    eugenics and genetics, 371
    health care practices, 370
    holy days and sacraments, 370

Religions *(Continued)*
    religious support system, 371
    social activities, 370
    substance use, 370
  Buddhist churches of America
    addendum, 373
    beliefs and religious practices, 372
    Buddhism, 371
    death and dying, 373
    diet, 372
    health care practices, 372–373
    holy days, 372
    medications, 373
    religious support system for, 373
    sacraments, 372
  Catholicism
    abortion, 375
    amniocentesis, 375
    autopsy and donation of body, 376
    beliefs and religious practices, 373–374
    birth control, 375
    church organizations, 376
    diet, 374
    disposal of body, 376
    Eucharist, 374
    euthanasia, 376
    health care practices, 375
    holy days, 374
    medical and surgical interventions, 375
    religious support system for, 375–376
    right to die, 376
    social activities, 374
    stem cell research, 375
    sterility tests and artificial insemination, 375
    substance use, 374
    titles of religious representatives, 376
  Christian science, 376
    addendum, 379
    beliefs and religious practices, 377
    death and dying, 379
    faith healing, 377
    health care practices, 377–378
    holy days, 377
    medications, 378
    reproduction, 378
    sacraments, 377
    social activities, 377
    support system for, 378–379
  Church of Jesus Christ of Latter-Day Saints, 379
    abortion, 380
    amniocentesis, 380
    beliefs and religious practices, 379
    birth control, 380
    church organizations to, 381
    death and dying, 381

    diet, 379–380
    health care practices, 380
    holy days/special days, 379
    medications, 380
    sacraments, 379
    social activities, 380
    sterility/fertility testing, 381
    substance use, 380
    support system for, 381
    title of religious representative, 381
  consequential dimension, 353
  contributions of, 362–365
  dimensions of, 352
  Hinduism
    beliefs and religious practices, 381–382
    birth control, 382
    Brahman, 382
    caste system, 382
    death and dying, 382
    diet, 382
    health care practices, 382
    holy days, 382
    support system for, 382
    Vedas, 381
  human behavior, 352
  ideologic dimension, 352
  intellectual dimension, 353
  internet websites for, 364*b*–365*b*
  Islam
    abortion, 385
    artificial insemination, 385
    beliefs and religious practices, 383
    death and dying, 385–386
    diet and substance use, 384
    health care practices, 385
    holidays, 383–384
    medications, 385
    muslim/moslem, 383
    reproduction, 385
    sects of Islam, 383
    support system for, 385
  Jehovah's Witnesses, 386–387
  Judaism, 387–391
  Mennonite Church, 391–392
  Native North American Churches, 392–393
  Protestantism, 393–394
  relation to health and illness, 353–354
  ritualistic dimension, 352
  Seventh-Day Adventists, 394–396
  and spiritual nursing care, 354–361
    for dying, 357–361
    ethnoreligious, assessment of, 355–356
    for ill children, 356–357
    spiritual concerns, 355
    spiritual health, 355

Unitarian Universalist Church, 396–397
in United States and Canada, 361–362
Religious affiliations
of United States and Canada, 362*t*
Religious body, membership for, 363*t*
Religious ideology/philosophical
beliefs, 337, 458, 461, 464
Religious/nonreligious holidays
in United States and Canada, 398*b*–400*b*
Rights, 406
Roman Catholic Saint Martin De Porres, 357*f*
Roman Catholic tradition, children, 374*f*
Rural Amish community, 152
Ruth May Harnar, 434*b*–435*b*

S

Sacrament of Sick, 375
Same-sex relationships
Nigerian American woman, 30
Sandwich generation, 159
Selected culture-bound syndromes, 45*t*
Self-management of diabetes mellitus
political and economic contexts of, 412*e*
Sex-role behavior, 137
Sexually transmitted infections (STIs)
treatment of, 432
Sick role behavior, 33, 78
Situational crises, 160
Situational transitions, 167
Skin, dryness, 150
Social age, definition of, 159
Social amnesia, 328
Social factors, 461
Social harmony, Asian American clients, 27
Social justice, 406
Social life, 457–458
Social networks, 454
Social responsibilities, 178
Social roles, 160
Social support, 303
Society, relation, groups of people, 20*b*–23*b*
Sociocultural factors, 159
Specialized community interventions, 278
Spiritual assessment, 356
Spiritual beliefs, 175
Spiritual distress, 355
Spiritual health, 355
Spirituality, 270, 397*c*–398*c*, 455
in lives of older adults, 119–120
and religious practices, 270
and transcultural mental health nursing, 270–271
Spiritual needs, in clients, 356*b*
Spiritual nursing care, 355
Standards and sources of evidence, address
culture, 215*b*–216*b*

Stereotyping, of patients, 245
Stress, 174
Stroke belt, 172
Suicide prevention, youth, 304*e*
Symbolic frame, 221
Symptoms, 40
client's perception, 41
of depression, 258
for psychologic issues, 266

T

Taboos, 103
Technology, 460–461
Teens grow
friends, from different cultures, 144*f*
Tertiary prevention, 305
cultural competence in, 305
goal of, 311
for traditional African American population, 312*b*
Time orientation, 335
Traditional African American population
cultural factors to consider in planning
tertiary prevention, 312*b*
Traditional beliefs
influencing factors, 297*b*
vs. modern medicine
AK's story, 439*c*
Traditional healing, components of, 464
Traditional health beliefs and practices, 282
Traditional peoples, culture, 261*f*
Transcultural mental health nursing, 264*e*
communication, important factors, 268–270
and spirituality, 270–271
Transcultural nursing, 3, 245*f*
administration, 325
definition of, 211
Andrews/Boyle transcultural nursing
assessment guide, 8, 9
assessment guide
for groups and communities, 39
for individuals and families, 39
biocultural variations, 54
Campinha-Bacote model of cultural competence, 8
certification, 13–14
exam, 13
critical analysis of, 9–11
Giger and Davidhizar transcultural assessment model, 6
history of, 5–6
importance of, 5
Madeleine Leininger
contributions of, 7*t*, 9
sunrise, 8
psychomotor skills, 24*b*
Purnell model, for cultural competence, 6

Transcultural nursing *(Continued)*
  resources for, 12*t*–13*t*
  standards for, 11–13
Transcultural Nursing Assessment Guide for Groups
        and Communities, 39
Transcultural Nursing Assessment Guide
      for Individuals and Families, 39
Transcultural perspectives
  on health history, 39
    biographic data, 40
    culture-bound syndromes, 41
    current medications, 41–44
    dosage modifications, 51
    family and social history, 54
    medication administration, 51–54
    plant-derived medications, 44–51
    present and past illnesses, 41
    reason for seeking care, 40–41
    review of systems, 54
  laboratory tests, 67–69
  on physical examination, biocultural variations, 54
    body proportions, 55
    in body secretions, 59
    cyanosis, 57
    ears, 60
    ecchymoses, 58–59
    erythema, 58
    eyes, 60
    in general appearance, 55–56
    hair, 59–60
    height, 55
    hyperpigmentation, 57
    in illness, 67
    jaundice, 57–58
    leukoedema, 61
    in mammary venous plexus, 61
    mongolian spots, 56–57
    mouth, 60–61
    in musculoskeletal system, 61–67
    normal age-related skin changes, 59
    pallor, 58
    petechiae, 58
    in skin, 56
    teeth, 61
    in vital signs, 55
    vitiligo, 57
    weight, 55
Translators, 33*e*–35*e*
Truth telling, 408

U

Underrepresented in mental health
        research (USDHHS), 257
UN High Commissioner for Refugees (UNHCR), 427
United Nations Children's Fund (UNICEF), 428
United Nations Development Program (UNDP), 427
The Universal Declaration of Human
        Rights (UDHR), 406
The U.S. Department of Health and Human
        Services (DHHS), 403
Utilitarianism, 407

V

Values orientation, 455–456
Vedas, 381
Ventricular septal defects (VSDs), 140
Veracity, principle of, 408
Verbal communication, 150

W

Wedding, of family member
      women of the South African Xhosa tribe, 411*f*
Western biomedicine, 45, 83
White, Anglo-Saxon, Protestant (WASP) views, 161
Women, Infants, and Children (WIC)
        Program, 306
Word of Wisdom, 379
World Bank, 146

Y

Yin and yang, 77
Young adult, 160

CCS0811